ACLS: Certification Preparation and A Comprehensive Review

Second Edition

Ken Grauer, M.D., F.A.A.F.P.

Associate Professor, Department of
 Community Health and Family Medicine,
Assistant Director, Family Practice Residency
 Program,
ACLS Affiliate Faculty for Florida,
University of Florida, College of Medicine,
 Gainesville, Florida

Daniel L. Cavallaro, NREMT

Assistant in Surgery,
Clinical Instructor of Medicine,
University of South Florida, College of
 Medicine,
Tampa, Florida.
Research Coordinator, Tampa Emergency
 Associates for Medicine
ACLS National Affiliate Faculty

with 477 illustrations

The C.V. Mosby Company

ST. LOUIS   *   TORONTO   *   WASHINGTON, D.C.   1987

Executive Editor: David T. Culverwell
Senior Editor: Richard A. Weimer
Production Coordinator: Lisa G. Cunninghis
Copy Editor: Gladys Layton
Cover: Dan Beisel, Medical Art Design
Interior art: Dan Beisel, Medical Art Design
Index: Leah Kramer

SECOND EDITION
Copyright © 1987 by The C.V. Mosby Company

Printed in the United States of America

The C.V. Mosby Company
11830 Westline Industrial Drive, St. Louis, Missouri 63146

Library of Congress Cataloging-in-Publication Data

Grauer, Ken.
  ACLS : certification preparation and a comprehensive review.
  Rev. ed. of: Study guide for advanced life support. 1984.
  Includes bibliographies and index.
  1. Cardiac arrest—Treatment—Problems, exercises, etc.   2. Cardiac resuscitation—Problems, exercises, etc.   I. Cavallaro, Daniel.   II. Grauer, Ken. Study guide for advanced life support.   III. Title. [DNLM: 1. Heart Arrest—examination questions. 2. Life support Care—examination questions.   3. Resuscitation—examination questions.   WG 18 G774a]
RC685.C173G73   1987   616.1′206   87-11155

UG/VH/VH 9   8   7   6   5   4   3   2   1   03/D/327

ABOUT THE AUTHORS

Ken Grauer, M.D., F.A.A.F.P., is an associate professor in the Department of Community Health and Family Medicine, College of Medicine, University of Florida and assistant director of the Family Practice Residency Program in Gainesville. He is board certified in family practice, and is an ACLS affiliate faculty member for the state of Florida. He has lectured widely and written numerous articles on cardiology for family physicians. He is the principal author of a book, "Clinical Electrocardiography: A Primary Care Approach" (Medical Economics Books, 1986) and with Dr. R. Whitney Curry, Jr., writes an "ECG of the Month" column in Cardiovascular Reviews & Reports. Dr. Grauer is well known throughout Florida for teaching ACLS courses and ECG/dysrhythmia workshops to physicians in practice, physicians in training, medical students, nurses, and other paramedical personnel, simplifying otherwise complicated topics into a concise, practical, and easy-to-remember format.

Daniel L. Cavallaro, NREMT, is an assistant in surgery and clinical instructor of medicine at the University of South Florida, College of Medicine. He is also research coordinator for Tampa Emergency Associates for Medicine. As a Nationally Registered Emergency Medical Technician, he has been extremely active developing and participating in courses on pre-hospital care and emergency medicine for the past decade, and has taught in well over 100 ACLS courses during that time. He is a newly appointed ACLS National Affiliate Faculty member.

To Michelle
for her patience, love, and support during
the seemingly endless hours of my second
consecutive "vacation" at the Macintosh.

FOREWORD

Advanced cardiac life support (ACLS) is a program designed by the American Heart Association for teaching health care professionals a systematic approach to the treatment of cardiac arrest and other acute cardiac-related problems. The tremendous success of this program nationally is evident from the continued demand for ACLS training, with well over 25,000 health care professionals being taught annually.

The participant of an ACLS course is expected to assimilate a large amount of material in a short period of time. Even though the American Heart Association ACLS textbook is distributed well in advance, it has not solved the problem of preparing the student for the intensive course to follow. Although extensive in scope, material in the ACLS textbook is not organized into a decision-making format for patient care, and practice exercises in arrhythmia interpretation and management of cardiac arrest are entirely lacking.

ACLS: Certification Preparation and A Comprehensive Review by Grauer and Cavallaro has been developed in an attempt to meet this need. In this the authors succeed even more masterfully than they had in their first edition published in 1984. In addition to a comprehensive discussion of the new guidelines put forth by the American Heart Association, chapters on airway management, IV access, pediatrics and medicolegal issues are included in this expanded second edition. As before, numerous exercises on arrhythmia interpretation and management of simulated cardiac arrest sequences provide the reader with more than ample practice in preparing for the ACLS course.

This book should be of interest to anyone taking the ACLS course and will serve as an extremely useful reference for those involved in emergency cardiac care. It is stimulating, informative, and an invaluable complement to the American Heart Association ACLS Textbook.

RICHARD J. MELKER, M.D., Ph.D
    National ACLS Affiliate Faculty
    Associate Professor
    Surgery, Anesthesiology, Pediatrics
    University of Florida
    College of Medicine
    Gainesville, Florida

PREFACE TO THE SECOND EDITION: HOW TO USE THIS BOOK

In the 3 short years since publication of the first edition of this book (previously titled "*Study Guide for Advanced Life Support: Problem Solving in Cardiac Arrest*"), numerous advances have been made in the field of cardiopulmonary resuscitation. In response to these advances, to the new standards and guidelines published by the American Heart Association in June 1986, and to feedback received from readers of our first edition, the need was felt to revise this book.

The second edition is double the size of the first edition and is completely updated. Although the title has changed (to "*ACLS: Certification Preparation and A Comprehensive Review*"), our goals have not varied from those of the first edition—we still intend the book as a study guide to prepare for the ACLS course and as a complement to the American Heart Association Textbook. In addition, we now feel it merits being called a *comprehensive review* with new sections on airway management (Chapter 7), achieving intravenous access (Chapter 8), pediatrics (Chapter 17), and medicolegal issues (Chapter 18). Sections on pitfalls in management of cardiac arrest (Chapter 9), new developments in CPR (Chapter 10), and lidocaine (Chapter 13) have been expanded and updated. Chapters on sudden cardiac death (Chapter 11) and acute myocardial infarction (Chapter 12) have been added, with the content of each reflecting a synthesis of current practice and state-of-the-art knowledge on the subject.

Part V has been added for those desiring to move even more "beyond the core" of the usual ACLS provider course curriculum. Contained herein is a drug compendium of additional agents used in emergency cardiac care (Chapter 14) and several challenging chapters that explore more advanced concepts in arrhythmia interpretation. Differentiation between ventricular ectopy and aberrant conduction is thoroughly discussed in Chapter 15, while pearls for diagnosing the more difficult forms of tachyarrhythmias and AV block are covered in Chapter 16. Numerous clinical examples illustrate important points that are made.

Despite the comprehensive nature of these latter portions of the text, the beginning of this book focuses on certification preparation. In this the text serves as a basic *study guide* for ACLS. Part I begins with the algorithms for treatment that summarize a suggested protocol for management of cardiac arrest (Chapter 1), complete with a step-by-step analysis that details each recommendation and highlights points of interest. Actions, indications, doses, and adverse effects of the most frequently used drugs in ACLS are discussed in Chapter 2. Calculation of intravenous infusion rates is thoroughly explained, and a method to facilitate remembering how to set up intravenous infusions is presented. (A condensed version of the algorithms with doses for the essential drugs is reproduced as A Pocket Guide at the back of the book.) Finally, the role of key therapeutic modalities such as the precordial thump, defibrillation, cardioversion, and cardiac pacemakers is discussed.

Basic dysrhythmia interpretation is addressed in Chapter 3. Material is presented in an easy-to-follow informative style that actively recruits the participation of the reader. Clinical relevancy is stressed, and numerous practice examples with explained answers are included.

Principles discussed in these first three chapters are applied in the MEGA CODE simulations that constitute Chapter 4. Additional practice for taking the ACLS course is provided by the case study vignettes presented in Chapter 5 and the written questions of Chapter 6. General knowledge of the subject is tested, while detailed answers based on the new guidelines furnish the reader with constructive feedback.

An invaluable feature of this book is its ability to lend itself to the needs of the reader. For those with only a limited time to prepare for an ACLS course, the study guide section (Part I) contains the essential material to concentrate on. *This may be done almost to the exclusion of other parts of the book.* Mastery of these first six chapters (and familiarity with Chapters 7 and 8 on airway management and IV access) should go a long way toward increasing reader confidence in managing cardiac arrest and assuring successful completion of the ACLS course. With more time available, or after completion of the ACLS course, the wealth of material contained in the rest of the book should prove interesting and serve as a useful reference for all those involved in emergency cardiac care.

Authors' Note

Although our recommendations are generally very consistent with those put forth by the American Heart Association, we do not always adhere strictly to their guidelines. In such cases we clearly state the rationale for our views and appropriately reference any points of contention. We do *not* feel such differences of opinion represent a departure from the objectives of the American Heart Association, since this agency freely acknowledges that their algorithms for treatment are not all inclusive:

" . . . Some patients may require care not specified herein. Th(ese) algorithm(s) should not be construed as prohibiting such flexibility" (JAMA Supplement, 1986*).

On the contrary, we firmly believe that acknowledging areas of controversy and presenting alternative approaches for selected situations is beneficial and may lead to improved emergency care.

Acknowledgments

I am indebted to the following people whose contributions were instrumental to the preparation of this book:

Dan Cavallaro, whose expertise has enriched my knowledge for the past seven years, and whose friendship and enthusiasm helped make the project fun. His contributions to this second edition have been invaluable to me.

Jim Hillman, M.D. and Paul Michlin, M.D. for allowing Dan the time and providing him with the freedom and support to assist me in the preparation of this manuscript.

Paul Augereau, M.D., Arlene Copenhaver, R.N., Jerry Diehr, M.D., Jim Hillman, M.D., Larry Kravitz, M.D., and Harry Sernaker, M.D., for helping me write selected portions of the text.

Helen Dalton, R.N., Jane Freeman, R.N., Holly Jensen, R.N., and James E. Jernigan, M.D., for reviewing the majority of the manuscript and "keeping me honest."

Rick Weimer, Lisa Cunninghis, and Susan Lawson of the C.V. Mosby Company, for their unlimited enthusiasm and skillful guidance of the project.

The Apple Macintosh Computer, without which I would still be typing this manuscript.

My father, Samuel Grauer, without whom this book would not have been possible.

Robyn Lyemance for her kindness and wonderful patience in the endless photographic sessions needed to prepare the chapters on airway management and IV access.

Pat, Kay, and the crew at Sonny's for their excellent service, and for providing me with a peaceful and pleasant environment for writing and reviewing much of the text.

Lee Crandall, Ph.D., Helen Dalton, R.N., Eric Diamond, Ph.D., Jane Freeman, R.N., Holly Jensen, R.N., James A. Jernigan, M.D., Lisa Moliter, R.N., Ray Moseley, Ph.D., and Martin Smith, for their assistance with the chapter on medicolegal aspects.

---

*American Heart Association Subcommittee on Emergency Cardiac Care: *Standards and guidelines for cardiopulmonary resuscitation (CPR) and emergency cardiac care (ECC).* JAMA (Supplement) 255:2905–2992, 1986.

Richard Bucciarelli, M.D., Greg Gaar, M.D., John Hellrung, M.D., John Santamaria M.D., and Bonnie Sharen, for their assistance with the chapters on pediatrics.

J. Daniel Robinson, Pharm. D. for contributing the SIMKIN figures which I modified in the chapter on lidocaine, and John Gums, Pharm. D. for his expert input on pharmacologic aspects of the text.

Betty Arnette, REMT-P, Phyllis Barks, PA-C, MPH, George Corey, M.D., Karen Curran, M.D., R. Whitney Curry, Jr., M.D., Eloise Harman, M.D., Phil Irwin, PA-C, Larry Kravitz, M.D., and Lou Kuritzky, M.D., for constructive commentary on selected portions of the text.

The residents, medical students, paramedics, physician assistant students, and nurses who have allowed us to learn by teaching them.

All those who have knowingly (and unknowingly) provided me with tracings.

The many excellent cardiologists who have inspired me and from whom I have learned.

We are particularly grateful to the American Academy of Family Physicians that allowed us to modify and reproduce the following figures from our Monograph #47, Interpreting ECGs: A Workbook 1983, one of a continuing series of monographs from the AAFP Home Study Self-Assessment Program: Figures 3A-1, 3A-2, 3A-16, 3A-18, 3B-16, 3C-9, 3C-11, 3C-11A, 16A-1, 16A–17A. In addition we reproduced Figures 3D-9 and 3D-17 from "Early Management of Myocardial Infarction," American Family Physician 28:162–170, 1983; and Table D-1 from New Trends in the Management of Cardiac Arrest, American Family Physician 29:223–236, 1984.

We are also grateful to Continuing Education for the Family Physician (Le Jacq Publishing Inc) for allowing us to modify and reproduce the following figures from articles and the "ECG of the Month" series that we wrote for their journal: Figure 3B-3, 3B-15, 3B-17, 3B-20, 3B-21, 16B-3, 16B-3A, and Table 16A-2.

Finally we appreciate Medical Economics Books for allowing us to modify and reproduce the following figures from "Clinical Electrocardiography: A Primary Care Approach," Medical Economics Books, Oradell, 1986: Figures 3A-9, 3B-2, 3B-10, 3B-11, and 3B-12.

ACLS: Certification Preparation and A Comprehensive Review

Antiarrhythmic Agents
  Digoxin
  Procainamide
  Propranolol

Miscellaneous Drugs
  Furosemide
  Naloxone
  Corticosteroids
  Magnesium Sulfate

PART I

THE ESSENTIALS OF RUNNING A CODE

OVERALL APPROACH TO MANAGEMENT OF CARDIOPULMONARY ARREST: ALGORITHMS FOR TREATMENT

A: OVERVIEW OF CARDIAC ARREST

Introduction

This chapter provides a brief overview of the approach to the management of cardiopulmonary arrest and introduces the algorithms for treatment. At first glance, the thought of having to learn all the material contained herein may seem overwhelming. This need not be the case. If one breaks down cardiac arrest into the rhythms that are associated with the initial event (*primary* or precipitating mechanisms of the arrest) and the rhythms that may follow conversion out of ventricular fibrillation (*secondary* mechanisms or post-conversion rhythms), organization of the problem becomes much simpler (Fig. 1-1).

> Although it may seem that innumerable therapeutic options are available, the essentials of management can be summarized by the four basic treatment algorithms that are presented in this chapter. Thorough mastery of these algorithms will provide the emergency care provider with the needed information to effectively run most codes.

Another reason these algorithms are important is that they provide an overall perspective for the management of cardiac arrest. They are the foundation on which the building blocks of treatment are laid. While some may object to a dependence on algorithms on the grounds that they sometimes restrict thinking and do not always apply to the particular situation at hand, their use in training emergency care providers to manage cardiac arrest has definitely been shown to expedite clinical decision making. Perhaps nowhere in medicine does the ability to rapidly decide on a rational course of therapy have as much impact on survival as it does at the scene of a cardiopulmonary arrest.

With practice, recall of the algorithms becomes automatic. Such "automaticity" is extremely beneficial during an arrest situation because it prevents the emergency care provider from forgetting basic material that was so well known under less stressful circumstances. Algorithms are *not* meant to be a substitute for judgment. On the contrary, reflexive recall of the framework of management facilitates organization of one's thinking, setting priorities, and institution of an appropriate therapeutic approach. Algorithms do *not* account for all possible permutations of management. They are not meant to, since doing so would entail specification of an endless number of uncommonly used treatment alternatives that would only confuse the issue and defeat the original goals of the algorithm—namely, organization, simplicity, and practicality.

Overview Algorithm of Cardiac Arrest

Most cases of cardiopulmonary arrest occur outside the hospital. In this setting, the three principal mechanisms of cardiac arrest are ventricular tachycardia, ventricular fibrillation, and

Overview Algorithm of Cardiac Arrest

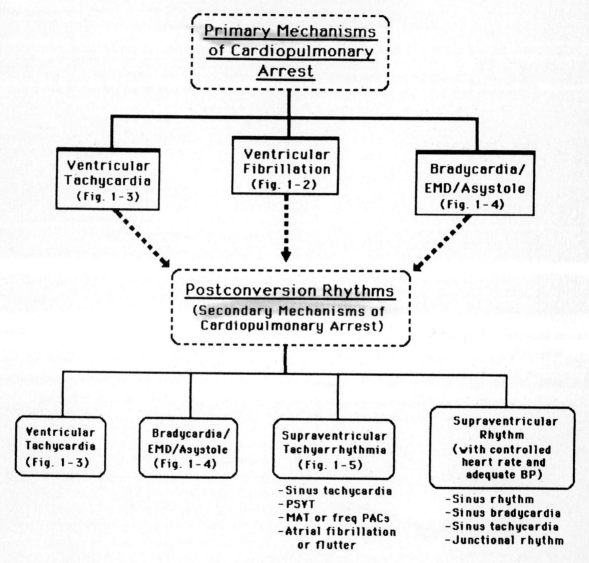

Figure 1-1

bradyarrythmias including electromechanical dissociation (EMD) and asystole **(Fig. 1-1)**. Of these, *ventricular fibrillation* is by far the most common, occurring in almost two thirds of cases. Ventricular tachycardia is a relatively in-frequent mechanism of out-of-hospital cardiac arrest, occurring in only about 5–10% of cases. A bradyarrhythmia (including EMD or asystole) accounts for the remainder.

Ventricular tachycardia appears to be a much

more common precipitating mechanism for cardiac arrests that occur in the hospital. Perhaps this is simply because the time from onset of the arrest until discovery by trained personnel is significantly less in a hospitalized setting. *Primary respiratory arrest* also becomes an important precipitating mechanism in hospitalized patients. Again, the reason is probably that earlier discovery and correction of respiratory arrest in the hospital prevents progression to the full cardiopulmonary arrest that is seen with the longer delays that occur outside of the hospital. Management of the three principal cardiac mechanisms of arrest is outlined by the treatment algorithms shown in Figures 1-2, 1-3, and 1-4 and is discussed in detail in its respective section in this chapter.

If the patient is successfully converted out of ventricular fibrillation, one of the four *secondary* mechanisms of cardiac arrest shown in Figure 1-1 may result. Treatment of ventricular tachycardia and bradycardia/EMD/asystole is similar to that recommended for these rhythms when they arise as the primary mechanism of the arrest (see Figures 1-3 and 1-4). If the patient is converted out of ventricular fibrillation to a supraventricular rhythm, the need for treatment will depend on the hemodynamic stability of the patient. If heart rate is controlled and blood pressure is adequate, no treatment may be necessary. If instead a rapid supraventricular rhythm is present, management according to the treatment algorithm shown in Figure 1-5 is suggested.

The ABCs of Cardiopulmonary Resuscitation

The key to survival from cardiopulmonary arrest lies with early recognition of the clinical state of unresponsiveness associated with apnea and/or pulselessness, initiation of basic life support by the lay public, and activation of emergency medical system (EMS) personnel capable of providing ACLS. Assessment and management of the unconscious victim begin with the ABCs. The following sequence should be mastered.

i) Establish unresponsiveness.
ii) Call for help.
iii) Position the victim and open the **A**irway.
iv) Check for the existence and adequacy of spontaneous **B**reathing.
v) Perform rescue breathing if needed. Start with two full breaths.
vi) Assess **C**irculation by establishing whether a pulse is present.
vii) Activate the EMS system.
viii) Begin external chest compression. Combine this with rescue breathing and continue until EMS personnel arrive.

Once providers capable of administering advanced life support arrive, attention may be directed to delivery of more definitive care. As soon as the prevailing mechanism of the arrest can be identified, treatment may be prescribed according to the appropriate algorithm.

B: VENTRICULAR FIBRILLATION

Algorithm for Ventricular Fibrillation

The recommended sequence for management of ventricular fibrillation is shown in **Figure 1-2.** By far the most important treatment modality is immediate defibrillation. Studies have shown that if EMS personnel are able to do nothing other than to defibrillate the patient, the likelihood of survival is significantly increased. The same urgency for prompt defibrillation carries over to the occurrence of ventricular fibrillation in the hospitalized setting. Endotracheal intubation, establishment of intravenous access, and administration of medications all play a secondary role.

Time is of the essence. The chances of converting a patient out of ventricular fibrillation are inversely proportional to the amount of time

Algorithm for Ventricular Fibrillation

Identification of V Fib and initial therapy:

Verify cardiopulmonary arrest — call for help —
initiate CPR — use quick-look paddles to verify V Fib

1) DEFIBRILLATE (Use **200** Joules for this 1st attempt)

If the patient is still in V Fib:

Verify pulselessness — resume CPR while recharging
defibrillator

2) DEFIBRILLATE (Use **300** Joules for this 2nd attempt)

If the patient is still in V Fib:

Verify pulselessness — resume CPR while recharging
defibrillator

3) DEFIBRILLATE (Use **360** Joules for this 3rd attempt)

If the patient is still in V Fib:

Verify pulselessness — resume CPR — intubate the patient
and establish IV access — apply monitor leads

4) EPINEPHRINE (1 mg IV or ET)
5) Consider **SODIUM BICARBONATE**
   (At this point, sodium bicarbonate should probably
   not be given unless the period of arrest has been
   extended {>5-10 min}, or if the patient has an
   underlying metabolic acidosis)
6) DEFIBRILLATE (Use **360** Joules)

If the patient is converted out of V Fib:

1) Treat further according to appropriate algorithm
2) If not already done, administer bolus of **LIDOCAINE** (50-100 mg) and begin IV infusion {Mix 1 g in 250 cc D5W, and run at 30 drops/min (= 2mg/min)}

If the patient is still in V Fib:

Verify pulselessness

7) LIDOCAINE (Give 50-100 mg IV bolus. Consider
   starting an IV infusion {Mix 1 g in 250 cc D5W and run
   at 30 drops/min (= 2mg/min)})
8) DEFIBRILLATE (Use **360** Joules)

If the patient is still in V Fib:

Verify pulselessness — look for potentially reversible
cause of V Fib

9) Repeat **EPINEPHRINE** (1 mg IV or ET) as appropriate
10) Consider **SODIUM BICARBONATE**
11) Repeat **LIDOCAINE** bolus (up to 225 mg maximum)
   or
   Give ≈1 amp (= 500 mg) of **BRETYLIUM** by IV bolus.
   May then give 10 mg/kg (= 1-2 amps) after defibrillation.
   Repeat thereafter q 15-30 min up to 30 mg/kg
12) DEFIBRILLATE (Use **360** Joules)

Figure 1-2

6

from the onset of this arrhythmia until counter-shock is applied. Consequently, all efforts must be directed toward rapid establishment of the diagnosis followed by immediate defibrillation.

> *Quick look paddles* facilitate this process. They should be applied *before* attempts are made at intubation or securing intravenous access. This holds true not only for cardiopulmonary arrests that occur in the field but also for those that take place in the hospital or emergency department when the patient is not being monitored. Immediate application of quick look paddles by hospital personnel may save precious seconds that determine whether resuscitation will be successful.

1) First Defibrillation Attempt

The preferred energy level for the first defibrillation attempt in adults is *200 joules*. This recommendation is based on the studies by Weaver et al. in Seattle that demonstrate fewer complications (heart block, asystole) but comparable conversion and survival rates for patients defibrillated with low (175 joules) versus high (320 joules) energy shocks.

2) Second Defibrillation Attempt

If pulselessness persists after the first shock and the patient remains in ventricular fibrillation, CPR should be resumed as the defibrillator is being recharged. Minimizing the time between countershock attempts lowers transthoracic resistance and allows a greater amount of *current* to pass through the heart on the second defibrillation attempt.

Whereas previous recommendations advised the use of similar energies for the first two defibrillation attempts, the new guidelines favor increasing the energy level for the second attempt to *300 joules*. By both increasing the energy level *and* minimizing the time between successive countershocks, one ensures that a greater amount of current flows through the heart on the second attempt. This enhances the chances for successful electrical conversion.

3) Third Defibrillation Attempt

If ventricular fibrillation persists, a third countershock with maximal energy *(360 joules)* should be delivered. The addition of a third

shock represents a change from previous guidelines that recommended only two countershock attempts before turning to other modalities.

4) Epinephrine

If ventricular fibrillation is still present after the third countershock, one should resume CPR, attempt to intubate the patient, establish intravenous access, and hook the patient up to a monitor. A trial of medications is now in order.

Epinephrine is the drug of choice. It may be administered either *intravenously (IV)* or *endotracheally (ET)*, depending on which route is established first. The dose is *1 mg* (1 ampule) of a 1:10,000 solution. Epinephrine is by far the most important pharmacologic agent used during cardiac arrest. In addition to its potent chronotropic and inotropic properties, it is the only one of the commonly employed agents to favor blood flow to the heart and brain during cardiac arrest.

5) Consider Sodium Bicarbonate

Although sodium bicarbonate has been liberally used during cardiac arrest in the past, recent data strongly question this practice. It is now becoming clear that the acidosis that occurs in this setting is predominantly respiratory in nature (due to hypoventilation) during the early minutes of the arrest. A metabolic component probably does not develop until *at least* 5 (if not 10) minutes after the collapse of the patient.

> Because the acidosis of cardiopulmonary arrest is primarily respiratory, treatment should be aimed at improving oxygenation and ventilation rather than trying to raise the pH by sodium bicarbonate administration. In fact, inappropriate focus on the latter measure can be detrimental since it may result in a paradoxical intracellular acidosis in myocardial and cerebral cells, depressing their function further. In view of this, the new guidelines favor *withholding* sodium bicarbonate unless the period of arrest has been extended (at least 5 to 10 minutes) or the patient is known to have had an underlying metabolic acidosis that may have precipitated the arrest.

6) Defibrillation

If ventricular fibrillation still persists following epinephrine administration, another countershock attempt with maximal energy *(360 joules)* should be delivered.

7) Lidocaine

Ventricular fibrillation not responding to the above measures is referred to as *refractory* and should prompt trial of an *antifibrillatory* agent. Whereas previous guidelines favored bretylium tosylate for this purpose, the new guidelines advocate *lidocaine*. Studies to date have failed to demonstrate a clear superiority of one of these agents over the other. Since lidocaine is a safer agent, and most emergency care providers are more familiar and comfortable with its use, it is now recommended as the agent of choice for refractory ventricular fibrillation.

> The loading dose of lidocaine is *50–100 mg* (1 mg/kg). In the spontaneously beating heart, an intravenous infusion (at a rate of 2 mg/min) is usually begun immediately after giving the bolus to maintain a therapeutic level of the drug. The effects of the bolus last only a short time and if an infusion is not started, additional boluses would be needed at least every 10 minutes to continue the action of the drug. In contrast, the pharmacokinetics of lidocaine in the arrested heart are somewhat unpredictable. Clearance of the drug is markedly decreased, and as little as one or two boluses of lidocaine may be adequate to maintain therapeutic lidocaine levels. Consequently, some emergency care providers choose to withhold the infusion until the patient is converted out of ventricular fibrillation. *If you do not start an IV infusion of lidocaine at this point, it is* **imperative** *that you remember to do so as soon as the patient is converted out of ventricular fibrillation.*

8) Defibrillation

Following administration of lidocaine, one should perform CPR for about 1–2 minutes to allow the drug a chance to reach the central circulation. Then *defibrillate* the patient again with full energy *(360 joules)*.

9) Repeat Epinephrine as Appropriate

Lack of response to the above measures should prompt the emergency care provider to scrutinize the circumstances leading up to the arrest, including a review of the pertinent medical history of the patient. Strong consideration should be given to whether any potentially reversible causes of refractory ventricular fibrillation may be present, such as volume depletion, inadequate ventilation, persistent severe metabolic acidosis, and/or electrolyte abnormalities. If no such causes appear to be operative, *epinephrine* should be repeated at least every 5 minutes by either the intravenous or the endotracheal route.

10) Consider Sodium Bicarbonate

By now, sufficient time may have passed for development of a metabolic component to the acidosis. Thus, one may reconsider whether to give *sodium bicarbonate*. The initial recommended dose is 1 mEq/kg (approximately 1–2 ampules). In a hospital setting, the results of arterial blood gas studies (ABGs) can help guide sodium bicarbonate therapy. It is extremely important *not* to overshoot correction of the acidosis since the body is much less adept at functioning in the presence of alkalosis than it is with a mild acidosis. In general, pH values between 7.25 and 7.35 are perfectly acceptable in the setting of cardiac arrest. Administration of sodium bicarbonate is rarely warranted unless the pH falls *below* 7.20.

11) Repeat Lidocaine Bolus or Administer Bretylium

An additional antifibrillatory agent should be administered. The new guidelines give the emergency care provider two options in this regard. The first is to repeat *lidocaine*. A second IV bolus of 50–75 mg of drug may be administered and possibly repeated in 5–10 minutes as needed (until a maximum dose of 225 mg). *As mentioned earlier, due to the altered pharmacokinetics of lidocaine in the arrested heart, less aggressive loading (repeating the bolus only once) may be desirable.*

Alternatively, a switch may be made to *bretylium tosylate*. The initial recommended dose of this drug for refractory ventricular fibrillation is 5 mg/kg (or approximately the contents of *1 ampule*) delivered as an IV bolus. The drug should be circulated (with CPR) for about 2 minutes before reattempting defibrillation. If there is no response, 10 mg/kg (1–2 ampules) may now be given, circulated, and followed by defibrillation. Additional 10 mg/kg boluses may be repeated at 15–30 minute intervals until a total of 30 mg/kg has been administered.

Although the *antifibrillatory* effect of bretylium is frequently seen within a few minutes after administration, a delay of up to 15 minutes may occur before the drug begins to work. Therefore, one should *not* terminate resuscitative efforts until adequate time has been allowed for this agent to take effect.

12) Defibrillation

Following each administration of the chosen antifibrillatory agent, CPR should be performed for at least 2 minutes to allow adequate time for the agent to reach the central circulation. *Defibrillation* should then be repeated with an energy of *360 joules*.

Repetition of Steps 9 through 12

There is *no limit* to the number of times a patient can be defibrillated. As long as ventricular fibrillation persists, a potentially treatable situation is present. Attention should be redirected to assessing the adequacy of ventilation and oxygenation (by physical examination and ABGs) and looking for underlying exacerbating factors. Epinephrine should be liberally repeated, sodium bicarbonate may be required, and maximum antifibrillatory treatment should be tried.

> Although still a matter of controversy, it is possible that the effects of lidocaine and bretylium in refractory ventricular fibrillation may be additive. Even if maximal doses of one agent don't work, the other drug may still be effective. It is also possible that addition of the second drug could result in a combination of agents that may now work. Therefore, it may be necessary to repeat steps 9 through 12 a number of times until all therapeutic options have been exhausted.

Conversion out of Ventricular Fibrillation

If at any time during the above protocol the patient is converted out of ventricular fibrillation, *prophylactic therapy* with *lidocaine* should be started in the hope of preventing a recurrence.

If bolus therapy has not yet been given or if more than 5 minutes have elapsed since the time of the last dose, an IV bolus should be administered and an infusion set up to run at 2 mg/min.

SPECIAL POINTS TO CONSIDER:

i) The **precordial thump** has become a "second class citizen" when defibrillation or cardioversion is an option. Because the procedure itself may result in a deterioration of the rhythm, the thump at present is indicated *only* for pulseless rhythms.

ii) The emergency care provider should *always* check for the presence of a **pulse** after each and every intervention. Forgetting to do so may result in iatrogenic defibrillation of a patient in sinus rhythm whose monitor leads fell off. (*It will also probably result in your failure of the ACLS course!!!*)

iii) Should a patient be converted out of ventricular fibrillation, to be followed a short while later by a *recurrence* of this rhythm, it may be reasonable to lower the energy level to 200 joules for the next defibrillation attempt. If this is not successful, maximal energy (360 joules) should then be used for subsequent attempts.

iv) The use of **sodium bicarbonate** has been greatly discouraged. Because of the potential deleterious effects of this drug, some clinicians question whether it should ever be given even if a pre-existing metabolic acidosis is known to be present.

C: VENTRICULAR TACHYCARDIA

Algorithm for Sustained Ventricular Tachycardia

The key to management of sustained ventricular tachycardia hinges on assessment of the patient's hemodynamic status. This is reflected in the recommendations shown in **Figure 1-3** for treatment of this condition.

If There Is No Pulse

Ventricular tachycardia without a pulse should be treated similar to ventricular fibrilla-

Algorithm for Sustained
Ventricular Tachycardia

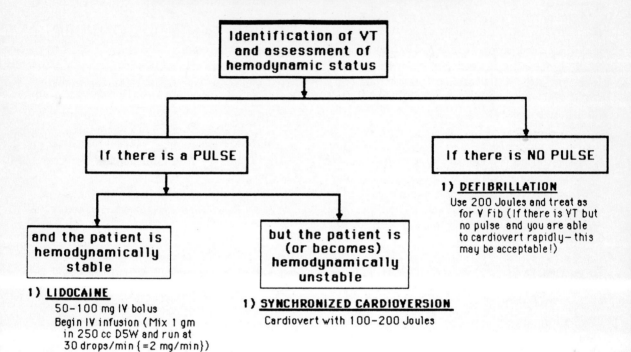

Identification of VT and assessment of hemodynamic status

If there is a PULSE

If there is NO PULSE

1) **DEFIBRILLATION**
Use 200 Joules and treat as
for V Fib (If there is VT but
no pulse and you are able
to cardiovert rapidly— this
may be acceptable!)

and the patient is hemodynamically stable

but the patient is (or becomes) hemodynamically unstable

1) **LIDOCAINE**
50-100 mg IV bolus
Begin IV infusion (Mix 1 gm
in 250 cc D5W and run at
30 drops/min {=2 mg/min})
May repeat lidocaine bolus if
needed up to a 225 mg loading
dose

2) **PROCAINAMIDE**
100 mg IV q 5 min up to 1 gm
loading dose
(An alternate loading protocol
is to mix 500-1000 mg in
100 cc D5W and infuse over
30-60 min)
If successful, an infusion may
be started at 2 mg/min

3) **BRETYLIUM**
Mix 500 mg in 50 cc D5W and
infuse over 10 min
This may be followed by an infusion
(Mix 1 gm in 250 cc D5W and run at
15-30 drops/min {1-2 mg/min})

4) **SYNCHRONIZED CARDIOVERSION**
Sedate the patient
Call anesthesia to the bedside
Cardiovert with 50-100-200 Joules

1) **SYNCHRONIZED CARDIOVERSION**
Cardiovert with 100-200 Joules

Figure 1-3

10

tion—by immediate countershock (*unsynchronized* defibrillation).

If There Is a Pulse and the Patient Is Hemodynamically Stable:

1) Lidocaine

If the patient is hemodynamically stable, antiarrhythmic therapy should be tried before attempting cardioversion. The drug of choice is *lidocaine*. An initial loading dose of *50–100 mg* (1 mg/kg) should be given, and an *IV infusion* started at *2 mg/min*. Additional 50–75 mg IV boluses should follow every 5–10 minutes as needed, or until a total loading dose of 225 mg has been given.

> Although some clinicans prefer to increase the infusion rate with each additional bolus of lidocaine, this is *not* essential during the period of lidocaine loading, and it may unnecessarily increase the risk of toxicity. On the other hand, if the ventricular arrhythmia resolves initially, only to recur after steady state conditions have been achieved at an infusion rate of 2 mg/min, an additional 50 mg bolus and an increase in the infusion rate to 3 mg/min may be warranted. (See Chapter 13, "Use of Lidocaine," for a more detailed discussion of the subject.)

2) Procainamide

The second-line agent for treatment of ventricular tachycardia is *procainamide.* The drug may be administered IV in 100 mg increments every 5 minutes (at a rate not to exceed 20 mg/min) until the arrhythmia is suppressed, hypotension occurs, the QRS complex widens by ≥50%, or a total loading dose of 1000 mg has been given. Alternatively, 500–1000 mg of drug may be mixed in 100 cc of D5W and infused over 30–60 minutes.

Following loading, a continuous infusion at 2 mg/min (1–4 mg/min range) may be needed to maintain the effect.

3) Bretylium

Bretylium has become a third line agent (*after* lidocaine and procainamide) for treatment of sustained ventricular tachycardia. This represents a change from previous guidelines that gave bretylium higher priority for treatment of ventricular arrhythmias. The drug appears to be more effective as an *antifibrillatory* agent than as an *antiarrhythmic* agent. The most common long-term adverse effect from bretylium therapy is hypotension which further limits its use.

For treatment of ventricular tachycardia, bretylium should be administered as an IV loading infusion. One ampule (500 mg) of the drug is mixed in 50 cc of D5W and infused over 10 minutes. Following loading, a continuous infusion at 1–2 mg/min may be needed to maintain the effect.

4) Synchronized Cardioversion

In the event that antiarrhythmic therapy is unsuccessful in converting the patient out of sustained ventricular tachycardia, *synchronized cardioversion* is indicated. If the patient shows no signs of hemodynamic compromise, this may be carried out under "semi-elective" circumstances. Sedation is advised to minimize patient discomfort from the procedure. In a hospital setting, an anesthesiologist may be called to the bedside for assistance. (In this way, qualified personnel can attend to the airway should the patient decompensate, leaving you free to concentrate on directing resuscitation and managing arrhythmias.)

An initial energy level of 50 joules may be chosen for the first attempt at synchronized cardioversion. If this is unsuccessful, increase the energy level to 100 and then 200 joules.

If There Is a Pulse but the Patient Is (or Becomes) Hemodynamically Unstable

If the patient has a pulse but is hemodynamically unstable, *immediate* cardioversion must take precedence over antiarrhythmic therapy. Delay for the several minutes needed to draw up and administer medications is unacceptable in this urgent situation. An energy level of at least 100 joules should probably be chosen for emergency cardioversion.

It should be emphasized that if the patient shows signs of hemodynamic compromise at any point during antiarrhythmic therapy, synchronized cardioversion must be *immediately* performed.

SPECIAL POINTS TO CONSIDER

i) A patient is said to be **"hemodynamically stable"** when blood pressure is adequate (≥90 mm Hg systolic) and no symptoms (chest pain, dyspnea, altered mental status) are present. It is important to remember that *not all patients with sustained ventricular tachycardia are (or immediately become) hemodynamically unstable!* A patient in ventricular tachycardia with a moderate ventricular response (140–170 beats/min) may remain alert and maintain an adequate blood pressure for minutes or even *hours* before showing any signs of decompensation.

ii) The **precordial thump** should only be given for pulseless ventricular tachycardia when a defibrillator is not available. The reason for deemphasizing the thump is that although this maneuver may occasionally convert ventricular tachycardia to sinus rhythm, it is equally likely (if not more so) to convert it to ventricular fibrillation, asystole, or pulseless idioventricular rhythm. If synchronized cardioversion is readily available, this is far preferable to delivery of 2–5 joules at a random (and possibly vulnerable) point in the cardiac cycle as provided by the thump.

iii) Don't forget about **cough version!!!** Whether the mechanism for cough version is improved coronary perfusion (from the increase in intrathoracic pressure generated by the cough), activation of the autonomic nervous system, or conversion of mechanical energy from the cough into an electrical depolarization is unknown. What has been shown, however, is that the cough may effectively convert ventricular tachycardia to normal sinus rhythm in a surprising number of cases. The technique is vastly underutilized. It should probably be the first intervention in treatment of the conscious, hemodynamically stable patient in sustained ventricular tachycardia.

iv) The recommended treatment for **ventricular tachycardia without a pulse** is unsynchronized defibrillation. However, if you are familiar enough with your equipment to activate the synchronizer switch in the same time it would take you to deliver an unsynchronized countershock, it may be reasonable to attempt synchronized cardioversion instead.

A word of caution is in order. The reason unsynchronized countershock has been recommended when no pulse is present is that at the more rapid rates of ventricular tachycardia usually associated with these unstable patients, distinction between the QRS complex and the T wave often becomes exceedingly difficult (if not impossible). Under such circumstances, delivery of a "synchronized" discharge becomes equally likely to fall on a T wave (during the vulnerable period) as not. Delivery of unsynchronized countershock for pulseless ventricular tachycardia may obviate the need for you (and the defibrillator) to try to make such a distinction.

v) While ventricular tachycardia frequently responds to cardioversion with energies as low as 20 joules, utilization of *at least* 100 joules may be preferable for the hemodynamically compromised patient. With a more stable patient, time is less critical and trials at lower energy levels may be reasonable.

D: BRADYARRHYTHMIAS, EMD, AND ASYSTOLE

The bradyarrhythmias encompass a wide range of rhythm disturbances ranging from the often innocent sinus bradycardia to the usually lethal asystole and electromechanical dissociation (EMD). Prognosis and treatment depend on the rhythm, the clinical setting, and the patient's hemodynamic status. Recommendations for management are summarized in the treatment algorithm shown in **Figure 1-4.**

Algorithm for Sinus Bradycardia

IF THERE IS A PULSE AND AN ADEQUATE BLOOD PRESSURE

No specific treatment other than routine supportive measures (ie, observation, oxygen, intravenous access) are needed for sinus bradycardia when a pulse is present and the patient has an adequate blood pressure.

Algorithm for Bradyarrhythmias, EMD & Asystole

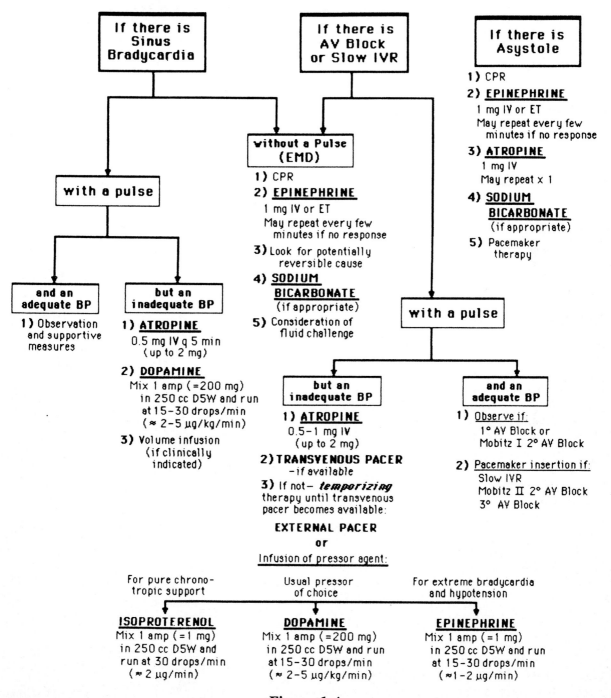

If there is Sinus Bradycardia

If there is AV Block or Slow IVR

If there is Asystole
1) CPR
2) **EPINEPHRINE**
   1 mg IV or ET
   May repeat every few minutes if no response
3) **ATROPINE**
   1 mg IV
   May repeat x 1
4) **SODIUM BICARBONATE**
   (if appropriate)
5) Pacemaker therapy

without a Pulse (EMD)
1) CPR
2) **EPINEPHRINE**
   1 mg IV or ET
   May repeat every few minutes if no response
3) Look for potentially reversible cause
4) **SODIUM BICARBONATE**
   (if appropriate)
5) Consideration of fluid challenge

with a pulse

and an adequate BP
1) Observation and supportive measures

but an inadequate BP
1) **ATROPINE**
   0.5 mg IV q 5 min
   (up to 2 mg)
2) **DOPAMINE**
   Mix 1 amp (=200 mg) in 250 cc D5W and run at 15-30 drops/min
   ($\approx$ 2-5 µg/kg/min)
3) Volume infusion (if clinically indicated)

with a pulse

but an inadequate BP
1) **ATROPINE**
   0.5-1 mg IV
   (up to 2 mg)
2) **TRANSVENOUS PACER**
   – if available
3) If not – *temporizing* therapy until transvenous pacer becomes available:

EXTERNAL PACER
or
Infusion of pressor agent:

and an adequate BP
1) Observe if:
   1° AV Block or
   Mobitz I 2° AV Block
2) Pacemaker insertion if:
   Slow IVR
   Mobitz II 2° AV Block
   3° AV Block

For pure chronotropic support

ISOPROTERENOL
Mix 1 amp (=1 mg) in 250 cc D5W and run at 30 drops/min
($\approx$ 2 µg/min)

Usual pressor of choice

DOPAMINE
Mix 1 amp (=200 mg) in 250 cc D5W and run at 15-30 drops/min
($\approx$ 2-5 µg/kg/min)

For extreme bradycardia and hypotension

EPINEPHRINE
Mix 1 amp (=1 mg) in 250 cc D5W and run at 15-30 drops/min
($\approx$ 1-2 µg/min)

Figure 1-4

IF THERE IS A PULSE BUT AN INADEQUATE BLOOD PRESSURE

If a pulse is present but the patient's blood pressure is insufficient (<90 mm Hg) to maintain adequate perfusion, *hemodynamic compromise* is said to exist and treatment is in order:

1) Atropine

The new guidelines have continued to deemphasize the use of atropine. The drug should *not* be used for the asymptomatic individual with bradycardia. Instead it is to be reserved for *symptomatic* bradycardia (associated with chest pain or dyspnea) or bradycardia accompanied by signs of *hemodynamic compromise* (hypotension, congestive heart failure, ventricular ectopy, or altered mental status).

The recommended initial dose of *atropine* for sinus bradycardia is *0.5 mg IV*. This may be repeated every 5 minutes until either a favorable clinical response occurs or a total of 2 mg have been administered.

2) Dopamine

If the patient's volume status is judged to be adequate and atropine has not been effective in achieving the desired clinical response, a *dopamine infusion* should be started. This may be prepared by mixing 1 ampule (200 mg) of drug in 250 cc of D5W and beginning the infusion at 15–30 drops/min ($\approx$2–5 μg/kg/min). The infusion may then be titrated to clinical effect.

3) Volume Infusion

The patient with bradycardia and hypotension may be volume depleted, either through volume loss (hemorrhage, dehydration) or inappropriate vasodilatation (acute myocardial infarction, septic or neurogenic shock). While in general most individuals with hypotension are *tachycardic*, this is not always the case. In particular, patients with acute inferior infarction frequently manifest excessive parasympathetic tone resulting in bradycardia and hypotension. Placing the patient in Trendelenburg position and starting careful volume infusion is the treatment of choice.

IF THERE IS SINUS BRADYCARDIA WITHOUT A PULSE (EMD)

If sinus bradycardia is present on the monitor (*electrical* activity) but no pulse is present (lack of *mechanical* activity), the patient is in *EMD*. The first priority in managing this condition is to resume CPR, since by definition this is a *nonperfusing* rhythm. Although epinephrine is the drug of choice, one usually will not be able to convert EMD to a perfusing rhythm unless an underlying precipitating cause of the disorder can be discovered and corrected. Thus, suggested management for EMD should include:

1) Resuming CPR

2) Epinephrine

The dose of *epinephrine* for EMD is the same as that for treatment of ventricular fibrillation—*1 mg* (1 ampule) of a 1:10,000 solution of the drug is given either IV or ET. This amount should be liberally repeated *at least* every 5 minutes.

> The principle reason for recommending epinephrine as the drug of choice for EMD is that this is the one drug that favors blood flow to the heart and brain. Development of EMD usually occurs *secondary* to some underlying precipitating factor. The potent chronotropic and inotropic effect of epinephrine may buy needed time until this causative factor can be identified and corrected. Occasionally, however, EMD is not secondary to any precipitating cause but is *primary* and due to inadequate coronary perfusion. In such instances, epinephrine's preferential shunting of blood to the coronary circulation may be lifesaving.

3) Look for a Potentially Reversible Cause

The most common potentially *reversible* causes of EMD to consider are:

—*inadequate ventilation* (intubation of the right mainstem bronchus, tension pneumothorax)

—*inadequate perfusion* (pericardial tamponade, hypovolemia)

—*metabolic abnormalities* (persistent severe acidosis, hyperkalemia).

4) Sodium Bicarbonate if Appropriate

In the event that lactic acidosis or diabetic ketoacidosis are present, administration of *sodium bicarbonate* may be needed (sometimes in large doses). In such cases, therapy should be guided by the results of ABGs. In the absence of an underlying acidosis, however, sodium bicarbonate is probably *not* indicated unless the period of arrest has been extended.

5) Consideration of a Fluid Challenge

Hypovolemia (from acute blood loss or septic, neurogenic or cardiogenic shock) is one of the most common and most easily correctable causes of EMD. Even without an obvious reason for hypovolemia, a trial of fluid infusion is probably indicated if EMD fails to respond to epinephrine.

Algorithm for Atrioventricular (AV) Block or Slow Idioventricular Rhythm (IVR)

IF THERE IS A PULSE AND AN ADEQUATE BP

No pharmacologic treatment is needed if AV block or slow IVR occur in a patient who is hemodynamically stable. Instead, the principal question is whether to insert a pacemaker. Pacemaker therapy is generally not needed for 1° AV block or 2° AV block Mobitz type I (Wenckebach). In contrast, 2° AV block Mobitz type II, high grade or complete (3°) AV block, and slow IVR signal much more severe conduction disturbances. In the setting of cardiac arrest, each of these conduction defects is an indication for

pacemaker insertion *regardless* of whether the patient is hemodynamically stable or not.

IF THERE IS A PULSE BUT AN INADEQUATE BP

Immediate treatment is indicated for the individual with any of the above conduction disorders when there is accompanying hypotension.

1) Atropine

As discussed above, the new guidelines favor the use of atropine *only* for bradyarrhythmias accompanied by signs of hemodynamic compromise. A dosing schedule of 0.5 mg IV every 5 minutes up to a total of 2 mg may not be practical for treatment of conduction disorders if the heart rate is extremely slow (under 40 beats/min) and the blood pressure very low (less than 80 mm Hg systolic). This is because such dosing would take no less than *15 minutes* to administer the full 2 mg of atropine. It may therefore be preferable in such instances to administer 1 mg of atropine at a time, repeating the dose in several minutes if the desired clinical response is not achieved.

2) Transvenous Pacemaker

The treatment of choice for AV block or slow IVR with associated hypotension in the setting of cardiac arrest is *transvenous pacemaker* insertion, provided that the necessary equipment, facilities and personnel are readily available. In general, external pacing and/or administration of a pressor agent should be viewed *only* as *temporizing* therapy that may be helpful in maintaining the patient until a transvenous pacemaker insertion may be accomplished.

3) Temporizing Therapy

An exciting advance in pacemaker therapy has been development of the *external pacemaker*. Obvious advantages of this device are speed of application and the fact that it is entirely noninvasive. This may be the temporizing measure of choice in the event that a transvenous pacemaker cannot be immediately inserted.

If there has been no response to full doses of atropine and pacemaker therapy is not immediately available, a trial with a *pressor agent* is indicated. It should again be emphasized that when hypotension accompanies AV block or slow IVR in the setting of cardiac arrest, pressor agents are to be used *only* as a stopgap measure to tide the patient over until more definitive (pacemaker) therapy can be initiated.

Under most circumstances, *dopamine* is the pressor agent of choice. Adjustment of the rate of infusion allows manipulation of dopaminergic, beta-adrenergic, and alpha-adrenergic receptor activity for optimal clinical effect. (Dosing of dopamine has been described above.)

Because of its propensity to increase myocardial oxygen consumption and cause peripheral vasodilatation, the indications for *isoproterenol* are limited. At low infusion rates, this drug provides effective *chronotropic* support. However, in the presence of accompanying hypotension (as is usually the case), one of the other agents is preferred. An isoproterenol infusion may be prepared by mixing 1 mg of drug (1 ampule) in 250 cc of D5W and beginning the drip at 30 drops/min (2 μg/min). The rate should not exceed 10 μg/min.

Epinephrine as an *infusion* is useful in treating extreme bradyarrhythmias that are accompanied by marked hypotension. With less severe degrees of hemodynamic compromise, dopamine is preferable. An epinephrine infusion may be prepared in a similar manner to an isoproterenol infusion: mix 1 mg of drug (1 ampule) in 250 cc of D5W. The drip should be started at 15–30 drops/min (1–2 μg/min) and titrated to clinical effect. The lowest effective dose should be used.

IF THERE IS NO PULSE (EMD)

The presence of AV block or slow IVR without a palpable pulse means that the rhythm is EMD. The treatment approach is identical to that outlined above for sinus bradycardia without a pulse.

Algorithm for Asystole

Although the prognosis for asystole is never good, the outlook for this arrhythmia when it develops during cardiac arrest that occurs *in* the hospital is not necessarily as bleak as when asystole is the primary mechanism of a cardiac arrest occurring *outside* of the hospital. Asystole in this latter setting is most often a preterminal rhythm that arises after ventricular fibrillation deteriorates. In contrast, asystole occurring in a hospital setting may occasionally result from massive parasympathetic discharge and, consequently, may be surprisingly responsive to atropine therapy. This phenomenon is most likely to be associated with certain operative procedures (endoscopy, cardiac catheterization), anesthesia, toxic drug reactions, vasovagal episodes, or heart block from acute inferior infarction. Another factor accounting for the better prognosis seen with asystole that occurs within the hospital is that the time elapsed from the onset of this arrhythmia until discovery of the patient by trained personnel tends to be much less than when the rhythm occurs on the outside.

The treatment approach to asystole should include:

1) Resuming CPR

Obviously there is no perfusion with asystole. CPR must be performed.

2) Epinephrine

Since *epinephrine* is the one agent that favors blood flow to the arrested heart and brain, this drug should be used *liberally* in asystole. An initial dose of *1 mg* is given *IV* or *ET* and continually repeated every few minutes.

3) Atropine

As mentioned above, asystole will occasionally result from massive parasympathetic discharge. Consequently, treatment with *atropine* should always be tried. The initial dose is *1 mg*, which should be repeated in *several* minutes if there has been no response.

4) Sodium Bicarbonate

The value of sodium bicarbonate during cardiac arrest has been seriously questioned since it appears that the acidosis developing in this setting is primarily respiratory for the first 5–10 minutes of the arrest. Consequently, sodium bicarbonate should probably *not* be administered for asystole unless the period of arrest has been extended or the patient is known to have a severe underlying acidosis that may have precipitated the arrest.

5) Pacemaker Therapy

In general, pacemaker therapy is *not* effective unless myocardial function has been preserved. It will usually *not* be helpful in asystole. Nevertheless, a trial of pacing may be warranted for the asystolic patient who has not responded to any of the above measures.

SPECIAL POINTS TO CONSIDER:

i) Fine ventricular fibrillation may occasionally masquerade as asystole. This can occur if the vector of the fibrillation wavefront happens to fall *perpendicular* to the plane of the lead being monitored. In view of this, one should *always* inspect more than one lead before concluding that a flat line represents asystole. If using quick look paddles, rotating paddle placement by 90° allows one to view the fibrillation wavefront from another direction. If the monitor again shows a flat line, it is safe to conclude that the rhythm is truly asystole. (Some observers believe this phenomenon explains anecdotal reports in the literature that claim successful defibrillation of "asystole." In such cases, the true rhythm was probably ventricular fibrillation that simulated asystole in the lead that was monitored.)

ii) **Atropine** is usually administered until either the desired clinical response is obtained or a total dose of 2 mg has been given. In most individuals, 2 mg is the full atropinization dose. However, occasionally up to *3 mg* may be needed in order to obtain the maximal effect of this drug. (Most emergency care providers still prefer to turn to a pressor agent when treating a symptomatic bradyarrhythmia that has not responded to the usual 2 mg dose of atropine.)

Administration of 0.5 mg IV every 5 minutes until the total dose of 2 mg has been given may not be practical if the heart rate is extremely slow and the blood pressure is markedly reduced. This is because it would take *no less* than 15 minutes to administer the full 2 mg of drug by this regimen. Thus, it may be preferable to give 1 mg of the drug at a time under such circumstances. In contrast, with less severe degrees of bradycardia and hemodynamic compromise, the lower dose (0.5 mg) should be used. Administering the 1 mg dose in this latter setting may result in overshoot tachycardia, with accompanying increased myocardial oxygen consumption and even possible deterioration to ventricular tachycardia or fibrillation. Atropine is not a totally benign drug, and its use should not be taken lightly.

iii) In the past, **calcium chloride** has been recommended for treatment of asystole and EMD. Recent studies, however, have demonstrated unacceptable mortality figures associated with the use of this agent. As a result, the new guidelines *no longer* recommend calcium chloride for treatment of either asystole or EMD. The *only* remaining indications for this agent at present are:

—hypocalcemia
—hyperkalemia
—asystole that develops following administration of a calcium channel blocking agent (as may occur when verapamil is given for treatment of a supraventricular tachyarrhythmia).

iv) **Epinephrine** is perhaps the most commonly used drug in cardiopulmonary resuscitation. It is the pharmacologic treatment of choice for ventricular fibrillation, asystole and EMD. Although best known for its potent chronotropic and inotropic effects, it is the alpha-adrenergic or vasoconstrictor effect of the drug that is more important in the setting of cardiac arrest. By this action, aortic diastolic pressure is increased, favoring circulation to the heart, and preferential shunting of blood occurs from the external to the internal carotid artery, favoring circulation to the brain.

The recommended dose of epinephrine is 0.5–1.0 mg IV every 5 minutes during the resuscitation effort. However, because of its beneficial action favoring myocardial and cerebral circulation in the arrested heart and the fact that rhythms of asystole and EMD are almost always fatal without such treatment, some observers have advocated much higher doses of epinephrine be used. Feeling that the above conditions represent "no lose" situations, *they recommend repetition of the 1 mg dose as often as every 2–3 minutes until 5 mg (and more) of the drug have been given for asystole and EMD.* Once again, the virtual impossibility of conducting prospective blinded and controlled studies in *man* on the effect of a treatment modality in cardiac arrest leaves the emergency care provider without incontestable data on which to base conclusions.

v) The new guidelines no longer recommend **isoproterenol** for treatment in the arrested heart. This is because of the pure beta-adrenergic action of this drug which results in peripheral vasodilatation. As opposed to epinephrine, isoproterenol lowers aortic diastolic blood pressure and consequently reduces myocardial and cerebral blood flow. Therefore its use should be *contraindicated* in ventricular fibrillation, asystole and EMD.

Isoproterenol is still recommended as a stopgap measure until pacemaker therapy can be initiated for hemodynamically significant bradyarrhythmias that have not responded to atropine. However, because of isoproterenol's vasodilatory effect (lowering peripheral vascular resistance), infusions of either **epinephrine** or **dopamine** are preferable when the bradyarrhythmia is associated with hypotension.

vi) When **epinephrine** is used to treat rhythms with a pulse (IVR or high-degree heart block with a slow ventricular response and marked hypotension), it should be administered as a *continuous IV infusion* rather than as a bolus. This allows moment-to-moment titration of the dose of the drug to clinical effect. In contrast, once a bolus of a drug has been given, *it cannot be taken back* and hemodynamic effects persist until the action of the drug wears off.

On the other hand, with rhythms such as ventricular fibrillation, asystole and EMD, higher levels of drug are likely to be obtained by bolus injection. Alternatively, if an epinephrine infusion has already been set up, turning it wide open may achieve the same effect as bolus administration.

E: SUPRAVENTRICULAR TACHYARRHYTHMIAS

Algorithm for Supraventricular Tachyarrhythmias

The multitude of supraventricular tachyarrhythmias encountered in emergency cardiac care may at times be intimidating to the emergency care provider. On the positive side, comfort can be taken in the fact that conversion of a patient out of one of the primary mechanisms of cardiac arrest and into a supraventricular tachyarrhythmia is usually a *good* sign associated with a high probability of successful resuscitation. Patients are likely to be hemodynamically stable with these arrhythmias, and most of the time heart rate control can be achieved with medication.

The supraventricular tachyarrhythmias most commonly seen in emergency cardiac care and suggested recommendations for their treatment are summarized in **Figure 1-5.**

IF THE PATIENT IS HEMODYNAMICALLY UNSTABLE

As for ventricular tachycardia, the *most* important facet of management to be assessed *before* the emergency care provider even begins to think about what a particular rhythm may be is the patient's hemodynamic status. If a patient with a rapid rhythm becomes acutely symptomatic (as indicated by hypotension, development of chest pain, dyspnea, or altered mental status), differential diagnosis of the tachyarrhythmia must take second place to stabilizing the patient.

1) Synchronized Cardioversion

The treatment of choice for hemodynamically significant supraventricular (or ventricular)

Algorithm for
Supraventricular Tachyarrhythmias

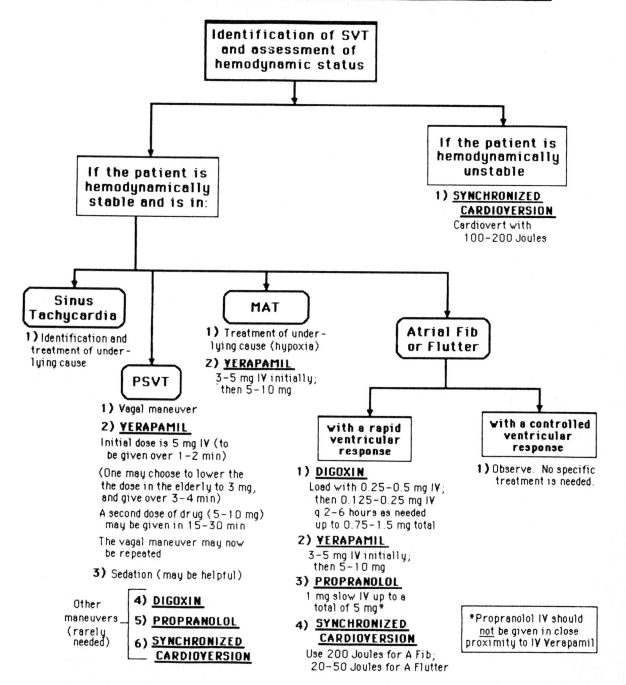

Figure 1-5

tachyarrhythmias is *synchronized cardioversion.* Certain arrhythmias such as atrial flutter are particularly sensitive to this modality, and conversion is usually possible with energy levels as low as 10–20 joules. Other arrhythmias such as atrial fibrillation are much more resistant to the effects of cardioversion and may require energy levels as high as 200 joules for success.

An even more important factor to consider when determining the initial energy level for the procedure is the *urgency* of the situation. When treating a patient in extremis, it may be preferable to maximize the chance for successful conversion of the rhythm on the first attempt by selecting a higher energy level (100–200 joules) than one would under more controlled circumstances.

IF THE PATIENT IS HEMODYNAMICALLY STABLE

If the patient with a supraventricular tachyarrhythmia is relatively comfortable and has an acceptable blood pressure, accurate diagnosis of the arrhythmia now takes on a much more important role in guiding therapy. Suggestions for treatment of supraventricular tachyarrhythmias follow below.

Sinus Tachycardia

No specific treatment is indicated for sinus tachycardia per se. Instead, treatment should focus on detection and correction of any underlying conditions (congestive heart failure, hypovolemia, shock) that may have brought about this arrhythmia.

Paroxysmal Supraventricular Tachycardia (PSVT)

The mechanism of PSVT in adults is almost always one of *reentry* into the AV node after the supraventricular impulse has been conducted to the ventricles. A reentry circuit is set up whereby the impulse is caught returning (in retrograde fashion) to the AV node, before being conducted back down again to the ventricles in what becomes a perpetual cycle. The goal of therapy is simply to interrupt this cycle in the hope that a normal rhythm may then take over.

1) Vagal Maneuvers

Vagal maneuvers act by transiently increasing parasympathetic tone. This slows conduction through supraventricular and AV nodal tissues. One hopes to delay AV nodal conduction just long enough to interrupt the reentry circuit of PSVT and terminate the arrhythmia.

Vagal maneuvers include carotid sinus massage, activation of the gag reflex, facial submersion in ice, eyeball pressure, squatting, and performing a Valsalva maneuver. Patients with recurrent episodes of PSVT have often instinctively learned how to perform one of these maneuvers on their own to terminate their arrhythmia.

In an emergency setting, *carotid sinus massage* is the vagal maneuver performed most often for treatment. Under constant ECG monitoring, the patient's head is turned to the left and the area of the right carotid bifurcation near the angle of the jaw is gently but firmly massaged for 5 seconds at a time. If right carotid massage is ineffective, the left side may be tried. (One should *never* massage both sides simultaneously.)

Carotid sinus massage may also be helpful diagnostically in distinguishing between PSVT, sinus tachycardia, and atrial flutter. PSVT will either be converted by the maneuver, or nothing will happen. In contrast, with sinus tachycardia or atrial flutter, transient slowing of the ventricular response during massage often allows telltale atrial activity to become apparent.

2) Verapamil

The drug of choice for treatment of PSVT is *verapamil.* It is effective over 90% of the time in converting this reentry tachyarrhythmia. The initial dose is *5 mg* IV given over 1–2 minutes. (In the *elderly,* one may want to give *less* of the drug [3 mg] over a somewhat *longer* period of time [3–4 min] to minimize the incidence of hypotension and/or excessive heart rate slowing.)

If there is no response to verapamil in 15 minutes, a second dose (of 5–10 mg) may be given. This can be followed in several minutes by another attempt at a vagal maneuver, since the effect of the drug and the maneuver are often synergistic.

> It has recently been shown that pretreatment with IV infusion of calcium chloride (infusing 1 gram over 5–10 minutes) virtually eliminates the hypotensive response of verapamil without diminishing the drug's efficacy in converting or controlling the ventricular response of patients with supraventricular tachyarrhythmias. Such pretreatment might be considered for patients with a borderline hemodynamic status (ie, systolic blood pressure < 100 mm Hg).

3) Sedation

In addition to relieving the anxiety that so often accompanies PSVT, sedation lowers sympathetic tone. This may help convert the arrhythmia by slowing conduction through the AV node.

4) Other Measures

Although *digoxin, propranolol,* and *synchronized cardioversion* were frequently used in the past to treat this arrhythmia, the tremendous success of verapamil has dramatically decreased the need for these therapies. As in the treatment of any tachyarrhythmia, however, if signs of hemodynamic compromise develop at any time with PSVT, one should forego medical treatment and immediately cardiovert the patient.

Multifocal Atrial Tachycardia (MAT)

MAT is most often seen in the setting of chronic obstructive pulmonary disease (COPD) and is associated with hypoxemia. It is important not to confuse this arrhythmia with atrial fibrillation since the treatments are different. Digoxin is the drug of choice for treatment of atrial fibrillation, with a rapid ventricular response. In contrast, MAT does not respond well to such therapy, and digitalis toxicity is likely to develop if multiple doses of this medication are given in an attempt to control the ventricular rate.

1) Improving Oxygenation

The treatment of choice of MAT is correction of the underlying cause of this rhythm disturbance. For patients with COPD, this entails oxygen therapy and bronchodilators.

2) Verapamil

When pharmacologic therapy is needed to control the ventricular rate with MAT, *verapamil* should be the drug of choice. Small doses of digoxin may be used, and when combined with verapamil a synergistic effect may be noted. However, large doses of digoxin should be avoided with this rhythm disturbance since they readily lead to toxicity.

Atrial Fibrillation or Flutter

IF THE VENTRICULAR RESPONSE IS CONTROLLED

Atrial fibrillation with a controlled ventricular response is often a very stable rhythm. No specific treatment is needed in the asymptomatic patient. Although atrial flutter is a less stable rhythm, it need not be treated either if the patient is asymptomatic and the ventricular response is controlled.

IF THERE IS A RAPID VENTRICULAR RESPONSE

In contrast, when the ventricular response to these arrhythmias is rapid, treatment is indicated. If the patient is tolerating the rapid rate, pharmacologic therapy may be tried first. If at any time hemodynamic compromise develops, immediate cardioversion should be performed.

1) Digoxin

Digoxin has been the pharmacologic agent preferred by most clinicians for treating these tachyarrhythmias. In a patient not previously taking this medication, one may administer a *loading dose of 0.25–0.5 mg IV* and follow this with *incremental doses* of *0.125–0.25 mg IV every 2–6 hours* as needed (depending on the ventricular response) until a total of 0.75–1.5 mg of drug has been given.

In the absence of hyperthyroidism, hypoxemia, acute myocardial infarction, and electrolyte disturbance, the ventricular response to the above therapy provides a fairly accurate indicator of the adequacy of digitalization. Thus, if the rate remains rapid after several boluses have been given, it suggests that additional digoxin may be needed. On the other hand, if any of these conditions are present, lower doses of the drug should be used.

2) Verapamil

Although verapamil is successful only about 30% of the time in converting atrial fibrillation or flutter to sinus rhythm, the drug is almost always effective in slowing the ventricular response to these tachyarrhythmias. Also, it may act synergistically when combined with digoxin.

3) Propranolol

Intravenous propranolol is currently used much less frequently than it was in the past for emergency treatment of supraventricular tachyarrhythmias. This is probably due to the tremendous efficacy of verapamil in these situations. One must remember that once IV verapamil is given, IV propranolol must *not* be administered for *at least* 30 minutes thereafter because the combination of these agents may produce marked slowing of the arrhythmia and even asystole.

4) Synchronized Cardioversion

As emphasized above, pharmacologic agents may be tried for the initial treatment of atrial fibrillation or flutter with a rapid ventricular response if the patient is not acutely unstable. If drugs are not effective, *cardioversion* will usually work. For atrial flutter, low energy levels (ie, 20–50 joules) are frequently all that are needed. In contrast, higher energy levels (100–200 joules) are often necessary for atrial fibrillation.

If hemodynamic compromise develops at any time during the above therapeutic sequence, immediate cardioversion with 100–200 joules should be performed.

SPECIAL POINTS TO CONSIDER:

i) Management according to the treatment algorithms shown in Figure 1-5 assumes that one has correctly diagnosed the tachyarrhythmia as **supraventricular**! Although distinction between supraventricular tachyarrhythmias and ventricular tachycardia is usually evident from inspection of the tracing, this will *not* always be the case. (See the chapter on "Diagnosis of Tachyarrhythmias" for further discussion on the subject.)

ii) It is important to emphasize that **carotid sinus massage** is *not* a totally benign maneuver, particularly in older individuals. It has been associated with syncope, stroke, sinus arrest, high-grade AV block, prolonged asystole, and ventricular tachyarrhythmias in patients with digitalis intoxication. As a result, it should probably *not* be attempted in patients with a history of sick sinus syndrome, cervical bruits, or cerebrovascular disease or when the possibility of digitalis intoxication exists.

CHAPTER 2

ESSENTIAL DRUGS AND TREATMENT MODALITIES

A: OVERVIEW

Introduction

The armamentarium of drugs and treatment modalities for cardiopulmonary resuscitation and emergency cardiac care is ever expanding. This situation could easily be overwhelming, especially for the ACLS provider who does not work with these drugs and modalities on a daily basis. In view of this and considering that the reader's need (and/or desire) to know about this material is likely to vary greatly, we have organized our presentation of the subject in as practical a format as possible. In this introductory section, we address the importance of the autonomic nervous system, adrenergic receptors, determinants of cardiac performance, and considerations that go into choosing a pressor agent. Although this material may be basic and/or review for some readers, we have included it in the hope that it may lay the groundwork for the description of drugs and treatment modalities to follow.

For each drug that is covered, we include dispensing and dosing information, indications for current use, and changes that have been made since the previous guidelines were published. Fortunately, the number of truly *essential* medications that one must be thoroughly familiar with in order to effectively manage a cardiac arrest is limited. These **"Key Drugs"** (the ones you need to master to pass the ACLS course) are discussed in Section B of this chapter. In Section C, we present an easy-to-learn method for **Simplified Calculation of IV Infusions** for the commonly used medications in emergency car-

diac care. This is followed in Section D by a brief discussion of the basic **Key Treatment Modalities** (for example, defibrillation, cardioversion, pacing).

The new guidelines have facilitated our task by deemphasizing or eliminating a number of agents that were previously recommended for use. These include sodium bicarbonate, isoproterenol, calcium chloride, and bretylium tosylate. Although there are still some indications for the use of each of these agents, these **Deemphasized Drugs** (discussed in Section E) are no longer viewed as *essential* in the management of cardiopulmonary arrest. Familiarity with their use may therefore be looked on as *optional,* particularly for the reader with only a limited time to prepare for the ACLS course. Similarly, drugs discussed in Chapter 14 comprise material "beyond the core" of what one needs to know to pass the course. It may be useful for those exposed to cardiology and acute care medicine on a regular basis and helpful as a reference to those who are not.

The Autonomic Nervous System

The **autonomic nervous system** is the *involuntary* nervous system of the body. It is made up of a series of reflex arcs which regulate functions of the body that are not under conscious control. Such functions include modulation of heart rate, control of blood pressure, intestinal motility, bladder function, and release of glandular secretions. Because it innervates the vis-

viscera, the autonomic nervous system is sometimes referred to as the *visceral* nervous system. Fibers from the autonomic nervous system are distributed to smooth muscles in all parts of the body. In contrast, the central nervous system per se supplies areas of the body that are under conscious control (or everything except the viscera).

The autonomic nervous system is divided into two major branches: the **sympathetic nervous system (SNS)** and the **parasympathetic nervous system (PNS).** A series of intricate interconnections exists between the central nervous system, efferent nerve fibers of the SNS and the PNS, autonomic ganglia, and the various target tissues and organs innervated by the autonomic nervous system.

> *Preganglionic* fibers of the autonomic nervous system transmit nerve signals from the central nervous system to the autonomic ganglia. Preganglionic fibers of both the SNS and the PNS stimulate nerve cells in these ganglia by releasing acetylcholine and, therefore, are said to be *cholinergic.*
>
> *Postganglionic* fibers of the autonomic nervous system emanate from the ganglia and go on to innervate their respective target organs. Postganglionic fibers of the SNS are **adrenergic** (with the exception of those nerves stimulating sweat glands and portions of skeletal muscle). They are so called because they mediate their effects on target organs by releasing *norepinephrine*. In contrast, postganglionic fibers of the PNS are cholinergic. Like preganglionic fibers of both branches of the autonomic system, they mediate their effects by releasing acetylcholine.

Generalized activation of the SNS results in a "fight or flight" reaction. In addition to adrenergic stimulation and release of the neurotransmitter norepinephrine, the adrenal gland is stimulated to release endogenous epinephrine. Heart rate and blood pressure increase, the pupils dilate, the individual perspires, bronchodilation occurs, intestinal peristalsis and glandular secretion are inhibited, and the anal sphincter contracts. In contrast, the PNS is the "repose and repair" system. Its activation results in slowing of the heart rate, a fall in blood pressure, and resumption of glandular secretion and peristalsis.

Adrenergic Receptors of the Autonomic Nervous System

The autonomic nervous system exerts an extremely important influence on cardiac function. As is the case for other internal organs of the body, the heart is doubly innervated by both sympathetic and parasympathetic nerve fibers. (In contrast, blood vessels have only sympathetic innervation.)

Impulses from the PNS are transmitted to the heart via the **vagus nerve.** The vagus innervates the sinoatrial and atrioventricular nodes and primarily exerts an *inhibitory* effect on the heart. Its stimulation therefore results in slowing of the heart rate and delay in atrioventricular (AV) conduction. As a result of optimal conditioning, young athletes often exhibit significant vagal tone at rest. They may, therefore, demonstrate a fairly marked sinus bradycardia and/or arrhythmia, first-degree AV block, and/or second-degree AV block Mobitz type I as *normal phenomena* that simply reflect the presence of marked vagotonia. On the other hand, excessive vagal discharge may also be commonly noted in association with acute inferior myocardial infarction. In this latter setting, the accompanying bradycardia, hypotension, and AV conduction disturbances are clearly pathologic.

> Adrenergic fibers of the SNS innervate the myocardium and primarily exert an *excitatory* effect. This results in acceleration of the heart rate (enhanced *chronotropy*) and increased contractility (positive *inotropic* effect). Adrenergic innervation is also present in the respiratory system and in vascular smooth muscle. Stimulation of these fibers may result in bronchodilatation or changes in vasomotor tone (vasoconstriction or vasodilatation, depending on the predominant type of adrenergic receptor activity).

Adrenergic activation is mediated by **alpha-** and **beta-adrenergic receptors** that are located on cellular surfaces. These receptors are of two subtypes: alpha-1 and alpha-2 and beta-1 and beta-2, respectively.

Beta-1 receptors are predominantly located in the myocardium. Adrenergic stimulation of these receptors is responsible for enhanced chronotropy and positive inotropy of the heart.

Beta-2 receptors are predominantly located in respiratory and vascular smooth muscle. Stimulation of these receptors results in bronchodilation and vasodilation.

Alpha-1 receptors are postsynaptic and are located on vascular smooth muscle. Their activation results in vasoconstriction.

Alpha-2 receptors are presynaptic and are located primarily in sympathetic nerve terminals. When stimulated, they prevent further release of the neurotransmitter norepinephrine. They thus act as a feedback mechanism to alpha-1 receptor activation.

As an aid to remembering what each beta-adrenergic receptor does, you may find it helpful to think of *"one heart, two lungs"*:
 —*beta-1 receptors* act on the *heart*
 —*beta-2 receptors* act on the *lungs*

> Thus beta-2 agonists (activators) such as terbutaline are very useful in treatment of asthma because of the bronchodilation they produce. On the other hand, an adverse effect of beta-blockers is that they may precipitate bronchospasm.

With respect to cardiac resuscitation, vasoconstriction is the *alpha*-adrenergic receptor activity with which we are most concerned. Unless otherwise specified, use of the general term *alpha-adrenergic stimulation* will therefore refer to stimulation of *alpha-1* adrenergic receptors.

> In our subsequent discussion of vasoactive drugs, note will be made of their degree of alpha- and beta-adrenergic receptor activity. For example, *isoproterenol* is a pure beta-adrenergic receptor stimulator. It therefore exerts a potent chronotropic and inotropic effect on the heart (beta-1 action), as well as causing bronchodilatation and peripheral vasodilatation (beta-2 effect).
>
> In contrast, *epinephrine* possesses *both* alpha- and beta-adrenergic activity. Its beta-1 effects produce enhanced chronotropy and inotropy in a similar manner as does isoproterenol. Its vasoactive action, however, will be somewhat dose dependent. At low doses, the beta-2 effects predominate and the result

is vasodilatation. With higher doses (as are used in emergency cardiac care), the alpha-adrenergic (vasoconstrictor) effect overrides the beta-2 (vasodilatory) action of the drug. It is this vasoconstrictor action of epinephrine that becomes so vitally important in maintaining coronary blood flow during cardiopulmonary resuscitation.

Under normal circumstances, *circulating* catecholamines (principally endogenous epinephrine, and to a lesser extent norepinephrine) exert little influence on cardiac function. Instead, cardiac tone and function are mediated by the autonomic nervous system. However, with chronic stress-inducing conditions (such as congestive heart failure), myocardial catecholamine stores may become depleted. In such situations, circulating catecholamines probably assume a much more important role.

> Administered medication with adrenergic stimulating properties may exert profound chronotropic and inotropic effects on the heart. In contrast, administration of a beta-blocking agent (such as propranolol) may dramatically depress myocardial function in patients who become dependent on circulating catecholamines to stimulate cardiac contraction.

Determinants of Cardiac Performance

The principal parameter for assessing cardiac performance is **cardiac output (CO).** This is simply a measurement of the volume of blood pumped out by the heart each minute. It is equal to stroke volume **(SV)** times heart rate **(HR)** as expressed by the following equation:

$$CO = HR \times SV$$

> where **SV** reflects the average amount of blood ejected from the heart with each contraction.

HEART RATE is a reflection of the interaction between *sympathetic* and *parasympathetic* tone of the autonomic nervous system. It is important to remember that the resting heart is normally under the influence of *both* of these divisions of the autonomic nervous system. Parasympathetic tone usually predominates. This is especially true for the case of the young well-trained athlete who, as was mentioned earlier, frequently manifests sinus bradycardia as the result of marked vagotonia. A certain amount of resting sympathetic tone is *also* usually present in most individuals. This is evidenced by experiments that demonstrate an increase in heart rate following parasympathetic denervation that far exceeds the original resting heart rate.

> Clinically, this becomes important when atropine is administered for treatment of hemodynamically significant bradyarrhythmias. Especially when a large dose of the drug (such as 1 mg at a time) is given, blockade of parasympathetic discharge may unmask underlying sympathetic hyperactivity (that previously had been held in check), with potentially deleterious effects (tachycardia, increased myocardial oxygen consumption, or tachyarrhythmias).

The second determinant of cardiac output in the above equation is **stroke volume.** The amount of blood ejected from the heart with each contraction depends on the interplay between three factors:

   i) **Preload**–which reflects the degree of passive "stretch" exerted on myocardial fibers

   ii) **Afterload**–or the resistance against which the heart must pump

   iii) **Contractility**–the force with which contraction takes place.

Clinically, *preload* is determined by left ventricular end diastolic volume (LVEDP). Under normal circumstances, the greater the LVEDP, the more the heart is stretched, and the stronger it will contract. This is the **Frank-Starling** principle. It explains why a failing heart requires a higher left ventricular filling pressure in order to perform the same amount of work as does a normal ventricle. Unless adequate myocardial "stretch" occurs, the heart will simply not contract forcefully enough to adequately eject blood. Thus, one frequently tries to achieve slightly higher than normal filling pressures in patients with acute myocardial infarction in an attempt to improve cardiac function. However, because too high filling pressures result in deterioration of cardiac function (as the heart will be unable to contract if there is too much "stretch"), careful hemodynamic monitoring

(with a Swan-Ganz catheter) is essential when manipulations are made in adjusting preload.

The other principal manner of improving cardiac output with acute infarction is to reduce *afterload*. Blood pressure control becomes vitally important in this setting. What would normally be a mild-to-moderate elevation in blood pressure (a blood pressure of 150–160 mm Hg systolic and 90–100 mm Hg diastolic) might severely overload an infarcting ventricle and precipitate overt cardiac decompensation. Agents such as nitroglycerin are ideal under such circumstances since they improve cardiac function by both decreasing preload *and* also reducing afterload in the patient in whom LVEDP is too high.

A very fine balance must be sought so as to maximize cardiac function without adversely affecting hemodynamics. Producing too potent an inotropic effect may disproportionately increase myocardial oxygen consumption and become deleterious. For this reason, agents that increase *contractility* (such as isoproterenol) are usually avoided in acute infarction. On the other hand, agents that produce too great an increase in peripheral vascular resistance (increasing afterload) may place too great a strain on the heart and also result in a reduction of cardiac output. Thus, in order to select the optimal agent for a given patient in a particular situation, a host of factors must be kept in mind.

Selection of a Pressor Agent

The cardiovascular drugs used in emergency cardiac care each affect one or more of the above determinants of myocardial performance. Adrenergic receptor agents with beta-1 stimulating properties (ie, isoproterenol, epinephrine, dopamine, dobutamine) increase heart rate and myocardial contractility. Those which also possess beta-2 stimulating properties (isoproterenol, low-dose epinephrine) vasodilate. Finally, those with alpha-adrenergic stimulating properties (moderate-to-high doses of epinephrine and dopamine, nonrepinephrine) vasoconstrict.

Collectively such drugs are frequently referred to as "pressor" agents. In light of the fact that isoproterenol and dobutamine produce little vasoconstriction per se, this is probably *not* the most appropriate term. Instead it may be better to think of these agents with regard to whether they provide *chronotropic* and/or *inotropic support* (act to improve cardiac output by increasing rate and force of contraction) or *pressor support* (increase peripheral vascular resistance and blood pressure). Drugs such as dopamine may do all of these things, depending on the dose of administration. At low-to-moderate infusion rates, dopamine increases cardiac output by its predominant beta-adrenergic effect, often with little change in blood pressure. At higher infusion rates, the vasoconstrictor effect of the drug (alpha-adrenergic effect) predominates and the pressor effect takes over. At this higher dose range, dopamine acts very much like epinephrine.

Which drug one selects for a particular situation depends primarily on the needs of that situation. In the case of the arrested heart, this means that the main concern must be to get the heart going and to maintain adequate coronary and cerebral circulation until a spontaneous perfusing rhythm takes over (**Table 2-1**). The drug of choice in this situation is *epinephrine*. Its alpha-adrenergic action favors coronary blood flow (by raising aortic diastolic blood pressure) and cerebral blood flow (by causing blood to be shunted from the external to the internal carotid artery), while its beta-adrenergic effect stimulates contractility. High-dose *dopamine* will probably provide similar success. In contrast, although *isoproterenol* offers potent chronotropic and inotropic activity, its pure beta-adrenergic stimulation may result in vasodilatation, lowering peripheral vascular resistance, aortic diastolic pressure, and coronary blood flow. Isoproterenol is contraindicated in the arrested heart.

Once the heart has been restarted and a *perfusing* rhythm is obtained, priorities change (**Table 2-1**). Achievement of high aortic diastolic pressures is no longer essential to maintain the coronary circulation. The goal of therapy now becomes improvement of cardiac output and

TABLE 2-1 SELECTION OF A PRESSOR AGENT IN THE ARRESTED HEART AND THE PERIOD IMMEDIATELY AFTER

	In the Arrested Heart (ventricular fibrillation, asystole)	**Once the Heart Has Been Restarted**
Needs of Therapy	Restart the heart Maintain coronary and cerebral perfusion	Improvement of cardiac output and peripheral perfusion
Drug of Choice	**Epinephrine** by bolus or infusion	Low-to-moderate dose **dopamine**
Alternative Agent(s)	Moderate-to-high dose **dopamine**	**Epinephrine** by infusion (for the slow idioventricular rhythm with a low blood pressure) **Isoproterenol** (if only chronotropic support is needed, and blood pressure is adequate)
Drugs that are Contraindicated	Isoproterenol	**Epinephrine** by bolus

peripheral perfusion. *Dopamine* administration at low-to-moderate infusion rates is probably the drug of choice. *Epinephrine by bolus* is contraindicated. *Epinephrine by infusion* may be effective and is often chosen for treatment of slow idioventricular rhythms with extremely low blood pressures. However, in the patient with a supraventricular rhythm and less-marked hypotension, epinephrine may be deleterious if it increases afterload to a greater extent than it improves cardiac output. *Isoproterenol* may be effective for treatment of hemodynamically significant bradyarrhythmias if *chronotropic support* is the primary need (if the heart rate is slow but the blood pressure is adequate). However, if hypotension accompanies the bradycardia, as is usually the case, use of isoproterenol runs the risk of exacerbating the situation by producing further vasodilatation.

Use of other "pressor" agents (dobutamine, norepinephrine, and amrinone) is much less frequent in the arrest or immediately postarrest period. We have therefore reserved our discussion of these drugs for the specific section under each agent.

B: KEY DRUGS

EPINEPHRINE

How Dispensed: 1 mg per 10 ml syringe

Dose and Route of Administration

IV Bolus: 0.5–1.0 mg IV (5–10 ml of a 1:10,000 solution)—may repeat at least every 5 min as needed.

IV Infusion: Mix 1 mg in 250 ml D5W and begin drip at 15 drops/min (1 μg/min). Usual range of infusion = 1–4 μg/min (15–60 drops/min). Higher doses may be used.

Endotracheal Instillation: Inject the contents of 1 ampule (1 mg diluted in 10 cc) down the endotracheal tube and follow by several forceful insufflations of the Ambu bag.

Intracardiac Injection: Essentially contraindicated.

Comments

The importance of epinephrine in the management of cardiac arrest has been known since 1896. Ninety years later the drug is still regarded as the most useful agent in the pharmacologic treatment of cardiovascular collapse, albeit by a different mechanism than is generally appreciated.

Epinephrine is an endogenous catecholamine with both *alpha-* and *beta*-adrenergic stimulating properties. The latter are responsible for the drug's potent *chronotropic* and *inotropic* effects, acting to increase the rate and force of myocardial contraction. Theoretically, epinephrine may facilitate conversion of ventricular fibrillation by countershock because it increases conduction velocity and shortens repolarization. This results in a reduction of dispersion for the refractory periods of individual myocardial cells. With greater uniformity during repolarization, the impetus for perpetuating ventricular fibrillation (persistence of multiple disorganized reentry circuits) is less, enhancing the chance of sustaining sinus rhythm following defibrillation.

However, the *alpha-adrenergic* effect of the drug appears to be a much more important attribute in the setting of cardiac arrest. This effect promotes peripheral vasoconstriction. The result is an increase in aortic diastolic pressure. The importance of aortic diastolic pressure in the arrested heart is that it determines the gradient for blood flow to the coronary arteries. Pure beta-adrenergic agents such as isoproterenol vasodilate, lowering peripheral vascular resistance and aortic diastolic pressure. They are contraindicated in cardiac arrest (Ralston, 1984). In contrast, the vasoconstrictor effect of epinephrine maintains coronary flow while CPR is in progress (Otto et al., 1981b; Parmley et al., 1982; Redding, 1979). Maintenance of adequate coronary flow during CPR is essential for preserving the chances of survival from ventricular fibrillation, asystole, and EMD.

Epinephrine also preserves blood flow to the brain. When CPR is performed in the absence of pharmacologic therapy, most of the blood flow from the common carotid artery goes to the external carotid. Very little is directed into the internal carotid artery. Thus, blood flow to the tongue and facial musculature is preserved, while cerebral flow is minimal during ordinary CPR (*"the tongue lives forever, but the brain dies"*). With the addition of sophisticated CPR techniques (ie, SCV-CPR or simultaneous compression-ventilation CPR), blood flow to the common carotid artery may dramatically increase. However, in the absence of pharmacologic therapy, the overwhelming majority of this increase continues to be directed to the external carotid branch. It is only after an agent with alpha-adrenergic properties (such as epinephrine) is added that blood flow is shunted from the external to the internal carotid artery, and a significant increase in cerebral blood flow occurs (Michael et al., 1984; Koehler et al., 1985).

> Epinephrine is not unique in its cardiac actions, and pure alpha-adrenergic agents such as methoxamine or phenylephrine also preserve myocardial blood flow by their vasoconstrictor properties (Otto et al., 1984). However, animal studies demonstrate that cerebral blood flow is not nearly as effective with phenylephrine (a pure alpha-adrenergic agent) as with epinephrine (Brown et al., 1986). This suggests that it is the combination of epinephrine's alpha- *and* beta-adrenergic properties that make it the drug of choice in cardiac arrest.

The recommended dose of epinephrine for treating ventricular fibrillation, asystole, and EMD is 0.5–1.0 mg IV. Because this is the one drug that favors coronary and cerebral blood flow, *we favor the higher dose in cardiopulmonary collapse.* If an initial 1 mg IV bolus of epinephrine proves to be ineffective, the recommendation is to repeat the drug at 5 minute intervals. *Especially in asystole, we favor more liberal repetition at 2–3 minute intervals until up to 5 mg (and more) of the drug have been given.*

Epinephrine should be given as soon as pos-

sible during cardiac arrest (Ralston, 1984). The reason for this is that with prolonged tissue hypoxia comes a loss in peripheral vascular tone. Since epinephrine's beneficial action during cardiac arrest stems from its vasoconstrictor effect, delayed administration of the drug in the setting of prolonged hypoxia often reduces vascular responsiveness to its actions.

> Epinephrine may also be given as an IV infusion. This has been suggested by some as an alternative to dopamine or isoproterenol for treatment of hemodynamically significant bradyarrhythmias that have not responded to atropine. Other clinicans prefer to administer epinephrine as an IV infusion for ventricular fibrillation or asystole. The advantage of this method of administration is that it allows moment-to-moment titration in dose that is not possible with IV injection of the drug. If initial infusion rates are unsuccessful, the drip is increased. As soon as the desired clinical response is obtained, the drip should be immediately turned down.
>
> In general it is probably easier to go with bolus therapy for treatment of ventricular fibrillation, asystole, and EMD, and most emergency care providers choose this route. With respect to treatment of rhythms *after* the heart has been restarted (for treatment of hemodynamically significant bradyarrhythmias), dopamine is probably a better agent than epinephrine by infusion.

Epinephrine is rapidly absorbed across bronchotracheal structures. Following intratracheal administration, the effect is sustained for at least as long as after IV injection. However, peak concentrations of the drug are not as high by the ET route (Roberts et al., 1979; Ralston et al., 1985). Consequently, the new guidelines recommend a dose of *at least* 1 mg if the ET route is used. Overall, the data suggest that endotracheal administration of epinephrine is a more than adequate route for drug delivery if a central line or large bore IV is not available. It is probably superior to giving the drug through a small bore peripheral IV from a distal site (dorsum of wrist, foot).

Intracardiac injection is fraught with hazard and is contraindicated under most circumstances. It should be resorted to only when all else fails.

LIDOCAINE

How Dispensed

IV Bolus: 100 mg per 10 ml syringe
IV Infusion: 1 g per 25 ml syringe

Dose and Route of Administration

IV Bolus: Give $\approx$ 1 mg/kg (50–100 mg) for
the initial IV bolus. Repeat boluses of
50–75 mg may be given every 5–10 minutes up to a total loading dose of 225 mg.

IV Infusion: Mix 1 g in 250 ml D5W and
begin drip at 30 drops/min (2 mg/min).
Usual range of infusion = 0.5–4 mg/
min.

ET Tube: 100 mg (the contents of a 10 ml
syringe) followed by several forceful insufflations of the Ambu bag.

Comments

Lidocaine has long been accepted as the antiarrhythmic agent of choice for the treatment
of PVCs in the setting of acute ischemia. However, it is only recently that the routine use of
this drug has been recommended as a prophylactic measure to prevent primary ventricular fibrillation in patients suspected of having acute
infarction even when they do not manifest ventricular ectopy.

Patients at greatest risk of developing ventricular fibrillation with acute myocardial infarction
are those seen within the first few hours of the
onset of symptoms and in whom a high clinical
index of suspicion for infarction exists. This is
the group most suited to receive prophylactic
treatment with lidocaine. Treatment of patients
over 70 years of age is probably not as essential,
since the incidence of primary ventricular fibrillation is less in this age group and the risk of
toxicity is significantly greater (Goldman et al.,
1979; Lie et al., 1974).

Recently lidocaine has also been advocated
for use as an antifibrillatory agent for patients
with refractory ventricular fibrillation (White,
1984; JAMA Suppl., 1986). Studies to date have
not demonstrated a significant difference in the
clinical efficacy between this drug and bretylium

in this setting. Because lidocaine is probably a
safer agent and most emergency care providers
are more comfortable with its use, the new
guidelines now favor this drug over bretylium
for refractory ventricular fibrillation.

Dosing of IV lidocaine is discussed in detail in
the Chapter 13 on "Use of Lidocaine." Several pertinent points are reemphasized here. When used
prophylactically (in the absence of PVCs) for suspected acute myocardial infarction, aggressive
loading is probably not needed and may unnecessarily increase the risk of toxicity. Usually 1–2 boluses of drug and constant infusion at a rate of 2
mg/min is adequate to ensure lidocaine's protective effect. Even if some ventricular ectopy is present, more than 2 boluses and higher infusion rates
may not be needed as long as repetitive forms (ventricular couplets or salvos) are infrequent. Elimination of every PVC is *not* essential for protection
against ventricular fibrillation.

Lidocaine toxicity is prone to develop in patients
with congestive heart failure or shock, the elderly,
subjects of lower body weight, and with concomitant use of propranolol or cimetidine. In such patients, infusion rates as low as 0.5–1 mg/min
should probably be used.

Because lidocaine pharmacokinetics during cardiac arrest are somewhat unpredictable, the new
guidelines suggest that only bolus therapy be used
in this setting. Less frequent administration of
loading boluses may be needed during this low-flow
state (McDonald, 1985). Once the patient has been
converted out of ventricular fibrillation, however,
clearance of the drug may markedly increase and
resumption of a normal dosing schedule (rebolus
and institution of a maintenance infusion) is
indicated.

Finally, although lidocaine may be administered
by the endotracheal route, it appears to be errati-
cally absorbed when given by this method during
cardiac arrest. Peak concentrations of drug are
often delayed for up to 10 minutes following intratracheal instillation (McDonald, 1985). Therefore,
if IV access is available, this route is definitely preferred for administration of lidocaine.

ATROPINE SULFATE

How Dispensed: 1 mg per 10 ml syringe

Dose and Route of Administration

IV Bolus: 0.5 mg IV every 5 minutes up to
a maximum dose of 2 mg. (For marked

bradycardia and/or hypotension, 1.0 mg of atropine may be given at a time.)

ET Tube: 1 mg at a time, followed by several forceful insufflations of the Ambu bag.

Comments

Atropine is a parasympathetic blocking agent that has been recommended for use in treatment of bradyarrhythmias. The drug, however, is not without adverse effects. Because it also enhances the rate of discharge from the sinus node, atropine may produce atrial tachyarrhythmias. Moreover, by blocking parasympathetic output, it may unmask underlying enhanced sympathetic activity and lead as well to ventricular tachyarrhythmias. Myocardial oxygen consumption may be increased and angina precipitated. Case reports of ventricular tachycardia or ventricular fibrillation following atropine administration have been noted (Massumi et al., 1977; Scheinman et al., 1975). As a result, only *hemodynamically significant* bradyarrhythmias or bradyarrhythmias associated with frequent PVCs should be treated.

In addition to the vagolytic effect of atropine, the drug also improves conduction through the AV node. This explains its beneficial effect in the treatment of second- and third-degree AV block *during the early hours* of acute inferior infarction at a time when these conduction defects often reflect excessive vagal tone. The drug is not expected to work as well *after* the first few hours of inferior infarction or with anterior infarction since excessive parasympathetic tone is less of a causative factor.

Again, one should remember that the effects of atropine may act as a double-edged sword. The fact that the drug enhances the rate of sinus node discharge may actually *counteract* its beneficial action on AV nodal conduction. For example, in the setting of acute inferior infarction, the AV node may be able to conduct every sinus impulse to the ventricles at a heart rate of 50 beats/min. However, acceleration of the heart rate to 80 beats/min (as frequently occurs following atropine administration) may be too rapid a rate for an ischemic AV node to continue with 1:1 AV conduction. Were

the AV node only able to conduct every *other* sinus impulse at this heart rate, then for an atrial rate of 80 the ventricular response would be only 40 beats/min (2:1 AV conduction). *In this theoretical example, administration of atropine would actually have made the patient's condition worse by decreasing the ventricular response from 50 to 40 beats/min.* The message is clear. Atropine is *not* benign. Its use should be reserved for *hemodynamically significant* bradyarrhythmias or bradyarrhythmias associated with frequent ventricular ectopy.

Atropine has also been recommended for treatment of asystole. The rationale for its use in this setting is that certain individuals have been shown to demonstrate parasympathetic innervation of the ventricles. Although prognosis for asystole is never good, it is important to emphasize that the outlook for this condition is not nearly as poor when it occurs *in* the hospital as when it occurs *outside* the hospital. Asystole in this latter setting is most often a preterminal event that results after prolonged cardiopulmonary arrest and which followed deterioration of ventricular fibrillation. On a cellular level, this type of asystole is associated with tissue hypoxia, acidosis, and cellular disruption (Coon et al., 1981; Niemann et al., 1985). Response to treatment is dismal (Stueven et al., 1984; Myerburg et al., 1982).

In contrast, asystole occurring in a hospital setting can sometimes be due to massive parasympathetic discharge. This may occur in association with certain operative or diagnostic procedures, anesthesia, toxic drug reactions, vasovagal episodes, or heart block from acute inferior infarction. In addition, the time from onset of asystole until discovery by trained personnel is usually significantly less in the hospital than when the condition occurs on the outside. As a result, asystole in this setting may respond surprisingly well for a "prelethal" arrhythmia to atropine therapy (Coon et al., 1981).

The recommended dose of atropine is 0.5 mg IV every 5 minutes until a total dose of 2 mg has been given. However, this dosing schedule may not be practical for treatment of conduction disorders if the heart rate is extremely slow (under 40 beats/min) and the blood pressure very low (ie, less than 80 mm Hg systolic). This is because it would take no less than *15 minutes* to administer the full 2 mg of drug. It may therefore be preferable under such circumstances to administer 1 mg of atropine at a time, repeating the dose in several minutes if the desired clinical response has not been observed.

On the other hand, when symptoms produced by the bradyarrhythmia are less severe (for mild bradycardia associated with minimal signs of hemodynamic compromise), *only* 0.5 mg increments of IV atropine should be given at the recommended 5 minute intervals, since larger doses may be associated with an unacceptable incidence of adverse effects (Scheinman et al., 1975).

> The reason doses less than 0.5 mg should not be used in adults is that paradoxical slowing of the heart rate may result.
>
> Although in most individuals, 2 mg is the full atropinization dose, occasionally up to 0.04 mg/kg (up to 3 mg or more) of the drug may be needed in order to obtain maximal effect (Jose et al., 1969). In general, most emergency care providers prefer to turn to a pressor agent when a symptomatic bradyarrhythmia has not responded to the usual 2 mg dose of atropine.

Cardiovascular effects of atropine last an estimated 2–4 hours. Other systemic effects (including pupillary dilatation) may persist much longer (Kaiser et al., 1970; Thomas and Woodgate, 1966).

Atropine may be given by the ET route. Although there is much less experience in administering the drug by this method than there is for epinephrine, absorption across tracheobronchial structures appears to be good and substantial atropine levels are achieved within 10 minutes of dosing (Greenberg, 1982). A dose of at least 1 mg at a time is advised when using atropine by the ET route.

DOPAMINE (INTROPIN)

How Dispensed: 200 mg per 5 ml ampule

Dose and Route of Administration

IV Infusion: Mix 1 ampule (200 mg) in 250 ml D5W and begin drip at 15–30 drops/ min ($\approx$ 2–5 μg/kg/min in an average-sized person). Titrate drip upward and adjust for the lowest infusion rate that maintains the desired clinical response.

Dopamine is a chemical precursor of norepinephrine with dopaminergic, alpha- and beta-adrenergic receptor stimulating properties. Which of these pharmacologic actions predominates depends principally on the rate of infusion of the drug:

At Low Infusion Rates (1–2 μg/kg/min), the dopaminergic effect prevails. This produces dilatation of renal and mesenteric blood vessels. Heart rate and blood pressure are often not affected at this low infusion rate.

At Moderate Infusion Rates (2–10 μg/kg/min), the beta-adrenergic receptor stimulating action prevails. This results in an increase in cardiac output without necessarily raising the blood pressure.

At High Infusion Rates (>10 μg/kg/min), the alpha-adrenergic receptor stimulating effect predominates. Peripheral vasoconstriction results. The initial dilatation of the renal and mesenteric vasculature reverses itself at higher doses.

> At moderate-to-high doses the drug resembles epinephrine. As the infusion rate is increased even further (to 15–20 μg/kg/min), it becomes more and more like norepinephrine.

Dopamine is indicated for the medical treatment of hemodynamically significant bradyarrhythmias and cardiogenic shock. It is probably the most commonly used pressor agent for this purpose. It also has been used with success to maintain coronary perfusion in the arrested heart (Otto et al., 1981a). Its appeal lies in its flexibility which allows this one drug to be used for both management of cardiac arrest and blood pressure maintenance with vital organ perfusion during the immediate postresuscitation period.

As with all pressor agents, dopamine may cause tachyarrhythmias, necessitating a reduction in the infusion rate.

OXYGEN

Dose and Route of Administration

Nasal Canula: 24–40% O_2 can be delivered with flow rates of 6 L/min.

Face Mask: Up to 50% O_2 can be delivered with flow rates of 10 L/min.

Venturi Mask: Fixed O_2 concentrations of 24%, 28%, 35%, and 40% may be delivered with flow rates of 4–8 L/min.

Pocket Mask: 50% O_2 can be delivered with flow rates of 10 L/min.

Bag-Valve-Mask Devices: May deliver room air or up to 90% O_2 with a high-flow oxygen source and attached reservoir.

Non-Rebreathing Oxygen Mask: A superior device for delivering high oxygen concentrations of up to 90%.

Comments

Oxygen *is* one of the truly essential drugs in cardiopulmonary resuscitation and emergency cardiac care. It is the treatment of choice for suspected hypoxemia of any cause (cardiopulmonary arrest, myocardial infarction), and should *not* be withheld for fear of causing carbon dioxide retention in the emergency situation. Delivery systems for oxygen are discussed in detail in the chapter on Airway Management (Part II: Chapter 7).

MORPHINE SULFATE

How Dispensed: 5, 10, or 15 mg per ampule.

Dose and Route of Administration:

2–5 mg IV. This may be repeated every 5–30 minutes as needed.

Comments

Morphine sulfate is a drug that has withstood the test of time. Even today it remains an ideal agent for treatment of acute ischemic chest pain and pulmonary edema.

Morphine works in a number of different ways. In addition to its extremely potent analgesic effect, it also allays anxiety in patients with acute chest pain or air hunger from pulmonary edema. Hemodynamically, the drug markedly increases venous capacitance. This significantly reduces preload by decreasing venous return. Morphine also induces mild arterial vasodilation which improves cardiac performance by lowering afterload.

> Caution has been urged when using morphine sulfate for treatment of acute inferior infarction because of concern that the drug might induce heart block, excessive bradycardia, or hypotension. Many authorities have even advocated substituting another analgesic agent (such as IV meperidine) for use in this setting rather than risk an adverse reaction to morphine. This degree of concern may *not* be necessary. In the largest study to date on the subject, 184 patients who presented with chest pain of suspected acute myocardial infarction, and who were treated with morphine sulfate, were examined (Semenkovich and Jaffe, 1985). Eighty-five per cent of these patients went on to develop a documented infarction. Adverse effects from morphine sulfate administration occurred in only 4 patients (*less* than 3% of the study group). These consisted of hypotension and heart rate slowing, suggesting a vasovagal influence contributed to the reaction. Three of the patients responded promptly to atropine and/or fluid administration, and hypotension spontaneously resolved within 1 minute in the other. Each of the 4 patients went on to receive an additional 8–31 mg of IV morphine over the next 12–48 hours *without* additional sequelae.

Thus, it appears that adverse reactions to morphine sulfate administered for acute ischemic chest pain have been overemphasized in the past and probably are much *less* common than is generally thought. When they do occur, they most often follow administration of the first dose and in *no way* preclude cautious additional use of the drug. In this study, the adverse reactions encountered in the 4 patients consisted of hypotension and/or heart rate slowing. Conduction system defects were *not* seen. Adverse reactions promptly resolved with treatment (atropine and/or fluid administration) or spontaneously. Finally, only 1 of the 4 patients had inferior or posterior infarction, contradicting the previous notion that the adverse effects from morphine were more common with this type of injury.

Optimal use of morphine sulfate entails dosing by small IV increments (2–5 mg) at frequent intervals (q 5–30 minutes) according to the patient's symptoms and clinical response. In addition to occasional bradycardia and hypotension, the drug may cause oversedation, nausea, and respiratory depression. The latter may be quickly reversed with 0.4 mg IV naloxone (Narcan). As noted above, vagotonic actions of the drug are reversed by either atropine or saline infusion.

VERAPAMIL

How Dispensed: 5 mg per 2 ml ampule.

Dose and Route of Administration:

IV Dosing: 3–5 mg IV to be given over a 1–2 min period (or over 3–4 min in the elderly). May give up to 10 mg in a dose and repeat once in 30 min if needed.

Comments

Verapamil is the pharmacologic agent of choice for the treatment of paroxysmal supraventricular tachycardia (PSVT). It is also a favored drug for treatment of atrial fibrillation and flutter with a rapid ventricular response and recently has become the drug of choice for multifocal atrial tachycardia (MAT). Verapamil exerts its primary effect on AV nodal tissue, slowing conduction and prolonging the effective refractory period within the AV node. As a result, this calcium channel blocking agent is extremely effective in terminating PSVT by interrupting the reentrant pathway. With other supraventricular tachyarrthythmias it works by slowing the ventricular response.

PSVT should first be treated by attempting to increase vagal tone with either carotid sinus massage (provided there is no history of carotid disease or neck bruits on exam) or the Valsalva maneuver. If these vagal maneuvers are not effective, *verapamil* becomes the drug of choice. The usual adult dose is 5 mg, which should be given IV over a 1–2 minute period. Lower doses (3 mg) given more slowly (over 3–4 minutes) are advised in the elderly.

Verapamil usually works within minutes. It successfully converts more than 90% of cases of PSVT. There may be gradual slowing of the tachyarrhythmia, and then sudden conversion to sinus rhythm. If the initial dose of the drug does not produce the desired effect, a second dose (of 5–10 mg IV) may be given 15–30 min later.

Verapamil is also a useful agent for treatment of atrial fibrillation and flutter. Although conversion to sinus rhythm occurs only about a third of the time, the drug effectively slows the ventricular response to both of these tachyarrhythmias.

Even though verapamil is an extremely useful agent for treatment of atrial fibrillation with a rapid ventricular response in the usual patient, the drug should *not* be used to treat this arrhythmia if Wolff-Parkinson-White syndrome is present. In such cases verapamil may accelerate conduction down the accessory pathway. Deterioration of the rhythm to ventricular fibrillation commonly follows (McGovern et al., 1986).

Combining small doses of IV digoxin with IV verapamil may produce a synergistic effect when treating atrial fibrillation or flutter with a rapid ventricular response. For patients controlled by this regimen in the acute phase, maintenance therapy with oral verapamil is often effective for long-term maintenance.

Recently, MAT has been shown to respond to verapamil. This arrhythmia is most often seen in acutely ill patients, especially when underlying pulmonary disease is present. While improving oxygenation is probably the most important therapeutic intervention, verapamil becomes the drug of choice when pharmacologic treatment is needed to slow down the ventricular rate (Levine et al., 1985). Although the mechanism of MAT is not clear, it appears that increased atrial automaticity due in part to intracellular calcium overload plays a contributing role. Verapamil may work by improving intracellular homeostasis. Thus, in addition to slowing the ventricular response by its effect on the AV node, verapamil probably also works in MAT by a direct depressant effect on atrial automaticity that reduces the number of ectopic atrial impulses (Levine et al., 1985). The drug is definitely preferable to digoxin for treatment of this arrhythmia.

Several words of caution regarding the use of verapamil are in order. The drug should not be used to slow the heart rate of a patient in sinus tachycardia for whom the rapid heart rate may be needed to sustain cardiac output. Instead, treatment of sinus tachycardia must be directed toward the underlying cause. Because of the drug's depressant effect on sinoatrial (SA) and atrioventricular (AV) conduction, it should be used very cautiously in patients with evidence of sinus node disease (ie, sick sinus syndrome) or in connection with digitalis, which also slows AV nodal conduction. For the same reason, verapamil should probably not be administered within 30 minutes of IV propranolol. Because of its negative inotropic effects, the drug is relatively contraindicated for use in patients with congestive heart failure. Occasionally a transient reduction in arterial blood pressure is noted after verapamil administration, especially if the drug is injected too rapidly or if given to overly sensitive elderly individuals. Slower administration and use of lower doses are advised in such cases.

> Recently Haft and Habbab have shown (1986) that pretreatment with calcium chloride virtually eliminates the hypotensive response of verapamil without diminishing verapamil's efficacy in converting or controlling the ventricular rate of patients with supraventricular tachyarrhythmias. One ampule of calcium chloride (1 gram) is infused IV over 5–10 minutes. Too rapid infusion may produce a generalized sensation of heat in the patient. Conversion of the rhythm or slowing of the ventricular response occasionally results from calcium infusion alone even before verapamil is administered.
>
> Consideration of pretreatment with calcium infusion would seem to be most suitable for patients with supraventricular tachyarrhythmias when hemodynamic status is borderline (ie, systolic blood pressure <100 mm Hg). In patients with supraventricular tachyarrhythmias who are given verapamil without such pretreatment, one should not forget that IV infusion of calcium chloride may effectively reverse hypotension should it occur.

Verapamil does *not* have any role in the treatment of ventricular arrhythmias. This point *cannot* be too strongly emphasized! It *must* not be given indiscriminately as a diagnostic and/or therapeutic trial to patients with regular, wide QRS complex tachyarrhythmias of uncertain etiology because of the disastrous consequences the drug usually has if the rhythm turns out to be ventricular tachycardia. This word of caution was well borne out in a study by McGovern et al. (1986) in which 39% of patients presenting with wide complex tachycardias were misdiagnosed as having PSVT when they in fact had ventricular tachycardia. Hemodynamic deterioration occurred in *all* 13 of the patients who received verapamil. Instead of reflexively administering verapamil to such patients when the etiology of the tachyarrhythmia is unclear, one should further examine the patient and ECG for subtle clues (which we discuss in detail in Chapter 15) and/or consider IV procainamide, which may be effective treatment for both supraventricular and ventricular tachycardia without being nearly as likely to cause hemodynamic disaster if the rhythm turns out to be VT (Wellens, 1986).

C: SIMPLIFIED CALCULATION OF IV INFUSIONS

For the uninitiated, calculation of IV infusions may appear to be a formidable task that requires a minimum of a Masters degree in mathematics to attain proficiency. In real life, calculation of IV infusions is performed most often by those assigned the chore of caring for intravenous lines that have already been established—namely, by nurses and paramedics. Physicians rarely go beyond giving the order to "mix up a drip of drug X and run the infusion as fast as we need to." In most settings, experienced nurses have the infusion ready to go long before the physician has even asked for the drug. Occasionally, however, the team leader may find himself/herself working with code team members who are unfamiliar with how to mix IV infusions. It is therefore essential for *all* ACLS providers to be able to order IV infusions for the drugs commonly used in emergency cardiac care.

You will probably need to know how to order IV infusions to pass the ACLS Course. A simplified method known as the **"Rule of 250 ml"** can facilitate this task.

The *Rule of 250 ml* is as follows:

Mix 1 *unit** of whatever drug you are using in *250 ml* of D5W and set the infusion to run at 15–30 *drops/min*.

Using this rule, you will arrive at an appropriate *initial* IV infusion rate for virtually any of the drugs administered by infusion for emergency cardiac care.

Examples

Lidocaine—Mix 1 g in 250 ml D5W (or 2 g in 500 ml) and set drip to run at 30 drops/min (2 mg/min).

Procainamide—Mix 1 g in 250 ml D5W (or 2 g in 500 ml) and set drip to run at 30 drops/min (2 mg/min).

Bretylium—Mix 1 g in 250 ml D5W (or 2 g in 500 ml) and set drip to run at 30 drops/min (2 mg/min). *One usually begins a bretylium infusion at 1 mg/min, so the drip should initially be set to infuse at 15 drips/min.*

Isoproterenol—Mix 1 mg (1 vial) in 250 ml D5W and set drip to run at 30 drops/min (2 μg/min).

Epinephrine—Mix 1 mg (1 ampule) in 250 ml D5W and set drip to run at 30 drops/min (2 μg/min). *One usually begins an epinephrine infusion at 1 μg/min, so the drip should initially be set to infuse at 15 drops/min.*

Dopamine—Mix 200 mg (1 ampule) in 250 ml D5W and set drip to run at 30 drops/min to infuse about 5 μg/kg/min (400 μg/

min for an 80 kg patient). *If the patient weighs significantly less than 80 kg or if you prefer initially to preferentially increase blood flow to the renal vascular bed, you may choose to begin the infusion at 15 drops/min.*

Calculation of the IV infusion rate for each of these drugs is shown below. With the exception of dobutamine, nitroprusside, and nitroglycerin, the rule of 250 ml is closely adhered to.

Note that most of the following manipulations involve *unit conversions*. The key to coming up with the correct answer is to carefully maintain units throughout!

Problem: **Make up a *lidocaine* infusion. How fast should the drip be set to infuse 2 mg of lidocaine per minute?**

Answer: Mix 1 g of lidocaine in 250 ml (or 2 g in 500 ml) of D5W:

$$\frac{1 \text{ g}}{250 \text{ ml}} \left(\text{or } \frac{2 \text{ g}}{500 \text{ ml}} \right) = \frac{4 \text{ g}}{1000 \text{ ml}}$$

$$= \frac{4000 \text{ mg}}{1000 \text{ ml}} = \frac{4 \text{ mg}}{\text{ml}} = \frac{2 \text{ mg}}{0.5 \text{ ml}}$$

This gives a concentration of 4 mg of lidocaine per ml or 2 mg of lidocaine per 0.5 ml.

To run an infusion at a rate of 2 mg/min implies that 0.5 ml/min of lidocaine must be infused.

---

1 ml = 60 *drops* for a *microdrip*
0.5 ml/min = 30 drops/min

Set the infusion at a rate of 30 drops/min. ✓

—a rate of 15 drops/min infuses 1 mg/min
—a rate of 30 drops/min infuses 2 mg/min
—a rate of 45 drops/min infuses 3 mg/min
—a rate of 60 drops/min infuses 4 mg/min

---

*The Rule of 250 ml depends on the amount of drug contained in one unit. The contents of a vial or an ampule may vary slightly from one hospital to the next so that you need to be familiar with the drug formulary used in your hospital. Calculations in this section assume the following:

1 g of lidocaine
1 g of procainamide ⎬ = 1 unit of drug
1 g of bretylium

1 mg (1 vial) of isoproterenol
1 mg (1 ampule) of epinephrine ⎬ = 1 unit of drug

200 mg (1 ampule) of dopamine] = 1 unit of drug

50 mg (1 vial) of sodium nitroprusside
50 mg of nitroglycerin ⎬ = 1 unit of drug

Problem: **Make up a *procainamide* infusion.**

Answer: Same method as for lidocaine.
Mix 1 g of procainamide in 250 ml of D5W (or 2 g in 500 ml) and set the drip to run at 30 drops/min to infuse 2 mg/min.

Problem: **Make up a *bretylium* infusion.**

Answer: Same method as for lidocaine.
Mix 1 g of bretylium in 250 ml of D5W (or 2 g in 500 ml) and set the drip to run at 30 drops/min to infuse 2 mg/min.
One usually begins a bretylium infusion at 1 mg/min; therefore, the drip should initially be set to infuse at 15 drops/min.

Problem: **Make up an *isoproterenol* infusion. How fast should the drip be set to achieve an initial infusion rate of 2 µg/min?**

Answer: Mix 1 mg (1 vial) of isoproterenol in 250 ml of D5W:

$$\frac{1 \text{ mg}}{250 \text{ ml}} = \frac{4 \text{ mg}}{1000 \text{ ml}} = \frac{4000 \text{ µg}}{1000 \text{ ml}}$$

$$= \frac{4 \text{ µg}}{\text{ml}} = \frac{2 \text{ µg}}{0.5 \text{ ml}}$$

This gives a concentration of 4 µg of isoproterenol per ml (or 2 µg of isoproterenol per 0.5 ml).
To begin an infusion at a rate of 2 µg/min, 0.5 ml/min must be infused. Therefore, the drip should be started at a rate of 30 drops/min.

Problem: **Make up an *epinephrine* infusion.**

Answer: Same method as for isoproterenol.
Mix 1 mg of epinephrine in 250 ml of D5W and set the drip to run at 30 drops/min to infuse 2 µg/min. *Usually one begins an epinephrine infusion at 1 µg/min, so the drip should be started at 15 drops/min.*

Problem: **Make up a *dopamine* infusion. How fast should the drip be set to achieve an initial rate of 5 µg/kg/min?**

Answer: Mix 200 mg (1 ampule) of dopamine in 250 ml of D5W:

$$\frac{200 \text{ mg}}{250 \text{ ml}} = \frac{800 \text{ mg}}{1000 \text{ ml}} = \frac{800,000 \text{ µg}}{1000 \text{ ml}}$$

$$= \frac{800 \text{ µg}}{\text{ml}} = \frac{400 \text{ µg}}{0.5 \text{ ml}}$$

This gives a concentration of 800 µg of dopamine per ml (or 400 µg of dopamine per 0.5 ml).
Dopamine exerts its most beneficial effects at an infusion rate of 2–10 µg/kg/min. Beginning the infusion rate at 5 µg/kg/min, an 80 kg patient would require 400 µg/min (ie, 5 × 80), which means that 0.5 ml/min must be infused. Begin the infusion at 30 drops/min. *If the patient weighs significantly less than 80 kg or if you prefer initially to preferentially increase blood flow to the renal vascular bed, you may choose to begin the infusion at 15 drops/min.*

Problem: **Make up a *dobutamine* infusion. How fast should the drip be set to achieve an initial infusion rate of 2.5 µg/kg/min with an 80 kg patient?**

Answer: Mix 250 mg (1 vial) of dobutamine in 250 ml of D5W:

$$\frac{250 \text{ mg}}{250 \text{ ml}} = \frac{1000 \text{ mg}}{1000 \text{ ml}} = \frac{1 \text{ mg}}{1 \text{ ml}} = \frac{1000 \text{ µg}}{1 \text{ ml}}$$

$$= \text{concentration of the drip}$$

Beginning the infusion at a rate of 2.5 µg/kg/min with an 80 kg patient, would mean that 200 µg/min (2.5 × 80) must be infused.
[If we wanted to infuse 1000 µg/min, the drip would have to be set at 60 drops/min (since 60 drops = 1 ml with a microdrip).] Because we want to infuse only 200 µg/min, we have to set the drip at 12 drops/min (60 ÷ 5). (This drug does *not* obey the Rule of 250 ml.)

Problem: **Make up an infusion of *sodium nitroprusside* and determine the speed of infu-**

sion needed to begin the drip at a rate of 10 µg/min.

Answer: Mix 50 mg (1 vial) of nitroprusside in 250 ml of D5W:

$$\frac{50 \text{ mg}}{250 \text{ ml}} = \frac{200 \text{ mg}}{1000 \text{ ml}} = \frac{200{,}000 \text{ µg}}{1000 \text{ ml}} = \frac{200 \text{ µg}}{1 \text{ ml}}$$

= concentration of the drip

Beginning the infusion at 10 µg/min implies that 1/20 ml/min must be infused.

Since 60 drops equal 1 ml with a microdrip, set the drip at 3 drops/min (60 ÷ 20) to begin the infusion rate at 10 µg/min.

Problem: **By how many drops per minute should the drip be increased to infuse an additional 10 µg each minute?**

Answer: Since a rate of 3 drops/min infuses 10 µg/min, one would have to increase the drip by 3 drops each minute to infuse an additional 10 µg each minute. Thus to infuse 20 µg/min the drip should be set at a rate of 6 drops/min, to infuse 30 µg/min the drip should be set at a rate of 9 drops/min, and so forth.

Problem: **What is the maximum infusion rate recommended for an 80 kg patient?**

Answer: The maximum recommended infusion rate is 8 µg/kg/min, which equals 80 × 8 or 640 µg/min.

At a concentration of 200 µg/ml, the maximum recommended infusion rate would be 3.2 ml/min (640 ÷ 200), which equals 192 drops/min (60 × 3.2).

Problem: **Calculate an infusion of IV** *nitroglycerin.*

Answer: Same method and doses as for sodium nitroprusside.

Mix 50 mg of nitroglycerin in 250 ml of D5W and set the drip to run at 3 drops/min to begin the infusion at 10 µg/min; increase the drip by 3 drops/min (10 µg/min) as needed to obtain the desired clinical response.

(Note that both sodium nitroprusside and nitroglycerin follow the Rule of 250 ml for pre-

paring the concentration of infusions, but drips for these agents should be initially set at 3 drops/min (*not* 30 drops/min).

The Rule of 250 ml is practical as well as being easy to learn and remember. It works. It is also all you'll need to know to pass the ACLS Course.

For those with a need (or desire) to be more specific in their calculation of infusions based on a microgram per kilogram per minute (µg/kg/min) schedule, the **"Rule of 150 mg in 250 ml"** is made to order. This rule is particularly helpful in determining the rate of infusion for drugs such as dopamine or dobutamine.

The *Rule of 150 mg in 250 ml* is as follows:

Mix *150 mg* of whatever drug you are using in *250 ml* of D5W. This will provide a drip concentration that contains 10 µg of drug for each 1 drop of IV solution.

$$\frac{150 \text{ mg}}{250 \text{ ml}} = \frac{600 \text{ mg}}{1000 \text{ ml}}$$

$$= \frac{600 \text{ µg}}{1 \text{ ml}} \times \frac{1 \text{ ml}}{60 \text{ drops}} = \frac{10 \text{ µg}}{1 \text{ drop}}$$

With this concentration, one can now easily calculate the number of drops per minute at which to set the infusion by the following formula:

$$\frac{\textbf{(Desired µg/kg/min)} \times \textbf{(bodyweight in kg)}}{\textbf{10}}$$

= Number of drops/min

Examples:

Problem: **Make up a *dopamine* infusion. How fast should the drip be set to achieve an initial rate of 3 µg/kg/min in a 60 kg woman?**

Answer: Mix 150 mg of dopamine in 250 ml of D5W.

$$\frac{\text{(Desired µg/kg/min)} \times \text{(bodyweight in kg)}}{10}$$

= Number of drops/min

$$\frac{(3 \ \mu g/kg/min) \times (60 \ kg)}{10}$$

$$= 18 \ drops/min$$

With a mixture of 150 mg of dopamine in 250 ml of D5W, the infusion rate should be set at 18 drops/min to infuse 3 $\mu g/kg/min$ for a 60 kg woman.

Problem: **Make up a *dobutamine* infusion. How fast should the drip be set to achieve an initial rate of 7 $\mu g/kg/min$ in a 90 kg man?**

Answer: Mix 150 mg of dobutamine in 250 ml of D5W.

$$\frac{(Desired \ \mu g/kg/min) \times (bodyweight \ in \ kg)}{10}$$

$$= Number \ of \ drops/min$$

$$\frac{(7 \ \mu g/kg/min) \times (90 \ kg)}{10}$$

$$= 63 \ drops/min$$

With a mixture of 150 mg of dobutamine in 250 ml of D5W, the infusion rate should be set at 63 drops/min to infuse 7 $\mu g/kg/min$ for a 90 kg man.

D: KEY TREATMENT MODALITIES

Precordial Thump

Technique: The precordial thump is a sharp, quick blow that is delivered with the fleshy part of the fist (hypothenar eminence) from a distance of 8–12 inches above the chest to the midportion of the sternum. It should *not* be so forceful as to break any ribs.

Indications: Pulseless rhythms in the absence of a defibrillator.

Comments

The history of the precordial thump dates back to 1920 when Schott first used the proce-

dure on a patient having Stokes-Adams attacks. Reports in the literature on the use of the thump since then were limited until the 1970s. The group of Morgera et al. (1979) were the most enthusiastic, reporting a success rate of almost 50% when the thump was applied to cases of ventricular tachycardia occurring in a hospital setting.

Less favorable results were obtained by Miller et al. (1984), who reported on their experience with the use of the thump in a prehospital setting. Among the 50 patients included in their study, the thump was applied for ventricular fibrillation in 23 cases and for ventricular tachycardia in 27 cases. None of those in ventricular fibrillation were converted out of this rhythm by the thump. The maneuver was successful in converting 3 of the 27 patients (12%) in ventricular tachycardia to a supraventricular rhythm with a pulse. However, the thump had no effect on 12 patients (44%), and in the remaining 12 patients (44%) it resulted in deterioration of the rhythm to ventricular fibrillation, pulseless idioventricular rhythm, or asystole. This study showed clearly that *the thump is not a benign procedure!* In contrast to the in-hospital experience of Morgera these authors found the thump to be detrimental more often than helpful, and advocated against its routine use in a prehospital setting.

Recent work by others caused the pendulum to swing back again. Such investigators have shown that the thump *could* be effective in converting patients out of ventricular fibrillation and even out of *asystole* (Patros and Goren, 1983; Caldwell et al., 1985).

What is the mechanism of the thump? Why should it be effective in some patients but detrimental in others? How best should the emergency care provider apply the procedure in the acute care setting?

The thump appears to be most effective in terminating rhythms dependent on a reentrant pathway. The mechanical stimulation it produces probably results in an electrical depolarization (of 2–5 joules) that is able to interrupt a reentrant pathway if delivered at an opportune moment in the cardiac cycle. On the other hand, if the thump occurs during the vulnerable period, it may precipitate ventricular fibrillation in much the same way that the ''R-on-T'' phenomenon does. Since ventricular tachycardia may frequently be cardioverted with energies of less than 10 joules, it is logical that it be the rhythm most susceptible to the effects of the thump.

Although no one has demonstrated precisely how energy requirements for defibrillation change with time, it is thought that exceedingly low energies (of a little as 5–10 joules) may be effective in terminating ventricular fibrillation if delivered *early* enough after the onset of this rhythm (Lown, 1980; Caldwell et al., 1985). Energy requirements for defibrillation appear to increase dramatically within seconds. Thus for the thump to be effective in terminating ventricular fibrillation, it must be delivered *as soon as possible after the onset of this rhythm.* How the thump works for asystole is unknown.

Our Recommendations for Use

In the past, recommendations for the thump were to employ the maneuver for ventricular tachycardia and fibrillation when the onset of these rhythms was monitored. However, concern for the potential of the procedure to worsen the arrhythmia led to deemphasis of the thump.

We suggest that the thump be thought of as a *''no lose''* procedure. Reserve it for patients presenting with *pulseless* rhythms, particularly when a defibrillator is not available. If delivered within the early moments of an arrest, it may on occasion convert a patient out of pulseless ventricular tachycardia, ventricular fibrillation, or even asystole. If out in the field and without access to a defibrillator, there is really *nothing to lose* (and everything to gain) by attempting the maneuver. The patient will die without it. If the thump is used in the prehospital setting, *don't delay* since the energy requirements for converting a patient out of ventricular fibrillation increase rapidly!

On the other hand, if a patient develops ventricular tachycardia or fibrillation and a defibrillator is readily available, use of this device is preferable to the thump. Should the defibrillator be ''moments away'' (as is usually the case when someone arrests in the intensive care unit or in an emergency department), the option of whether to thump should be at the discretion of the rescuer on the scene. The thump offers the advantage of *speed* but has the drawback of delivering its mechanical input at an unpredictable point in the cardiac cycle.

Finally, if the patient is in ventricular tachycardia *with* a pulse, do *not* use the thump!!! Because of the substantial chance of converting this rhythm to a more malignant one, there is simply too much to lose by attempting the thump in this situation. If the patient in sustained ventricular tachycardia is hemodynamically stable, a trial of medical therapy is reasonable. If the patient is unstable, delivery of an electrical impulse at a predictable point in the cardiac cycle (the upstroke of the R wave) with synchronized cardioversion is much safer and offers a far greater chance for successful conversion to sinus rhythm than does the random delivery of electrical output provided by the thump.

Cough Version:

Description: The patient is instructed to ''Cough hard and keep coughing!'' as soon as the arrhythmia is noted (Schultz and Olivas, 1986).

Indications: At the onset of ventricular tachycardia, ventricular fibrillation, or asystole before consciousness is lost.

Comments

As we will discuss in Chapter 10 (New Developments in CPR), the main mechanism for blood flow with CPR is not due to a ''squeezing'' of the heart between the sternum and vertebral column as was previously thought, but rather to increases in intrathoracic pressure with resultant development of a pressure gradient between the intrathoracic and extrathoracic compartments. Much of the impetus for advancing this theory was provided by Criley et al. (1976) from work performed in the cardiac catheterization laboratory. Criley observed that forceful and repetitive coughing (Cough CPR) could sustain consciousness for periods of up to 90 seconds in patients with pulseless ventricular tachycardia, ventricular fibrillation, or asystole! Intrathoracic pressures of up to 140 mm Hg were generated by such coughing and somehow resulted in adequate blood flow despite the presence of a nonperfusing rhythm.

It is not known whether the mechanism for cough version is improved coronary perfusion, activation of the autonomic nervous system, or conversion of mechanical energy from the cough into an electrical depolarization (up to 25 joules of kinetic energy may be generated by a cough!). What is known is that the cough may occasionally convert malignant arrythmias to normal sinus rhythm (Caldwell et al., 1985; Schultz and Olivas, 1986).

Since Criley's description of cough CPR, instructing patients to cough at the onset of nonperfusing rhythms has become standard procedure in many cardiac catheterization laboratories. However, the technique has been largely ignored by the rest of the medical community, who rarely invoke coughing at the onset of a malignant arrhythmia.

Our Recommendations for Use

Don't forget about **cough version!!!!** Consider using it at the bedside or in the field for any patient who goes into a sustained malignant arrhythmia. Clinically, the most commonly encountered situation in which cough version may be applied is for patients in ventricular tachycardia with a pulse. However, the procedure is also indicated for pulseless ventricular tachycardia, ventricular fibrillation, and asystole. Practically speaking because consciousness is so rapidly lost with these latter rhythms, it is usually impossible for the rescuer to react in time to instruct the patient to initiate coughing. However, for the individual subject to repeated episodes of ventricular tachycardia, one might consider formulating a prearranged signal with the patient to indicate that immediate coughing (at 1–3 second intervals) must begin. If cough version is successful, it will either convert the rhythm or "buy time" (maintain perfusion) until definitive therapy can be administered.

Defibrillation

Indications: Ventricular fibrillation, pulseless ventricular tachycardia, asystole (if the possibility exists that the rhythm may really be fine ventricular fibrillation).

Recommended Energy Levels for Adults:

Initial defibrillation attempt—200 joules
2nd defibrillation attempt—300 joules
3rd defibrillation attempt—360 joules
Subsequent defibrillation attempts—360 joules
    (although it may be reasonable to drop back to 200 joules at a later point in the code).

Comments

Electrical defibrillation is by far the most important treatment modality for the patient in ventricular fibrillation. Convincing studies have shown that if emergency medical service personnel are allowed to do nothing other than defibrillate victims of cardiac arrest, lives will be saved.

The history of electrical defibrillation dates back to 1899 when Prevost and Battelli first used the technique on laboratory animals. Although studied by researchers at Consolidated Edison in the 1920s, defibrillation was not successfully performed in humans for another quarter century. Then in 1947 Beck defibrillated a patient with the open-chest technique, and 9 years later in 1956 Zoll published the first report of successful closed-chest defibrillation in men.

The theory of electrical defibrillation is simple: in an attempt to eliminate the chaotic asynchronous activity of ventricular fibrillation, a current is passed through the heart. If defibrillation is successful, individual cardiac cells will be depolarized and then repolarize in a uniform manner with resumption of organized, coordinated contractile activity.

It appears that a *"critical mass"* of myocardium is required to sustain ventricular fibrillation. Thus spontaneous resolution of ventricular fibrillation may occasionally be seen in the neonate and in previously healthy adults with otherwise normal hearts. In contrast, ventricular fibrillation in diseased hearts is much more likely to be self-perpetuating since the initial asynchrony of the fibrillating heart propagates further asynchrony (Ewy, 1982).

In view of the above, it appears that depolarization of the entire myocardium is *not* necessary for successful defibrillation. Instead, all that is needed is to depolarize enough cardiac cells so that a critical mass of fibrillating cells no longer exists. This may explain why relatively lower energy levels can be effective in defibrilation.

The strength (energy) of a defibrillation countershock is most often expressed in *joules* (or *watt-seconds*), where:

Energy = Power × Duration
(joules)   (watts)   (seconds)

$$\text{Power} = \text{Potential} \times \text{Current}$$
$$\text{(watts)} \qquad \text{(volts)} \qquad \text{(amperes)}$$

In the early days of defibrillation, it was of paramount importance to distinguish between the amount of electrical energy *stored* in a machine and the actual amount delivered with each countershock (*delivered* energy). Variability between these two parameters was so great that a defibrillator indicating 400 joules might deliver from 155 to 400 joules (Parmley et al., 1982)! Defibrillator efficiency has markedly increased since then. Although a discrepancy often still exists between "stored" and "delivered" energy (due to internal resistance of the defibrillator), the difference is much less than in the past.

One should appreciate that it is *current* (*not* voltage) that defibrillates! The relationship between current, voltage, and resistance is as follows:

$$\text{Current (amperes)} = \frac{\text{Potential (volts)}}{\text{Resistance (ohms)}}$$

Thus the amount of current flowing through a circuit for any given voltage will depend on the electrical resistance (or *impedance*) of the circuit. If resistance increases, less current flows through the circuit.

The same holds true for electrical defibrillation. The amount of current penetrating the chest wall to defibrillate the heart depends on the *transthoracic resistance (TTR)* to the passage of that current.

Despite the fact that current defibrillates, convention holds that defibrillators continue to be calibrated in units of energy (watt-seconds or joules). The emergency care provider must therefore consider the effect that certain factors have on TTR, since this will determine how much current actually penetrates the heart with each defibrillation attempt.

Factors known to affect TTR include:

i) Defibrillating energy
ii) The time interval between successive shocks
iii) The total number of shocks delivered
iv) Size of the paddle electrodes
v) The interface used between the electrodes and the chest wall
vi) Chest wall configuration
vii) The pressure of the electrodes against the chest wall
viii) The phase of ventilation of the patient

The higher the energy used for countershock, the lower the TTR. This raises the question of what the optimal energy for defibrillation should be? Much controversy centered around this point during the 1970s, and significant effort was devoted to making defibrillators capable of delivering well over 400 joules per countershock attempt. Although a *dose-weight* relationship (that lower defibrillation energies are needed to defibrillate lower weight individuals) appears to exist in animals, infants, and small children, it is likely that body weight per se is *not* a major determinant of the energy needed to defibrillate *adults!* (Kerber et al., 1981, Ewy, 1982). In animal studies, body weight often varies by a factor of 10; in adults, it varies by a factor of only 2 or at most 3. Thus, the current feeling is that countershock attempts with lower energy levels (≤ 300 joules) are often equally effective in converting adults out of ventricular fibrillation and carry much less risk of producing cardiac injury.

Weaver et al. (1982) found that defibrillation with 175 joules was equally effective in converting patients out of ventricular fibrillation as was 320 joules but was associated with a lower incidence of conduction system damage (heart block, asystole). The recommendation to use 200 joules for the initial defibrillation attempt in adults is based to a large extent on this work.

The effect of the number of shocks delivered on TTR is *cumulative*. In addition, TTR is also affected by the time interval between successive shocks. This latter finding led to the recommendation that time be minimized between the initial and second countershock attempt.

In reality, it appears that only a modest reduction in TTR occurs between successive countershock attempts (Kerber et al., 1981). Consequently, the new guidelines recommend that energy levels be raised to 300 joules for the second countershock if an initial attempt with 200 joules is unsuccessful. In this way, one can at least be sure that a greater amount of current passes through the heart with the second attempt.

The reason for increasing the energy level to

maximum output (usually 360 joules) for the third countershock attempt is to account for the possibility that certain individuals will require maximum energy for defibrillation.

Current recommendations are that "if fibrillation recurs during the arrest sequence (rather than persists), defibrillation should be reinitiated at the energy level that had previously resulted in successful defibrillation" (JAMA Suppl, 1986).

Because of the *cumulative* (albeit modest) reduction in TTR with successive countershock attempts, and the host of impossible-to-control-for patient-specific variables (such as metabolic condition and state of oxygenation) that may change during the resuscitation effort, it may be reasonable to drop back to 200 joules should ventricular fibrillation recur later on in the code. Then if this is not successful, subsequent attempts should be with 360 joules.

Other factors affecting TTR include paddle size, placement, pressure, and interface. Up to a point, TTR decreases with increasing electrode paddle size. A greater than 20% reduction may be noted when paddles with a 12.5 cm diameter instead of the standard 8 cm paddles are used to defibrillate adults (Ewy, 1982).

Another reason for selecting optimal paddle size is that larger paddles are less likely to concentrate current and produce conduction system damage. (In children, optimal paddle size is determined by choosing the largest electrode diameter that will allow good skin contact with the entire paddle surface.)

The recommended position for paddle placement is to put one paddle under the right clavicle just to the right of the sternum and put the other lateral to the left nipple in the anterior axillary line. Exerting firm pressure (of 25 pounds) on each paddle may further lower TTR by up to 25% (Kerber et al., 1980).

TTR appears to be lowest when countershock is performed during the expiratory phase of respiration. This is because the distance between paddle electrodes and the heart is least at this moment. Air (in the inflated lung) is not a good conductor of electricity. Exerting firm pressure on the paddles probably also acts to lower TTR by assuring forced expiration of the victim.

Chest configuration (particularly *chest width*) plays a role in determining TTR (Kerber et al., 1981).

Clinically this may become important when a low energy is selected to defibrillate a patient with a large chest diameter, since TTR is greatest in such individuals. High outputs (maximal energy of 360 joules) may be needed for successful defibrillation of these patients.

The final factor to consider regarding TTR is the paddle-skin interface. The skin acts as a potent electrical resistor between electrode paddles and the heart. Defibrillation without the use of a suitable interface is likely to result in a burn of the skin surface and a lack of penetration of the defibrillator current.

A number of electrode gels are commercially available to optimize conductivity. One should take pains to assure that too much gel is not applied to the paddles, however, since this may result in bridging of current when the patient is defibrillated. Excess gel also leaves a slippery residue that makes it more difficult to perform CPR.

Saline-soaked gauze pads may be used as a substitute for conductive medium, although they are not quite as effective as clear electrode gel. (Alcohol-soaked sponges must *NEVER* be used, since vaporized alcohol may ignite from the defibrillation shock.)

Recently, disposable electrode pads have been introduced as a third option. While this product provides less conductivity than do most commercial gels, it eliminates the problems of bridging and of leaving a slippery residue on the patient's chest.

Despite meticulous attention to all of the above factors, in many instances successful defibrillation may not be possible. Impossible-to-control-for factors include the underlying condition of the patient, the precipitating cause of ventricular fibrillation, and the duration of time until countershock is applied. Particularly in cases where a prolonged period of time has elapsed before arrival of the defibrillator, the chance for successful defibrillation dramatically decreases. In such individuals, a bradyarrhythmia or asystole is often the precipitating mechanism of arrest, and ventricular fibrillation resistant to all forms of treatment develops only as the terminal event (Kerber et al., 1983). *Promptness* in defibrillation must therefore again be stressed as the *most* important factor in determining the likelihood for successful resuscitation.

Synchronized Cardioversion

Terminology: Confusion often arises regarding the terminology used to describe this procedure. Many emergency care providers incorrectly interchange the term cardioversion with defibrillation and countershock.

As discussed in the previous section, *defibrillation* is the process of passing an electric current through the heart with the intent of depolarizing myocardial cells. The electrical discharge is delivered randomly (in an *unsynchronized* manner) with respect to the cardiac cycle.

> We use the term *countershock* synonymously with defibrillation and reserve both of these terms for discussion of the treatment of ventricular fibrillation.

In contrast, the term *cardioversion* implies that the electrical discharge has been timed to occur at a specific point in the cardiac cycle. This treatment modality is used for attempting to convert tachyarrhythmias to normal sinus rhythm. To avoid any possible confusion about the mode of delivery of the electrical discharge, we will often refer to the procedure as *synchronized* cardioversion.

Indications and Recommended Energy Levels for *Emergency* Cardioversion:

Ventricular tachycardia that is hemodynamically unstable or which has not responded to antiarrhythmic therapy:

> Although ventricular tachycardia may respond to synchronized cardioversion with as little as 1 joule and up to 90% of cases may be reverted with ≤10 joules (Lown and DeSilva, 1982), our recommendation is to let the urgency of the situation be the guide for the amount of energy to use. Thus one might consider using 100–200 joules for the acutely decompensating patient. Under somewhat less urgent circumstances (the hemodynamically stable patient who has not responded to a trial of

antiarrhythmic therapy), lower energies (50 joules) should be tried.

Supraventricular tachyarrhythmias that are hemodynamically unstable:

> *Atrial flutter* is the tachyarrhythmia most responsive to cardioversion. Energies of 25–50 joules are recommended for the emergency situation and will almost always be successful in converting this arrhythmia to sinus rhythm. Although energies of ≤10 joules may also be effective, there is a significant chance of converting atrial flutter to atrial fibrillation instead of sinus rhythm when energies this low are used (Lown and DeSilva, 1982).
>
> Patients with *PSVT* usually do not require cardioversion, because this tachyarrhythmia will almost always respond to pharmacologic treatment (verapamil) and/or vagal maneuvers. When cardioversion is required, an energy of 75–100 joules is recommended for the initial attempt. If unsuccessful, increase the energy to 200 joules.
>
> *Atrial fibrillation* may be relatively resistant to cardioversion. We recommend an initial energy of 100–200 joules.

Comments

Synchronized cardioversion was born out of necessity. Following the successful use of closed-chest defibrillation in 1956, it became apparent that a therapeutic modality was needed for treatment of hemodynamically significant tachyarrhythmias that did not respond to pharmacologic therapy (Alexander, 1986). Use of original defibrillating machines was unsafe for this purpose since the prolonged (150–250 msec) alternating current (AC) discharge they delivered was extremely likely to produce postconversion arrhythmias, asystole, or myocardial damage. Development of direct current (DC) capacitors (able to deliver the electrical impulse in as little as 4–30 msec) and the ability to *synchronize* the discharge to the nonvulnerable period of the cardiac cycle made cardioversion a reality (Lown et al., 1962).

> The *vulnerable period* is the time during the cardiac cycle when the heart is most susceptible to developing ventricular fibrillation if excited by an electrical stimulus. It is approximately 30 msec in duration and just precedes the apex of the T wave on the surface ECG. By synchronizing the electrical impulse to the height of the R wave (before the vulnerable period), the risk of inducing a more malignant arrhythmia is minimized.

Cardioversion is most effective against arrhythmias due to a *reentry* mechanism such as atrial flutter, fibrillation, PSVT, and ventricular tachycardia. It produces a single, brief electrical impulse that terminates the arrhythmia by interrupting the reentrant circuit.

The procedure may be employed electively or on an urgent or emergent basis. Discussion of the former topic is beyond the scope of this book. The use of *emergent* cardioversion is indicated for treatment of tachyarrhythmias in a patient who is acutely decompensating. Most often this will be for ventricular tachycardia. Time is at a premium. The procedure is as follows:

Monitor the ECG in a lead with a tall R wave configuration. Apply conductive medium to the electrode paddles (or use disposable electrode pads) and place the paddles on the patient's chest in the same manner as for unsynchronized defibrillation. Turn on the "synch" switch and verify that the defibrillator is sensing the QRS complex. Charge the defibrillator, make sure everyone is clear from the bed, and then simultaneously depress the buttons on each paddle. Unlike the case for defibrillation, *the buttons on each paddle must remain depressed until the machine has discharged.* Recheck the patient, the pulse, and the ECG monitor. Repeat the process if necessary.

If the patient is awake and time permits, administer a sedative. Diazepam, 5–20 mg IV is usually adequate for this purpose. Also if time allows, a bedboard should be placed under the patient prior to the procedure in the event that CPR may be needed.

In the less emergent situation (the hemodynamically stable patient in ventricular tachycardia who has not responded to antiarrhythmic therapy), it may be advisable to call an anesthesiologist to the bedside. In this way qualified personnel can attend to the airway if the patient decompensates, leaving you free to concentrate on directing resuscitation and managing arrhythmias.

SPECIAL CONSIDERATIONS

Prior to performing any procedure, it is always helpful to anticipate potential problems that might be encountered. Occasionally cardioversion can precipitate malignant arrhythmias (including ventricular fibrillation) or asystole. Therefore, a fully equipped crash cart should be in the room. Should the patient go into ventricular fibrillation, simply turn off the synchronizer switch and immediately defibrillate with 200 joules.

When ventricular tachycardia is very rapid (usually >200 beats/min) and the QRS complex is particularly wide, it may be extremely difficult to differentiate between the QRS and the T wave. If you find yourself unable to make this distinction, it will probably also be impossible for the defibrillator to do so. Synchronization then becomes equally likely to fall on a T wave (the vulnerable period) as not. Under such circumstances, delivery of an unsynchronized countershock is preferable to cardioversion.

A warning is frequently cited not to cardiovert patients on digitalis. Such precaution may not be essential, as there appears to be no increased risk of postconversion arrhythmias when cardioversion is performed on patients with *therapeutic* digoxin blood levels (Mann et al., 1985). On the other hand, cardioversion most definitely should be avoided (if at all possible) in patients suspected of having digitalis *toxicity* (Lown and DeSilva, 1982).

Cardiac Pacemakers

Indications in the Setting of Acute Myocardial Infarction

—Mobitz II 2° AV block
—3° AV block with anterior myocardial infarction
—New bifascicular bundle branch block
—New unifascicular bundle branch block (controversial)

—Severe sinus bradycardia
—Mobitz I 2° AV block
—3° AV block with inferior myocardial infarction
} When hemodynamically significant and resistant to medical therapy

Indications in the Setting of Cardiac Arrest

—Mobitz II 2° AV block
—3° AV block
—Slow idioventricular escape rhythm
—Asystole

—Severe sinus bradycardia
—Mobitz I 2° AV block
} When hemodynamically significant and resistant to medical therapy

—Refractory tachyarrhythmias including torsade de pointes (overdrive pacing)

Comments

The topic of cardiac pacing is a comprehensive one that extends well beyond the scope of this book. We will therefore limit our comments in this section to those aspects of cardiac pacing that are pertinent to the emergency care provider in charge of an acutely unstable patient or in the setting of cardiac arrest. We add to this discussion in Chapter 12 with a brief commentary on indications for insertion of a temporary transvenous pacemaker in the setting of acute mycardial infarction.

Practically speaking, the prinicpal indication for emergency cardiac pacing can be summarized as symptomatic or hemodynamically significant bradycardia (be this from marked sinus bradycardia, high-degree or complete AV block, or other conduction disturbance). In most instances, drug therapy is a *temporizing measure* that is used only until preparations for pacing can be made.

Three types of cardiac pacemakers may be used in the emergency care setting: transvenous pacemakers, transthoracic pacemakers, and transcutaneous (external) pacemakers.

A **transvenous pacemaker** is inserted through either the brachial, subclavian, internal jugular, or femoral vein. The pacemaking wire is advanced by means of a flow-directed balloon-tipped catheter with electrocardiographic monitoring or under fluoroscipic guidance if time permits and skilled personnel and equipment are on hand. In its final position, it lies in the right ventricular apex. Transvenous pacing is the most reliable of the three types of emergency pacemakers. It is the procedure of choice when time permits and an operator skilled in the technique is available.

For years, the **transthoracic pacemaker** was used when rapid pacing was urgently needed. The procedure is simple: a transthoracic needle is inserted just to the left of the subxiphoid notch. After entering the skin at a 30°–45° angle, the needle is advanced aiming for the sternal notch. When about three fourths of its length has been inserted, the inner trocar of the needle is withdrawn. Aspiration of blood with a syringe confirms correct placement within the right ventricular cavity. The pacing wire can then be introduced and hookup made to the external energy source.

The advantage of transthoracic pacing is speed of insertion—it can be performed in less than 1 minute. The drawbacks include complications (pneumothorax, hemothorax, hemopericardium), interference with external chest compression, and unreliable pacing. In most instances this procedure is reserved as a "last ditch effort" when all else has failed.

The most exciting advance in pacemaker therapy has been development of the **transcutaneous (external) pacemaker.** First introduced by Zoll in 1952, this device fell out of favor when transvenous pacing became popular during the 1960s. Problems caused by the original external pacemaker were severe patient discomfort (from cutaneous sensory nerve and skeletal muscle stimulation) and significant stimulus artifact (from involuntary skeletal muscle contraction) that made interpretation of the surface ECG exceedingly difficult.

The device was modified and reintroduced in 1981. The improved model minimized patient discomfort from cutaneous sensory nerve stimulation and skeletal muscle contraction and produces an easily interpretable ECG recording. Several features make it extremely attractive as an emergency pacing procedure:

  i) It is entirely noninvasive.
 ii) It is easily and rapidly applied.
iii) It produces effective cardiac pacing in a majority of cases.

It is important to emphasize that the external pacemaker is only a *temporizing* measure. Transvenous pacing is still the treatment of choice for patients who develop a severe conduction disorder in the setting of cardiac arrest. However, if transvenous pacing is not readily available, transcutaneous pacing may be preferable to pharmacologic therapy. Moreover, in certain instances when the need for transvenous pacing is questionable (for example, 3° AV block with an acceptable junctional escape pacemaker in the setting of inferior infarction and acute unifascicular block with acute infarction), insertion of a transvenous pacemaker as a *prophylactic* measure may no longer be needed if the rescuer knows that external pacing is available as a backup should the patient decompensate.

SPECIAL CONSIDERATIONS

Practically speaking, pacemaker therapy is rarely a lifesaving procedure in the setting of cardiac arrest. Insertion of a pacemaker is ineffective for EMD since the problem with this disorder is not the lack of electrical activity but rather the inability of the myocardium to generate effective contraction.

Patients who have received emergency pacing for bradyasystolic cardiac arrest also have a dismal prognosis (Niemann et al., 1986; Syverud et al., 1986). However, most studies reported in the literature have been conducted retrospectively, and pacemaker insertion was only performed after prolonged resuscitation and lack of response to other therapeutic modalities. One could not reasonably expect any intervention to work under such circumstances.

Resurgence of a noninvasive, rapidly applied, external method of cardiac pacing holds promise of improving on these dismal statistics by offering the patient definitive care sooner—hopefully before irreversibility has set in (Zoll and Zoll, 1985).

E: DRUGS THAT HAVE BEEN DEEMPHASIZED

SODIUM BICARBONATE

How Dispensed: 44.6 to 50 mEq per 50 ml ampule

Dose and Route of Administration

IV Bolus: If sodium bicarbonate is indicated at all, an initial dose of 1 mEq/kg ($\approx$1–1.5 ampules) has been recommended. No more than half this amount should be given every 10 min. In the postresuscitation phase, sodium bicarbonate administration should be guided by ABG measurements.

Comments

Despite the intuitive logic that administration of sodium bicarbonate to buffer acid should be beneficial in cardiopulmonary arrest, there is very little data to back this up (Niemann et al., 1984; Sanders et al., 1984). During the early minutes of an arrest, the primary acid-base disturbance appears to be respiratory acidosis. This results from hypoventilation. If a victim of cardiopulmonary arrest can be adequately ventilated and perfused, the need for sodium bicarbonate should be minimal.

Significant metabolic acidosis may *not* develop in cardiopulmonary arrest for some time (at least 5–15 minutes?) after patient collapse (Sanders et al., 1984; Weil et al., 1984; Grundler et al., 1985). Since the primary abnormality in the inital minutes is hypoventilation (respiratory acidosis), it would therefore seem far more appropriate to correct the acidosis of cardiac arrest by improving ventilation (by hyperventilating the patient) than by administering sodium bicarbonate.

Sodium bicarbonate therapy is *not* benign. Adverse effects of excessive administration of this agent include extreme alkalosis, hyperosmolality, hypokalemia, sodium overload, shifting of the oxyhemoglobin dissociation curve leftward with consequent impaired oxygen release to the tissues, and precipitation of convulsions and/or arrhythmias. Moreover, unless adequate ventilation is achieved, carbon dioxide (CO_2) will tend to accumulate. Since CO_2 is freely diffusable across cellular and organ membranes, it readily enters the brain and heart where it may further depress function by producing a *paradoxical intracellular acidosis* (Grundler et al., 1985). Administration of sodium bicarbonate only aggravates this acidosis.

The manner in which the paradoxical intracellular acidosis is aggravated by sodium bicarbonate therapy can best be understood by examining the following equation:

$$H^+ + HCO_3^- \leftrightarrow H_2CO_3 \leftrightarrow H_2O + CO_2$$

Loading one side of the equation drives the reaction to the other side.

In the presence of acidosis, bicarbonate ion (HCO_3^-) in the form of sodium bicarbonate is administered in an attempt to neutralize acid (H^+). A weak acid (carbonic acid = H_2CO_3) is formed, which subsequently breaks down into water (H_2O) and carbon dioxide (CO_2). The freely diffusable CO_2 readily crosses cellular membranes. Once inside the cell, it combines with H_2O and the above equation moves back to the left. Extra H^+ ions are then formed, intracellular pH is lowered, and the paradoxical intracellular acidosis is produced.

The old standby, arterial blood gas (ABG) studies, is *not* the dependable predictor of *intra*-cellular acid-base status that we used to think (Weil et al., 1986, Relman, 1986). Instead, pH of mixed *venous* blood much more closely reflects the pH inside the cell. Studies have shown that a significant discrepancy (of up to several pH units) rapidly develops in cardiopulmonary arrest between arterial and mixed venous blood (Weil et al., 1984 and 1985; Grundler et al., 1984). Suprisingly severe venous hypercarbia and acidosis may coexist with simultaneous arterial alkalosis. Fortunately, mixed venous acidosis (which reflects intracellular acidosis) can be rapidly corrected by hyperventilation. This eliminates residual CO_2 and prevents the above equation from moving to the left. Unfortunately, the emergency care provider all too often reflexively orders one or more ampules of sodium bicarbonate at the onset of cardiopulmonary arrest and repeats the drug liberally thereafter. While this may correct arterial pH (and make the emergency care provider feel better when he/she sees "nice" ABG values), it only aggravates the intracellular acidosis. Intravenously administered sodium bicarbonate generates additional CO_2 (by the above equation) which readily diffuses into cells and leads to depressed myocardial and cerebral function.

In summary, with the usual scenario that occurs during cardiopulmonary arrest, the acidosis that develops appears to be primarily respiratory in nature during the early minutes after patient collapse. Appropriate initial therapy must therefore be directed toward improving ventilation. Sodium bicarbonate is probably *not* indicated for *at least* the first 5–10 min of the resuscitation effort and may in fact be deleterious by aggravating intracellular acidosis (and further depressing myocardial and cerebral function).

The only exception to the above generality is if a *preexisting* metabolic acidosis is present before the arrest (as in a patient with diabetic ketoacidosis) and may have contributed to causing the arrest. Even in such situations the value of sodium bicarbonate is now being questioned, and some investigators feel it should probably *never* be given regardless of the pH because of its potential deleterious effects (Morris et al, 1986; Stacpoole, 1986).

Standard ABG studies may mislead the clinician because *arterial* pH does *not* reflect the state of intracellular homeostasis. Thus the practice of obtaining ABGs to guide sodium bicarbonate therapy in the setting of cardiopulmonary arrest is being seriously questioned. It may be that arterial blood gas studies should only be used to monitor the state of oxygenation of blood being delivered to the tissues until the spontaneous circulation has been restored (Relman, 1986).

Measurement of mixed *venous* blood gases appears to be a much more reliable indicator of intracellular acid-base status (Weil et al., 1986). Unfortunately, there is no practical way to monitor this parameter during most cases of cardiopulmonary arrest. Even if mixed venous blood gas studies were routinely available, one would still be faced with the dilemma of knowing that intravenous sodium bicarbonate administration may paradoxically exacerbate the intracellular acidosis of cardiopulmonary arrest.

Many questions remain, and more work will have to be done before firm recommendations can be made regarding the use of sodium bicarbonate in cardiopulmonary arrest. At the moment the main point that has become clear is that in the arrested heart *much less sodium bicarbonate should be used than in the past*. One should probably resist the urge to administer this drug for *at least* the first 5–10 minutes of an arrest (and perhaps thereafter), and strive to correct acid-base abnormalities by improving ventilation.

BRETYLIUM TOSYLATE
How Dispensed: 500 mg per 10 ml ampule

Dose and Route of Administration

IV Bolus: 5 mg/kg initially ($\approx$ 1 ampule). Defibrillate. If patient is still in ventricular fibrillation, give a second dose of 10 mg/kg (1–2 ampules). This may be repeated every 15–30 minutes up to a total loading dose of 30 mg/kg.

IV Maintenance Infusion: Mix 1 g in 250 ml D5W and begin drip at 15–30 drops/min (1–2 mg/min).

IV Loading Infusion for VT: Dilute 500 mg in 50 ml of D5W and infuse over 10 minutes. This may be followed with an IV infusion at 1–2 mg/min.

Comments

Bretylium is a quaternary ammonium compound that was initially used in the 1950s as an antihypertensive agent. The drug has a complex mechanism of action including adrenergic stimulation that results in an initial release of norepinephrine, followed several minutes later by adrenergic blockade in which uptake of norepinephrine and epinephrine into postganglionic adrenergic nerve endings is prevented. This latter effect becomes the predominant one and accounts for the fact that following an initial increase in blood pressure, hypotension commonly occurs. This hypotension has a particularly strong orthostatic component and is a major factor limiting use of this drug for ventricular tachycardia. Another result of the adrenergic blockade is that hypersensitivity to infused catecholamines (such as epinephrine, norepinephrine, dopamine) may develop.

Bretylium is an effective agent for treatment of *refractory ventricular fibrillation*. The drug exerts and *antifibrillatory* effect that facilitates subsequent electrical conversion. For this indication, the initial dose is an IV bolus of at least 5 mg/kg ($\approx$ 1 ampule). *Chemical* conversion (spontaneous conversion of ventricular fibrillation by the drug itself) is rare. It is therefore important to continue CPR for at least 1–2 minutes after giving bretylium to allow adequate time for the drug to reach the central circulation. Then defibrillate. If there is no response, a second dose

of 10 mg/kg (1–2 ampules) of drug should be given, circulated, then followed again by defibrillation.

The onset of action of bretylium following bolus injection is variable. Although the drug often begins to exert its antifibrillatory effect within 2 minutes (Koch-Weser, 1979; Nowak et al., 1981), delays of up to 10–15 minutes have been encountered (Dhurandhar et al., 1980; Haynes et al., 1981; Holder et al., 1977). This makes it imperative that resuscitation efforts *not* be abandoned until one has given the drug adequate time to take effect. Following the second dose of bretylium, additional 10 mg/kg boluses of the drug may be administered at 15–30 minute intervals until a maximum of 30 mg/kg has been given.

The duration of action of a bretylium bolus is between 2–6 hours. Thus, some protection against recurrence of ventricular fibrillation is provided by this form of administration. As extra insurance, one should probably begin a prophylactic maintenance infusion of either bretylium or lidocaine as soon as the patient is converted to a normal rhythm.

> The new guidelines have demphasized bretylium and made it a *second-line* agent to lidocaine for treatment of refractory ventricular fibrillation. The reason for this is the lack of clear evidence that one agent is superior to the other in decreasing mortality from cardiac arrest (Haynes et al., 1981; White, 1984; Olson et al., 1984). Theoretically, administration of bretylium may be counterproductive in the arrested heart since the vasodilatation it produces may adversely affect aortic diastolic pressure and coronary blood flow. Lidocaine may thus be a safer drug and because most emergency care providers are much more comfortable and familiar with its use, it has been given precedence over bretylium. If a patient in refractory ventricular fibrillation does not respond to an initial bolus of lidocaine, however, the new guidelines allow the emergency care provider the option of either repeating the lidocaine bolus or changing to bretylium (Step 11 of the Algorithm for Ventricular Fibrillation shown in Figure 1-2).

The use of bretylium for treatment of ventricular tachycardia has been deemphasized. The new guidelines have made it a *third-line* agent that probably should *not* be tried unless optimal doses of procainamide and lidocaine have failed. When used to treat *ventricular tachycardia,* the drug is best administered as a slow IV loading infusion to minimize hypotension and nausea and vomiting (in the awake patient) that may occur if the drug is injected too rapidly. One can dilute 500 mg in 50 ml of D5W and set up a drip to run in over a 10 minute period. If successful, IV loading may be followed by a maintenance infusion of the drug at 1–2 mg/min. Torresani (1984) has suggested that slower loading (over 30 min) and lowering the rate of the maintenance infusion (to 0.5 mg/min) further minimizes adverse effects from this drug.

> It is important to emphasize that bretylium is *not* a drug of first choice for treatment of PVCs. Instead, it appears to be much more potent an as *antifibrillatory* agent than as an *antiectopic* agent (Castle, 1984; Lucchesi, 1984). PVCs may actually be made *worse* when bretylium is first administered, due to the initial adrenergic stimulation (and release of norepinephrine) it causes. Lidocaine and procainamide are therefore better agents for treating ventricular ectopy. Only if malignant ventricular arrhythmias persist despite optimal administration of these two agents is a trial of bretylium warranted.

CALCIUM CHLORIDE

How Dispensed: The 10% solution contains 1000 mg (13.6 mEq) of calcium per 10 ml syringe.

Dose and Route of Administration

IV Bolus: 500 mg (5 ml) IV. May repeat once in 10 minutes.

Comments

In the past, calcium chloride had been recommended for treatment of asystole and EMD. No longer. The new guidelines have toally dropped these indications for the drug because of the absence of clinical data supporting the efficacy of this agent. Previous reports were largely anecdotal (Harrison and Amey, 1984; Stueven, 1984). Some were of surgical patients (who were likely hypocalcemic from multiple blood transfusions), while others were of patients who presented with pulseless intraventricular conduction defects that were due to hyper-

kalemia. Both conditions would be expected to respond to calcium administration. On the contrary, more recent work on the use of calcium chloride for patients with prehospital cardiovascular collapse and asystole show the drug to be associated with an unfavorable outcome in a significant percentage of patients (Stueven et al., 1983; Stueven, 1984).

> There are several reasons calcium may be deleterious. The drug had been recommended in the past because it was felt that "the inotropic state of the heart is dependent on calcium" (Redding et al., 1983). But calcium increases ventricular excitability and suppresses sinus impulse formation. Given too rapidly or in excess amount, it may produce marked bradycardia or even asystole. Studies have shown that routine adminsitration of a 500 mg IV bolus of the drug results in dangerously high elevations of the serum calcium level (to a mean value of 15 mg/100 ml). Levels remain elevated for an average of 15 min after the drug is given (Dembo, 1981; Resnekov, 1981). Moreover, administration of calcium may induce spasm of the cerebral microvasculature, leading to cerebral hypoperfusion (White et al., 1983; Redding et al., 1983). Preliminary work suggests that administration of calcium antagonists improves cerebral blood flow and neurologic recovery when given during cardiac arrest (Winegar et al., 1983; White et al., 1982). If calcium antagonists act to improve cerebral blood flow (and *save* the brain), calcium chloride might well be expected to do the opposite.

For all of these reasons, the use of calcium chloride is not *contraindicated* for asystole and EMD. The *only* special stiuations remaining as indications for its use are:

i) Hypocalcemia
ii) Hyperkalemia
iii) Asystole that occurs following the use of a calcium antagonist (such as may occur when verapamil is used to treat PSVT).
iv) Pretreatment of patients with supraventricular tachyarrhythmias prior to administration of verapamil.

ISOPROTERENOL

How Dispensed: 1 mg vials

Dose and Route of Administration

IV Infusion: Mix 1 mg in 250 ml D5W and begin drip at 30 drops/min (2 μg/min).

Titrate infusion to clinical effect. Rate of infusion should not exceed 10 μg/min.

Comments

Isoproterenol is a pure beta-adrenergic receptor stimulating agent with potent chronotropic and inotropic properties. The new guidelines have greatly deemphasized its use. The drug is now *contraindicated* for asystole, EMD, and ventricular fibrillation. Presently, its *only* use is as a stopgap measure (until pacemake therapy can be initiated) for hemodynamically significant bradyarrhythmias that have not responded to atropine. In this setting, low-dose infusion of the drug effectively provides *chronotropic* support. However, when used in higher doses, myocardial oxygen consumption is increased, ventricular arrhythmias develop, and the drug's beta-2 adrenergic (vasodilator) effect becomes much more prominent. As a result, peripheral vascular resistance is lowered. During cardiac arrest, such vasodilation leads to a lowering of aortic diastolic pressure, causing coronary blood flow to drop to extremely low values. In contrast, the alpha-adrenergic effect of drugs such as epinephrine maintains (or raises) peripheral vascular resistance and increases coronary blood flow. When confronted with a patient in asystole or with a hemodynamically significant bradyarrhythmia necessitating CPR, the use of epinephrine and dopamine, respectively, is far preferable to isoproterenol (Otto et al., 1981b; Parmley et al., 1982; Redding, 1979).

REFERENCES

Alexander S: The new era of cardioversion. JAMA 256:628–629, 1986.

American Heart Association Subcommittee on Emergency Cardiac Care: Standards and guidleines for cardiopulmonary resuscitation (CPR) and emergency cardiac care (ECC). JAMA (Supplement) 255:2905–2992, 1986.

Auerbach PS, Budassi SA (Ed): Cardiac Arrest and CPR. Aspen Systems Corp. Rockville, MD, 1983.

Brown CG, Werman HA, Davis EA, Katz S, Hamlin RL: Effect of High-Dose Phenylephrine versus Epinephrine on Regional Cerebral Blood Flow During Cardiopulmonary Resuscitation. (Abstract). Ann Emerg Med 15:14–15, 1986.

Caldwell G, Millar G, Quinn E, Vincent R, Chamberlain DA: Simple mechanical methods for cardioversion: Defense of the precordial thump and cough version. Br Med J 291:627–630, 1985.

Castle L: Therapy of ventricular tachycardia. Am J Cardiol 54:26A–33A, 1984.

Colucci WS, Wright RF, Braunwald E: New positive inotropic agents in the treatment of congestive heart failure. N Engl J Med 314:290–299 (Part I); 349–358 (Part II), 1986.

Coon GA, Clinton JE, Ruiz E: Use of atropine for brady-asystolic prehospital cardiac arrest. Ann Emerg Med 10:462–467, 1981.

Criley JM, Blaufuss AH, Kissel GL: Cough-induced cardiac compression: Self-administered form of cardiopulmonary resuscitation. JAMA 236:1246–1250, 1976.

Dalsey WC, Barsan WG, Joyce SM, Hedges JR, Lukes SJ, Doan LA: Comparison of superior vena cava vs inferior vena cava access for delivery of drugs using a radioisotope technique during normal perfusion and CPR (abstract). Ann Emerg Med 12:247–248, 1983.

Dembo DH: Calcium in advanced life support. Crit Care Med 9:358–359, 1981.

Dhurandhar RW, Pickron J, Goldman AM: Bretylium tosylate in the management of recurrent ventricular fibrillation complicating acute myocardial infarction. Heart Lung 9:265–270, 1980.

Ewy GA: Defibrillation. In Harwood AL (Ed): Cardiopulmonary Resuscitation. Williams & Wilkins, Baltimore, 1982, pp 89–126.

Ewy GA: Ventricular fibrillation masquerading as asystole. Ann Emerg Med 13:811–812, 1984.

Falk RH, Jacobs L, Sinclair A, Madigan-McNeil C: External noninvasive cardiac pacing in out-of-hospital cardiac arrest. Crit Care Med 11:779–782, 1983.

Falk RH, Zoll PM, Zoll RH: Safety and efficacy of noninvasive cardiac pacing: A preliminary report. N Engl J Med 309:1166–1168, 1983.

Goldman L, Batsford WF: Risk-benefit stratification as a guide to lidocaine prophylaxis of primary ventricular fibrillation in acute myocardial infarction: An analytic review. Yale J Biol Med 52:455–466, 1979.

Grauer K: Should prophylactic lidocaine be routinely used in patients suspected of acute myocardial infarction? J Fla Med Assoc 69:377–379, 1982.

Greenberg MI, Mayeda DV, Chrzanowski R, Brumwell D, Baskin SI, Roberts JR: Endotracheal adminsitration of atropine sulfate. Ann Emerg Med 11:546–548, 1982.

Grundler W, Weil MH, Yamaguchi M, Michaels S: The paradox of venous acidosis and arterial alkalosis during CPR (abstract). Chest 86:262, 1984.

Grundler W, Weil MH, Rackow EC, Falk JL, Bisera J, Miller JM, Michaels S: Selective acidosis in venous blood during human cardiopulmonary resuscitation: A preliminary report. Crit Care Med 13:886–887, 1985.

Haft JI, Habbab MA: Treatment of atrial arrhythmias: Effectiveness of verapamil when preceded by calcium infusion. Arch Intern med 146: 1085–1089, 1986.

Harrison EE, Amey BD: Use of calcium in electromechanical dissociation. Ann Emerg Med 13:844–845, 1984.

Haynes RE, Chinn TL, Copass MK, Cobb LA: Comparison of Bretylium Tosylate and Lidocaine in Management of Out of Hospital Ventricular Fibrillation: A Randomized Clinical Trial. Am J Cardiol 48:353–356, 1981.

Hedges JR, Syverud SA, Dalsey WC: Developments in transcutaneous and transthoracic pacing during bradyasystolic arrest. Ann Emerg Med 13:822–827, 1984.

Heissenbuttel RH, Bigger JT: Bretylium tosylate: A newly available antiarrhythmic drug for ventricular arrhythmias. Ann Intern Med 91:229–238, 1979.

Holder DA, Sniderman AD, Fraser G, Fallen EL: Experience with bretylium tosylate by a hospital arrest team. Circulation 55:541–544, 1977.

Jose AD, Taylor RR: Autonomic blockage by propranolol and atropine to study intrinsic myocardial function in man. J Clin Invest 48:2019–2031, 1969.

Kaiser SC, McLain PL: Atropine metabolism in man. Clin Pharmacol Ther 11:214–227, 1970.

Kerber RE: External defibrillation: New technologies. Ann Emerg Med 13:794–797, 1984.

Kerber RE, Grayzel J, Hoyt R, et al: Transthoracic resistance in human defibrillation: Effect of body weight, chest size, serial same energy shocks, paddle size, and paddle contact pressure. Med Instrum 14:52–56, 1980.

Kerber RE, Grayzel J, Hoyt R, Marcus M, Kennedy J: Transthoracic resistance in human defibrillation: Influence of body weight, chest size, serial shocks, paddle size and paddle contact pressure. Circulation 63:676–682, 1981.

Kerber RE, Jensen SR, Gascho JA, Grayzel J, Hoyt R, Kennedy J: Determinants of defibrillation: Prospective analysis of 183 patients. Am J Cardiol 52:739–745, 1983.

Koch-Weser J: Bretylium. N Engl J Med 300:473–477, 1979.

Koehler RC, Michael JR, Guerci AD, Chandra N, Schleien CL, Dean JM, Rogers MC, Weisfeldt ML, Traystman RJ: Beneficial effect of epinephrine infusion on cerebral and myocardial blood flows during CPR. Ann Emerg Med 14:744–749, 1985.

Kuhn GJ, White BC, Swetnam RE, Mumey JF, Rydesky MF, Tintinalli JE, Krome RL, Hoehner PJ: Peripheral vs central circulation times during CPR: A pilot study. Ann Emerg Med 10:417–419, 1981.

Levine JH, Michael JR, Guarnieri T: Treatment of multifocal atrial tachycardia with verapamil. N Engl J Med 312:21–25, 1985.

Lie KI, Wellens HJ, van Capelle FJ, Durrer D: Lidocaine in prevention of primary ventricular fibrillation. N Engl J Med 291:1324–1326, 1974.

Lown B, Amarasingham R, Neuman J: New method of terminating cardiac arrhythmias: Use of synchronized capacitor discharge. JAMA 182:548–555, 1962.

Lown B: Cardiovascular collapse and sudden cardiac death. In Braunwald E (Ed): Heart Disease. W. B. Saunders Co., Philadelphia, 1980, pp 778–817.

Lown B, DeSilva RA: The technique of cardioversion. In Hurst JW (Ed): The Heart. McGraw-Hill, New York, 1982, pp. 1752–1756.

Lucchesi BR: *Rationale of therapy in the patient with acute myocardial infarction and life-threatening arrhythmias: A focus on bretylium.* Am J Cardiol 54:14A–19A, 1984.

Mann DL, Maisel AS, et al: Absence of cardioversion-induced ventricular arrhythmias in patients with therapeutic dioxin levels. J Am Coll Cardiol 5:882–888, 1985.

Massumi RA, Mason DT, Amsterdam EA, DeMaria A, Miller RR, Scheinman MM, Zelis R: Ventricular fibrillation and tachycardia after intravenous atropine for treatment of bradycardias. N Engl J Med 287:336–338, 1977.

McDonald JL: Serum lidocaine levels during cardiopulmonary resuscitation after intravenous and endotracheal administration. Crit Care Med 13:914–915, 1985.

McGovern B, Garan H, Ruskin JN: Precipitation of cardiac arrest by verapamil in patients with Wolff-Parkinson-White symdrome. Ann Intern Med 104:791–794, 1986.

McNeil EL: Successful resuscitation using external cardiac pacing. Ann Emerg Med 14:1230–1232, 1985.

Michael JR, Guerci AD, Koehler RC, Shi AY, Tsitlik J, Chandra N, Niedermeyer E, Rogers MC, Traystman RJ, Weisfeldt ML: Mechanisms By Which Epinephrine Augments Cerebral and mYocardial Perfusion During Cardiopulmonary Resuscitation in Dogs. Circulation 69:822–835, 1984.

Miller J, Tresch D, Harwitz L, Thompson BM, Aprahamian C, Darin JC: The precordial thump. Ann Emerg Med 13:791–794, 1984.

Moncure AC, McEnany MT: Cardiovascular emergencies. In Wilkins (Ed): MGH Textbook of Emergency Medicine. Williams & Wilkins, Baltimore, 1978, pp. 377–381.

Morgera T, Baldi N, Chersevan D, Medugro G, Camerini F: Chest thump and ventricular tachycardia. PACE 2:69–75, 1979.

Morris LR, Murphy MB, Kitabchi AE: Bicarbonate therapy in severe diabetic ketoacidosis. Ann Int Med 105:834–840, 1986.

Myerburg RJ, Kessler KM, Zaman L, Conde CA, Castellanos A: Survivors of prehospital cardiac arrest. JAMA 247:1485–1490, 1982.

Niemann JT, Rosborough JP: Effects of acidemia and sodium bicarbonate therapy in advanced cardiac life support. Ann Emerg Med 13:781–784, 1984.

Niemann JT, Adomian GE, Garner D, Rosborough JP: Endocardial and transcutaneous cardiac pacing, calcium chloride, and epinephrine in postcountershock asystole and bradycardias. Crit Care Med 13:699–704, 1985.

Niemann JT, Haynes KS, Garner D, Rennie CJ, Jagels G: Postcountershock pulseless rhythms: Response to CPR, artificial cardiac pacing, and adrenergic agonists. Ann Emerg Med 15:112–120, 1986.

Nowak RM, Bodnar TJ, Dronen S, Gentzkow G, Tomlanovich MC: Bretylium tosylate as initial treatment for cardiopulmonary arrest: Randomized comparison with placebo. Ann Emerg Med 10:404–407, 1981.

Olson DW, Thompson BM, Darin JC, Milbrath MH: A randomized comparison study of bretylium tosylate and lidocaine in resuscitation of patients from out-of-hospital ventricular fibrillation in a paramedic system. Ann Emerg Med 13:807–810, 1984.

O'Rourke GW, Greene NM: Autonomic blockade and the resting heart rate in man. Am Heart J 80:469–474, 1970.

Otto CW, Yakaitis RW, Blitt CD: Mechanism of action of epinephrine in resuscitation from asphyxial arrest. Crit Care Med 9:321–324, 1981.

Otto CW, Yakaitis RW, Redding JS, Blitt CD: Comparison of dopamine, dobutamine, and epinephrine in CPR. Crit Care Med 9:640–643, 1981.

Otto CW, Yakaitis RW: The role of epinephrine in CPR: A reappraisal. Ann Emerg Med 13:840–843, 1984.

Parmley WW, Hatcher CR, Ewy GA, Furman S, Redding J, Weisfeldt ML: Task Force V: Physical Interventions and Adjunctive Therapy. Thirteenth Bethesda Conference on Emergency Cardiac Care. Am J Cardiol 50:409–420, 1982.

Patros RJ, Goren CC: The precordial thump: An adjunct to emergency medicine. Heart Lung 12:61–64, 1983.

Ralston SH: Alpha agonist drug usage during CPR. Ann Emerg Med 13:786–789, 1984.

Ralston WH, Tacker WA, Showen L, Carter A, Babbs CF: Endotracheal versus intravenous epinephrine during electromechanical dissociation with CPR in dogs. Ann Emerg Med 14:1044–1048, 1985.

Redding JS: Cardiopulmonary resuscitation: An algorithm and some common pitfalls. Am Heart J 98:788–797, 1979.

Redding JS: Commentary on the proceedings: Second Wolf Creek Conference on CPR. Crit Care Med 9:432–435, 1981.

Redding JS, Haynes RR, Thomas JD: Drug therapy in resuscitation from electromechanical dissociation. Crit Care Med 11:681–684, 1983.

Relman AS: "Blood Gases": Arterial or venous? N Engl J Med 315:187–188, 1986.

Resnekov L: Calcium antagonist drugs—Myocardial preservation and reduced vulnerability ventricular fibrillation during CPR. Crit Care Med 9:360–361, 1981.

Roberts JR, Greenberg MI: Emergency transthoracic pacemaker. Ann Emerg Med 10:600–612, 1981.

Roberts JR, Greenberg MI, Knaub MA, Kendrick ZY, Baskin SI: Blood levels following intravenous and endotracheal epinephrine administration. JACEP 8:53–56, 1979.

Sanders AB, Ewy GA, Taft TY: Resuscitation and arterial blood gas abnormalities during prolonged cardiopulmonary resuscitation. Ann Emerg Med 13:676–679, 1984.

Scheinman MM, Thorburn D, Abbott JA: Use of atropine in patients with acute myocardial infarction and sinus bradycardia. Circulation 52:627–635, 1975.

Schott E: Uber ventrikelstillstand (Adams-Stokes sche Anfalle) nebste Bemerkungen uber Anderstartige Arhymien Passagerer. Natur Dtsch Kin Med: 131:211–215, 1920.

Schultz DD, Olivas GS: The use of cough cardiopulmonary resuscitation in clinical practice. Heart Lung 15:273–280, 1986.

Semenkovich CF, Jaffe AS: Adverse effects due to morphine sulfate: Challenge to previous clinical doctrine. Am J Med 79:325–330, 1985.

Stacpoole P: Lactic acidosis: The case against bicarbonate therapy. Ann Int Med 105:276–279, 1986.

Stewart RB, Bardy GH, Greene HL: Wide complex tachycardia: Misdiagnosis and outcome after emergent therapy. Ann Med Intern 104:766–771, 1986.

Stueven H, Thompson BM, Aprahamian C, Darin JC: Use of calcium in prehospital cardiac arrest. Ann Emerg Med 12:136–139, 1983.

Stueven HA: Calcium chloride: Reassessment of use in asystole. Ann Emerg Med 13:820–822, 1984.

Stueven HA, Tonsfeldt DJ, Thompson BM, Whitcomb J, Kastenson E, Aprahamian C: Atropine in asystole: Human studies. Ann Emerg Med 13:815–817, 1984.

Syverud SA, Dalsey WC, Hedges JR: Transcutaneous and transvenous cardiac pacing for early bradyasystolic cardiac arrest. Ann Emerg Med 15:121–124, 1986.

Syverud SA, Daisey WC, Hedges JR, Kicklighter E, Barsan WG, Joyce SM, van der Bel-Kahn JM, Levy RC: Transcutaneous cardiac pacing: Determination of myocardial injury in a canine model. Ann Emerg Med 12:745–748, 1983.

Thomas M, Woodgate D: Effect of atropine on bradycardia and hypotension in acute myocardial infarction. Br Heart J 28:409–413, 1966.

Torresani J: Bretylium tosylate in patients with acute myocardial infarction. Am J Cardiol 54:21A–25A, 1984.

Weaver WD, Cobb LA, Compass MK, Hallstrom AP: Ventricular defibrillation—A comparative trial using 175-J and 320-J shocks. N Engl J Med 307:1101–1106, 1982.

Weaver WD, Cobb LA, Dennis D, Ray R, Hallstrom AP, Copass MK: Amplitude of ventricular fibrillation waveform and outcome after cardiac arrest. Ann Med Intern 102:53–55, 1985.

Weaver WD, Copass MK, Cobb LA, Hill D, Newman BH: A new compact, automatic, external defibrillator designed for layperson use (Abstract). JACC 5:457, 1985.

Weil MH, Grundler W, Rackow EC, Bisera J, Miller JM, Michaels S: Blood gas measurements in human patients during CPR. (abstract). Chest 86:282, 1984.

Weil MH, Grundler, W, Yamaguchi M, Michaels S, Rackow EC: Arterial blood gases fail to reflect acid-base status during cardiopulmonary resuscitation: A preliminary report. Crit Care Med 13:884–885, 1985.

Weil MH, Rackow EC, Trevino R, Grundler W, Falk JL, Griffel MI: Difference in acid-base state between venous and arterial blood during cardiopulmonary resuscitation. N Engl J Med 315:153–156, 1986.

Weil MH, Ruiz CE, Michaels S, Rackow EC: Acid-base determinants of survival after cardiopulmonary resuscitation. Crit Care Med 13:888–892, 1985.

Wellens HJJ: The wide QRS tachycardia. Ann Med Intern 104:879, 1986.

White BC, Winegar CD, Wilson RF, Hoehner PJ, Prombley JH: Possible role of calcium blockers in cerebral resuscitation: A review of the literature and synthesis for future studies. Crit Care Med 11:202–207, 1983.

White BC, Gadzinski DS, Hoehner PJ, Krome C, Hoehner T, White SD, Trombley JH: Effect of flunarizine on canine cerebral cortical blood flow and vascular resistance post cardiac arrest. Ann Emerg Med 11:119–126, 1982.

White RD: Antifibrillatory drugs: The case for lidocaine and procainamide. Ann Emerg Med 13:802–804, 1984.

Winegar CP, Henderson O, White BC, Jackson RE, O'Hara T, Krause GS, Vigor DN, Kontry R, Wilson W, Shelby-Lane C: Early amelioration of neurologic deficit by lidoflazine after fifteen minutes of cardiopulmonary arrest in dogs. Ann Emerg Med 12:471–477, 1983.

Wyman MG, Gore S: Lidocaine prophylaxis in myocardial infarction: A concept whose time has come. Heart Lung 12:358–361, 1983.

Zoll PM, Zoll RH: Noninvasive temporary cardiac stimulation. Crit Care Med 13:925–926, 1985.

CHAPTER 3

BASIC ARRHYTHMIA INTERPRETATION

A: BASIC PRINCIPLES AND SYSTEMATIC APPROACH

In order to effectively manage a cardiac arrest, one has to be able to rapidly and accurately diagnose cardiac arrhythmias. The goal of this chapter is to present a readily mastered approach to aid in rapid recognition. We will then run through the gamut of arrhythmias that are likely to be encountered during a cardiac arrest and show how the method may be applied.

HEART RATE

Before tackling the intricacies of rhythm analysis, it is important to feel comfortable calculating heart rate. Many methods exist for doing this. Perhaps the easiest to master is simply to *take 300 and divide it by the number of boxes in the R-R interval.* Explanation of this method is as follows. The dimensions of small and large boxes on ECG grid paper are 1 mm and 5 mm, respectively. Since the usual speed of recording is 25 mm/second, the amount of time needed to travel the distance represented by each small box (1 mm) is $\frac{1}{25th}$ (0.04) of a second (**Fig. 3A-1**). Similarly, the amount of time needed to travel the distance represented by each large box (5 mm) is $5 \times 0.4 = 0.20$ seconds.

If a QRS complex were to occur every large box (every 0.20 sec) as shown in **Figure 3A-1** then 5 QRS complexes would occur in 1 second ($5 \times 0.20 = 1.0$ sec). Since there are 60 seconds in a minute, the heart rate would be 300 beats per minute (5 beats/sec $\times$ 60 sec = 300 beats/min). Thus, if a QRS complex occurs every large box, the heart rate will be 300 beats/min. If the rate were only half as fast (if a QRS complex occurred every 2 large boxes), it would be 150

beats/min ($300 \div 2 = 150$ beats/min). A heart rate one third as fast (a QRS occurring every 3 large boxes) reflects a rate of 100 beats/min ($300 \div 3$); a QRS complex every 4 large boxes, a rate of 75 beats/min ($300 \div 4$); and so forth (**Fig. 3A-2**).

PROBLEM   **Apply this method in calculating the heart rate of the examples shown in** <u>Figures 3A-3</u> **through** <u>3A-6</u> **on page 58.**

Before calculating the heart rate of any arrhythmia, it is important to determine if the rhythm is *regular*. Although this can usually be done quite adequately by inspection, at times subtle variations in regularity may easily be missed by this method. When in doubt, regularity of the rhythm may be confirmed by measuring each R-R interval with a pair of calipers (or by marking down the R-R interval on a sheet of paper and checking to see if each beat is on time).

When the rhythm is regular, the easiest way to determine the R-R interval is to select a QRS complex that begins on a *heavy* line and to count over to where the next QRS complex occurs.

ANSWER TO FIGURE 3A-3   The

rhythm is regular. The upstroke of the R wave of beat no. 5 occurs on a heavy line. The R wave of beat no. 6 is a little over 4 large boxes away. Thus the R-R interval is between 4 and 5 large boxes and slightly closer to the former. If it were exactly 4 large boxes, the rate would be 75 beats/min. If it were 5 large boxes, the rate would be 60 beats/min. The rate is about 70 beats/min.

ANSWER TO FIGURE 3A-4   Again the

rhythm is regular. Using beat no. 1 (which falls on a heavy line) as a starting point and counting over, the R-R interval is just less than 3 large boxes. If it were exactly 3 large boxes, then the

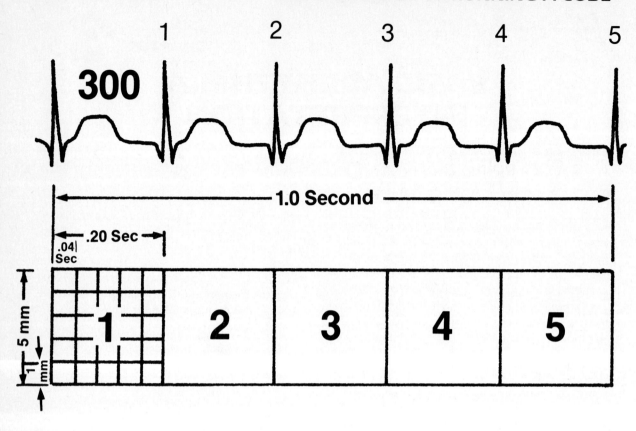

Figure 3A-1

rate would be 100 beats/min. Since it is a little faster than this, the rate is about 105 beats/min.

ANSWER TO FIGURE 3A-5   The rhythm is *slow* but regular. The R-R interval is between 8 and 9 large boxes. If it were 8 boxes, the heart rate would be 38 beats/min (300 ÷ 8). If it were 10 boxes, the rate would be 30 beats/min (300 ÷ 10). The heart rate is therefore about 35 beats/min.

ANSWER TO FIGURE 3A-6   The rhythm is *rapid* but regular. Using beat no. 6 as a starting point and counting over, the R-R interval is just over 2 large boxes. Thus the rate is just under 150 beats/min, or about 140 beats/min.

> When the heart rate is extremely rapid (between 150 and 300 beats/min), accurate estimation becomes difficult, since minor discrepancies in how one measures the R-R interval may exert a dispro-

portionately large effect on the calculated rate. Not accounting for the thickness of one's calipers (or even of the QRS complex itself) may throw the estimate off by as much as 30 beats per minute!

PROBLEM   Calculate the heart rate in Figure 3A-7 on page 59. Is it above or below 200 beats/min?

ANSWER TO FIGURE 3A-7   The rhythm is extremely rapid but regular. Since the R-R interval is between 1 and 2 large boxes, the heart rate must be between 150 and 300 beats/min. However, it is hard to tell by the method just presented whether the rate is above or below 200 beats/min.

Figure 3A-8 illustrates a handy trick for overcoming this difficulty. When the rate is fast and regular, simply measure the R-R interval of every other beat. Dividing 300 by this number will yield *one half* the actual rate.

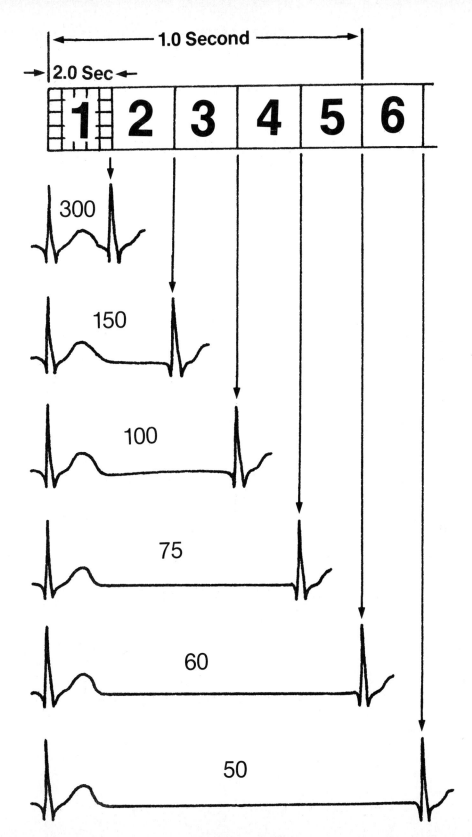

Figure 3A-2

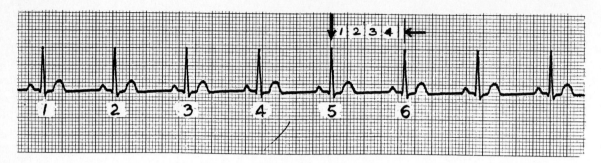

Figure 3A-3:

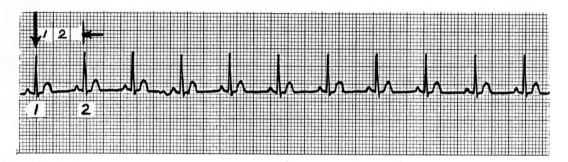

Figure 3A-4

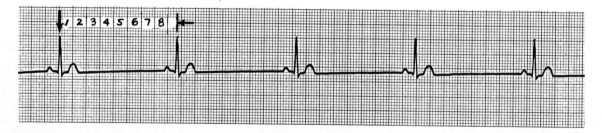

Figure 3A-5

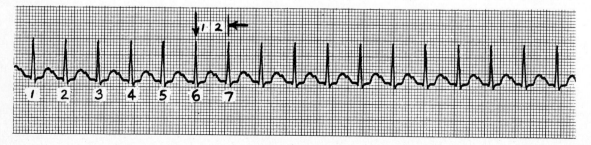

Figure 3A-6

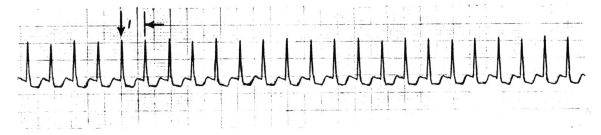

Figure 3A-7

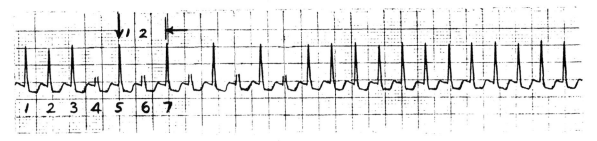

Figure 3A-8

If one picks a QRS complex that falls on a heavy line (beat no. 5 will do), it can be seen that the R-R interval of every other beat in Figure 3A-8 is just under 3 large boxes. Thus *half the rate* must be a little more than 100 beats/min ($\approx$ 105 beats/min). The actual rate in Figure 3A-8 is therefore about 210 beats/min.

> As stated above, the R-R interval of the rhythm in Figure 3A-8 is between 1 and 2 large boxes. If it were exactly 1 large box (5 small boxes), the heart rate would be 300 beats/min. If it were exactly 2 large boxes (10 small boxes), the rate would be 150 beats/min. One might reason that if an R-R interval of 5 small boxes reflects a heart rate of 300 beats/min and one of 10 small boxes reflects a rate of 150 beats/min, each small box should represent an increment of 30 beats/min. Similarly, an R-R interval of 1.5 large boxes (7.5 small boxes) should represent a heart rate that is midway between 300 and 150 beats/min, or 225 beats/min.
>
> Unfortunately, calculation of heart rate is not quite so simple. The incremental increase in heart rate for each small box is *not* equal. This concept is illustrated in **Figure 3A-9.**
>
> Note in Figure 3A-9 that there is a 50 beat/min decrement in heart rate (from 300 to 250 beats/min) when the R-R interval lengthens from 5 to 6 small boxes, but only a 17 beat/min decrement (from 167 to 150 beats/min) when it lengthens

> from 9 to 10 small boxes. Decrements become nearly equal once the heart rate drops below 100 beats/min.

PROBLEM   **Return to Figure 3A-6 and determine the number of small boxes in the R-R interval. Refer to Figure 3A-9 to determine the heart rate.**

ANSWER   The upstroke of the R wave of the 6th QRS complex in Figure 3A-6 occurs on a heavy line. Counting over, the R-R interval is 11 small boxes in duration. According to Figure 3A-9, the heart rate should be 136 beats/min.

> In practice, estimating heart rate by dividing 300 by the number of large boxes in the R-R interval will *almost always* be accurate enough for our purposes. For those interested in more precise estimation, particularly in the presence of rapid heart rates, referral to Figure 3A-9 may be helpful.

RHYTHM DETERMINATION

The key to dysrhythmia interpretation is to apply a *systematic* approach. In addition to estimating heart rate, four basic points must be assessed with every arrhythmia that is analyzed. These points have been incorporated into the *four basic questions* (**Table 3A-1**).

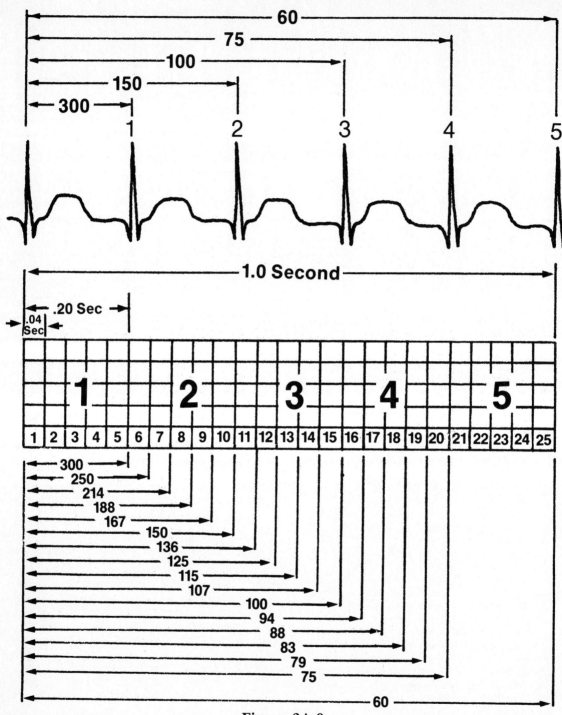

Figure 3A-9

Approach to Rhythm Analysis

A) RATE
B) RHYTHM
    1) Is the rhythm regular?
    2) Are there P waves?
    3) Is the QRS wide or narrow?
    4) Is there a relationship between P waves
       and the QRS complex?

1) Is the Rhythm Regular?

Regularity of the rhythm is usually easy to assess from inspection. One should be aware of the fact that slight irregularity may not be readily apparent with extremely rapid rhythms. In these cases, calipers should be used to verify regularity.

2) Are There P Waves?

Detection of *P waves* is the cornerstone of rhythm analysis. By definition, the P wave should *always* be upright in standard lead II with normal sinus rhythm. This is because orientation of the electrical impulse as it travels from the

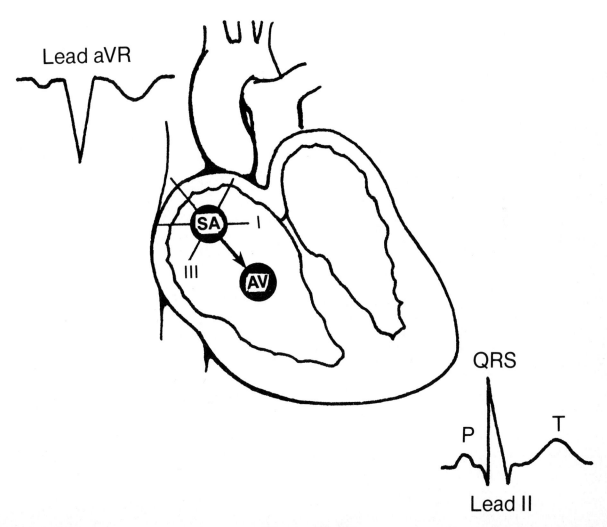

Figure 3A-10

sinoatrial (SA) node to the atrioventricular (AV) node is virtually parallel to lead II (Fig. 3A-10). Under normal circumstances, *if the P wave is not upright in lead II, normal sinus rhythm cannot be present!*

3) Is the QRS Complex Wide or Narrow?

Width of the QRS complex is a most helpful determinant of the site of origin of the electrical impulse. The usual upper limit of normal for duration of the QRS complex in adults is 0.10 seconds. A QRS duration of 0.11 seconds is borderline, while one of 0.12 seconds or greater is definitely prolonged.

> A caveat to keep in mind when assessing QRS duration is that occasionally a portion of the QRS complex may be *isoelectric* (lie on the baseline). When this happens one may get the false impression that in a particular lead the QRS complex is shorter than it really is. To avoid this pitfall, whenever possible one should try to survey the ECG in more than one lead.

When the QRS complex is *narrow* (≤0.10 seconds), the electrical impulse almost always has a *supraventricular* origin. That is, the impulse originates from the SA node, the AV node, or from elsewhere in the atria (from anywhere above the dotted line in **Figure 3A-11.** Rarely it may arise from a site low down in the conduction system (below the dotted line) such as the bundle of His or one of the bundle branches.

On the other hand, when the QRS complex is *widened* (≥0.12 seconds), the site of origin may not be so certain. Although widening of the QRS complex suggests a ventricular site of origin, the impulse may still be supraventricular if something has happened to alter ventricular conduction.

The Pathway of Normal Conduction

> With normal sinus rhythm, the electrical impulse originates in the SA node, the principal pacemaker of the heart. From there it spreads through the right and left atria on its way to the AV node. The impulse then enters the ventricular conduction system, from which it will be carried to all parts of the ventricles (Fig. 3A-11).
> When the ventricular conduction system is functioning normally, the time required for conduction

of the electrical impulse from the SA node throughout the ventricular myocardium is short. Such conduction results in a narrow QRS complex. Should the impulse originate from another supraventricular site instead of the SA node (from either the right or left atria or from the AV node), it will still pass through the ventricular conduction system en route to activating the ventricles. Therefore, under normal circumstances the QRS complex will be narrow and of identical morphology for normal sinus beats, AV nodal beats, or beats originating from elsewhere in the atria since the same conduction pathway through the ventricles will have been used.

Should there be a defect in ventricular conduction (should bundle branch block exist) or should ventricular conduction be abnormal (aberrant) due to incomplete recovery of a portion of the conduction system following a premature beat, both the path and the time for the electrical impulse to travel through the ventricles will be altered. In such cases, the QRS complex may change in morphology and become *widened* despite a supraventricular origin.

4) Is There a Relationship between P Waves and the QRS Complex?

Determination of the relationship between P waves and QRS complexes is critical to rhythm analysis. In analyzing any given rhythm strip, it is probably easiest to first identify QRS complexes. Then look to see if P waves precede each QRS. If they do, are the P waves related (*"married"*) to their respective QRS complex?

With *normal sinus rhythm,* every QRS complex is preceded by a P wave with a *constant* PR interval. That is, each atrial impulse is conducted to the ventricles. If AV conduction is normal, the PR interval will be ≤0.20 seconds. With 1° AV block, each atrial impulse is still conducted to the ventricles with a constant PR interval, but AV conduction is prolonged to ≥0.21 seconds. With more advanced degrees of AV block, conduction of one or more atrial impulses to the ventricles is prevented (*"blocked"*), and the relationship between P waves and QRS complexes is altered.

> Regarding the four questions, it doesn't matter in which order they are asked. In fact it will often be advantageous to alter the order. What *is* important is to *always* ask *each* of these questions when analyzing *any* arrhythmia. Even when the answer is

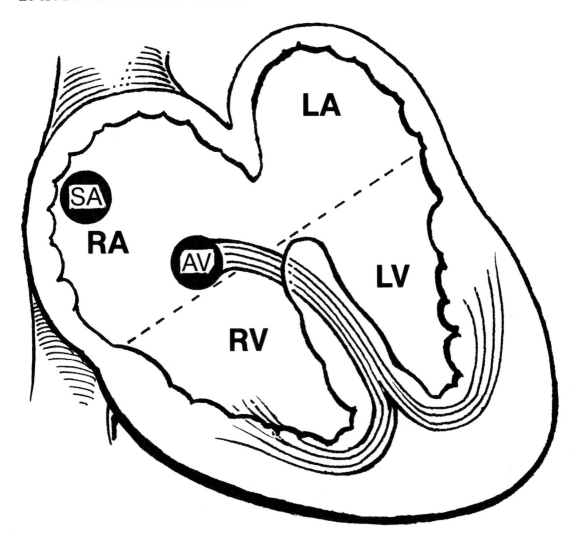

Figure 3A-11

obvious, mentally checking off these four points as a matter of routine will be extremely helpful in organizing one's approach to dysrhythmia interpretation. Especially when confronted with more difficult arrhythmias, adherence to this systematic method will go a long way toward narrowing the list of diagnostic possibilities.

PROBLEM Return to **Figures 3A-3** and **3A-4**. Analyze these rhythms by the four question approach.

ANSWER TO FIGURE 3A-3 The rhythm is regular and the heart rate is 70 beats/min. The QRS complex is narrow (≤0.10 sec).

Each QRS is preceded by a P wave with a constant, normal (≤0.20 sec) PR interval. Thus this is *normal sinus rhythm*.

Normal Sinus Rhythm

By convention, we define normal sinus rhythm in the adult to have a rate between 60 and 100 beats/min. Sinus conduction with a faster ventricular rate is termed *sinus tachycardia*, while a slower rate is sinus bradycardia. Neither sinus bradycardia nor sinus tachycardia necessarily represents a disease state, and both are commonly found among normal individuals.

ANSWER TO FIGURE 3A-4   The rhythm is regular and the heart rate is 105 beats/min. The QRS complex is narrow, and each beat is preceded by a P wave with a constant PR interval. This is *sinus tachycardia*.

PROBLEM   **What about the rhythm shown in Figure 3A-12? In what way does this arrhythmia differ from those we have examined up to now?**

though sinus arrhythmia may also occur normally in the elderly, it is usually not related to respiration in this age group and sometimes is the precursor of *sick sinus syndrome*.

The rate of even "normal sinus rhythm" will often vary slightly from beat to beat. In order to diagnose sinus *arrhythmia* and to distinguish it from the slight normal variation in rate that occurs with normal sinus rhythm, there should be a difference of *at least* 0.08 seconds between the shortest and longest R-R intervals. Despite the existence of this criterion, the presence of sinus arrhythmia is fre-

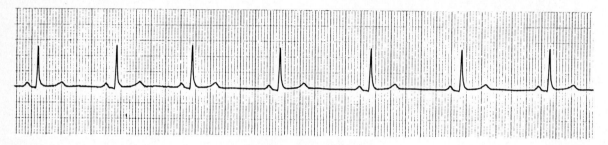

Figure 3A-12

ANSWER TO FIGURE 3A-12   Although at first glance this rhythm may appear to be regular, measurement with calipers reveals a slight but definite irregularity. The R-R interval is between 5 and 6 large boxes, putting the rate between 50 and 60 beats/min. Each QRS complex is preceded by a P wave, and the PR interval is normal. This is *sinus bradycardia* and *arrhythmia*.

Sinus Arrhythmia

Sinus arrhythmia is an extremely common normal finding among children and young adults, in whom heart rate often varies with respiration. Al-

quently not noted in practice since subtle differences in heart rate are easy to overlook unless one meticulously measures each R-R interval on every tracing. Clinically, sinus arrhythmia is usually of little significance. More marked variations in the R-R interval (>0.20 sec), however, should probably be noted.

PROBLEM   **Examine the rhythm shown in Figure 3A-13. From where in the conduction system would you expect this rhythm to arise?**

ANSWER TO FIGURE 3A-13   The rhythm is regular, and the R-R interval is between 5 and 6 large boxes. Thus, the heart rate

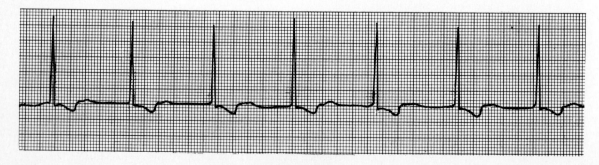

Figure 3A-13

is about 55 beats/min. The QRS complex is of normal duration, but there are no P waves! This is *AV nodal (or junctional) rhythm.*

Junctional (AV Nodal) Rhythm

We have already stated that the SA node is the principal pacemaker of the heart and that with normal sinus rhythm it usually fires at a rate of between 60 and 100 beats/min. Should something happen to the SA node's pacesetting ability, other areas of the heart with inherent automaticity may take over the pacemaking function. With an inherent rate of 40–60 beats/min, the AV node is usually next in line. Should the AV nodal pacemaker also fail, a ventricular pacemaker at a rate of between 30 and 40 beats/min may take over. In the event that no other area of the heart takes over the pacesetting function, asystole will result.

An additional point to be made about junctional rhythms deals with the atrial activity that one is likely to see with this rhythm. In Figure 3A-10, we showed how with normal sinus rhythm the P wave must always be upright in lead II. This is because orientation of the electrical impulse as it travels from its origin in the SA node toward the AV node is virtually parallel to lead II.

PROBLEM   **What would you expect P waves to look like in lead II if the electrical impulse originated from the AV node instead of the SA node?**

ANSWER   With junctional rhythm, P waves tend to be inverted and may either occur before the QRS complex, after the QRS, or be hidden within it. This concept is illustrated in the *laddergram* shown below (**Fig. 3A-14**). Panel A represents normal sinus rhythm. The impulse

originates from the SA node and travels sequentially through the atria, AV node, and ventricles. In contrast, with *junctional rhythm* (panels **B, C,** and **D**), the electrical impulse originates from the AV node. P waves now travel backward *(retrograde)* from the AV node to depolarize the atria. Consequently, atrial activity (P waves) are negative (inverted) in lead II. If retrograde conduction is extremely rapid, inverted P waves will *precede* the QRS complex (Fig. 3A-14 panel B). If retrograde conduction is slow, the atria will not be depolarized until *after* the ventricles, and retrograde P waves will *follow* the QRS complex (Fig. 3A-14 panel D). However, if the speed of retrograde conduction is about equal to the speed of forward *(antegrade)* conduction through the ventricles, the inverted P waves will occur *simultaneously* with the QRS complex and be hidden within it (Fig. 3A-14 panel C).

PROBLEM   **Examine Figure 3A-15. Note that P waves are absent. Is this likely to be a junctional rhythm?**

ANSWER TO FIGURE 3A-15   The rhythm is regular at a rate of 130 beats/min (the R-R interval is between 2 and 3 boxes and is closer to the former). The QRS complex is *wide* (≥ 0.12 sec), and no P waves are evident. Although this could be a junctional tachycardia (with the wide QRS complex being due to either preexisting bundle branch block or aberrant conduction), one has to assume *ventricular tachycardia* until proven otherwise!

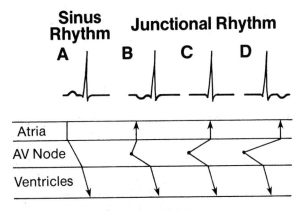

Figure 3A-14

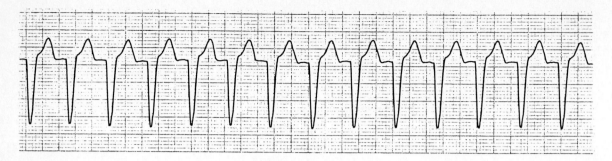

Figure 3A-15

Regular Wide QRS Complex Tachycardias

An extremely common and critically important problem in managing cardiac arrest is determining the cause of regular wide QRS complex tachycardias. *Five* entities should always come to mind:

    i) VENTRICULAR TACHYCARDIA
    ii) VENTRICULAR TACHYCARDIA
    iii) VENTRICULAR TACHYCARDIA
    iv) Supraventricular tachycardia with preexisting bundle branch block
    v) Supraventricular tachycardia with aberrant conduction.

The onus of proof must always be to show that a wide QRS complex tachycardia is not ventricular tachycardia, rather than the other way around. Although the QRS complex in the above example does not appear to be particularly bizarre, it *is* wide and evidence of atrial activity is lacking. QRS morphology with junctional rhythms is similar (if not identical) to QRS morphology with normal sinus rhythm. Usually the QRS is narrow. Statistically, the overwhelming majority of wide QRS complex tachycardias are ventricular in origin. Therefore, unless previous rhythm strips demonstrate sinus conduction with identical QRS morphology, or there is unequivocal evidence of aberrancy, one has to assume that the rhythm in Figure 3A-15 is ventricular tachycardia.

PROBLEM **From where in the conduction system do you suppose the three dysrhythmias shown in Figures 3A-16 through 3A-18 come from?**

ANSWER TO FIGURE 3A-16 The rhythm is regular, and the R-R interval is a little over 6 large boxes. The rate is therefore just under 50 beats/min. No P waves are seen, and the QRS complex is wide. Although a junctional rhythm with a preexisting bundle branch block cannot absolutely be ruled out, one should once again assume a ventricular etiology. This rhythm is known as an *accelerated idioventricular rhythm (AIVR)*.

Accelerated Idioventricular Rhythm (AIVR)

AIVR is an *escape rhythm* that usually arises when the sinus pacemaker fails. The ventricular rate is

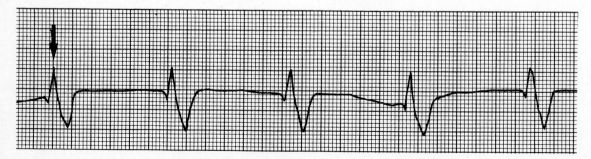

Figure 3A-16

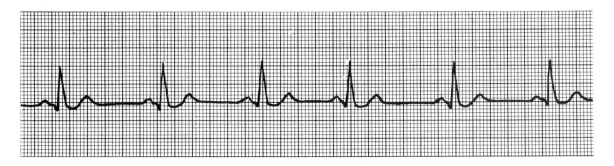

Figure 3A-17

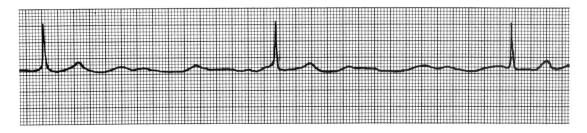

Figure 3A-18

between 50 and 110 beats/min. This is termed *accelerated* because it is faster than the usual idioventricular rate of 30–40 beats/min.

In general, AIVR is a *benign* rhythm that only rarely degenerates to rapid ventricular tachycardia. It is commonly seen in the setting of acute myocardial infarction. Frequently the patient is asymptomatic and does not need to be treated. However, if the rhythm is accompanied by hypotension, measures should be taken to speed up the rate.

ANSWER TO FIGURE 3A-17
The R-R interval is slightly irregular and averages out to between 5 and 6 boxes. Thus the rate is between 50 and 60 beats/min. Close inspection of the QRS complex reveals it to be wide; it is almost 3 small boxes in duration (0.11 to 0.12 sec). Yet unlike the rhythm in Figure 3A-16, each QRS complex is preceded by a normal-appearing P wave with a constant PR interval. Clearly a sinus mechanism is operative here. *Sinus bradycardia* is present, since the rate is under 60 beats/min, and there is *sinus arrhythmia*, since the R-R interval varies. The QRS prolongation can be explained by the existence of a

preexisting intraventricular conduction delay (bundle branch block).

ANSWER TO FIGURE 3A-18
This is an excellent example of how our method for calculation of heart rate works even when the rhythm is exceedingly slow. The R-R interval is almost 15 boxes. Dividing 300 by 15, we can estimate the heart rate to be about 20 beats/min.

Although one may be tempted to call many of the small undulations in the baseline of this tracing P waves, *no definite atrial activity is present!* The undulations seen here are commonly noted in tracings taken while cardiopulmonary resuscitation is in progress and are probably due to movement of the bed and/or the patient being resuscitated.

Despite the slow rate, the QRS complex is narrow! This makes the rhythm less likely to arise from a ventricular focus. Sinus mechanism is precluded by the fact that atrial activity is absent. Thus Figure 3A-18 probably represents an *escape rhythm* that arises from somewhere in the conduction system.

The combination of the exceedingly slow rate shown on page 67, the lack of atrial activity, and the narrow QRS complex suggests that the escape focus is probably low down in the conduction system (in the His or bundle branches). Regardless of where the escape focus arises, however, treatment will be the same—acceleration of the heart rate in an attempt to improve hemodynamic status.

ATRIAL ACTIVITY

Let us now concentrate on the presence of P waves and their meaning.

PROBLEM　　**Examine the rhythms shown in Figures 3A-19, 3A-20, and 3A-21. What is the mechanism of these arrhythmias? Are P waves present? Are they related to the QRS complex?**

Since the heart rate is over 100 beats/min, Figure 3A-19 is either an *accelerated* junctional rhythm or a low atrial *tachycardia*. It is impossible to tell which from the rhythm strip alone. Clinically, distinction between these two entities is of little importance.

ANSWER TO FIGURE 3A-20　　A slow, slightly irregular rhythm is present with a heart rate of about 35 beats/min (the R-R interval is between 8 and 9 boxes; $300 \div 8.5 \approx 35$). The QRS complex is narrow, and an upright P wave with a constant PR interval precedes each QRS complex, indicating sinus mechanism. This is *sinus bradycardia* and *sinus arrhythmia*.

The PR interval in this example is about 0.19 second. This is still within normal limits. In order for

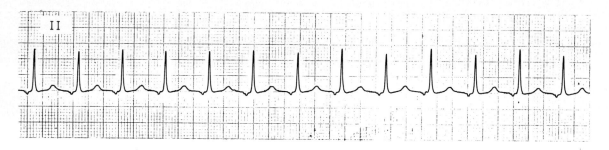

Figure 3A-19

ANSWER TO FIGURE 3A-19　　The rhythm is regular at a rate of 105 beats/min. The QRS complex is narrow. Although P waves with a constant PR interval are present, these P waves are *negative* in this standard lead II monitoring lead. This means that *the rhythm cannot be arising from the sinus node.* It must be either *junctional* or a *low atrial rhythm.*

1° *AV block* to be present, the PR interval must be *greater* than 0.20 second.

ANSWER TO FIGURE 3A-21　　The tracing in Figure 3A-21 is taken from the same patient as was tracing Figure 3A-20. Sinus rhythm at a rate of about 60 beats/min is seen for the first 3 beats, after which long pauses precede the next 2 QRS complexes. However, the

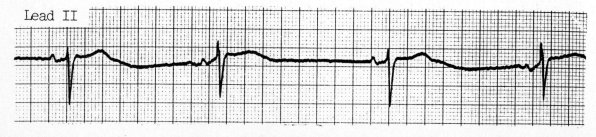

Figure 3A-20

Lead II

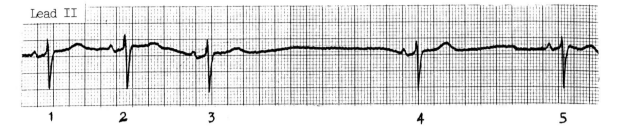

Figure 3A-21

QRS configuration of beats no. 4 and 5 is identical to that of the first 3 beats, and sinus P waves with a constant PR interval precede all 5 QRS complexes in the rhythm strip. The basic rhythm is therefore *sinus*. *Sinus pauses* follow beats no. 3 and 4. The combination of sinus arrhythmia, bradycardia, and sinus pauses seen in Figures 3A-20 and 3A-21 suggest that the patient has *sick sinus syndrome*.

Sick Sinus Syndrome (SSS)

SSS is a commonly encountered entity among the elderly. The syndrome encompasses a wide variety of cardiac arrhythmias that result from progressive deterioration of sinoatrial (SA) node function. These include persistent *sinus bradycardia* (which is the most common and often the earliest manifestation of SSS) *sinus arrhythmia,* and *sinus pauses.* As the disease develops, sinus pauses may become progressively more prolonged, until eventually sinus node activity ceases *(sinus arrest).* When this happens, some other escape focus must take over or asystole will result. Escape rhythms may arise from elsewhere in the atria (ectopic or low atrial rhythm), from the AV node (junctional rhythm), or from the ventricles (AIVR). Alternatively, atrial fibrillation (which we will discuss in the next section) may supervene. Because patients with SSS frequently have

AV nodal disease, the ventricular response to atrial fibrillation is often slow.

In addition to the bradyarrhythmias noted above, many patients with SSS intermittently manifest tachyarrhythmias. These include paroxysmal-supraventricular tachycardia (PSVT), atrial fibrillation or flutter, and ventricular tachycardia.

The course of SSS is highly variable. Development of the full electrocardiographic picture often takes years. Despite extremely slow heart rates, symptoms are minimal or absent in a surprising number of individuals. Underlying etiologies of SSS include myocardial infarction and coronary artery disease, degenerative disease of the conduction system, and hypothyroidism. Iatrogenic causes of the disorder (for example excessive use of medications such as digoxin, B-blockers, or verapamil) must be ruled out. Permanent pacemaker implantation is recommended once patients become symptomatic.

PROBLEM **Let us conclude this section by analyzing the rhythm shown in Figure 3A-22, taken from another patient with SSS. Can you explain the irregularity in the rhythm?**

ANSWER TO FIGURE 3A-22 The QRS complex remains narrow (≤ 0.10 sec) in this rhythm strip, suggesting that all 5 beats arise

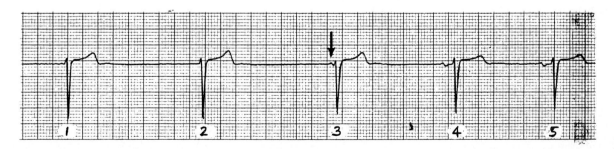

Figure 3A-22

at or above the AV node. Beats no. 4 and 5 are clearly sinus conducted. Each is preceded by a P wave with a fixed PR interval of 0.16 second. In contrast, no P wave precedes beats no. 1 and 2. These are *junctional (AV nodal) escape beats* that (fortunately) arise in response to the lack of atrial activity.

PROBLEM   **What is the rate of the AV nodal escape pacemaker in this example?**

ANSWER   One can determine the rate of the AV nodal escape pacemaker by calculating the R-R interval between successive junctional beats. Approximately 9 boxes separate beats no. 1 and 2. Therefore, the AV nodal rate is about 33 beats/min ($300 \div 9$) in this example.

PROBLEM   **A P wave is seen immediately preceding beat no. 3 (arrow). Do you suppose it is conducted?**

ANSWER   The PR interval of the P wave preceding beat no. 3 is exceedingly short. Normally, *at least* 0.12 second is required for normal conduction (from the SA node through the AV node) to occur. In this particular example, we know from beats no. 4 and 5 that 0.16 second is needed for normal conduction (since this is the PR interval of these sinus conducted beats). Therefore, *the P wave that precedes beat no. 3 is too short to conduct!*

PROBLEM   **Then what type of beat (sinus? junctional? ventricular?) is beat no. 3?**

ANSWER   Since the PR interval of beat no. 3 is too short to conduct, it cannot be coming from the SA node. Beat no. 3 is not ventricular because the QRS complex is narrow and looks very much like the other supraventricular complexes in this rhythm strip. By the process of elimination, beat no. 3 must arise from the AV node.

Further support for this assumption comes from the observation that the R-R interval between beats no. 2 and 3 is equal to the R-R interval between beats no. 1 and 2. Marked sinus slowing occurred prior to the onset of this rhythm strip. This led to the emergence of a junctional escape rhythm (beats no. 1 and 2) at a rate of 33 beats/min. Atrial activity then resumed with the P wave (arrow) preceding

beat no. 3. Acceleration of atrial activity finally leads to resumption of sinus rhythm by the end of the strip (beats no. 4 and 5).

An appreciation of the rhythms encountered in SSS may be worthwhile for the emergency care provider since many of the same arrhythmias are frequently seen acutely during cardiac arrest.

B: PREMATURE BEATS AND TACHYARRHYTHMIAS

PREMATURE BEATS

Recognition of premature beats is an essential component of cardiac monitoring. Three different types exist:

  i) Premature *atrial* contractions (PACs)
 ii) Premature *junctional* contractions (PJCs)
iii) Premature *ventricular* contractions (PVCs)

Clinically, the importance in emergency cardiac care of distinguishing between these three lies in the fact that PVCs frequently warrant treatment whereas premature *supraventricular* contractions (PACs and PJCs) most often do not.

Recognition of the different types of *premature* beats is usually easy. As implied in their name, PACs, PJCs, and PVCs all occur early. Under normal circumstances (as discussed in Fig. 3A-11), the QRS complex of premature supraventricular beats will be narrow and identical (or nearly identical) in morphology to normal sinus beats. In contrast, the QRS complex of PVCs should be wide (≥ 0.12 sec) and markedly different from normal sinus beats in morphology.

Theoretically, PACs should always be preceded by a premature P wave. Usually this P wave is readily apparent. Occasionally, however, it may be hard to identify and represent no more than subtle notching of the preceding T wave.

PJCs are uncommon. It is frequently difficult to distinguish them from PACs since the QRS complex looks the same for both. As noted in Figure 3A-14, P waves tend to be *inverted* with junctional beats. Inverted P waves may precede the QRS complex (usually with a short PR interval), follow the QRS complex, or be hidden within it. Because there is no difference in the clinical significance of PACs and PJCs, distinction between these two types of premature beats is primarily of academic interest.

PROBLEM Examine the tracing shown in <u>Figure 3B-1</u>. Beat nos. 3, 6, and 10 all occur

mature beats is narrow and virtually identical to that of the sinus conducted beats, these premature beats must be *supraventricular* (PACs or PJCs).

PROBLEM Do you see a premature P wave preceding beats no. 3 and 6?

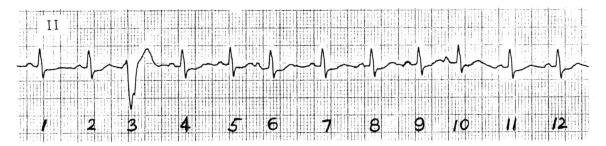

Figure 3B-1

early. Are these premature beats likely to be PACs, PJCs, or PVCs?

ANSWER TO FIGURE 3B-1 The underlying rhythm is sinus tachycardia at a rate of 100 beats/min. The QRS complex is narrow. As noted above, beat nos. 3, 6, and 10 all occur early. Beat no. 3 is clearly a PVC. It is bizarre in shape and much wider than the normally conducted sinus beats. In contrast, beat nos. 6 and 10 are PACs. Each is preceded by a premature P wave, and the QRS complex is virtually identical to that of the normally conducted beats.

PROBLEM Examine the rhythm shown in Fig. 3B-2. Identify the early beats.

ANSWER TO FIGURE 3B-2 The underlying rhythm is sinus. Beats no. 3 and 6 occur early. Because the QRS complex of these pre-

ANSWER Subtle notching of the T wave preceding beat nos. 3 and 6 is evident. This represents the premature P wave.

> Although impossible to be certain, one should assume beat nos. 3 and 6 in Figure 3B-2 are PACs rather than PJCs. In general, premature beats should probably not be interpreted as PJCs unless preceding atrial activity is definitely absent or the preceding P wave is clearly inverted and the PR interval is short.

PROBLEM Examine <u>Figure 3B-3</u>. Although beat no. 3 looks markedly different from the other QRS complexes, it is *not* a PVC. Why?

ANSWER TO FIGURE 3B-3 The underlying rhythm is sinus at a rate of 85 beats/min. Beats no. 3, 7, and 11 all occur early. The latter two are clearly PACs. This is because the

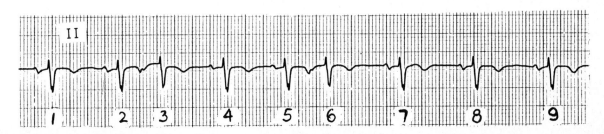

Figure 3B-2

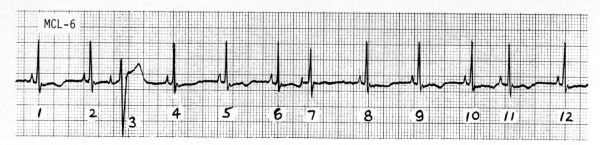

Figure 3B-3

QRS complex of these beats is narrow, similar in morphology to the sinus beats, and preceded by a premature P wave.

Although beat no. 3 is wide and bizarre, it too is clearly preceded by a premature P wave. Consequently, beat no. 3 must also be a PAC. The explanation for its different appearance is that this PAC is conducted with *aberrancy*.

Aberrant Conduction

Immediately following depolarization of a normal sinus impulse, the conduction system becomes *refractory*. Additional impulses, no matter how strong, cannot be conducted at this time. The *absolute refractory period (ARP)* lasts only a short while. It is followed by a *relative refractory period (RRP)* during which portions of the conduction system have recovered while others have not. Additional impulses may now be conducted but, because a part of the ventricular conduction system is still refractory, such conduction will not be normal. Instead it will be *aberrant*. QRS morphology may differ markedly from normal when premature impulses occur during the RRP. This is the case with beat no. 3 in Figure 3B-3.

It is of interest that the other premature beats in this tracing (nos. 7 and 11) are conducted with minimal degrees of aberrancy. Although similar in morphology to the normally conducted complexes, the S waves of these beats are slightly deeper than normal. The reason beat nos. 7 and 11 are *less aberrant* than beat no. 3 is that they are not quite as early (they occur at a time when a greater portion of the ventricular conduction system will have recovered).

The concept of aberrancy is rather complicated. For this reason we have deferred full discussion of this topic to the Advanced Arrhythmia Section (Chapter 15). For now, suffice it to say that not all wide complex premature beats are PVCs. While guidelines do exist for differentiating between aberrantly conducted supraventricular beats (PACs, PJCs) and PVCs, most of these are well beyond the scope of this chapter. However, one thing that can be looked for is a *premature* P wave preceding the anomalous complex. When seen (as it was in beat no. 3 above), this finding argues strongly for aberrancy. If doubt remains, *one should always consider a premature beat as guilty* (a PVC) *until proved otherwise.*

PROBLEM   **Examine Figure 3B-4. What would you say about beats no. 3 and 8?**

ANSWER TO FIGURE 3B-4   The underlying rhythm is sinus at a rate of 80 beats/min. The PR interval is at the upper limits of

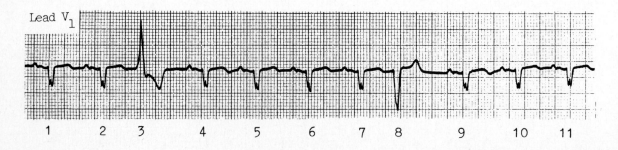

Figure 3B-4

normal (0.20 second). Beat nos. 3 and 8 are both premature. The former is definitely a PVC. It is wide and bizarre and is not preceded by a premature P wave. In contrast, beat no. 8 is not all that different in appearance from the normally conducted sinus beats. One might be tempted to call it a PAC (or PJC).

The point to remember is that when doubt exists, *a premature beat should always be considered as guilty (a PVC) until proven otherwise.* Careful inspection of the T wave preceding beat no. 8 does not reveal any deformity in the T wave suggestive of a premature P wave. One must therefore assume beat no. 8 is also a PVC.

> When PVCs of differing morphologies are seen (as they are in Fig. 3B-4), they are said to be *multiform*. In the past, such PVCs were called *multifocal* since it used to be thought that different morphologies indicated different ectopic *foci*. We now know that this is not necessarily the case. PVCs may arise from the same focus but use a different reentrant pathway, thus giving rise to a different morphology. As a result, it is more appropriate to use the term multiform rather than multifocal.

COMPLEX VENTRICULAR ECTOPY

In general, PVCs are cause for increasing concern as they become more frequent and complex in nature. Examples of *complex* forms of ventricular ectopy include:

i) *Multiform PVCs*
ii) *Couplets* (two PVCs in a row).
iii) *Salvos* (three PVCs in a row).
iv) Longer runs of *ventricular tachycardia*. (The definition of ventricular tachycardia is ≥3 PVCs in a row.)

PROBLEM   **Figures 3B-5 through 3B-8 were taken sequentially from a patient with acute myocardial infarction. What is happening?**

ANSWER   The underlying rhythm is sinus at a rate of 85 beats/min. Increasingly frequent and complex ventricular ectopy is noted. This would be particularly worrisome in the setting of acute infarction.

Single *uniform* (of similar morphology) PVCs are seen in Figure 3B-5 (Beats no. 2, 6, and 10). Repetitive PVCs are seen in the other rhythm strips. In Figure 3B-6, there are two ventricular *couplets* (beats no. 4 & 5, and 9 & 10). In Figure 3B-7, there is one couplet (beats no. 3 & 4), and one *salvo* (beats no. 7–9). Finally, a 6 beat run of *ventricular tachycardia (VT)* is seen (beats no. 3–8) in Figure 3B-8.

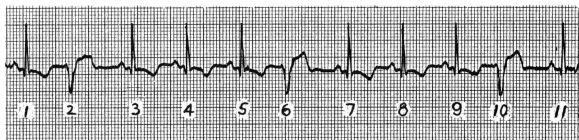

Figure 3B-5

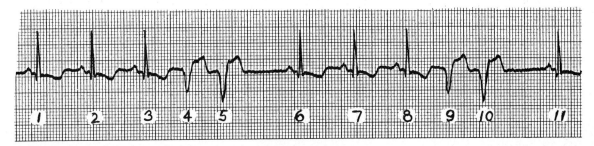

Figure 3B-6

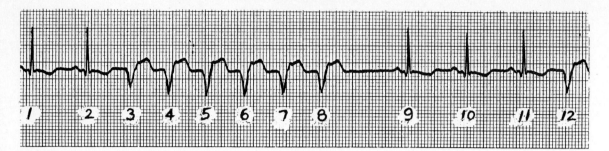

Figure 3B-7

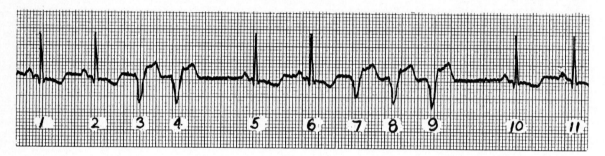

Figure 3B-8

In the acute care setting, frequent and repetitive ventricular ectopy (couplets, salvos, and nonsustained VT are frequent precursors of *sustained* VT (VT lasting more than 15 seconds) and ventricular fibrillation. Aggressive treatment is indicated.

With respect to PVC *frequency,* a wide range of definitions have been proposed. In patients with chronic ventricular ectopy, as few as 10 PVCs per hour (which comes out to a PVC every 6 minutes) is sometimes considered "frequent," since this incidence has been associated with an increased risk of sudden death in patients with underlying heart disease. Acutely, the term "frequent" is usually applied when PVCs number ≥5 per minute. In both instances when deciding whether to treat, far more

important than frequency is consideration of the clinical setting in which the ectopy occurs.

In Figure 3B-5, PVCs occur every fourth beat. This is known as ventricular *quadrigeminy.* (It is ventricular *trigeminy* if PVCs occur every third beat, and ventricular *bigeminy* if they occur every other beat.)

ATRIAL TACHYARRHYTHMIAS

Let us now turn our attention to the atrial tachyarrhythmias.

PROBLEM   **Examine Figures 3B-9 and 3B-10. Is there evidence of atrial activity?**

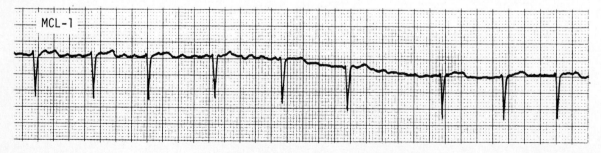

Figure 3B-9

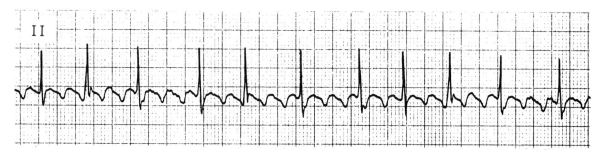

Figure 3B-10

ANSWER TO FIGURE 3B-9

The QRS complex is narrow. The rhythm is irregularly irregular (each R-R interval is different). Although there are undulations in the baseline, no definite P waves are present. This is *atrial fibrillation* by definition.

Atrial Fibrillation

Atrial fibrillation is recognized by the absence of P waves and the *irregular irregularity* of the rhythm. Although multiple atrial foci are firing at an extremely rapid rate (up to 600 times/minute), only a fraction of these atrial impulses are able to be conducted through the AV node.

Untreated, the ventricular response to atrial fibrillation is typically *rapid* (greater than 120 beats/min). Following treatment with digitalis, the ventricular response becomes more *"controlled"* and usually falls within the range of 60–110 beats/min. If too much digitalis is given (or in some cases of sick sinus syndrome or atrioventricular heart block), atrial fibrillation may manifest a *slow* ventricular response (less than 60 beats/min).

PROBLEM
What type of ventricular response is evident in **Figure 3B-9**?

ANSWER
The R-R interval throughout most of this rhythm strip is between 3 and 5 large boxes. Therefore, the heart rate varies between 60 and 100 beats/min. This is atrial fibrillation with a *controlled ventricular response.*

ANSWER TO FIGURE 3B-10
Once again the QRS complex is narrow and the rhythm is irregularly irregular. However, as opposed to Figure 3B-9, more definite evidence of atrial activity is present. A repetitive negative deflection is seen at a rate of 280 beats/min. This is *atrial flutter,* in this case with a *variable* ventricular response. The negative deflections are flutter waves.

Atrial Flutter

The atrial rate in flutter most often hovers around 300 beats/min (range 250–350 beats/min), except when it has been slowed by a medication such as quinidine. Fortunately, the AV node is unable to conduct each atrial impulse at this rapid a rate. If 1:1 AV conduction were possible, the ventricular response with atrial flutter would be about 300 beats/min, which is much too fast a rate to maintain effective cardiac pumping. As a protective mechanism, the AV node limits the number of atrial impulses that are conducted to the ventricles. Usually every other impulse is conducted, so that *the most common ventricular response in untreated atrial flutter is 2:1* (an atrial rate of 300 beats/min and a ventricular response of 150 beats/min). Less commonly there is 4:1 AV conduction or variable AV conduction (as in Fig. 3B-10).

PROBLEM
The rhythm strip shown in **Figure 3B-11** is taken from another patient in atrial flutter. How many flutter waves are present for every QRS complex?

ANSWER TO FIGURE 3B-11
The QRS complex is narrow, and the ventricular response is regular at a rate of about 80 beats/min. Atrial flutter waves are regular and occur in this V1 lead as upright deflections at a rate of about 320 beats/min. There are *four* flutter waves for each QRS complex (there is 4:1 AV conduction).

If you had difficulty spotting the fourth flutter wave, it makes up the terminal r′ of the QRS complex (**Fig. 3B-12**).

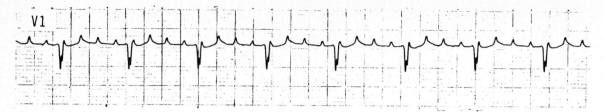

Figure 3B-11

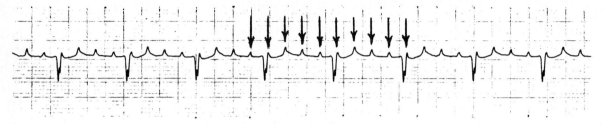

Figure 3B-12

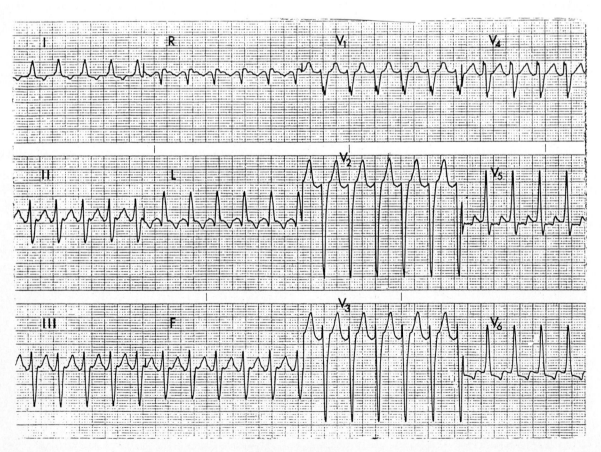

Figure 3B-13

When the characteristic sawtooth pattern of atrial flutter (seen in Fig. 3B-10) or distinct atrial activity at a rate approximating 300 beats/min (seen in Fig. 3B-11) are present, recognition of this arrhythmia poses no problem. However, flutter waves are often much more subtle in their appearance.

PROBLEM   **Examine the ECG shown in Figure 3B-13. Focus for a moment on lead II. A regular supraventricular tachycardia at a rate of 140 beats/min is present. Could this possibly be sinus tachycardia?**

ANSWER TO FIGURE 3B-13   No. Since normal upright P waves are not present in lead II, sinus tachycardia can be ruled out. The rhythm in Figure 3B-13 is again *atrial flutter*, al-

though the diagnosis is not at all obvious from this tracing. The only leads that even remotely hint at the presence of the characteristic saw-tooth pattern of flutter are the inferior leads (II, III, and aVF) (See Fig. 3B-14). Note in particular that evidence of atrial activity is totally lacking from leads I, V_{1-3}, and V_6.

Because flutter waves are frequently not apparent, the diagnosis is often overlooked. In order to avoid this pitfall, one must always maintain a high index of suspicion and *strongly consider the possibility of atrial flutter in the presence of any regular supraventricular tachycardia with a rate of between 140 and 160 beats per minute when normal atrial activity cannot be identified.*

PROBLEM   **Interpret the arrhythmias shown in Figures 3B-15 and 3B-16. Is atrial flutter likely to be present in either tracing?**

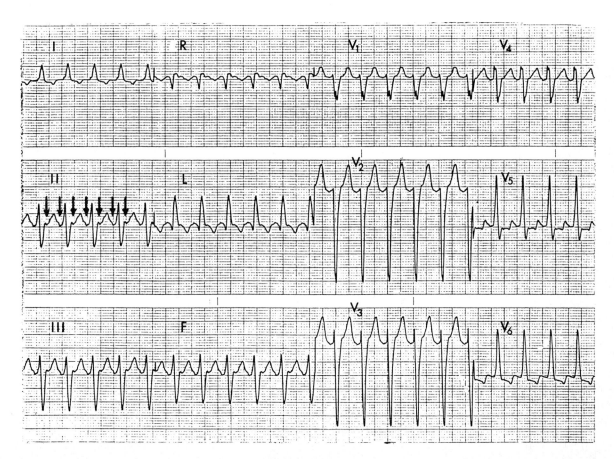

Figure 3B-14

Lead MCL₁

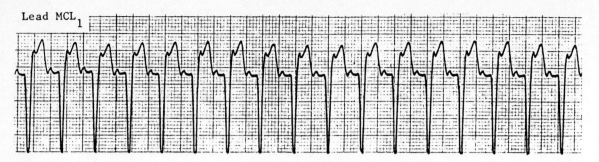

Figure 3B-15

Lead II

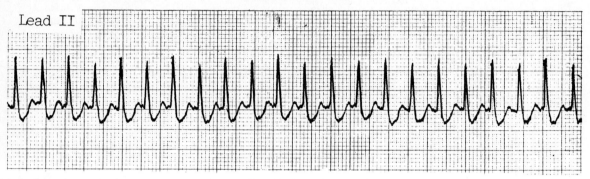

Figure 3B-16

ANSWER TO FIGURE 3B-15   A regular supraventricular tachyarrhythmia at a rate of 150 beats/min is present. Although a seemingly normal P wave is seen preceding each QRS complex, notching on the upstroke of each T wave suggests that there may actually be two P waves for each QRS complex.

When definitive diagnosis of a tachyarrhythmia is not apparent from inspection of a tracing, it may sometimes be made clear by slowing the ventricular response with a vagal maneuver such as carotid sinus massage. **Figure 3B-17** shows the effect of carotid massage on the rhythm in Figure 3B-15. The

degree of atrioventricular block has been increased by carotid massage, and atrial flutter waves at a rate of about 300 beats/min (arrows) are now evident.

ANSWER TO FIGURE 3B-16   Once again a regular supraventricular tachyarrhythmia is seen. The rate, however, is significantly faster than it was for Figure 3B-15. The R-R interval in this tracing is between 1 and 2 large boxes, making the rate between 150 and 300 beats/min. As suggested earlier, when the rate is regular and this rapid, a handy trick for calculating rate is to measure the R-R interval of

Lead MCL₁

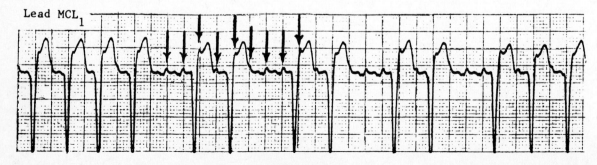

Figure 3B-17

every other beat. Here, the R-R interval for every other beat (half the rate) is a little less than 3 large boxes. Therefore, half the rate is 110 beats/min, and the actual rate is 220 beats/min.

Atrial flutter with 1:1 AV conduction would be unlikely at this rate unless the patient was being treated with a medication (such as quinidine) that might slow the atrial response. Atrial flutter with 2:1 AV conduction would also be unlikely, since this would require an atrial rate of 440 beats per minute, which is well beyond the usual range for flutter.

PROBLEM   Does the upright deflection seen between QRS complexes in <u>Figure 3B-16</u> represent atrial activity?

ANSWER   It is impossible to determine from Figure 3B-16 whether the upright deflection between QRS complexes represents the P wave, the T wave, or both. If it were the P wave, then the rhythm in Figure 3B-16 would be sinus tachycardia at a rate of 220 beats/min. Since sinus tachycardia rarely exceeds 160 beats/min in an adult, this diagnosis is unlikely. Thus, the upright deflection probably represents the T wave, and the rhythm is presumed to be *paroxysmal supraventricular tachycardia (PSVT)*.

Paroxysmal Supraventricular Tachycardia (PSVT)

PSVT is a commonly seen, extremely regular tachyarrhythmia that usually has a rate of between 150–250 beats/min. In the past, distinction was made between two types of PSVT, *paroxysmal atrial tachycardia (PAT)* and *paroxysmal junctional tachycardia (PJT)*. Such differentiation was probably more of academic interest than of clinical utility, since both tachyarrhythmias are thought to be due to similar *reentry* mechanisms involving the AV node. In reentry, the impulse travels through the AV node, enters the ventricular conduction system, and then somehow is conducted back to *(reenters)* the AV node. A continuous cycle in which the impulse is conducted down (to the ventricles) and back (to the AV node) is perpetuated, and rapid heart rates are attained.

The QRS complex is most often narrow with PSVT, unless bundle branch block or aberrant conduction exist. P waves are usually not evident. When present, they are frequently inverted and partially hidden in the terminal portion of the QRS complex.

A final point about PSVT should be made regarding terminology so that one does not confuse this entity with the more generally used term, supraventricular tachycardia. By definition, a *supraventricular tachycardia* is any tachycardia in which the impulse originates at or above the AV node. Examples include:

  i) Sinus tachycardia
 ii) Junctional tachycardia
iii) Atrial fibrillation
 iv) Atrial flutter
  v) Multifocal atrial tachycardia
 vi) Ectopic atrial tachycardia
vii) PSVT

The term PSVT implies that the mechanism of a particular tachyarrhythmia is reentry. A better term for these arrhythmias might simply be to call them *reentry tachycardias*. Thus, the rhythm in Figure 3B-15 is a *supraventricular* tachycardia, but it is not PSVT!

SUBTLE CLUES IN DIAGNOSIS OF TACHYARRHYTHMIAS

Let us conclude this section by putting together the concepts we have covered.

PROBLEM   Examine the tracings shown in <u>Figures 3B-18</u> through <u>3B-20</u>. Does the regularity of the rhythms and the width of the QRS complex supply clues to the etiology?

ANSWER TO FIGURE 3B-18   The rhythm is precisely regular at a rate of 190 beats/min. The QRS complex appears wide (at least 0.12 seconds in duration), and no atrial activity is evident.

PROBLEM   Could this tachyarrhythmia possibly be of supraventricular etiology?

ANSWER   Yes. As discussed in response to Figure 3A-15, whenever one is confronted by a regular wide complex tachyarrhythia, *five* entities must always be kept in mind:

  i) VENTRICULAR TACHYCARDIA
 ii) VENTRICULAR TACHYCARDIA

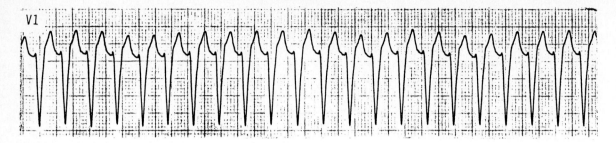

Figure 3B-18

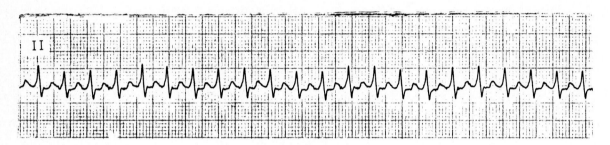

Figure 3B-19

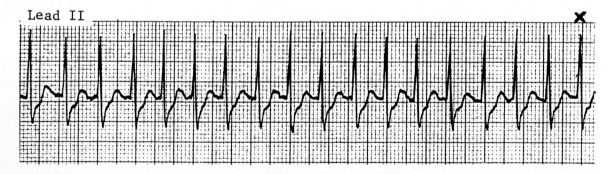

Figure 3B-20

iii) VENTRICULAR TACHYCARDIA
iv) Supraventricular tachycardia with preexisting bundle branch block
v) Supraventricular tachycardia with aberrant conduction

However, unless there is strong evidence to the contrary, ventricular tachycardia *must* always be assumed until proved otherwise.

ANSWER TO FIGURE 3B-19 This rhythm is also precisely regular at 190 beats/min. The QRS complex appears to be narrow,

and P waves seemingly precede each QRS complex. One might think this was sinus tachycardia.

Actually, the rhythms shown in Figures 3B-18 and 3B-19 were obtained *simultaneously* in the *same* patient! They emphasize the point previously stated that the QRS complex may appear deceptively narrow in certain leads when a portion of the QRS is isoelectric with the baseline. This patient was in *ventricular tachycardia!* The rate is much faster than one usually sees with sinus tachycardia in adults, and the upright deflection seen between QRS complexes in Figure 3B-19 represents the T wave, *not* the P wave!

ANSWER TO FIGURE 3B-20 The QRS complex appears to be narrow in this lead, and no definite P waves are seen. At first glance, the rhythm appears to be regular. If this were the case, then the differential diagnosis for this arrhythmia would be identical to that considered for the regular narrow complex tachyarrhythmia shown in Figure 3B-16—sinus tachycardia, atrial flutter, or PSVT.

PROBLEM   **Is the rhythm in Figure 3B-20 really regular?** *Be sure to verify your answer with calipers.*

ANSWER   Slight but definite irregularity of the R-R interval is present in Figure 3B-20.

Figure 3B-21 shows the continuation of this rhythm strip from the point marked **X.** The irregular irregularity of the rhythm becomes much more evident during the final beats of Figure 3B-21. Thus, the rhythm in Figure 3B-20 is *atrial fibrillation* with a *rapid ventricular response.*

This example highlights the difficulty in detecting the irregularity of atrial fibrillation when the ventricular response is rapid. Without calipers it would be extremely easy to mistake the rhythm shown in Figure 3B-20 as PSVT. This misdiagnosis might have important clinical implications. Although either digoxin or verapamil can be used to treat rapid atrial fibrillation and PSVT, many clinicians prefer digoxin for the former and verapamil for the latter.

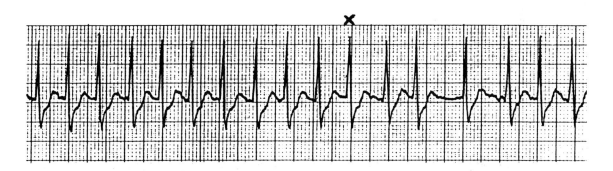

Figure 3B-21

C: ARRHYTHMIA REVIEW (1)

As review, apply the four question approach to arrhythmia interpretation in analyzing the following 20 tracings.

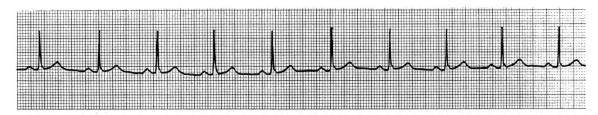

Figure 3C-1

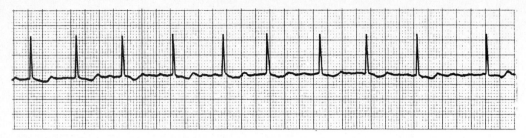

Figure 3C-2

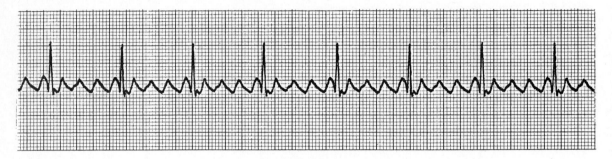

Figure 3C-3

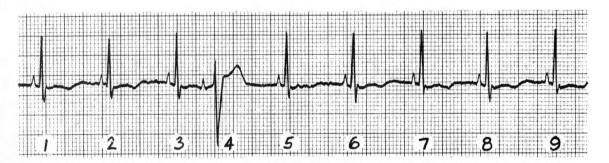

Figure 3C-4

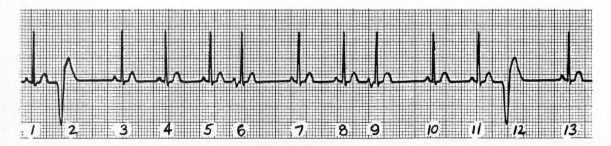

Figure 3C-5

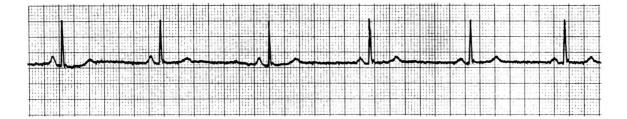

Figure 3C-6

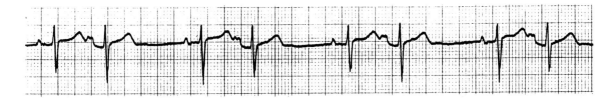

Figure 3C-7

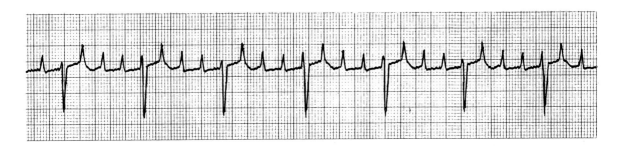

Figure 3C-8

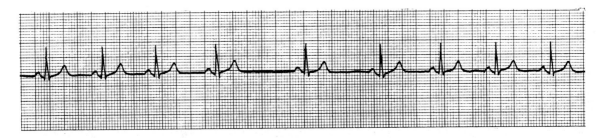

Figure 3C-9

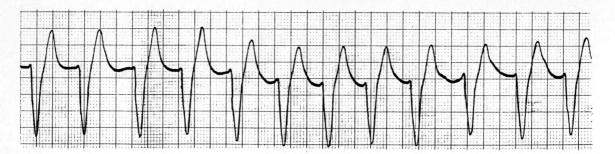

Figure 3C-10

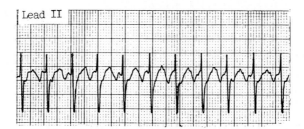

Figure 3C-11

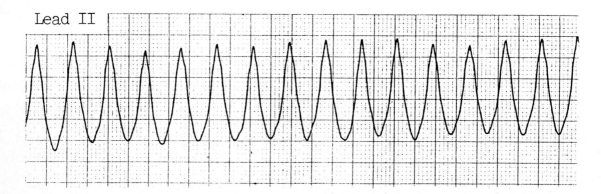

Figure 3C-12

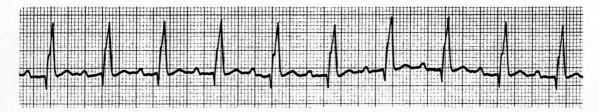

Figure 3C-13

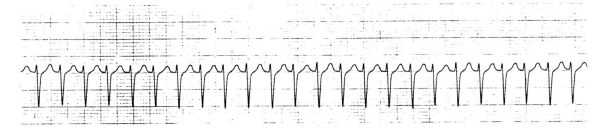

Figure 3C-14

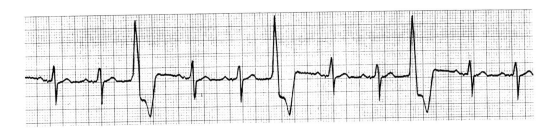

Figure 3C-15

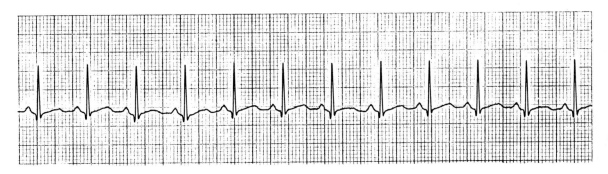

Figure 3C-16

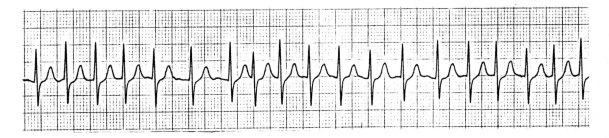

Figure 3C-17

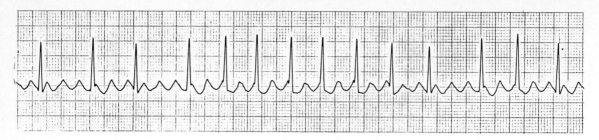

Figure 3C-18

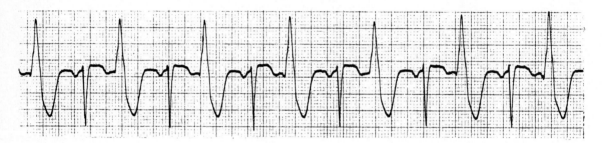

Figure 3C-19

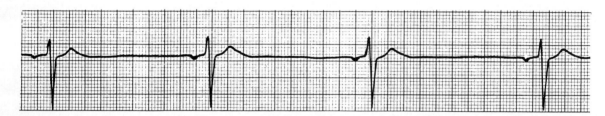

Figure 3C-20

ANSWERS TO ARRHYTHMIA REVIEW (1)

Answer to Figure 3C-1

Rhythm—regular
Rate—65–70 beats/min
PR interval—normal (0.18 second)
QRS complex—normal duration (≤0.10 second)
Impression: Normal sinus rhythm.

Answer to Figure 3C-2

Rhythm—irregularly irregular
P waves—none
QRS complex—normal duration
Impression: Atrial fibrillation with a controlled ventricular response
Comment: Although many undulations are seen along the baseline, no consistent atrial activity is present. Atrial fibrillation is diagnosed by the finding of an irregularly irregular rhythm and absence of P waves. The ventricular response averages out to be between 60 and 110 beats/min (*controlled* ventricular response).

Answer to Figure 3C-3

Rhythm—regular
Atrial rate—sawtooth flutter waves at 270 beats/min
Ventricular rate—65–70 beats/min
QRS complex—normal duration
Impression: Atrial flutter with 4:1 AV conduction
Comment: Untreated atrial flutter most commonly manifests 2:1 AV conduction (atrial rate $\approx$ 300 beats/min; ventricular rate $\approx$ 150 beats/min). The next most common conduction ratio is 4:1 as is shown here. It is uncommon to have atrial flutter with an odd number conduction ratio.

Answer to Figure 3C-4

Rhythm—essentially regular except for beat no. 4
Rate—85 beats/min
PR interval—a little short (0.10 second)
QRS complex—normal duration
Impression: Sinus rhythm with a PAC that conducts with aberrancy
Comment: Although beat no. 4 is much wider and looks quite different from the normal sinus beats, it *is* preceded by a *premature* P wave. This makes the beat a PAC that conducts with aberrancy.

Answer to Figure 3C-5

Rhythm—irregular
PR interval—normal for the sinus conducted beats
QRS complex—normal duration (except for beats no. 2 and no. 12)
Impression: Sinus tachycardia (at a rate of 100 beats/min) with PACs and PVCs
Comment: Beats no. 2 and 12 are clearly PVCs. They are wide, bizarre in appearance, and very much different from normally conducted beats. In contrast, beats no. 6 and 9 are PACs (both are preceded by a P wave, and the QRS looks identical to that for the normally conducted beats).

Answer to Figure 3C-6

Rhythm—slightly irregular
Rate—$\approx$45 beats/min
PR interval—normal
QRS complex—normal duration
Impression: Sinus bradycardia and arrhythmia. P wave morphology varies slightly.

Answer to Figure 3C-7

Rhythm—irregular
Atrial rate—irregular
QRS complex—normal duration
Impression: Atrial bigeminy
Comment: Every other beat is a PAC. Ectopic P waves are broader and notched compared to the more pointed sinus P waves.

Answer to Figure 3C-8

Atrial rate and rhythm—regular at about 230 beats/min
Ventricular rate and rhythm—regular at just under 60 beats/min
QRS complex—normal duration
Impression: Probable atrial flutter with 4:1 AV conduction (versus atrial tachycardia with 4:1 block)
Comment: Rapid and regular atrial activity is seen. However, the atrial rate is a little slower than the 250–350/min usually seen with flutter, and the typical sawtooth pattern (noted in Fig. 3C-3) is not evident in this particular lead (the baseline between P waves is isoelectric). This raises the possibility that the rhythm could be atrial tachycardia with 4:1 block. It is hard to be sure from this one tracing alone.

Answer to Figure 3C-9

Rhythm—irregular
P waves—precede each QRS complex with a constant PR interval
QRS complex—normal duration
Impression: Sinus arrhythmia.
Comment: Sinus arrhythmia is a common normal variant in children and young adults. In the elderly it may be a manifestation of sick sinus syndrome.

Answer to Figure 3C-10

Rhythm—slightly irregular
Rate—varies between 85 and 110 beats/min
P waves—none evident
QRS complex—wide (0.16 second)
Impression: Atrial fibrillation with preexisting bundle branch block (versus slow ventricular tachycardia).
Comment: It is hard to be certain of the etiology of this arrhythmia from this tracing alone. At first glance the R-R interval appears fairly constant. However, on close inspection, an *irregular irregularity* is definitely seen. In the absence of atrial activity, this degree of irregularity suggests atrial fibrillation. One would feel more comfortable with this diagnosis if it were known that the patient had a bundle branch block (wide QRS) on a baseline 12-lead ECG.

The other possibility to consider is an accelerated idioventricular rhythm ("slow VT"). The rhythm is usually more regular with this entity.

Answer to Figure 3C-11

Rhythm—regular
Rate—155 beats/min
QRS complex—normal duration
Impression: Regular supraventricular tachycardia at a rate of 155 beats/min, probable atrial flutter with 2:1 AV conduction.

Comment: One should always maintain a high index of suspicion for atrial flutter in the presence of any regular supraventricular tachycardia with a rate of about 150 beats (140–160) per minute. In this particular tracing, normal atrial activity is *not* present since P waves are *not* upright in lead II. If one sets a pair of calipers at precisely half the R-R interval, the negative deflection that precedes the QRS complex can be seen to notch the ST segment, further suggesting flutter. Confirmation is forthcoming with application of a vagal maneuver (**Fig. 3C-11A**).

The vagal maneuver slows AV conduction, permitting flutter waves to become more evident (arrows in Fig. 3C-11A).

Answer to Figure 3C-12

Rhythm—regular
Rate—170 beats/min
P waves—none
QRS complex—wide!
Impression: Ventricular tachycardia.
Comment: A regular wide complex tachycardia is seen. Although the differential includes supraventricular tachycardia with preexisting bundle branch block or aberrant conduction, ventricular tachycardia must be assumed until proved otherwise.

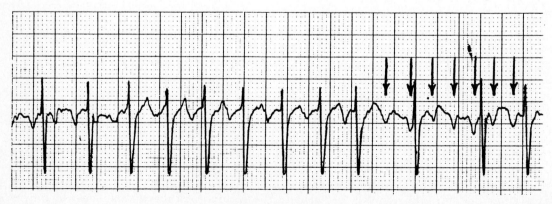

Figure 3C-11A

Answer to Figure 3C-13

Rhythm—regular
Rate—90 beats/min
PR interval—prolonged (0.24 second)
QRS complex—wide (0.13 second)
Impression: Sinus rhythm with 1° AV block.
Comment: Despite the fact that the QRS is wide, each complex is preceded by a P wave with a fixed (albeit prolonged) PR interval. Therefore the rhythm is sinus. QRS prolongation is due to preexisting bundle branch block.

Answer to Figure 3C-14

Rhythm—regular
Rate—210 beats/min
P waves—none
QRS complex—normal duration
Impression: PSVT
Comment: A regular supraventricular tachycardia is present at a rate of 210 beats/min. The differential includes sinus tachycardia, atrial flutter, and PSVT. In adults, sinus tachycardia usually does not exceed 160 beats/min. Atrial flutter is also unlikely, given that the ventricular response with this arrhythmia most commonly is about 150 beats/min. This leaves PSVT as the probable diagnosis.

Answer to Figure 3C-15

Rhythm—irregular
P waves—precede each of the sinus beats
PR interval—normal (0.20 second)
QRS complex—normal duration (0.10) for the sinus beats
Impression: Ventricular trigeminy
Comment: Every third beat is a PVC (wide, bizarre complex, oppositely directed T wave).

Answer to Figure 3C-16

Rhythm—regular
Rate—110 beats/min
PR interval—normal
QRS complex—normal duration
Impression: Sinus tachycardia.

Answer to Figure 3C-17

Rhythm—irregularly irregular
Rate—between 115–160 beats/min
P waves—none
QRS complex—normal duration
Impression: Atrial fibrillation with a rapid ventricular response.

Answer to Figure 3C-18

Rhythm—irregular
Rate—between 85–135 beats/min
P waves—sawtooth appearance
QRS complex—normal duration
Impression: Atrial flutter with a variable (moderately rapid) ventricular response.
Comment: As opposed to the irregular rhythm just discussed in Figure 3C-17, atrial activity *is* present in this tracing in the form of the typical sawtooth pattern characteristic of flutter. Although the ventricular response with atrial flutter most often is regular (usually with an even conduction ratio such as 2:1 or 4:1), it may occasionally be irregular as shown here.

Answer to Figure 3C-19

Rhythm—irregular
P waves—precede the sinus beats
PR interval—normal
QRS complex—normal duration for the sinus beats
Impression: Ventricular bigeminy
Comment: Every other beat is a PVC. Because two sinus beats never occur in a row, it is impossible to know the underlying sinus rate.

Clinically, PVCs that can be palpated in the peripheral pulse contribute to cardiac output. This explains why many patients are able to tolerate this arrhythmia for extended periods of time.

Answer to Figure 3C-20

Rhythm—fairly regular
Rate—about 30 beats/min
P waves—precede each QRS complex with a constant PR interval
PR interval—normal
QRS complex—normal duration
Impression: Marked sinus bradycardia (and slight sinus arrhythmia).

D: AV BLOCKS (BASIC CONCEPTS)

Diagnosis of the AV blocks is a common source of confusion for the emergency care provider not accustomed to dealing with these rhythm disturbances on a daily basis. Confusion begins with the terminology, encompasses diagnosis, and extends into therapeutic implications. To simplify our discussion, we have broken the topic down into two parts. In this initial chapter, we will simply define the three degrees of AV block, point out their clinical significance, and present basic examples of each type. We will also introduce the concept of AV dissociation. A more in-depth discussion of the AV blocks (sprinkled with pearls and pitfalls along the way) will follow in Section B of Chapter 16.

Classification of the AV Blocks

Table 3D-1 indicates the traditional classification of the AV blocks. Implicit in the division of these blocks into three degrees is the tacit assumption that 2° AV block portends a more ominous prognosis than does 1° AV block, and that 3° AV block portends the poorest prognosis of all. This is *not* necessarily the case.

In addition, there are a few terms that are "left over," such as *high-degree* or *high-grade heart block* and *AV dissociation*. These terms frequently hold different meanings to different emergency care providers. Particularly misunderstood is the concept of AV dissociation, which is often used synonymously with 3° AV block. The two are very different, as we shall see momentarily.

TABLE 3D-1

Classification of the AV Blocks
1 ° AV block
2 ° AV block
—Mobitz I (Wenckebach)
—Mobitz II
3 ° (complete) AV block
AV dissociation?
High-grade heart block?
High-degree block?

Overview

In Section A of this chapter we discussed how with normal sinus rhythm all QRS complexes are preceded by P waves with a *constant* PR interval. Each atrial impulse is conducted to the ventricles, and the PR interval is ≤0.20 seconds. With **1° AV block,** atrial impulses are still conducted to the ventricles with a constant PR interval, but atrioventricular (AV) conduction is delayed (to ≥0.21 second).

With more severe impairment of AV conduction (with **2° AV block**), conduction of one or more atrial impulses to the ventricles is prevented ("*blocked*"). P waves may precede and be related to at least some of the QRS complexes, but their relationship may not be readily apparent. This type of block is broken down further into **Mobitz I** and **Mobitz II** varieties (Table 3D-1).

Finally, with complete block of AV conduction (3° or **complete AV block**), none of the atrial impulses are conducted to the ventricles. In this case, both the atria and ventricles discharge at their own inherent rate. P waves may precede QRS complexes, but they are totally unrelated to them, and the PR interval continually changes.

Approach to Diagnosis

Application of the systematic four question approach to arrhythmia analysis presented earlier is all that is needed to diagnose the AV blocks. One looks for:

i) Regularity of the rhythm

ii) Evidence of atrial activity (P waves)

iii) QRS widening

iv) The relationship (if any) between P waves and the QRS complex

Not all conduction disturbances fall "neatly" into the three categories of AV block. However, careful attention to each of these four factors will be extremely helpful in narrowing down the possibilities and in describing the characteristics of the conduction disturbance in question.

A way to simplify classification of the AV blocks is the following:

i) Look first to see if 1° AV block is present. This is usually easy to recognize.

ii) Look next to see if 3° AV block is present. This is *also* usually easy to recognize.

iii) If the block is neither 1° nor 3°, but beats are being dropped due to AV block, the block must be 2°!

FIRST-DEGREE AV BLOCK

As alluded to above, *1° AV block* is easy to recognize. It is simply a sinus rhythm in which the PR interval is prolonged. All atrial impulses are conducted to the ventricles—they just take a little longer to arrive.

PROBLEM Examine **Figure 3D-1. Does it appear that the P waves in this rhythm strip are conducted?**

ANSWER The atrial and ventricular rates in this example are regular at 65 beats/min. Each QRS complex is preceded by a P wave, and it appears that these P waves *are* conducting

since the PR interval is constant. *First-degree AV block* is present because this PR interval is prolonged (to 0.34 second).

The PR interval varies with age. This becomes readily apparent with our discussion of pediatric arrhythmias in Chapter 17. (For example, a PR interval of 0.17 second in a 3-year-old child is definitely *prolonged* and constitutes 1° AV block for this age group.

On the other hand, advancing age normally causes AV conduction to take a little longer. Thus although 0.20 second is usually taken as the upper limit of normal for the PR interval in adults, a slightly longer interval is probably still normal in many older individuals. Practically speaking, the isolated occurrence of 1° AV block is rarely of clinical importance. Therefore our preference is *not* to call 1° AV block unless the PR interval is clearly prolonged to *at least* 0.22 second. For a similar reason we tend to avoid the term *borderline* 1° AV block (for PR intervals of 0.19–0.21 second), as this connotation rarely adds useful clinical information.

THIRD-DEGREE AV BLOCK

Third-degree (complete) AV block is also *usually* an easy conduction disturbance to recognize. Because none of the atrial impulses are able to penetrate through to the ventricles, atrial activity is separated from what occurs in the rest of the heart. As a result, the atria beat at their own inherent rate, an escape pacemaker (from the AV node or a site below) does the same, and "n'er the twain shall meet."

PROBLEM Analyze **Figure 3D-2 by the four question approach. Is there any apparent relationship between P waves and the QRS complex?**

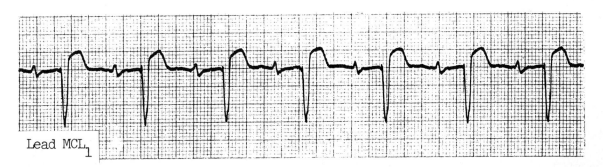

Figure 3D-1

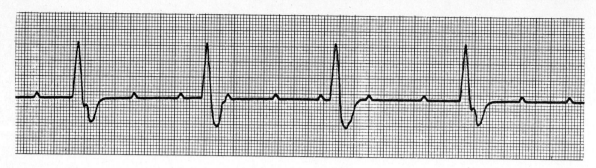

Figure 3D-2

ANSWER   Although both atrial and ventricular rates are fairly regular, P waves appear *unrelated* to (they "march through") the QRS complex. We describe this lack of relationship between atrial and ventricular activity as *AV dissociation*. It is easily recognized in this example by the *varying PR interval*.

This patient is in *3° AV block*. Despite the fact that P waves are given ample opportunity to conduct (they occur at every possible point in the R-R interval), they fail to do so.

With 3° AV block then, one expects to see:

i) A regular atrial rate (constant P-P interval)
ii) A regular ventricular rate (constant R-R interval)
iii) No relationship between the two (*complete AV dissociation*).

> *Most of the time the ventricular response will be regular with 3° degree AV block. This is a helpful point to keep in mind when sorting out AV conduction disturbances, since recognition of R-R irregularity makes it much less likely that complete AV block is present.*

We have already alluded to the fact that 3° AV block may occur at two levels: *at* the AV node or *below* the AV node.

PROBLEM   What would you expect the escape pacemaker to look like if the level of 3° AV block was *at* the AV node? What if it were *below* the AV node? (What is the probable level of block for the example shown in <u>Figure 3D-2</u>?)

ANSWER   If the level of 3° AV block was at the AV node, an *AV nodal* pacemaker should take over. One would therefore expect the QRS complex of the escape pacemaker to be narrow and discharge at a rate of between 40 and 60 beats/min.

If on the other hand the level of 3° AV block was below the AV node, an *idioventricular* escape pacemaker should take over. In this case the QRS complex would be wide, and the rate much slower (usually between 30 and 40 beats/min).

The fact that the QRS complex in Figure 3D-2 is markedly widened and the rate exceedingly slow (34 beats/min) suggests that the block occurs at a low level (below the AV node) in the conduction system.

PROBLEM   **Figure 3D-3 is taken from the same patient who was shown to be in 1° AV block in <u>Figure 3D-1</u>. Initially in this tracing the P waves appear to be totally unrelated to the QRS complex. Has the patient gone into 3° AV block?**

ANSWER   Resist the urge to comment on the dropped beats until you have systematically analyzed the tracing. The QRS complex is at the upper limit of normal (0.10 second), and the atrial rate is fairly regular. The last three beats of the tracing very much resemble the rhythm shown previously in Figure 3D-1—a P wave precedes the QRS complex of beat nos. 3, 4, and 5 with a fixed (albeit prolonged) PR interval. These P waves appear to be conducting—thus 3° AV block *cannot* be present! Instead there is *transient AV dissociation*. At least momentarily, atrial activity appears totally unrelated to the QRS complexes of beat nos. 1 and 2.

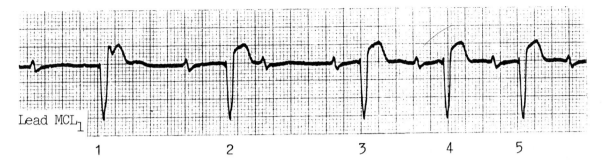

Lead MCL$_1$

Figure 3D-3

A way to recognize *at a glance* that 3° AV block is probably *not* present in Figure 3D-3 is to note that the ventricular rate does not remain constant! (See above.)

Note also in this figure that the atrial rate is not perfectly regular. Occasionally in the setting of AV block or AV dissociation with a slow escape rhythm, the atrial rate will vary slightly *(ventriculophasic sinus arrhythmia)*. The mechanism of this is not clear.

PROBLEM   Now examine **Figure 3D-4. Is atrial activity related to ventricular activity?**

ANSWER   The ventricular rate is regular at 53 beats/min. Atrial activity can be seen preceding each QRS complex (and deforming its initial upstroke; see arrows in Fig. 3D-5). However, none of the P waves are related in any consistent manner to the QRS complex (the PR interval keeps changing). *Complete AV dissociation* therefore is present.

PROBLEM   **Is there also 3° AV block in Figure 3D-5?**

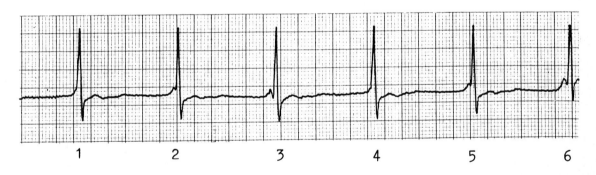

Figure 3D-4

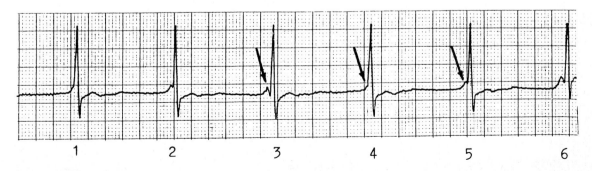

Figure 3D-5

ANSWER   There is no way to tell from this rhythm strip alone. The important point to make from this tracing is that, despite the presence of complete AV dissociation, *3° AV block cannot be diagnosed since none of the P waves were ever given a reasonable opportunity to conduct*. The PR interval throughout the rhythm strip simply remains too short to allow conduction. Without more information (a longer rhythm strip), there is simply no way to know if P waves could conduct were they given the chance.

We might therefore restate our criteria for diagnosing 3° AV block as the following:

    i) Atrial regularity
    ii) Ventricular regularity (usually)
    iii) Complete AV dissociation *(despite adequate opportunity for normal conduction to occur)*

> This last condition implies that the ventricular rate must be slow enough (and the rhythm strip long enough) for P waves to occur at all points of the R-R interval. *Usually this requires a ventricular rate of 45 beats/min or less.* Inclusion of this rate criterion helps avoid overdiagnosing AV dissociation as complete AV block.

PROBLEM   **Return to Figure 3D-2. Does it meet *all* of these criteria for diagnosing 3° AV block?**

ANSWER   Yes. The atrial and ventricular rates are regular, complete AV dissociation is present, and the ventricular rate is less than 45 beats/min. None of the P waves conduct despite having adequate opportunity to do so.

Second-Degree AV Block

Let us now turn our attention to the 2° AV blocks. If the atrial rate is *regular* and some atrial impulses are conducted to the ventricles but others are not, a type of 2° AV block (Mobitz I or II) is present.

> It is important to emphasize the need for *regularity of the atrial rate* in this definition. Awareness of this point helps differentiate 2° AV blocks from mimics such as blocked PACs and sinus pauses.
> In addition, consideration must be given to the appropriateness of the failed conduction. For example, the usual atrial rate in flutter is 300 beats/

min. One-to-one ventricular conduction under these circumstances would be incompatible with life. Fortunately, the AV node is able to protect the ventricles by limiting the number of atrial impulses it allows to pass through. Much of the time this entails conduction of every other atrial impulse. The result is that the most common ventricular response to atrial flutter is 2:1 conduction with a ventricular rate of approximately 150 beats/min. This rhythm should *not* be misclassified as 2:1 AV *block* since it really represents *physiologic* 2:1 AV conduction.

MOBITZ I (WENCKEBACH) 2° AV BLOCK

Mobitz I 2° AV block is characterized by progressive lengthening of the PR interval until a beat is dropped. This conduction disturbance is most often associated with acute inferior infarction. Anatomically, it is located at the level of the AV node. This accounts for the fact that QRS duration tends to be normal, and the PR interval may be prolonged (1° AV block). The junctional pacemaker is usually reliable, and observation of the patient until the conduction disturbance resolves is often all that is needed (**Table 3D-2**).

MOBITZ II 2° AV BLOCK

In contrast, *Mobitz II 2° AV block* is associated with anteroseptal myocardial infarction. The block lies at a lower anatomic level in the conduction system (it is *always* infranodal) than does Mobitz I block. As a result, the QRS complex is most often wide, and the escape focus much less reliable. In addition, Mobitz II has a disturbing tendency to develop into complete AV block, often with little (or no) warning. Because of this, *immediate* pacemaker insertion is essential as soon as this conduction disturbance is diagnosed. Clinically, this type of block is much less common than is Mobitz I, but it must be carefully watched for.

Electrocardiographically, Mobitz II 2° AV block is recognized by nonconduction of one or more atrial impulses despite maintenance of a constant PR interval. As for Mobitz I, the atrial rate remains fairly regular throughout (Table 3D-2).

TABLE 3D-2   Comparison of Mobitz I and Mobitz II 2° AV Block

	Mobitz I	Mobitz II
Clinical occurrence	Usually associated with inferior myocardial infarction Relatively frequent Usually transient	Usually associated with anteroseptal myocardial infarction Uncommon Often progresses to complete AV block
Anatomic level	At the AV node	Below the AV node
ECG characteristics	Gradually lengthening PR interval until a beat is dropped: —1° AV block is common —QRS is usually narrow	Constant PR interval until one or more beats are dropped: —PR interval is usually normal —QRS is usually wide
Treatment	Observation usually suffices, provided that ventricular response is adequate	Pacemaker insertion is required

PROBLEM   **Examine Figure 3D-6. What type of AV block is present—Mobitz I or Mobitz II? (Are P waves related to the QRS?)**

ANSWER   The atrial rate is regular at 65–70 beats/min. The QRS complex is narrow, and each QRS is preceded by a P wave. Even though the PR interval is not constant, P waves *are* related to the QRS complex (by progressive PR interval lengthening in each sequence [from 0.25 to 0.48 second] until a beat is dropped (**Fig. 3D-7**)). Therefore this is *Mobitz I* 2° AV block.

Several features characterize Mobitz I 2° AV block. Marriott has colorfully labeled these the "footprints of Wenckebach." They include:

i) Regularity of the atrial rate
ii) Group beating
iii) Progressive lengthening of the PR interval until a beat is dropped
iv) Duration of the pause (that contains the dropped beat) of less than twice the shortest R-R interval

All of these features are present in Figure 3D-7.

    The finding of *group beating* deserves special mention. Note in Figure 3D-6 that there is a *regular irregularity* to the rhythm (alternating short-long-short-long segments of the R-R interval). When a repetitive cadence to the R-R interval is noted, one

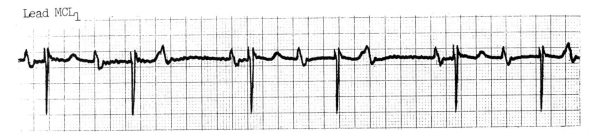

Lead MCL₁

Figure 3D-6

Lead MCL₁

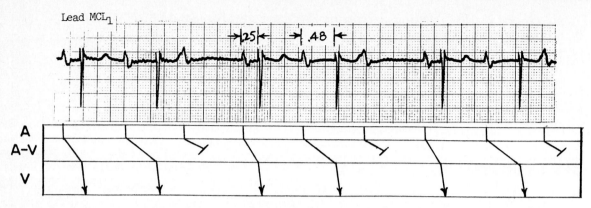

Figure 3D-7

should suspect that a Wenckebach block may be operative.

As noted previously, other features commonly associated with Mobitz I are normal QRS duration, 1° AV block, and accompanying acute inferior infarction.

PROBLEM   **Examine Figure 3D-8. Note the pause between beat nos. 8 and 9. Is this due to Wenckebach?**

ANSWER   Yes, although the diagnosis of Mobitz I in this example is not nearly as obvious as it was in Figure 3D-6. Eight consecutive beats are conducted (with 1° AV block) in this tracing until a beat is finally dropped. If one merely compared consecutive PR intervals during the run, it would not be at all apparent that the PR interval was progressively lengthening. Only by comparing the last PR interval just before the dropped beat (the PR interval of beat no. 8) with the PR interval at the start of the run (the PR interval of beat no. 1) can this relationship be established. With the onset of the next Wenck-

ebach cycle (beat no. 9), the PR interval has again shortened.

Figure 3D-8 effectively illustrates how with Wenckebach *the pause containing the dropped beat* (the R-R interval between beat nos. 8 and 9) *is less than twice the shortest R-R interval.* This finding is helpful in differentiating Wenckebach blocks from Mobitz II 2° AV block (in which the pause is precisely twice the regular R-R interval) and from sinus pauses (in which the interval including the dropped beat is often more than twice the regular R-R interval).

PROBLEM   **What type of conduction disturbance is present in Figure 3D-9?**

ANSWER   The atrial rate is fairly regular at 98–100 beats/min. Several atrial impulses are not conducted (the P waves following beat nos. 1, 3, 4, 6, and 8). The QRS appears to be wide, and P waves precede each complex. In contrast to the case in Mobitz I, the PR interval remains *constant* for beats that are conducted (**Fig. 3D-10**). This is *Mobitz II* 2° AV block.

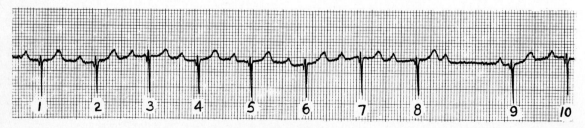

Figure 3D-8

Lead MCL₁

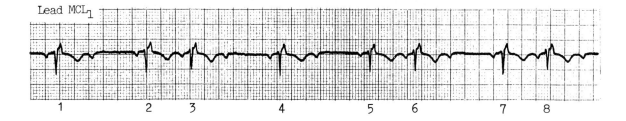

Figure 3D-9

Lead MCL₁

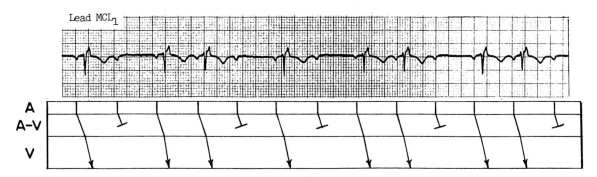

A
A-V
V

Figure 3D-10

Even though *group beating* is present here, this is one example when it is not due to Wenckebach.

2° AV BLOCK WITH 2:1 AV CONDUCTION

The presence of 2° AV block with 2:1 AV conduction poses an additional problem.

PROBLEM   **Consider Figure 3D-11, in which every other beat is conducted. Is this likely to represent the Mobitz I or Mobitz II type of 2° AV block?**

ANSWER   Both atrial and ventricular rates are regular (at 58 and 29 beats/min, re-spectively). Each QRS complex is preceded by a P wave with a constant PR interval, but only half the atrial impulses are conducted to the ventricles. This is 2° AV block with 2:1 AV conduction (since every other atrial impulse is blocked). Theoretically, *either* Mobitz I or Mobitz II could be present. Granted, a constant PR interval precedes each QRS complex (consistent with Mobitz II) but, since only one QRS complex at a time is conducted, the opportunity for the PR interval to lengthen before dropping a beat does not exist.

Two factors suggest that this rhythm is more likely to be Mobitz I—the normal duration of the

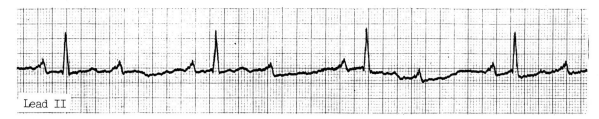

Lead II

Figure 3D-11

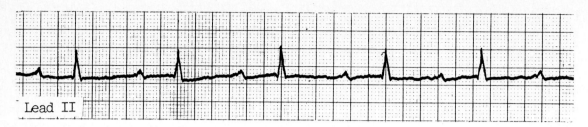

Lead II

Figure 3D-12

QRS complex and the presence of 1° AV block. However, *when there is 2:1 AV conduction, there is no way to be completely sure from the rhythm strip alone if this is due to Mobitz I or Mobitz II 2° AV block.*

PROBLEM   **The patient was medicated with 0.5 mg atropine. Shortly thereafter the rhythm shown in <u>Figure 3D-12</u> was observed. What has happened?**

ANSWER   Second-degree AV block is no longer present. Instead there is *sinus bradycardia* with *1° AV block.* This increases the likelihood that Figure 3D-11 represented Mobitz I 2° AV block, since one would not expect Mobitz II to respond so easily to medical treatment. The case for Mobitz I would be strengthened even more if it were known that the patient was having an acute *inferior* infarction.

> When the etiology of 2° AV block with 2:1 AV conduction is not clear, review of tracings obtained earlier may sometimes provide a helpful clue. Since it is distinctly unusual for Mobitz I and Mobitz II conduction to alternate in any given patient, documentation of Mobitz I on previous tracings would be presumptive evidence of its presence with 2:1 conduction.

Return to Figure 3D-11. Even though this conduction disturbance is "only" due to Mobitz I 2° AV block, it may nonetheless produce serious hemodynamic consequences as a result of the exceedingly slow ventricular response. Contrast this case with that of a patient in 3° AV block at the level of the AV node. In this latter instance one would expect the ventricular response to be between 40 and 60 beats/min (the inherent rate of a junctional escape pacemaker). *Much more important than the "degree" of AV block per se is the ventricular response.* A patient with 1° AV block and a sinus rate of 20 beats/min will need a pacemaker (if there is no response to medical therapy), while one with 2° (or even 3°) AV block may not if there are no symptoms and the ventricular response is adequate.

Apply the material covered up to now in evaluating the arrhythmias that follow. (**HINT:** AV block is *not* necessarily present in each of these tracings!)

PROBLEM   **Figure 3D-13.**

Lead MCL₁

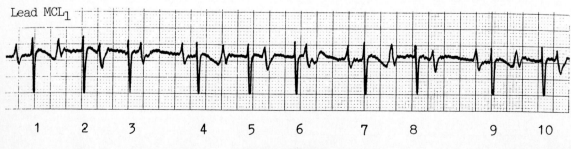

1   2   3   4   5   6   7   8   9   10

Figure 3D-13

ANSWER TO FIGURE 3D-13   The most striking finding about this tracing is *group beating* (initially groups of three beats [nos. 1, 2, 3 and nos. 4, 5, 6] followed by groups of two beats [nos. 7, 8 and nos. 9, 10]). This should immediately increase one's suspicion that Wenckebach may be present.

Although the ventricular rate is variable (with the *regular irregularity* of group beating), regular P waves continue throughout the tracing. The QRS complex is narrow and always preceded by a P wave. If one focuses on one of the groups (beat nos. 4–6 for example), it becomes apparent that the PR interval progressively lengthens until a beat is dropped (the P wave following beat no. 6 is not conducted). The cycle then resumes with beat no. 7. This is Mobitz I (Wenckebach) 2° AV block.

> For the groups represented by beats no. 1–3 and nos. 4–6, *four* P waves are present but only *three* are conducted. This is termed 4:3 AV conduction. For the other two groups (beats no. 7–8 and nos. 9–10), three P waves are present and two conduct (3:2 AV conduction).

This is not an easy tracing to interpret. However, it is a good example of how recognizing group beating can be extremely helpful in leading up to the correct diagnosis.

Another point well illustrated by this tracing is that *calipers* greatly facilitate the task of dysrhythmia interpretation. There is no other way to rapidly determine that the atrial rate in Figure 3D-13 is regular!

PROBLEM   Figure 3D-14.

ANSWER TO FIGURE 3D-14   Although there is also group beating in this tracing, the other *footprints* of Wenckebach are missing. Most notably, the atrial rate is not regular. Instead, beats no. 3 and 6 occur early—they are *premature* atrial contractions (PACs). The rhythm is, therefore, sinus bradycardia (at a rate of about 45 beats/min) with PACs. The QRS complex is normal in duration.

> In addition to occurring early, note that there is a subtle difference in morphology of the P waves preceding beats no. 3 and 6 (these P waves are notched) indicating their origin from a different atrial focus.

PROBLEM   Figure 3D-15.

ANSWER TO FIGURE 3D-15   Despite the fact that there are many more P waves than QRS complexes, 3° AV block is not present in this tracing. Both atrial and ventricular rates are regular (at 105 and 35 beats/min, respectively). Each QRS complex is preceded by a P wave with a *constant* PR interval. This rules out 3° AV block, because P waves *are* related to the QRS complex. By the process of elimination (since neither 1° nor 3° AV block is present), the rhythm in Figure 3D-15 must be a form of 2° AV block. We refer to it as a *high-grade* (or *high-degree*) AV block, as only one of every three atrial impulses is conducted to the ventricles.

> High-grade AV block is most often due to a conduction disturbance of the Mobitz II variety. In Figure 3D-15, however, this may not be the case considering that the QRS complex is narrow (it should be wide with Mobitz II). There are two possibilities:
>   **i)** A portion of the QRS complex may lie on the baseline in this particular monitoring lead, and the expected QRS widening may be readily apparent in other leads.
>   **ii)** This could be Mobitz I with 3:1 AV conduction.

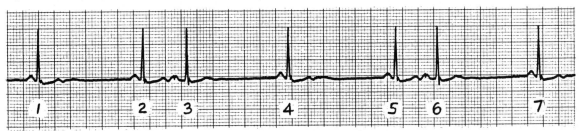

Figure 3D-14

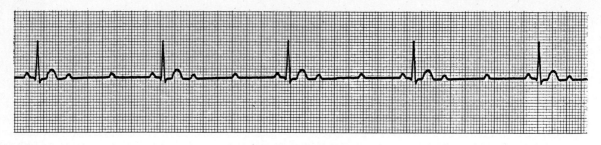

Figure 3D-15

The dilemma presented by the conduction disturbances shown in Figures 3D-11 and 3D-15 is due to the absence of *consecutively* conducted complexes on each tracing. In order to diagnose the type of 2° AV block with certainty, one must see *at least* two QRS complexes in a row before the dropped beat.

> Clinically, although the type of treatment may vary, the urgent need to increase the ventricular response in Figures 3D-11 and 3D-15 is the same regardless of whether the conduction disturbance is due to Mobitz I or Mobitz II.

PROBLEM   Figure 3D-16.

ANSWER TO FIGURE 3D-16   The QRS complex in this tracing is narrow, and the ventricular response is slightly irregular. Although atrial activity precedes the last four beats, it is absent from the first four. Thus *AV nodal rhythm* is present at the start of the tracing. As the junctional pacemaker slows down ever so slightly, P waves can be seen to emerge from the

QRS complex (beginning with the P wave that deforms the upstroke of the QRS complex of beat no. 5). This atrial pacemaker is set at 68 beats/min and ultimately takes over, but initially it is unrelated to the more rapid juntional pacemaker (the PR interval of beat no. 5 is *definitely* too short to conduct). Thus there is *transient AV dissociation,* in this case due to acceleration of the AV nodal pacemaker to 70 beats/min during the first portion of this rhythm strip.

> This tracing reemphasizes the point made earlier when discussing the rhythm shown in Figure 3D-4. That is, even though AV dissociation is present (transiently in this case), diagnosis of 3° AV block (or any degree of AV block for that matter) is *not* possible here, since P waves never occur at a point in the R-R interval when they would be expected to conduct.

PROBLEM   Figure 3D-17.

ANSWER TO FIGURE 3D-17   The ventricular rate is regular at about 34 beats/min. The atrial rate is also fairly regular; how-

Lead II

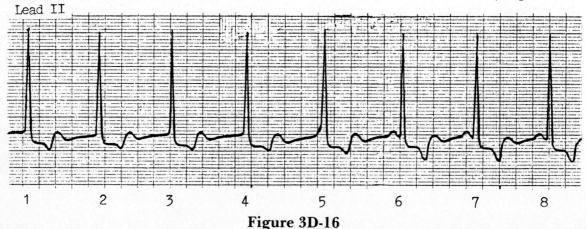

1   2   3   4   5   6   7   8

Figure 3D-16

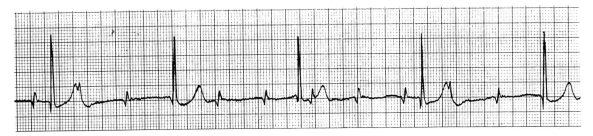

Figure 3D-17

ever, P waves are totally unrelated to the ventricular response (P waves "march" through the QRS). Thus there is *complete AV dissociation*. In addition, there is *complete AV block*. We can diagnose this with certainty because the ventricular response is slow *(<45 beats/min)* and the rhythm strip is long enough to demonstrate P waves occurring at many points in the R-R interval when conduction would be expected to occur.

> Note that the QRS complex is not really wide, suggesting that the level of the block is somewhere in the conduction system and not at the idioventricular level. Regardless of the level at which the block occurs, however, treatment must be directed at increasing the heart rate.

PROBLEM   **Figure 3D-18.**

ANSWER TO FIGURE 3D-18   The rhythm is regular at 70 beats/min. The QRS complex appears slightly widened. It is regularly preceded by a P wave with a constant (albeit markedly prolonged) PR interval (0.41 second). This is sinus rhythm with 1° AV block.

PROBLEM   **Figure 3D-19.**

ANSWER TO FIGURE 3D-19   The QRS complex is narrow. The rhythm is irregular and group beating is present. However, this is not Wenckebach since the PR interval remains constant instead of lengthening. P waves *are* related to QRS complexes in this example and

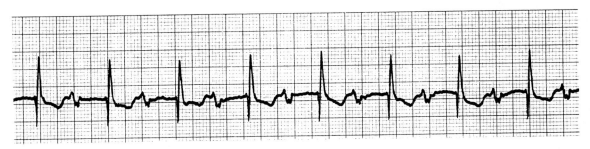

Figure 3D-18

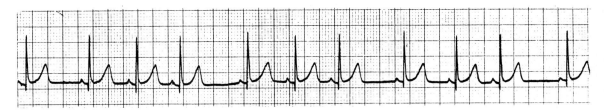

Figure 3D-19

conduct with a normal PR interval. This is *sinus arrhythmia,* in this case with respiratory variation producing the group beating.

PROBLEM   Figure 3D-20.

ANSWER TO FIGURE 3D-20   In this final example of group beating, Mobitz I (Wenckebach) 2° AV block (with 4:3 AV conduction) is present. All of the characteristic "footprints" are here:

  i) Group beating
  ii) Regularity of the atrial rate
  iii) Progressive lengthening of the PR interval until a beat is dropped
  iv) Duration of the pause being *less* than twice the shortest R-R interval

somewhat more complicated. Pacemaker insertion is routinely performed in patients who develop complete AV block as the result of acute *anterior* infarction. As we discussed, the escape pacemaker tends to be idioventricular (wide QRS complex) and is often associated with a slow heart rate and signs of hemodynamic compromise. On the other hand, complete AV block that develops with acute *inferior* infarction may occur with a stable junctional escape rhythm (narrow QRS complex) that is able to maintain the patient's hemodynamic status. The mechanism of AV block in this setting may simply reflect increased parasympathetic tone and/or ischemia of the AV node rather than irreversible myocardial damage. The conduction defect is usually transient. If the heart rate remains close

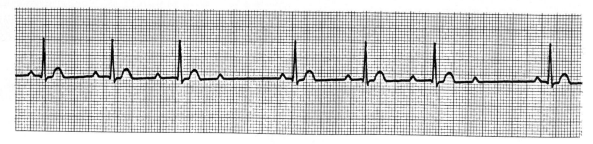

Figure 3D-20

Clinical Significance of the AV Blocks

Let us conclude this section by briefly reviewing the clinical significance of the conduction disturbances we have diagnosed. Hemodynamic status (as well as survival) of patients with 1° AV block and Mobitz I 2° AV block is generally not jeopardized by the conduction disturbance itself. As a result, no treatment other than observation is generally needed. In contrast, pacemaker insertion is strongly recommended for patients with Mobitz II 2° AV block, since this conduction disturbance has a disturbing tendency to rapidly (and suddenly) develop complete AV block.

The situation with 3° (complete) AV block is

to 60 beats/min, no treatment may be indicated. With slower heart rates, atropine may effectively accelerate the ventricular response and/or improve AV conduction. Pacemaker insertion is often not needed (**Table 3D-3**).

As we highlighted earlier, an important exception to these generalities is illustrated by the example shown in Figure 3D-11. Even though this conduction disturbance is "only" Mobitz I 2° AV block, the accompanying marked bradycardia would be likely to jeopardize the patient's hemodynamic status if it had not responded to atropine. *Clinical significance of the AV blocks often depends more on the ventricular response than on the "degree" of the block.*

The final concept to emphasize is that of AV dissociation. The rhythm shown in Figure 3D-16 is *not* due to 3° AV block. Instead it reflects what

TABLE 3D-3   Clinical Implications of 3° AV Block with Acute Myocardial Infarction

	Anterior Infarction	Inferior Infarction	
		Junctional escape focus (narrow QRS)	Idioventricular escape focus (wide QRS)
Rate of ventricular response	30–60 beats/min (depending on the site of the escape pacemaker)	40–60 beats/min	30–40 beats/min
Usual duration of conduction disturbance	Long-term	Transient	Long-term
Response to atropine	Poor	Good	Poor

Recommended treatment	Transvenous pacemaker insertion	Observation if hemodynamically stable
		
		Treat symptomatic bradycardia and/or hypotension with:
		1) Atropine
		2) External pacemaker
		    or
		  Dopamine, epinephrine, or isoproterenol
		3) Transvenous pacemaker insertion
			Transvenous pacemaker insertion

may happen when the AV nodal pacemaker accelerates to a rate that exceeds that of the underlying sinus rhythm. Pacemaker insertion is not indicated, as the resultant ventricular response is more than adequate to maintain hemodynamic stability.

Clinically accelerated junctional rhythms (and resultant AV dissociation) are commonly encountered in the setting of acute *inferior infarction* and *digitalis toxicity*. Recognition of the difference between AV dissociation and 3° AV block is essential in avoiding unnecessary treatment with pacemaker insertion.

E: RHYTHMS OF CARDIAC ARREST

In this section we apply the techniques we have covered to diagnosing the arrhythmias encountered during a typical cardiac arrest. The patient in question is a middle-aged man admitted for acute myocardial infarction. Imagine yourself as the emergency care provider assigned to watch the ECG monitor. At the time you arrive, the patient is awake but complaining of chest pain. His extremities are cold and clammy, and a systolic blood pressure of 90 mm Hg is recorded. Two sublingual nitroglycerin tablets and 5 mg of morphine sulfate have already been given.

PROBLEM   **The code director asks you to tell him the rhythm (Fig. 3E-1). How do you respond?**

PROBLEM   **What has happened (Fig. 3E-2)?**

ANSWER TO FIGURE 3E-2   Sinus tachycardia continues for the first three beats of Figure 3E-2. This is followed by a PVC (beat no. 4), another sinus beat, and then the abrupt onset of *ventricular fibrillation.*

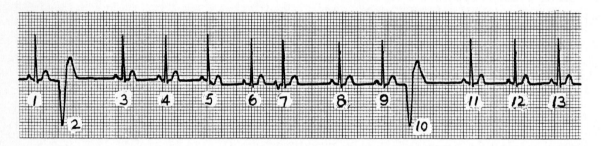

Figure 3E-1

ANSWER TO FIGURE 3E-1   The underlying rhythm is sinus tachycardia at a rate of 100 beats/min. Two PVCs (beats no. 2 and 10) and a PAC (beat no. 7) are seen.

    Although beats no. 2 and 10 are not quite as wide as one expects PVCs to be (they are not ≥ 0.12 seconds in duration), these beats are clearly much wider than the normally conducted sinus beats and are definitely very different in morphology. They must be considered PVCs. (It is possible that if other monitoring leads were obtained these beats might appear "wider.")

    The other early beat (beat no. 7) is identical in morphology to the normally conducted sinus beats and is preceded by a premature P wave. This is a PAC.

    The patient suddenly becomes unresponsive.

Ventricular Fibrillation

    Ventricular fibrillation is an extremely common inciting mechanism of cardiac arrest. Electrocardiographically, this rhythm is totally chaotic. The P wave, QRS complex, and T wave all are absent. Instead, an irregular zig-zag pattern is seen in which electrical waveforms continuously vary in size and shape.

    The patient is immediately defibrillated with 200 joules. This results in the rhythm shown in **Figure 3E-3.** A rapid but definite pulse is palpated at the bedside.

PROBLEM   **How would you interpret the rhythm shown in Figure 3E-3? What would you**

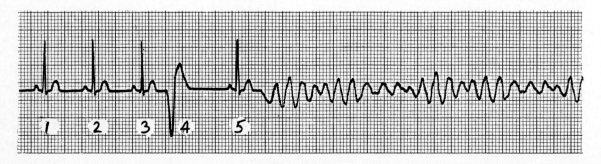

Figure 3E-2

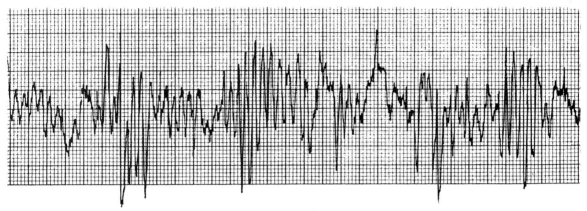

Figure 3E-3

suggest to the other members of the code team?

ANSWER TO FIGURE 3E-3
A bizarre series of vertical lines at an extremely rapid rate is noted. This rhythm is incompatible with the physical finding of a palpable pulse, and one should strongly suspect *artifact*. Ask the other team members if a monitor lead has fallen off.

Artifact

Artifactual rhythms are commonly seen during cardiopulmonary resuscitation. This should not be unexpected considering the large number of health care providers feverishly working at the bedside. Artifact-generating tasks performed include CPR, intubation, ventilation, defibrillation, intravenous cannulation, and drawing of arterial blood gases. In addition, monitor leads may frequently be knocked off. For these reasons one should always check for the presence of a pulse and patient responsiveness before defibrillating a patient based on the reading of the ECG monitor.

The disconnected monitor lead is reapplied. The rhythm shown in **Figure 3E-4** now flashes across the monitor. A rapid pulse is still palpated.

PROBLEM   What is the rhythm?

ANSWER TO FIGURE 3E-4
A *supraventricular tachycardia* at a rate of 150 beats/min is seen. The rhythm is regular. Although hard to be sure, P waves appear to be present (arrow). This suggests that the rhythm is *sinus tachycardia*.

> The usual differential for *regular* supraventricular tachyarrhythmias with a rate in the range of 150 beats/min is sinus tachycardia, atrial flutter, and PSVT. Much more important than the differential at this point during the code, however, is the patient's clinical status.

A normal blood pressure is obtained momentarily. Then the rhythm on the monitor suddenly changes (**Fig. 3E-5**).

PROBLEM   What has happened?

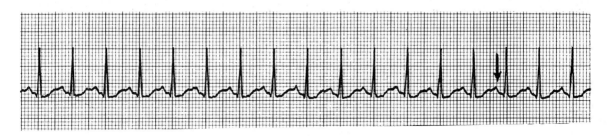

Figure 3E-4

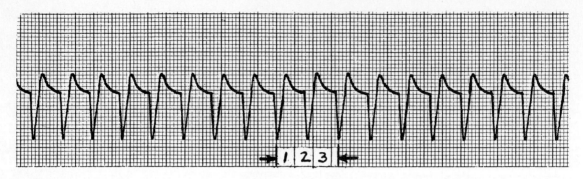

Figure 3E-5

ANSWER TO FIGURE 3E-5   A regular, wide complex tachycardia is seen at a rate of about 170 beats/min. This is *ventricular tachycardia*.

>   That the rate is approximately 170 beats/min can be determined by the method suggested earlier. Select a QRS complex that peaks on a heavy line. Then calculate the R-R interval for two beats. This is just over 3 boxes in this example (Fig. 3E-5). *Half the rate* is, therefore, about 85 beats/min. The actual rate must be twice this, or 170 beats/min.
>
>   Although the QRS complex of the tachycardia in this figure is not as wide as one expects for ventricular tachycardia (it is not ≥0.12 second), it is clearly wider than and dramatically different in morphology from the supraventricular rhythm that was just seen in Figure 3E-4. While one cannot absolutely rule out aberrant conduction, *one must assume ventricular tachycardia and treat accordingly!*
>
>   Another retrospective point in favor of VT is that the morphology of the QRS complex in Figure 3E-5 is identical to that of the PVCs identified earlier in Figure 3E-1.

A systolic blood pressure of only 70 mm Hg "palp" is obtained with the rhythm shown in Figure 3E-5. Synchronized cardioversion is ordered.

PROBLEM   **Synchronized cardioversion with 200 joules is delivered at the arrow in Figure 3E-6. What is the result?**

ANSWER TO FIGURE 3E-6   Synchronized cardioversion results in ventricular fibrillation.

   There is no longer any pulse. The patient is immediately defibrillated with 200 joules.

PROBLEM   **Defibrillation results in a rapidly changing sequence of events (Fig. 3E-7). How would you interpret this for the code director?**

ANSWER TO FIGURE 3E-7   Four beats of what appears to be VT at an extremely rapid rate is seen, followed by a 10 beat run of a supraventricular tachycardia (at a rate of about 210 beats/min), and then resumption of ventricular fibrillation.

   There is no pulse. Defibrillation is ordered.

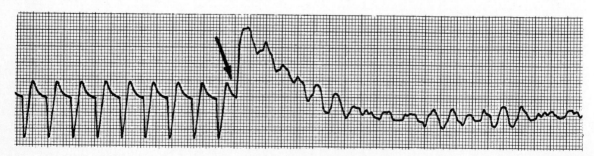

Figure 3E-6

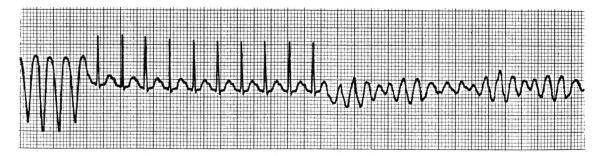

Figure 3E-7

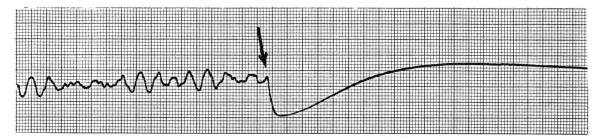

Figure 3E-8

PROBLEM   **Defibrillation with 300 joules is delivered at the arrow in Figure 3E-8. What does this lead to?**

ANSWER TO FIGURE 3E-8   Defibrillation leads to *asystole.*

There is no pulse. CPR is resumed and the patient is intubated. The code director asks you if there is any change in the rhythm?

PROBLEM   **What do you see on the monitor (Fig. 3E-9)?**

ANSWER TO FIGURE 3E-9   Extremely broad waveforms are seen separating rare *idioventricular complexes* (**X**).

PROBLEM   **Do you think that the broad waveforms in Figure 3E-9 might be due to CPR? Is there a way to tell?**

ANSWER   Yes. Stop CPR.

CPR is stopped and the rhythm shown in **Figure 3E-10** results. This confirms your previous suspicion.

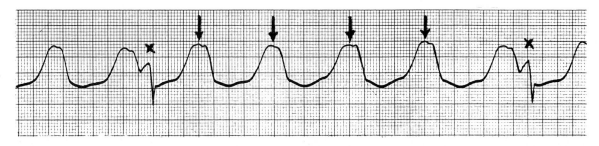

Figure 3E-9

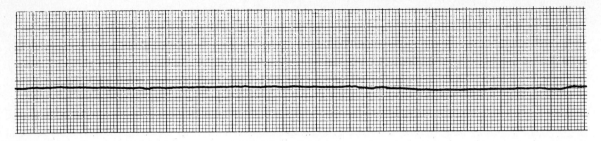

Figure 3E-10

PROBLEM   Could **Figure 3E-10** possibly represent *fine* ventricular fibrillation? Is there a way to tell?

ANSWER   Yes! Switch the ECG monitor to several other leads to see whether a flat line is still recorded.

The "Flat Line" Recording: Asystole or Ventricular Fibrillation?

On rare occasions, ventricular fibrillation may masquerade as asystole. Like any other electrocardiographic complex, the undulations of ventricular fibrillation possess a predominant vector of electrical activity. Should this vector be *perpendicular* to the monitor lead recorded, a flat line will be obtained. As a result, many clinicians advocate countershocking asystole on the remote chance that the rhythm may really be ventricular fibrillation in disguise. While hard to fault this practice (since realistically there is little to lose by shocking the patient at this point even if the rhythm is asystole), a simpler (though less dramatic) way to determine if ventricular fibrillation is masquerading as asystole is to switch the ECG monitor to several other monitoring leads. If ventricular fibrillation is present, this should be clearly evident in the other leads.

PROBLEM   Was CPR being performed *correctly* in **Figure 3E-9?**

ANSWER   The R-R interval of the broad waveforms in Figure 3E-9 is about 5 large boxes. This corresponds to a rate of 1 waveform (or external chest compression) per second and 60 compressions per minute. Although the recommended rate for external chest compression with 2-rescuer CPR used to be 60 per minute, new recommendations advocate higher rates (80–100 compressions per minute).

At this point (Fig. 3E-10), there is no pulse and the patient's rhythm is asystole. CPR is resumed (with a faster compression rate), and epinephrine is given by the intravenous route. A minute passes.

PROBLEM   How would you describe the rhythm now seen on the monitor (**Fig. 3E-11**)?

ANSWER TO FIGURE 3E-11   The rhythm is fairly regular, and the rate is just under 30 beats/min. P waves are absent, and the QRS complex appears to be wide. This is a slow *idioventricular escape rhythm*.

The R-R interval measures approximately 11 large boxes. If it were exactly 10 large boxes, the rate would be 30 beats/min (300 ÷ 10). The rate

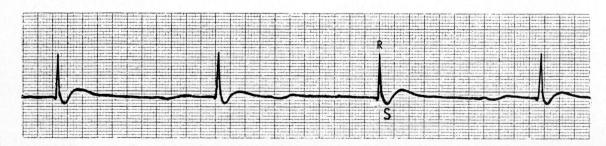

Figure 3E-11

must therefore be a little slower, or about 28 beats/min.

If one takes into account the deep S wave in measuring duration of the QRS complex in this example, there is no question that the QRS is wide. The difficulty lies in determining where the QRS really ends and the ST segment begins. There is really no way to be sure from this single monitoring lead alone. In this case, however, regardless of whether the QRS is wide, the escape rhythm is extremely slow and the treatment priority is the same—speed up the rate!

Slow Idioventricular Rhythm (IVR)

Slow IVR is a rhythm that is commonly encountered during cardiac arrest. It is seen more often than the AV blocks in this setting. As discussed earlier, the SA node usually acts as the principal pacemaker of the heart. With normal sinus rhythm it fires at a rate of between 60 and 100 beats/min. Should something happen to the SA node's pacesetting ability, other areas of the heart with inherent automaticity must take over. With an inherent rate of 40–60 beats/min, the AV node is usually next in line. However, should the AV nodal pacemaker also fail, the pacesetting function then falls to the ventricles. Hopefully an idioventricular escape rhythm will arise and be able to take over.

The inherent automaticity of slow IVR is usually between 30 and 40 beats/min. Electrocardiographically this rhythm is recognized as a fairly regular wide complex bradyarrhythmia. P waves are absent. Supportive treatment with positive chronotropic and inotropic agents is needed until an artificial pacemaker can be employed.

Epinephrine and sodium bicarbonate are both given for the rhythm shown in **Figure 3E-11**. Unfortunately, deterioration to the rhythm shown in **Figure 3E-12** results.

PROBLEM   Given that CPR is *not* being performed at the time Figure 3E-12 is recorded, how would you interpret this tracing?

ANSWER TO FIGURE 3E-12   The complexes in this rhythm are extremely wide (over 0.20 second in duration) and totally amorphous. This is an *agonal rhythm.*

Agonal Rhythm

In general, agonal rhythm (as its name implies) is a manifestation of a dying heart. Surprisingly, this sporadic electrical activity may continue for minutes (and up to hours) after meaningful cardiac function has ceased. Isolated and grouped idioventricular complexes, or the amorphous waveforms seen in Figure 3E-12 may appear, be interrupted by periods of asystole, and then reappear on the monitor. Clinically the significance of an agonal rhythm is similar to that of asystole.

CPR is continued. More epinephrine is given.

PROBLEM   Is there any change (Fig. 3E-13)?

ANSWER TO FIGURE 3E-13   Midway through the rhythm strip shown in Figure 3E-13 ventricular fibrillation develops.

This is one occasion when development of ventricular fibrillation should be viewed as a favorable response! The chance for potential reversibility is much greater for this rhythm than for agonal rhythm or asystole.

The patient is defibrillated with 360 joules. The rhythm shown in **Figure 3E-14** results.

PROBLEM   What has happened?

ANSWER TO FIGURE 3E-14   Idioventricular complexes begin and end this rhythm strip. In between, there is a long period of *ventricular standstill.* Slightly irregular atrial activity at a rate of ≈ 70 beats/min continues throughout.

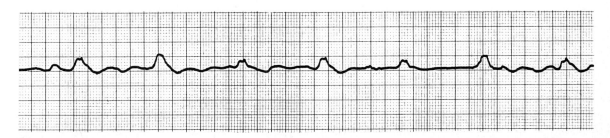

Figure 3E-12

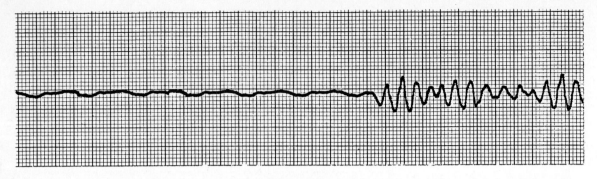

Figure 3E-13

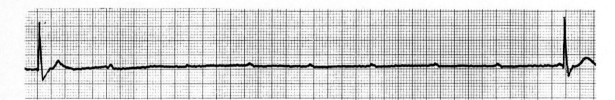

Figure 3E-14

None of the atrial impulses seen in this rhythm strip conduct, suggesting 3° (complete) AV block. However, more than heart block, the problem is the absence of an appropriate escape focus.

CPR is resumed. Arterial blood gases are drawn, and more epinephrine is administered.

PROBLEM   The monitor changes again (Fig. 3E-15). What has happened?

ANSWER TO FIGURE 3E-15   The patient has gone back into ventricular fibrillation. Waveform undulations are of small amplitude— this is *fine* ventricular fibrillation.

More epinephrine is given.

PROBLEM   Was the epinephrine successful (Fig. 3E-16)?

ANSWER TO FIGURE 3E-16   The fine ventricular fibrillation of Figure 3E-15 has now become *coarse*. Many clinicians view such coarsening as a beneficial therapeutic response to epinephrine that facilitates subsequent conversion to sinus rhythm when countershock is applied.

"Coarsening" may be artificially produced by manipulating the amplitude of the ECG monitor. In the same manner, "fine ventricular fibrillation" can be made to appear as asystole if the amplitude dial is turned all the way down. For this reason, it

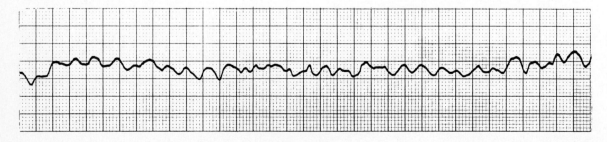

Figure 3E-15

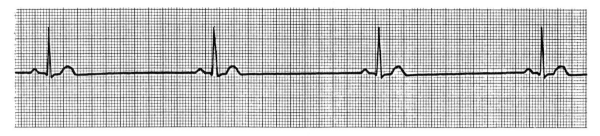

Figure 3E-16

is advantageous to hook up a 12-lead ECG machine at the bedside as soon as possible during any code.

Following defibrillation, the rhythm shown in **Figure 3E-17** is seen. This is associated with a slow, weak pulse.

PROBLEM   Is this another slow IVR?

ANSWER TO FIGURE 3E-17   The rhythm is regular and exceedingly slow. With an R-R interval of just under 12 large boxes, the heart rate is 25 beats/min (300 ÷ 12). However, this is not a slow IVR since P waves *are* present. They precede each QRS complex with a constant PR interval. This is *sinus bradycardia* with an extremely slow ventricular response.

> The PR interval is 0.20 second, which is still within the normal range. In order for 1° AV block to be present, the PR interval must be *greater* than 0.20 second.

Moments later the pulse is lost.

PROBLEM   What happened (Fig. 3E-18)?

ANSWER TO FIGURE 3E-18   An 11-beat run of ventricular tachycardia begins this rhythm strip at a rate of 210 beats/min. This deteriorates into ventricular fibrillation.

A *precordial thump* is delivered as the paddles are charged. The patient remains pulseless. Countershock with maximal energy is repeated.

A strong but irregular pulse is now palpable and associated with a blood pressure of 120/80 mm Hg. A bolus of lidocaine is given, and an intravenous infusion of this drug is started. The patient begins to wake up.

PROBLEM   How would you interpret the rhythm (Fig. 3E-19)?

ANSWER TO FIGURE 3E-19   The rhythm is irregularly irregular. Atrial activity is evident (there are undulations in the baseline), but there are no clear P waves. This is *atrial fibrillation* with a *controlled* ventricular response.

> Even though normal sinus rhythm has not been restored, the patient's hemodynamic status has stabilized and resuscitation is successful.

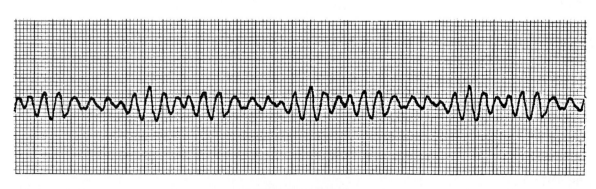

Figure 3E-17

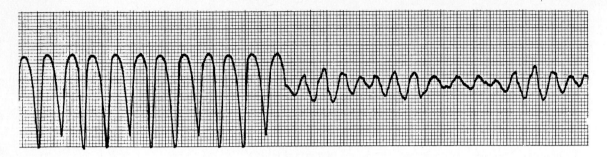

Figure 3E-18

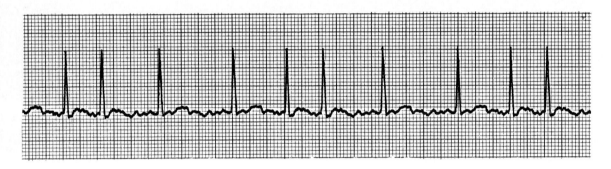

Figure 3E-19

This sequence of events is probably as complicated as any you will encounter in a real-life setting. Appreciation of the rationale presented here for arrhythmia recognition should make you much more comfortable performing both at the MEGA CODE station and in actual code situations.

F: ARRHYTHMIA OR DYSRHYTHMIA? . . . AND OTHER CONFUSING TERMS

A number of years ago, a Task Force was appointed with the specific goal of trying to standardize the terminology used in electrocardiographic interpretation (Surawicz et al., 1978). Controversy began with the attempt to define "normality" and persisted throughout the entire conference. Even among experts, wide discrepancies in the use of certain electrocardiographic terms are prevalent.

Examples of confusing terminology abound in the field of arrhythmia interpretation and advanced cardiac life support. Prior to delving into a detailed description of the various cardiac arrhythmias, it may therefore be helpful to clarify a number of points about terminology that commonly come up in discussion of cardiopulmonary resuscitation.

The opinions expressed in this section are our own. We fully acknowledge that they may not be shared by others in the field.

Arrhythmia versus Dysrhythmia

The two terms that have probably generated the most controversy are arrhythmia and dysrhythmia. Which one should be used?

The purist undoubtedly favors *dysrhythmia,* despite the fact that this word lacks both the tradition and phonetic facility of arrhythmia. He/she would contend that *arrhythmia* should literally mean "no rhythm" (or asystole), since attachment of the prefix "*a*" to any word implies an "absence of" the entity in question. These individuals prefer to add the prefix "*dys*" (meaning "a disorder of") to the word stem "rhythm." The result—*dysrhythmia*—"properly" connotes a disturbance of rhythm.

This line of reasoning is faulty. The prefix "*a*" is not limited to meaning an "absence of" the entity in question but may also be used to imply an "imperfection" of the entity. Furthermore, the root "rhythmos" is not restricted to meaning "a regular recurring motion" but instead has also been used to describe "an arrangement, a symmetry, or order"—and, "what could be more disorderly than atrial fibrillation?" (Marriott, 1984).

Were one to restrict words to their derivations and/or original meanings, much of the color and richness of the English language would be lost. Similarly, the evolutionary importance accrued from usage over the years would also be lost. We believe the dictionary definition of *arrhythmia*—"a variation from the normal rhythm, especially of the heart beat"—has withstood the test of time. We do not ascribe any difference to the meaning of arrhythmia and dysrhythmia and favor using these terms interchangeably.

Characteristics of Ideal Terminology

The ideal term should be easily pronounced, spelled, written, and remembered. It should not be ambiguous or likely to engender confusion in interpretation. If subject to abbreviation, the letters chosen for this should not be the same as other commonly used abbreviations. Finally, the term should not be one that promotes fear or panic when overheard by a patient with the disorder (Constant, 1978; Marriott, 1986).

Heart Block versus AV Block

"Heart block" is a poor term that disregards several of the above ground rules. One can easily imagine a patient becoming unduly alarmed on learning that his/her heart is "blocked." Technically, the term lacks specificity and fails to differentiate between the various types of heart block: atrioventricular (AV) block, bundle branch block, and fascicular (hemi-) block. When used to indicate a defect in atrioventricular conduction, it doesn't offer the listener the slightest clue as to whether 1°, 2°, or 3° AV block is present.

Classification of the types of AV blocks was discussed in detail in Section D of this chapter. Let us reemphasize the need for clearly defining conduction disturbances in as complete and specific a manner as possible. Referral to a disorder as "2° AV block, Mobitz Type I" is infinitely preferable to simply describing a rhythm as "Wenckebach."

PVCs, VPDs, and Ventricular Extrasystoles

Numerous terms have been used to define early-occurring beats of ventricular origin. These include:

  i) PVC (premature ventricular contraction)
  ii) VPC (ventricular premature complex)
  iii) VPD (ventricular premature depolarization)
  iv) VPB (ventricular premature beat)
  v) VEC (ventricular ectopic complex)
  vi) ventricular extrasystole

Which of these connotations is chosen depends less on any inherent benefits of the term than on how one was taught and what general custom prevails in one's area of practice. Semantic problems can be found with the use of *each* of these terms (Marriott, 1986). For example, a shortcoming of PVC (premature ventricular *contraction*) is that the word contraction implies a mechanical event, whereas the electrocardiographic manifestation of the phenomenon is purely electrical. Despite legitimate concerns about the appropriateness of this term, years of usage have accustomed us to "the PVC," and we use this connotation exclusively throughout this book.

Supraventricular Tachycardia, PAT, PJT, or PSVT?

As discussed in Section B of this chapter, the term *supraventricular tachycardia (SVT)* is a general one that encompasses all tachyarrhythmias in which the impulse originates at or above the AV node. Unless aberrant conduction or preexisting bundle branch block is present, the QRS complex will be narrow. Entities included within this definition are:

  i) Sinus tachycardia
 ii) Junctional tachycardia
iii) Atrial fibrillation or flutter with a moderately rapid or rapid ventricular response
 iv) Multifocal atrial tachycardia (MAT or chaotic atrial mechanism)
 vii) Ectopic atrial tachycardia
viii) Paroxysmal atrial or junctional tachycardia (PAT or PJT)
 ix) Paroxysmal supraventricular tachycardia (PSVT)

In the past, the term SVT was used synonymously with PAT or PJT. This practice is potentially misleading since arrhythmias such as sinus tachycardia constitute a form of SVT that is very different from ectopic atrial tachycardia, PAT, or PJT. Normal atrial activity (upright P waves in lead II) is seen with sinus tachycardia. In contrast, with ectopic tachycardia, another atrial focus (often recognized by unusual-looking P waves in lead II) takes over with enhanced automaticity. Finally, with PAT or PJT, the tachyarrhythmia is *paroxysmal* (of sudden onset) and due to a reentry phenomenon involving the AV node.

The usage we favor is to apply *supraventricular tachycardia* as the generic, all-encompassing term for any narrow QRS complex tachyarrhythmia (for example, sinus tachycardia, atrial fibrillation or flutter). We tend to avoid the abbreviation *SVT* because it is too easily confused with PSVT. We use this latter term *(PSVT)* to connote those regular supraventricular tachycardias that appear to operate by a *reentry* mechanism involving the AV node. This contrasts with the situation when ectopic P waves can be clearly identified. In such cases, the rhythm is most appropriately termed *atrial tachycardia* (with or without associated block at the AV node). Finally, we have discarded the terms *PAT* and *PJT* since these abbreviations imply more than we know about the mechanism and site of origin of the arrhythmia.

Surprising Origin of the P-QRS-T

We will close this section by commenting on the derivation of the lettering used to describe electrocardiographic morphology. Impetus for selecting the sequence of letters **P-Q-R-S-T-U** to denote various waveforms on the electrocardiogram actually has *nothing* to do with electrocardiography (Henson, 1971). Instead it dates back to the time of the great mathematician René Descartes, who lived in the mid 1600s. Descartes opted to choose the letter "P" as a convenient starting place in many of his mathematical series primarily because of its alliterative and pneumonic effects ("point P"). These effects operated in the Latin, French, Dutch, and German languages. Willem Einthoven (1860–1927), trained as a physician at the University of Utrecht in Holland, was heavily schooled in mathematics and physiology. It is felt that he adopted this sequence of letters as the nomenclature for electrocardiography as a result of his *mathematical* training!

G: ARRHYTHMIA REVIEW (II)

As a final review, interpret the following 30 tracings.

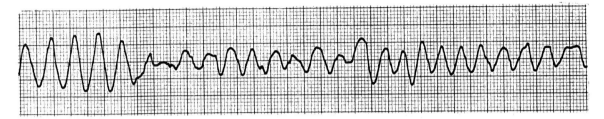

Figure 3G-1

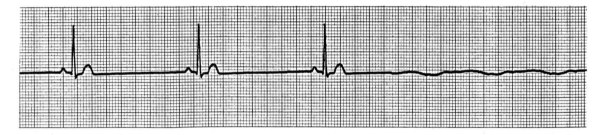

Figure 3G-2

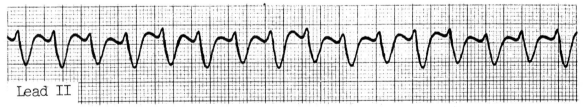

Figure 3G-3

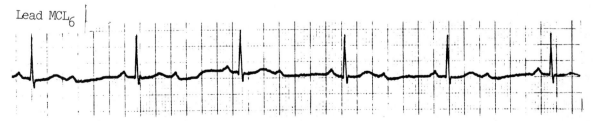

Figure 3G-4

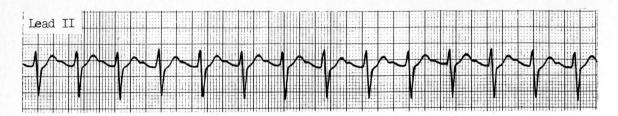

Figure 3G-5

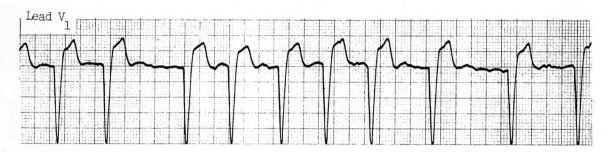

Figure 3G-6

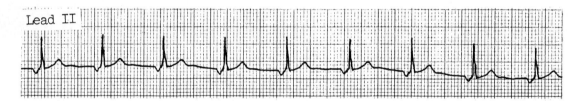

Figure 3G-7

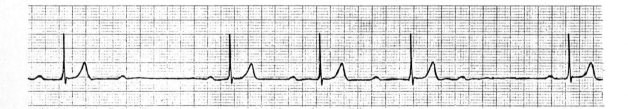

Figure 3G-8

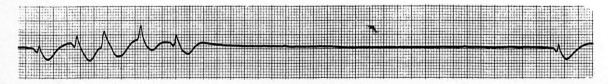

Figure 3G-9

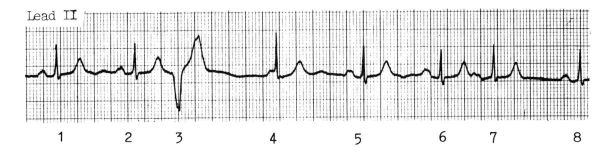

Lead II

1   2   3   4   5   6   7   8

Figure 3G-10

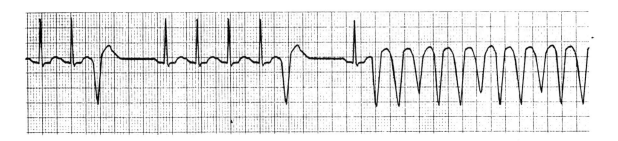

Figure 3G-11

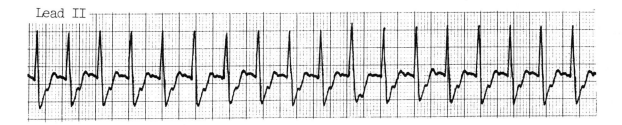

Lead II

Figure 3G-12

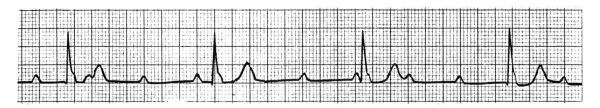

Figure 3G-13

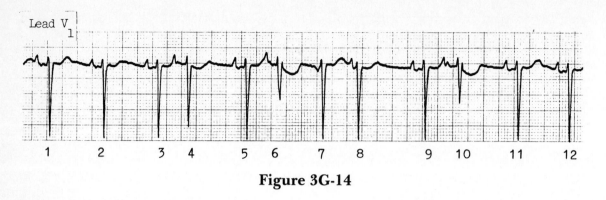

Figure 3G-14

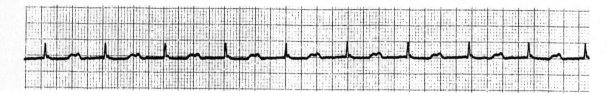

Figure 3G-15

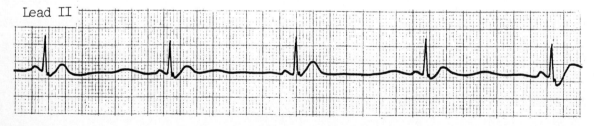

Figure 3G-16

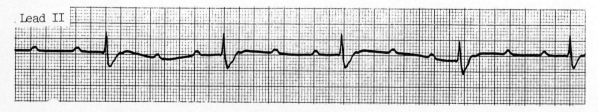

Figure 3G-17

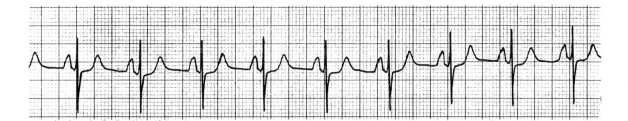

Figure 3G-18

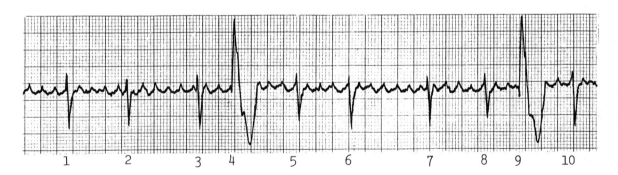

Lead V₁

Figure 3G-19

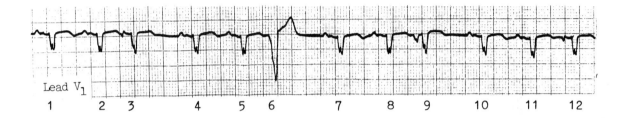

Figure 3G-20

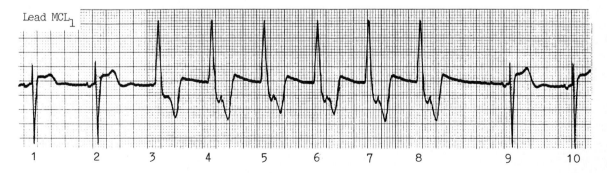

Lead MCL₁

Figure 3G-21

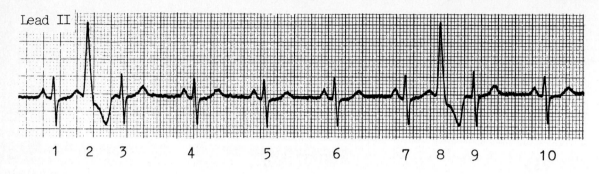

Figure 3G-22

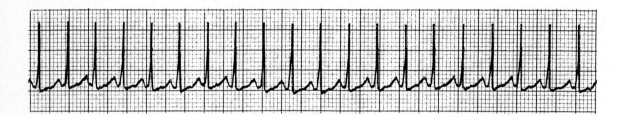

Figure 3G-23

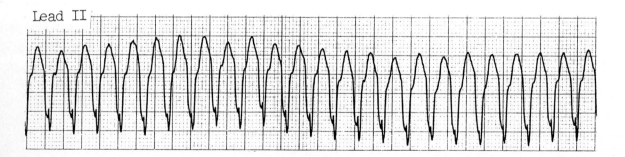

Figure 3G-24

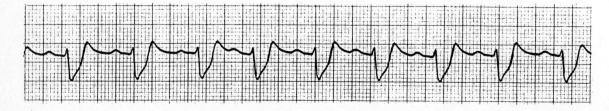

Figure 3G-25

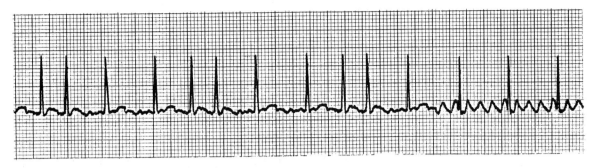

Figure 3G-26

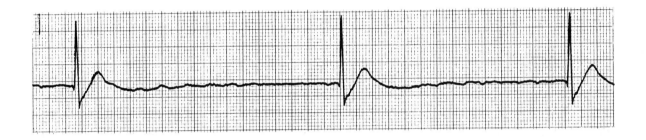

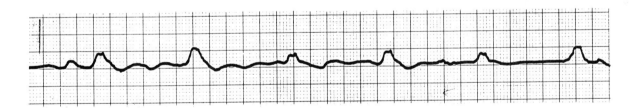

Figure 3G-28

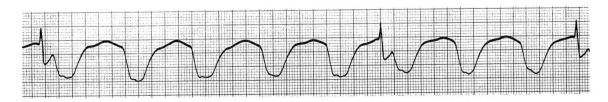

Figure 3G-29

Lead MCL$_1$

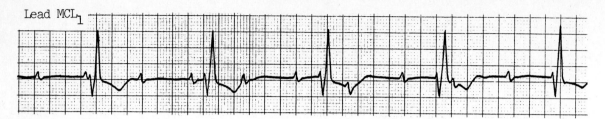

Figure 3G-30

ANSWERS TO ARRHYTHMIA REVIEW (II)

Answer to Figure 3G-1

Rhythm—irregular
Impression: Ventricular flutter rapidly degenerating to coarse ventricular fibrillation.

Answer to Figure 3G-2

Rhythm—regular for the first three beats, then flat line
Rate—35 beats/min initially
PR interval—normal
QRS complex—normal duration
Impression: Sinus bradycardia initially, then asystole.

Answer to Figure 3G-3

Rhythm—regular
Rate—155 beats/min
P waves—none evident
QRS complex—wide (0.18 second)
Impression: Ventricular tachycardia
Comment: Although this rhythm could possibly represent a supraventricular tachycardia with either aberrant conduction or preexisting bundle branch block, ventricular tachycardia must be assumed until proved otherwise.

Answer to Figure 3G-4

Rhythm—regular
Atrial rate—90 beats/min
Ventricular rate—45 beats/min
QRS complex—normal duration
Impression: 2° AV block with 2:1 AV conduction, either Mobitz I or II
Comment: One cannot absolutely differentiate between Mobitz I and II 2° AV block in the presence of 2:1 AV conduction. The normal QRS duration, however, strongly favors Mobitz I.

Answer to Figure 3G-5

Rhythm—regular
Rate—112 beats/min
PR interval—probably normal (0.20 second)
QRS complex—borderline prolongation (0.11 second)
Impression: Sinus tachycardia
Comment: Although not obvious, P waves follow each T wave (arrows in **Fig. 3G-5A**). Were the rate to speed up any more, the P waves would become buried in the T wave.

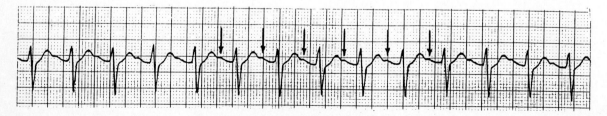

Figure 3G-5A

Answer to Figure 3G-6

Rhythm—irregularly irregular
P waves—none
QRS complex—wide (0.12 second)
Impression: Atrial fibrillation with a controlled ventricular response
Comment: Although low amplitude undulations are seen along the baseline, no consistent atrial activity is present. The QRS prolongation is caused by a preexisting left bundle branch block (LBBB).

Answer to Figure 3G-7

Rhythm—regular
Rate—80 beats/min
P waves—*inverted;* precede the QRS complex with a short PR interval
QRS complex—normal (≤0.10 second)
Impression: Accelerated junctional (AV nodal) rhythm
Comment: With junctional rhythm, P waves may precede the QRS complex as shown here, follow the QRS complex, or be hidden by their simultaneous occurrence with the QRS complex. Because of the retrograde activation of the atria from the junctional focus, P waves will be inverted in lead II. A low atrial rhythm may also manifest negative P waves in lead II, but the PR interval is usually longer than is shown here.

The heart rate in this tracing is somewhat faster than one characteristically sees with a junctional rhythm. If the patient was on digitalis, toxicity should be suspected.

A final possibility should be considered in this tracing. One cannot be absolutely sure from this one monitoring lead that the negative deflection preceding the QRS complex is a P wave. It could be part of the QRS. If this were the case, then the QRS complex would be wide, and this would be an accelerated idioventricular rhythm (AIVR). The importance of having more than one monitoring lead for diagnosing arrhythmias cannot be overstated.

Answer to Figure 3G-8

Ventricular rhythm—irregular
Atrial rate and rhythm—fairly regular (at 47–50 beats/min)
PR interval—progressively increases until a beat is dropped
QRS complex—normal duration
Impression: Mobitz I 2° AV block
Comment: This tracing was taken from an elderly patient who presented with syncopal spells. There was no acute infarction, and the patient was not on any cardioactive drugs. Despite the fact that this is "only Mobitz I," a permanent pacemaker was justifiably implanted because of the slow ventricular response and associated symptoms (syncope). *More important than the degree of AV block is the ventricular response and the hemodynamic status of the patient.*

Answer to Figure 3G-9

Rhythm—irregular
P waves—none
QRS complex—wide (0.16 second)
Impression: Agonal rhythm with a long period of asystole

Answer to Figure 3G-10

Rhythm—irregular
PR interval—normal
QRS complex—normal duration
Impression and Comment: The first two beats are sinus. Beat no. 3 is a PVC. It is wide, bizarre in shape, and demonstrates a QRS configuration that is oppositely directed to the normally conducted beats.

The P wave preceding beat no. 4 occurs on time but with a PR interval that is too short to conduct. Although beat no. 4 differs slightly in configuration from the other beats, it has a similar initial deflection, a similar T wave, and it is not really widened. It is a junctional escape beat that occurred before the P wave preceding it could be conducted to the ventricles. Beat no. 7 is a PAC.

Answer to Figure 3G-11

Rhythm—irregular

QRS complex—narrow initially, then QRS morphology changes and the complex widens

Impression: Sinus tachycardia with PVCs. The third PVC exhibits the "R-on-T" phenomenon and precipitates ventricular tachycardia at a rate of 210 beats/min.

Comment: The underlying rhythm is sinus tachycardia at a rate of 140 beats/min. P waves are not well seen during the supraventricular tachycardia (they are probably "notching" the terminal portion of the T wave) but become more apparent in front of QRS complexes that terminate the postectopic pauses.

Answer to Figure 3G-12

Rhythm—regular

Rate—155 beats/min

P waves—no well-defined P waves are seen, although notching of the baseline may represent atrial activity, possibly flutter

QRS complex—probably of normal duration, although one cannot be certain of where the QRS complex ends and the ST segment begins

Impression: Regular tachyarrhythmia at 155 beats/min.

Comment: This is a difficult tracing. Although the occurrence of a tachyarrhythmia at a rate of about 150 beats/min and the notching in the baseline suggest the possibility of atrial flutter, it would be presumptive to make this diagnosis based on this one tracing alone. The notching could be part of the QRS complex itself, in which case the rhythm might be ventricular tachycardia.

Assuming that the patient were hemodynamically stable, obtaining a 12-lead ECG might be helpful in resolving the issue. If the QRS complex were clearly of normal duration in other leads, then the differential would be one of a supraventricular tachycardia (PSVT, sinus tachycardia, or atrial flutter). Maneuvers to better elicit atrial activity (obtaining additional monitoring leads, carotid massage) might then prove diagnostic.

On the other hand, if the QRS complex appeared consistently wide in other leads of a 12-lead ECG, one would again be faced with having to differentiate between ventricular tachycardia and supraventricular tachycardia with either preexisting bundle branch block or aberrant conduction.

Answer to Figure 3G-13

Atrial rate and rhythm—regular at 100 beats/min

Ventricular rate and rhythm—regular at 37 beats/min

PR interval—variable (P waves "march" through the QRS complex)

QRS complex—wide (0.12 second)

Impression: Complete (3°) AV block

Comment: The diagnosis of 3° AV block can be confidently made here since the ventricular rate is slow (<45 beats/min) and P waves fail to conduct despite being given adequate opportunity to do so.

Answer to Figure 3G-14

Rhythm—irregular

PR interval—normal

QRS complex—normal duration

Impression: Sinus rhythm with PACs, most of which conduct with aberrancy

Comment: The first three beats demonstrate an underlying sinus rhythm at 80 beats/min. Beats no. 4, 6, 8, and 10 are all PACs.

Answer to Figure 3G-15

Rhythm—regular

Rate—75 beats/min

PR interval—markedly prolonged (0.39 second)

QRS complex—normal duration

Impression: Sinus rhythm with 1° AV block

Comment: Although one might interpret this as a junctional rhythm, the notch in the T wave is most likely the result of a P wave with a markedly prolonged PR interval.

Answer to Figure 3G-16

Rhythm—regular
Rate—40 beats/min
PR interval—normal
QRS complex—normal duration
Impression: Sinus bradycardia

Answer to Figure 3G-17

Atrial rate and rhythm—110 beats/min and fairly regular
Ventricular rate and rhythm—38 beats/min and fairly regular
QRS complex—wide (0.13 second)
Impression: High-grade 2° AV block, Mobitz II
Comment: Although severe impairment of AV conduction is present, each QRS complex is preceded by a P wave with a *constant* PR interval. Thus P waves *are* related to the QRS, and this cannot be 3° AV block.

Although high-grade block could theoretically be due to Mobitz I, it much more commonly is the result of Mobitz II. The QRS widening seen here strongly suggests this to be the case.

Answer to Figure 3G-18

Rhythm—regular
Rate—85 beats/min
PR interval—normal
QRS complex—normal duration
Impression: Sinus rhythm
Comment: The shape of the T wave resembles that of the P wave, suggesting that 2:1 AV conduction might exist. However, use of calipers to measure the P-T interval reveals that it differs from the T-P interval. Thus this is simply a sinus rhythm.

Answer to Figure 3G-19

Rhythm—irregular
PR interval—normal (0.20 second)
QRS complex—normal duration

Impression: Sinus rhythm with PACs and a PVC
Comment: Beats no. 3, 9, and 12 are clearly PACs. They occur early and are preceded by P waves, yet manifest a QRS configuration identical to that of the normally conducted beats.

Beat no. 6 is a PVC. It is wider, more bizarre in shape, and has an oppositely directed initial deflection to that of the normally conducted beats. (Beat no. 6 has a QS morphology that differs from the rS configuration of the normally conducted beats.)

Answer to Figure 3G-20

Rhythm—irregular
Atrial rate—sawtooth flutter waves at 360 beats/min
QRS complex—normal duration
Impression: Atrial flutter with a variable ventricular response. Uniform PVCs (beats no. 4 and 9).
Comment: The atrial rate in this example is somewhat faster than one usually sees with atrial flutter.

Answer to Figure 3G-21

Rhythm—irregular
Impression: Sinus rhythm interrupted by a run of accelerated idioventricular rhythm (beats no. 3–8).
Comment: Following two sinus beats, the QRS configuration changes with beat no. 3. This beat is not premature but is rather an escape beat that arises because of the slight slowing of the sinus pacemaker. Retrograde P waves notch the T waves of beats no. 4–8. After a short pause, sinus rhythm resumes with beat no. 9.

Beats no. 3–8 are *not* the result of aberration. There would be no reason for these beats to conduct aberrantly, since they occur so long after the refractory period of beat no. 2.

Answer to Figure 3G-22

Rhythm—regular except for beats no. 2 and 8
Rate—70 beats/min
PR interval—normal
QRS complex—normal duration
Impression: Sinus rhythm with two *(interpolated)* PVCs.
Comment: Beats no. 2 and 8 are PVCs, since they are wide and bizarre and are not preceded by a premature P wave. They are somewhat unusual in being sandwiched between two normally occurring QRS complexes without producing any postectopic pause (they are interpolated).

Answer to Figure 3G-23

Rhythm—regular
Rate—210 beats/min
P waves—impossible to determine if the positive deflection preceding each QRS complex is a P wave, a T wave, or both
QRS complex—normal duration
Impression: PSVT
Comment: Although the differential includes PSVT, sinus tachycardia, and atrial flutter, the latter two possibilities are much less likely. Sinus tachycardia rarely goes above 160 beats/min in an adult. The atrial rate in flutter is most often around 300 beats/min (range 250–350 beats/min). A rate of 210 beats/min would be slower than expected if there were 1:1 AV conduction and too fast if there were 2:1 AV conduction.

Answer to Figure 3G-24

Rhythm—regular
Rate—230 beats/min
P waves—none
QRS complex—wide (0.14 second)
Impression: Ventricular tachycardia
Comment: Once again, the presence of a wide complex tachyarrhythmia suggests the possibility of ventricular tachycardia or supraventricular tachycardia with either preexisting bundle branch block or aberrancy. Ventricular tachycardia must be assumed until proved otherwise.

Answer to Figure 3G-25

Rhythm—fairly regular
Rate—85 beats/min
PR interval—prolonged (0.22 second)
QRS complex—very wide (0.19 second)
Impression: Sinus rhythm with 1° AV block
Comment: Despite marked widening of the QRS complex, well-defined P waves precede each beat, identifying the rhythm as sinus.

Answer to Figure 3G-26

Rhythm—irregular
P waves—none, although a sawtooth pattern is evident toward the end of the tracing
QRS complex—normal duration
Impression: Atrial flutter/fibrillation with a controlled ventricular response
Comment: The rhythm is irregularly irregular. Low-amplitude undulations of the baseline (consistent with atrial fibrillation) give way to the sawtooth pattern characteristic of atrial flutter. To acknowledge that both of these atrial arrhythmias are seen, the rhythm may be designated as *atrial flutter/ fibrillation.*

Answer to Figure 3G-27

Rhythm—slightly irregular
Rate—≈ 20 beats/min
P waves—none
QRS complex—probably wide, although one cannot be certain where the QRS complex ends and the ST segment begins
Impression: slow idioventricular rhythm

Answer to Figure 3G-28

Rhythm—irregular
P waves—none
QRS complex—very wide (up to 0.30 second)
Impression: Agonal rhythm
Comment: Although this tracing superficially resembles an idioventricular rhythm, the QRS complexes are extremely wide and formless, suggesting a preterminal state. This is an agonal rhythm.

Answer to Figure 3G-29

Rhythm—irregular

P waves—none

QRS complex—probably of normal duration

Impression: CPR with underlying agonal rhythm

Comment: Apart from an occasional agonal complex, one is struck by the regular broad-based negative deflections in the baseline. These occur at a frequency of about 60/min and reflect ongoing CPR. (This tracing is *dated*—current standards recommend a chest compression rate of 80–100 times/min in adults!)

Answer to Figure 3G-30

Atrial rate and rhythm—88 beats/min and regular

Ventricular rate and rhythm—40 beats/min and regular

QRS complex—wide (0.16 second)

Impression: Complete (3°) AV block

Comment: In contrast to Figure 3G-17, the PR interval in this tracing continuously varies (the P wave "marches" through the QRS complex). This is complete AV block.

REFERENCES

Constant J: Solving nomenclature problems in cardiology. JAMA 240:868–871, 1978.

Grauer K, Curry RW: Practical electrocardiography: A primary care approach. Medical Economics Books, Oradell, 1986.

Henson JR: Descartes and the ECG lettering series. J Hist Med 26:181–186, 1971.

Marriott HJL: Arrhythmia versus dysrhythmia. Am J Cardiol 54:628, 1984.

Marriott HJL: More comments on proper terminology for the VPC (letter). Am J Cardiol 57:191–192, 1986.

Surawicz B, Uhley H, Borun R, Laks M, Crevasse L, Rosen K, Nelson W, Mandel W, Lawrence P, Jackson L, Flowers N, Clifton J, Greenfield J, Robles de Medine EO: Task Force I: Standardization of terminology and interpretation. Am J Cardiol 41:130–145, 1978.

CHAPTER 4

PUTTING IT ALL TOGETHER: PRACTICE FOR MEGA CODE

The essentials of running a code are contained within the algorithms presented in Chapter 1. The problem is that it is often difficult to memorize material presented in "algorithmic" form unless one has practice in applying it. As we often learn only too well (and too late), the ability to recite the exact sequence of an algorithm in the peace and quiet of one's own study facility in no way correlates with the ability to command instant recall of the same material in an emergency situation *(or when you are being tested at the MEGA CODE station)!*

The exercises in this chapter have been included to give you an opportunity to "put together" what has been covered previously. Four basic scenarios of cardiac arrest are presented. The rationale for treatment in these scenarios follows closely the protocols laid out in the algorithms and commentary in Chapter 1. The material is probably very similar to what you will be tested on at the MEGA CODE station. It also makes up the "bread and butter" of what you will encounter in a real code situation.

To obtain maximum benefit from these exercises, *try to put yourself at the bedside for each case.* Imagine the events transpiring before you as they might actually occur. Then assume the position of the code director and take over.

CASE STUDY A

You are working in the emergency department where a middle-aged man collapses. He cannot be aroused. A *code blue* is called, and a full complement of qualified assistants assemble around you waiting for your next command. How would you proceed?

PLAN

1) Confirm unresponsiveness.
2) Open the airway.
3) Verify apnea—then give 2 *slow,* full breaths.
4) Verify pulselessness—then begin CPR.
5) (There is no need to call for help, since you are surrounded by qualified assistants. They may be instructed to carry on CPR for you.)
6) Bring over the crash cart, turn on the defibrillator, and apply the quick-look paddles.

All of these steps are accomplished within 40 seconds, and you observe the rhythm shown in **Figure 4A-1.** What is this rhythm? How would you treat it?

ANALYSIS OF FIGURE 4A-1 AND PLAN

There is a total lack of organized electrical activity. Therefore, the rhythm is *ventricular fibrillation.*

7) Apply conductive medium to the paddles (or put on defibrillator pads), assure that no one is in contact with the patient, apply firm pressure to the paddles (pressing down with approximately 25 pounds of force), and <u>defibrillate</u> the patient with <u>200 joules</u> of delivered energy.

The patient remains pulseless and unresponsive. The quick-look paddles reveal the rhythm shown in **Figure 4A-2.** What would you do now?

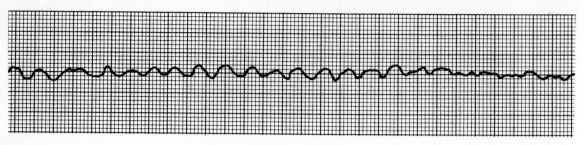

Figure 4A-1

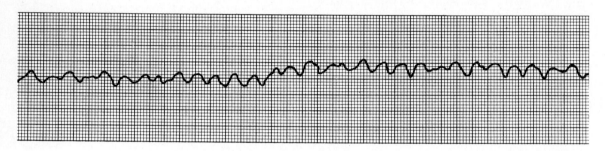

Figure 4A-2

ANALYSIS OF FIGURE 4A-2 AND PLAN

The patient is still in ventricular fibrillation.

8) Repeat <u>defibrillation</u> with <u>300 joules</u> as soon as possible.

Minimizing the time between these two electrical discharges lowers transthoracic resistance. This allows a greater amount of *current* to pass through the heart on this second countershock attempt. The new guidelines favor increasing the energy for the second defibrillation attempt to 300 joules which provides further assurance that a greater amount of current will be operating.

The patient fails to respond. He remains pulseless and in ventricular fibrillation. What should be done next?

PLAN

9) <u>Defibrillate</u> a *third* time, using full energy (<u>360 joules</u>) for this attempt.

The new guidelines have added a third countershock attempt to the suggested protocol for treatment of ventricular fibrillation. The rationale for this change is that some individuals may require maximal energy (360 joules) for conversion.

The patient remains in ventricular fibrillation. What next?

PLAN

10) Resume CPR.
11) Establish an airway and intubate the patient if possible.

Intubation is *not* recommended before the initial three defibrillation attempts, since it consumes valuable time and requires the cessation of CPR. Success at defibrillation is inversely proportional to the amount of time between the onset of ventricular fibrillation and the application of electrical countershock. (Intubation may not even be needed if defibrillation successfully restores an effective cardiac rhythm.)

12) Establish intravenous access.
13) Administer <u>1 mg</u> of <u>epinephrine</u> by either the intravenous (<u>IV</u>) or endotracheal (<u>ET</u>) route, depending on which is established first.

Administration of cardiac drugs for ventricular fibrillation is *not* recommended before the initial three countershocks if a defibrillator is available, since this would only delay the application of electrical countershock.

Note that we have not even mentioned considering **sodium bicarbonate** up to this point!!! The reason for this is that the acidosis that occurs during cardiac arrest appears to be primarily respiratory in nature (due to hyp**o**ventilation) for the first 5 to 10 minutes after patient collapse. Recommended treatment for this is to improve ventilation—*not* to give sodium bicarbonate. Sodium bicarbonate may actually worsen the situation by producing a *paradoxical* intracellular acidosis that further depresses myocardial function. Thus the new guidelines *discourage* the use of sodium bicarbonate in the usual code situation for *at least the first 10 minutes of the arrest!*

An exception to this rule may be if a preexisting metabolic acidosis was present at the time of the arrest (as in a patient with diabetic ketoacidosis or lactic acidosis) and possibly caused the arrest. However, recent data now question whether sodium bicarbonate should ever be given under such circumstances due to its potential deleterious effects.

The patient is intubated and IV access is secured with a large bore catheter inserted into the antecubital fossa. One milligram of epinephrine is given IV. This is followed by a 50 cc bolus of fluid to "flush" in the medication and by elevation of the arm to favor venous return.

It is important to secure **effective** IV access. While ideally this entails establishment of an upper torso central line (subclavian or internal jugular), a large bore IV catheter in a proximal upper extremity site such as the antecubital fossa may be almost as good when medications are "flushed" by a 50–100 cc bolus of fluid and the extremity is elevated to favor venous return.

The femoral line is no longer recommended, since we now know that blood flow below the diaphragm is minimal in the arrested heart. Establishment of a "butterfly" in a distal IV site (ie, dorsum of the wrist) is also unlikely to provide adequate access to the central circulation in a code situation.

Administration of epinephrine by the ET route is a good alternative if a large bore IV site is not available. Absorption is rapid and complete for epinephrine, although somewhat higher doses of the drug may be needed to achieve the same effects as from IV administration. At least 10 cc (= 1 mg = 1 ampule) should be injected down the ET tube and followed by several forceful insufflations of the Ambu bag.

CPR is continued. The respiratory therapist draws blood for a set of ABGs from the femoral pulse that is palpated with external chest compressions. What should you do at this point?

14) Have your assistants hook up monitoring leads or preferably an ECG machine to the patient.
15) Recheck the patient for responsiveness, the presence of a pulse, and a rhythm on the ECG.

The patient remains unresponsive. The rhythm is shown in **Figure 4A-3**. What is there to do now?

ANALYSIS OF FIGURE 4A-3 AND PLAN

Once again the rhythm is ventricular fibrillation.

16) Recheck the pulse.

It is imperative to check for a pulse after each intervention and/or whenever the rhythm changes on the monitor. Even though the rhythm

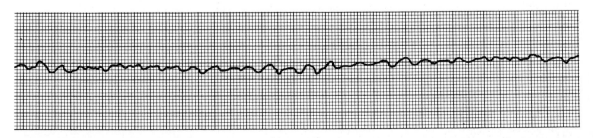

Figure 4A-3

in Figure 4A-3 still appears to be ventricular fibrillation, it is possible that a monitor lead fell off and the patient might not need defibrillation.

There is no pulse.

17) The patient should again be defibrillated since he is still in ventricular fibrillation. This fourth time, maximum delivered energy should again be used (360 joules).

The patient remains unresponsive, without a pulse, and in ventricular fibrillation. What to do?

PLAN

18) If the patient has not responded to the above measures, a trial of *antifibrillatory therapy* is indicated. Give a 50–100 mg IV bolus ($\approx$ 1 mg/kg) of lidocaine.

Whereas previous guidelines had given the nod to bretylium tosylate for this purpose, the new guidelines favor lidocaine. Studies to date have failed to demonstrate a clear superiority of one of these agents over the other. Since lidocaine may be a safer agent and most emergency care providers are more familiar and comfortable with its use, it is now recommended as the agent of choice for refractory ventricular fibrillation.

The duration of action of a lidocaine bolus in the arrested heart is significantly prolonged. Therefore one or at most two boluses of the drug are probably all that is needed. Similarly, there is no real need to begin a maintenance infusion until the spontaneous circulation is restored. However, if one chooses not to initiate a continuous IV infusion of lidocaine at this time, *it is imperative* that you remember to *do so as soon as the heart is restarted.*

19) Circulate the drug with CPR.

At least 1–2 minutes are needed to allow time for the lidocaine to reach the central circulation.

20) Defibrillate the patient again. Continue to use maximum energy (360 joules).

The patient remains in ventricular fibrillation. Unresponsive. No pulse. What next?

PLAN

21) *Look for reasons to explain the refractory ventricular fibrillation.* Was the **A**irway secure? Was mechanical **B**reathing effective? (Were good bilateral breath sounds pres-

ent? Was the Pa0$_2$ adequate?) Was **C**irculation reestablished? (Did CPR produce a pulse?) Was there some preexisting metabolic condition (diabetic ketoacidosis, hyperkalemia) that could have precipitated the arrest and which needs to be corrected?

These are some of the potentially reversible factors that might account for refractory ventricular fibrillation. Alternatively, the patient may have suffered a massive myocardial infarction or ruptured an aortic aneurysm, factors that would be extremely difficult to reverse at this point by any therapy.

22) Repeat epineprhine, giving 1 mg by either the IV or the ET route.

Epinephrine is the one drug that favors blood flow to the heart and the brain during ventricular fibrillation. It should be repeated liberally during a code situation.

23) *Consider* sodium bicarbonate.

By this time, it is likely that 10 minutes will have passed (which may be enough time for a metabolic component to the acidosis to develop), and the emergency care provider may wish to consider sodium bicarbonate administration. In a hospital situation, ABGs may help guide therapy, but one must remember that *arterial* pH is not a good reflection of *intracellular* acid-base homeostasis.

In general, sodium bicarbonate therapy is probably not warranted for a pH $\geq$ 7.15, and even then some investigators question its utility..

24) Repeat *antifibrillatory therapy.* At this point, one may either repeat a lidocaine bolus (of 50–70 mg) or turn to bretylium tosylate.

Bretylium is an effective antifibrillatory agent. Although administration of the drug rarely results in spontaneous conversion to sinus rhythm from ventricular fibrillation, it facilitates conversion with subsequent countershock. The antifibrillatory effect of the drug usually begins to work within a few minutes but occasionally is delayed for up to 10–15 minutes. Therefore, it is important not to terminate resuscitative efforts until adequate time has been allowed for the drug to work!

You choose to give bretylium and order administration of 1 ampule (500 mg) by IV bolus. The patient remains pulseless, unresponsive, and in ventricular fibrillation. What next?

PLAN

25) Resume CPR and circulate the drug for ≈ 2 minutes. Then defibrillate again.

26) If there is no response, give 10 mg/kg of bretylium (1–2 ampules), circulate the drug for ≈ 2 minutes, and defibrillate once more. Another 10 mg/kg IV bolus may be given and repeated each 15–30 minutes until a total dose of 30 mg/kg has been administered.

Following the second bolus of bretylium and the accompanying countershock, the rhythm shown in **Figure 4A-4** is noted. What to do?

ANALYSIS OF FIGURE 4A-4 AND PLAN

27) Check for a pulse!

If no pulse were present, the rhythm would be EMD! In this case, CPR would need to be resumed immediately.

A bounding pulse is present, blood pressure is 120/80 mm Hg, and the patient begins to open his eyes. What should be done before transferring the patient to the coronary care unit?

PLAN

28) Rebolus the patient with 50–75 mg of lidocaine and begin a maintenance infusion at 2 mg/min.

Discussion

This case illustrates the steps in the algorithm for resuscitation of a patient in ventricular fibrillation (see Fig. 1-2). Several points are deserving of special mention.

Notable for its absence is the precordial thump. The efficacy of this maneuver is a debatable issue. While there are reports in the literature of the thump converting patients in ventricular tachycardia and fibrillation to normal sinus rhythm, there are probably more reports showing further deterioration of the rhythm after the thump is given. On the positive side, the thump does deliver between 2 and 5 joules of energy, albeit at a random point in the cardiac cycle. At present, the thump is probably indicated only in a "no-lose" situation such as *monitored* ventricular fibrillation. That is when there is *little to lose* if the thump does not work. The thump is also indicated for witnessed cardiac arrests if a defibrillator is unavailable. This would include the situation in which an ACLS provider witnesses a patient collapse (in or out of the hospital), and there is *no pulse*. Again one would have nothing to lose by thumping, and there is a small but finite chance that the thump might provide definitive therapy. In contrast, one should *not* thump a patient who is in ventricular tachycardia if a pulse is palpable. This is because the chance that the thump might worsen the arrhythmia far outweighs any benefit that it might provide.

Thus, in this particular case study, a precordial thump was not given because the emergency care provider was on the scene with a defibrillator.

It is important to emphasize that the likelihood of successfully resuscitating a patient in cardiac arrest is inversely proportional to the interval between the onset of ventricular fibrillation and the application of countershock. Thus *all patients should be defibrillated as soon as the diagnosis of ventricular fibrillation has been estab-*

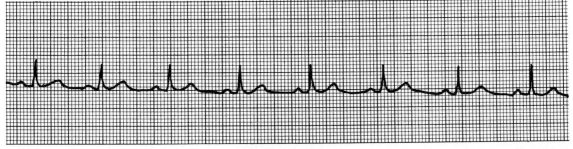

Figure 4A-4

lished. Delay for the purpose of intubation and/or starting an IV line to administer epinephrine is unwarranted and may adversely affect the chances for survival. To assure that diagnosis of ventricular fibrillation is established as soon as possible, it is advisable to always apply *quick-look paddles* as soon as the defibrillator arrives. This pertains *both* to arrests that occur inside and those that occur outside of the hospital. Application of quick-look paddles should take only seconds. If the patient is in ventricular fibrillation—countershock!

The final point is that *there is no limit to the number of times that the patient may be defibrillated!* As long as ventricular fibrillation is present, you have a *potentially* treatable rhythm. The patient in this case study was refractory to the usual treatment until after the second dose of bretylium was given. If he remained in ventricular fibrillation beyond this point, repetition of steps 21 through 26 in the above sequence would be in order. This would entail the additional use of epinephrine (and possibly sodium bicarbonate), a third dose of bretylium (and/or repetition of the lidocaine bolus), and further attempts at defibrillation until the patient was either converted out of ventricular fibrillation or cardiovascular unresponsiveness could be conclusively established.

CASE STUDY B

You are on call making your rounds when a *code blue* is called. You run to the room of the code and find numerous hospital personnel standing around the bed of an elderly woman who is awake and alert but a little bit short of breath. She is not having any chest pain. The ECG monitor reflects the rhythm shown in **Figure 4B-1.**

What is the rhythm? What should you do?

ANALYSIS OF FIGURE 4B-1 AND PLAN

The first thing to do is to take your own pulse! Although the rhythm on the monitor is extremely worrisome, the patient (at least for the moment) is awake, alert, and appears to be *hemodynamically stable!*

1) Check the patient's blood pressure.
2) Remember the four questions and systematically analyze the arrhythmia.

The patient's blood pressure is 90/60 mm Hg.

The rhythm in Figure 4B-1 is a wide complex tachycardia at a heart rate of about 150 beats/min. No P waves are evident. The differential should include **five** entities:

    i) VENTRICULAR TACHYCARDIA
    ii) VENTRICULAR TACHYCARDIA
    iii) VENTRICULAR TACHYCARDIA
    iv) Supraventricular tachycardia with a preexisting bundle branch block
    v) Supraventricular tachycardia with aberrant conduction

Although there is some irregularity to the rhythm and the patient is awake and alert, *VEN-*

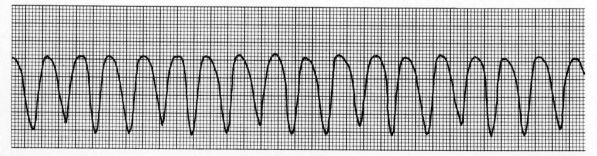

Figure 4B-1

TRICULAR TACHYCARDIA must be assumed until proved otherwise!

The point cannot be overemphasized that not everybody with ventricular tachycardia decompensates immediately. Patients may remain in sustained VT for minutes and even *hours* at a time. This is especially likely to occur if the rate of the VT is not excessively rapid, as is the case in this example. Hemodynamic decompensation develops much quicker with heart rates of ≥200 beats/min.

There are a number of diagnostic steps one may follow to help resolve the question of whether the above rhythm could possibly be supraventricular. One of the simplest measures is to look for a previous ECG recording from the patient to see what the QRS complex looks like when sinus rhythm is present. Other measures including QRS morphology and what to look for on physical examination are discussed in detail in Chapter 15. For now, *one must assume that a regular (or fairly regular) wide complex tachycardia is ventricular tachycardia until proved otherwise—and treat accordingly.*

3) Consider <u>cough version</u>.

Although the mechanism is not exactly clear, instructing a patient who is still conscious to forcefully cough at the onset of ventricular tachycardia will occasionally convert the tachyarrhythmia to sinus rhythm.

4) Administer a 50–100 mg IV bolus of <u>lidocaine</u>. Begin an infusion at 2 mg/min.
5) Think ahead. Anticipate the *worst* that could happen. (This would be for the patient to suddenly decompensate by a drop in blood pressure, a loss of pulse, and/or development of ventricular fibrillation.)

Anticipating what may happen may be helpful in two ways. First, it allows you to prepare the next line of medications and/or therapeutic modalities that you will turn to if your present therapy does not work. Second, and equally important, is that thinking ahead and being able to formulate your next plan of attack often has a calming effect and increases your confidence in being able to successfully manage the problem.

The lidocaine has not had any effect. The rhythm is unchanged. The patient is still alert, fairly comfortable, and has a blood pressure of 90/60 mm Hg. What to do now?

PLAN

6) Repeat the lidocaine bolus in several minutes. If there is no response, a third dose of this drug may be given in 5 more minutes.

Still no response. What are your options at this point?

PLAN

7) Try <u>procainamide</u>. One may administer this drug by giving 100 mg IV increments over a 5 minute period (at 20 mg/min) until the patient has received a loading dose of 500–1000 mg, the arrhythmia is suppressed, or hypotension or QRS widening occurs.

Alternatively, 500–1000 mg of procainamide may be diluted in 100 cc of D5W and infused over 30–60 minutes.

Following loading, a maintenance infusion of procainamide may be started at 2 mg/min.

8) Try <u>bretylium</u>. When used to treat ventricular tachycardia, the drug should be administered as a slow IV loading infusion. Mix 500 mg (1 ampule) in 50 cc of D5W and drip in over 10 minutes. If successful, this may be followed by a maintenance infusion at 1–2 mg/min.

Because of its propensity to cause hypotension, the new guidelines have deemphasized bretylium and made it a *third*-line agent for ventricular tachycardia that should probably only be tried if neither lidocaine nor procainamide is effective.

9) <u>Cardiovert</u> the patient. If the patient is still hemodynamically stable at this point, synchronized cardioversion may be carried out under "semielective" circumstances. This includes sedation (with Valium or another agent), calling anesthesia to the bedside to assist with intubation if needed (leaving you free to concentrate on managing the arrhythmia), and a trial at low energies (50 joules, then 100 joules, and then 200 joules).

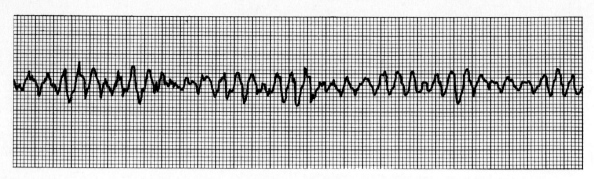

Figure 4B-2

If lidocaine is unsuccessful in converting the patient out of VT, the emergency care provider may choose to either cardiovert or give a trial to procainamide and/or bretylium. The choice of therapy will depend both on the clinical situation and personal preference.

The three boluses of lidocaine you have given have not been effective. You are about to begin administering procainamide when the patient suddenly loses consciousness. The pulse has weakened, yet the rhythm on the monitor remains unchanged. What should you do?

PLAN

10) One should carry out the plan formulated earlier. Since you are now dealing with ventricular tachycardia which has become *hemodynamically unstable,* immediate cardioversion is in order. There is no time (or need in an unconscious patient) for sedation. Use at least 100 joules.

Immediately following synchronized cardioversion with 200 joules, the rhythm shown in **Figure 4B-2** develops. The patient is unresponsive and there is no pulse. What is the rhythm? What do you do?

ANALYSIS OF FIGURE 4B-2 AND PLAN

The patient has gone into ventricular fibrillation.

11) Shut off the synchronized mode and immediately defibrillate the patient with maximum energy (360 joules).

Considering that the likelihood of successfully resuscitating a patient in ventricular fibrillation is inversely proportional to the interval between the onset of this rhythm and the application of countershock, this is probably the best chance you will ever have of converting a patient in ventricular fibrillation. You are right on the scene with a defibrillator and should be able to apply countershock immediately.

Your immediate defibrillation results in the rhythm shown in **Figure 4B-3.** What do you do now?

ANALYSIS OF FIGURE 4B-3 AND PLAN

Sinus tachycardia at a heart rate of 125 beats/min is seen on the monitor.

12) Check for a pulse and blood pressure.

The pulse is strong and the blood pressure is 140/80 mm Hg. The patient is regaining consciousness.

Note that the QRS morphology in this lead is very different from what it was during the wide complex tachycardia (Figure 4B-1). This rules out a preexisting bundle branch block as the etiology for the rhythm in Figure 4B-1 and adds credence to our previous assumption that ventricular tachycardia was present.

13) Maintain the patient on at least a lidocaine infusion.

Discussion

This case illustrates the steps in the algorithm for sustained ventricular tachycardia (see Fig. 1-3). The *key* factor resides in the first step: *iden-*

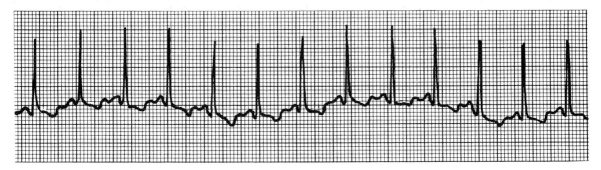

Figure 4B-3

tification of VT and assessment of hemodynamic status. If a patient is hemodynamically compromised, it matters little whether a tachyarrhythmia is supraventricular or not. The treatment is the same—emergency cardioversion to stabilize the patient. On the other hand, if the patient is stable one has the luxury of trying antiarrhythmic agents and/or synchronized cardioversion on a "semielective" basis. However, if decompensation occurs at any time during treatment, immediate cardioversion with at least 100 joules is in order.

CASE STUDY C

You are obtaining a history from a middle-aged man who has just been admitted to the coronary care unit for chest pain. He is still wearing a nitroglycerin patch on his chest which he had put on at home that morning. He has received two sublingual nitroglycerin tablets since arriving in the hospital. A peripheral IV of D5W at KVO has been inserted. Blood pressure is 110/70 mm Hg, the monitor shows sinus rhythm, and the patient is complaining of only mild chest discomfort when he suddenly collapses. You note the rhythm shown in **Figure 4C-1** on the monitor. What do you do?

ANALYSIS OF FIGURE 4C-1 AND PLAN

The patient is in *ventricular fibrillation.*

1) Confirm unresponsiveness. Verify pulselessness. Deliver a <u>precordial thump</u>. Then yell for help and begin CPR.

This is one indication for the precordial thump—the onset of ventricular fibrillation has been witnessed by an ACLS provider. There is little to lose (the patient is pulseless), and definitive backup in the form of a defibrillator will soon be on hand.

Several CCU nurses with a crash cart and defibrillator immediately join you in the room. What do you do next?

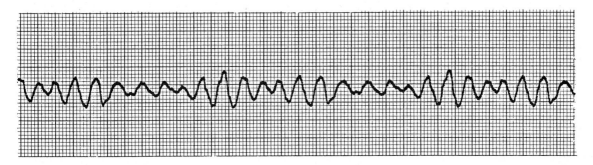

Figure 4C-1

PLAN

2) <u>Defibrillate</u> the patient with <u>200 joules</u> of delivered energy.

> As always before defibrillating, it is essential for the *code director* (YOU!) to verify that no one is in contact with the patient. Add conductive medium to the paddles and apply firm pressure to the paddles when discharging.

In this particular case, what else should have been done before defibrillating?

Answer

The patient's chest should have been wiped clean and the nitroglycerin patch removed *before* defibrillating. Nitroglycerin is an excellent conductive medium. If a patch is left on the chest of a patient who is defibrillated, sparks may fly (and/or much worse could happen).

Defibrillation is successful in producing the rhythm shown in **Figure 4C-2.** What is the rhythm? How would you proceed?

PLAN

3) Check for a pulse!

> Even before attempting to interpret the rhythm, it is essential to determine if a pulse is present. If not, this would be EMD which would mandate immediate resumption of CPR and a different therapeutic approach.

Despite the fact that the patient is unresponsive, a pulse is present and a palpable blood pressure of 60 mm Hg is obtained. What is the rhythm?

ANALYSIS OF FIGURE 4C-2

A bradyarrhythmia is seen in which the QRS complex is wide and the ventricular rate regular at 35–40 beats/min. The atrial rate is also fairly regular at about 90 beats/min. However, P waves "march through the QRS complex" and are totally unrelated to it (the PR interval constantly changes). This is *complete (3°) AV block*.

4) Administer <u>atropine</u>.

> The suggested protocol for administration of this drug is to give 0.5 mg IV every 5 minutes until a total dose of 2 mg has been given. At this slow heart rate and with this low blood pressure, an initial dose of 1 mg of atropine would be reasonable. Alternatively, considering the patient's unstable hemodynamic status, if one chose to give only 0.5 mg initially, one might repeat the dose in *less* than 5 minutes (that is, in 2–3 min) if the desired clinical response was not obtained.

5) Insert a <u>transvenous pacemaker</u>. This is the treatment of choice for hemodynamically significant 3° AV block that develops in the setting of cardiac arrest.

One milligram of atropine has had no effect. You request assistance from the cardiologist for pacemaker insertion, but it will be at least 10 minutes before the person on call can get there. What to do in the meantime?

PLAN

6) Intubate the patient.
7) Repeat the atropine. Give the second 1 mg dose.
8a) While you are doing this, have your nurse prepare the pressor agent of your choice in the event that the atropine is not effective.

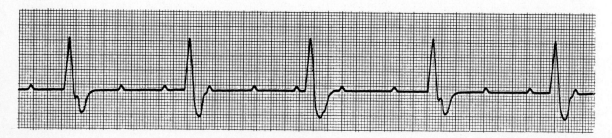

Figure 4C-2

Either dopamine or isoproterenol is commonly used in this setting. At low-to-moderate infusion rates (2–10 μg/kg/min), dopamine primarily exerts a beta-adrenergic effect which increases heart rate and stroke volume without necessarily increasing blood pressure. The alpha-adrenergic (vasoconstrictor) effect becomes more prominent at infusion rates of > 10 μg/kg/min. One usually begins the infusion at 2–5 μg/kg/min and titrates the rate to clinical response.

Isoproterenol provides *chronotropic* support. It does this by its potent pure beta-adrenergic effect. Cardiac output usually goes up—ideally not at the expense of excessive peripheral vasodilation and increase in myocardial oxygen consumption.

Epinephrine by infusion could also be chosen; however, because of its alpha-adrenergic activity (which acts to vasoconstrict and increase afterload), its use might better be reserved for slower bradyarrhythmias with more dire hemodynamic compromise.

Regardless of which drug is chosen, however, the point to emphasize is that use of a pressor agent for treatment of an atropine-resistant, hemodynamically significant bradyarrhythmia should be *only* as a stopgap measure until a transvenous pacemaker can be inserted.

or

8b) Set up an external pacemaker.

This noninvasive device may be effective *temporizing* therapy for use with hemodynamically significant bradyarrhythmias while awaiting more definitive treatment (insertion of a transvenous pacemaker). An obvious advantage over pharmacologic therapy is that the external pacemaker does not produce potentially adverse hemodynamic effects (uncontrolled tachycardia, arrhythmias, increased oxygen consumption). If a *reliable* unit is available, this may be the way to go.

The second milligram of atropine also has no effect. An isoproterenol infusion is begun. The response shown in **Figure 4C-3** occurred moments later. A weak pulse is present with this rhythm, but it is hard to obtain a blood pressure. The patient is unresponsive. What should you do?

ANALYSIS OF FIGURE 4C-3 AND PLAN

Halfway through the rhythm strip, *ventricular tachycardia* supervenes.

9) Stop the isoproterenol!

It is easy to lose track of what medications have been given during a code and what infusions are running. If initiation of an infusion of a pressor agent results in an adverse effect, the infusion must be stopped immediately!

10) Consider delivering a precordial thump.
11) And/or cardiovert the patient with 100–200 joules.

This would be another indication for the thump. When ventricular tachycardia is accompanied by a pulse, a thump should be delivered *only* if a defibrillator is *on hand,* so that in the event that the thump results in deterioration of the rhythm the patient can be immediately cardioverted. Alternatively, many emergency care providers prefer not to use the thump in this situation and go immediately instead to cardioversion. The ability to synchronize the electrical discharge at a precise point in the cardiac cycle is perhaps preferable to the random delivery of the small amount of energy that the thump provides.

Because of the unstable state of the above patient, cardioversion with *at least* 100 joules is ad-

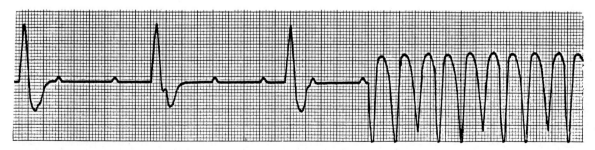

Figure 4C-3

vised. A trial of cardioversion with lower energy levels should probably be reserved for tachyarrhythmias that occur in a more stable patient.

You raise your clenched fist about a foot over the patient's chest and come down forcefully on his midsternum with a firm blow. **Figure 4C-4** shows the fruit of your labor. What to do?

ANALYSIS OF FIGURE 4C-4 AND PLAN

Your precordial thump has precipitated *ventricular fibrillation*.

12) Immediately defibrillate the patient. Use 200 joules.

> Since 200 joules was effective in converting the patient out of ventricular fibrillation at the onset of the code, this energy level should again be tried at this point.

The arrow in **Figure 4C-5** indicates the point at which the electrical discharge was delivered. What has happened?

ANALYSIS OF FIGURE 4C-5 AND PLAN

Defibrillation has resulted in *asystole*.

13) Verify pulselessness. Then resume CPR.
14) Administer 1 mg of epinephrine by either the IV or the ET route.

> You have already administered the usually complete vagolytic dose of atropine (ie, 2 mg). Sodium bicarbonate is *not* indicated at this point since you are adequately preforming CPR and ventilating the patient.

The 1 mg of epinephrine produces the rhythm shown in **Figure 4C-6.** What next?

ANALYSIS OF FIGURE 4C-6 AND PLAN

Ventricular fibrillation is again evident. Considering the patient was in asystole, this is a beneficial response. This is a rhythm you can treat!

15) Defibrillate the patient with 200 joules.

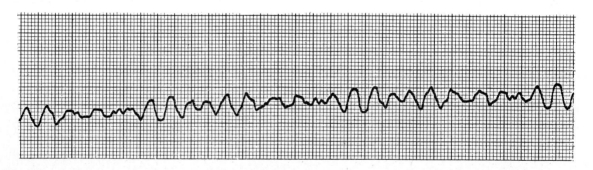

Figure 4C-4

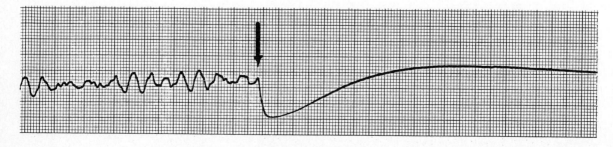

Figure 4C-5

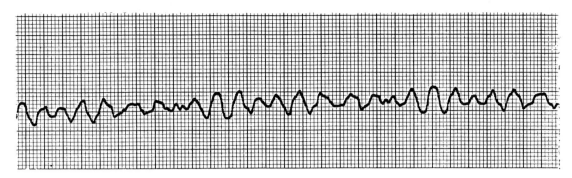

Figure 4C-6

Since the last defibrillation attempt produced asystole, it may be advisable to remain at the lower energy level of 200 joules for this attempt.

The result of defibrillation is shown in **Figure 4C-7.** What next?

ANALYSIS OF FIGURE 4C-7 AND PLAN

The monitor shows *normal sinus rhythm.*

16) Check for a pulse.

A strong pulse is present. Blood pressure is 130/85 mm Hg.

17) Verify again that good breath sounds are present bilaterally and that the isoproterenol infusion that you previously ordered is *off.* Obtain ABGs, a chest x-ray (for endotracheal tube placement), 12-lead ECG, and blood chemistries (as indicated),

and

18) Give <u>lidocaine</u>. Administer a 50–100 mg IV bolus and start a drip at 2 mg/min.

It is extremely important to remember to initiate prophylactic lidocaine as soon as a patient is converted out of ventricular fibrillation and into a stable rhythm to minimize the chance of recurrence.

Discussion

In addition to reviewing the early management of witnessed ventricular fibrillation and hemodynamically unstable ventricular tachycardia, this case illustrates many of the steps in the algorithm for treatment of bradyarrhythmias (see Fig. 1-4).

Despite reasonable treatment and a successful final outcome, things did not go quite as well as they might have. Initial defibrillation was carried out with a nitroglycerin patch still on the patient's chest. Administration of isoproterenol precipitated ventricular tachycardia. Delivery of the precordial thump caused this rhythm to deteriorate into ventricular fibrillation, and then countershock resulted in further deterioration to asystole.

While hindsight is 100% and one can never assure success even if a correct treatment se-

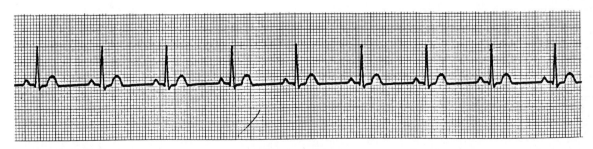

Figure 4C-7

quence is followed perfectly, thoughtful review of the events of a code immediately *after* the acute situation has passed may provide the emergency care provider with valuable insight that proves useful with future resuscitation efforts.

CASE STUDY D

You are called to the emergency department where a *code in progress* has just been brought in. The patient is an elderly woman who had been found at home unresponsive. The time from collapse until arrival of the EMS unit is unknown. CPR is being performed, the patient is intubated, and a large bore peripheral IV is in place. One ampule of sodium bicarbonate and two ampules of epinephrine have already been given. Nothing else has been done. The patient is unresponsive. There is no spontaneous pulse, and monitor leads reveal the rhythm shown in **Figure 4D-1.** What do you do?

ANALYSIS OF FIGURE 4D-1 AND PLAN

The patient is in *ventricular fibrillation*.

1) Defibrillate with 200 joules of delivered energy.

What should have been done before your arrival?

Answer

The patient should have been defibrillated!

Electrical defibrillation is by far the most important therapeutic intervention we have for treatment of ventricular fibrillation. Therefore, as soon as one documents the presence of this rhythm, the patient should be defibrillated. Delay for the purpose of intubating the patient and/or insertion of an IV is unacceptable. Quick-look paddles facilitate the process of documentation and save precious seconds that are wasted if time is taken to put monitor leads on.

There is no response. The rhythm shown in Figure 4D-1 persists. What next?

PLAN

2) Verify pulselessness, immediately recharge the defibrillator paddles, and defibrillate again—this time with 300 joules.

Once again there is no response. What next?

PLAN

3) Verify pulselessness, immediately recharge the defibrillator paddles, and defibrillate a third time—this time with 360 joules.

The patient is converted to the rhythm shown in **Figure 4D-2.** What next?

PLAN

4) Check for a pulse.

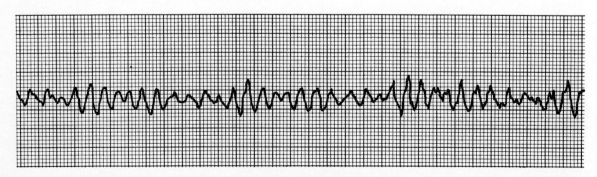

Figure 4D-1

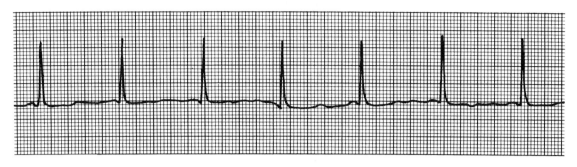

Figure 4D-2

There is *no pulse!!!*

What does this mean? What treatment is indicated?

ANALYSIS AND PLAN

By definition the patient is in EMD, since there is organized electrical activity (the rhythm shown in Figure 4D-2) but no effective mechanical contraction (the lack of a pulse).

5) Resume CPR.
6) Repeat the epinephrine.
7) Look for a *potentially reversible* cause of the EMD.

An ampule of epinephrine is given. Lung auscultation reveals no breath sounds on the left. After withdrawal of the endotracheal tube "a tad," bilateral breath sounds can be heard. Shortly thereafter, a weak pulse is felt. Blood pressure is 70 mm Hg systolic. What to do?

PLAN

8a) Begin dopamine.

> Prepare the drip by mixing 1 ampule of drug (200 mg) in 250 cc of D5W and begin the infusion at 15–30 drops/min ($\approx$2–5 μg/kg/min).

or

8b) Consider a trial of volume infusion.

Dopamine is begun and the blood pressure increases to 100/70 mm Hg. What should be done at this point? Sinus rhythm is still present on the monitor.

PLAN

9) Load the patient with a 50–100 mg IV bolus of lidocaine and begin an infusion at 2 mg/min.

> Once again, administration of lidocaine after a patient is converted out of ventricular fibirllation into a stable rhythm is strongly recommended as a prophylactic measure in the hope of preventing a recurrence of the event.

The patient is transferred to the coronary care unit.

Discussion

This case underscores the importance of *always* checking for a pulse after every intervention or change in the patient's status or cardiac rhythm. Production of an esthetic-looking sinus rhythm on the monitor means little when there is no accompanying pulse. EMD is then the diagnosis.

In most cases, EMD is *secondary* to some underlying disorder which must be discovered and corrected. **Table 4D-1** highlights the most common underlying etiologies to consider when confronted with a patient having this disorder.

Therapeutically, the first thing to do is to resume CPR, since by definition EMD is a *nonperfusing* rhythm. Following this, epinephrine should be given. The reason epinephrine is important is that it favors blood flow to the heart and brain. Some cases of EMD are thought to be *primary*—that is, due to diffuse myocardial ischemia (Ewy, 1984). This may develop as the

TABLE 4D-1:   UNDERLYING ETIOLOGIES OF ELECTROMECHANICAL DISSOCIATION*

Inadequate Ventilation
● Intubation of right mainstem bronchus ● Tension pneumothorax (trauma, asthma, patient on ventilator) ● Bilateral pneumothorax (trauma)
Inadequate Circulation

● Pericardial effusion with tamponade (trauma, pericarditis, uremia, too vigorous CPR)
● Myocardial rupture or rupture of aortic aneurysm
● Massive pulmonary embolism
● Hypovolemia due to:
   —Acute blood loss (trauma, GI bleeding)
   —Dehydration
   —Septic shock
   —Cardiogenic shock (acute myocardial infarction, myocardial contusion)
   —Anaphylactic shock
   —Neurogenic shock (cervical spine fracture)

Metabolic Disorders
● Persistent acidosis (diabetic ketoacidosis, lactic acidosis) ● Electrolyte disturbance (hyperkalemia, hypokalemia) ● Overdose of cardiac depressant drugs

*Reproduced with permission from Grauer K: New Trends in the Management of Cardiac Arrest. AFP **29:**223, 1984.

end point following prolonged and unsuccessful attempts at resuscitating ventricular fibrillation. Occasionally, however, inadequate coronary perfusion per se may precipitate EMD. In such instances, treatment directed at optimizing myocardial blood flow may be effective, and epinephrine is an ideal agent for accomplishing this (Nieman et al., 1986).

If a patient with EMD doesn't respond to epinephrine, a vigorous search for an underlying *secondary* etiology must be undertaken (Table 4D-1). If EMD is due to rupture of an aortic aneurysm or massive pulmonary embolism, there will be little one can do to save the patient. On the other hand, a number of *potentially reversible* causes of EMD are listed in the table. The first thing to check for is **adequacy of ventilation.** Absence of breath sounds on the left suggests intubation of the right mainstem bron-chus. Simply withdrawing the endotracheal tube a small distance should restore bilateral breath sounds (as it did in this case). If this maneuver is not successful and/or breath sounds are absent on the right and tracheal deviation is present, the possibility of tension pneumothorax should be considered. One's index of suspicion for tension pneumothorax should be further aroused in association with significant trauma and in patients with asthma or chronic obstructive pulmonary disease, particularly if they have been on a ventilator. If time does not allow for radiographic confirmation, a diagnostic and therapeutic tap with a large-bore needle (or Heimlich valve) should be performed in the second or third intercostal space. The needle should be inserted over the top of the rib (to avoid the intercostal vessels that run along the lower border of each rib) and in the midclavicular line (to avoid the internal mammary artery that lies medially). Air under tension produces a hissing sound, and prompt improvement of the patient's hemodynamic condition usually follows.

If inadequate ventilation is not the problem, attention should be directed to **assessing volume status.** Was the patient dehydrated on admission? Is there cardiogenic shock from a massive myocardial infarction? Was the patient at risk for throwing a pulmonary embolus? Was there a known aortic aneurysm? Could the patient have been in septic shock? Even without an obvious cause of hypovolemia, strong consideration should be given to administration of a fluid challenge at this point.

Other potentially reversible causes of EMD in a hospitalized patient include **persistent acidosis** (diabetic ketoacidosis, lactic acidosis) **electrolyte disturbance** (hyperkalemia, hypokalemia), and pericardial effusion with **tamponade.** Obtaining ABGs and serum electrolyte studies will aid in the investigation of the first two possibilities. If tamponade is suggested by the history (uremia, pericarditis, fractured ribs from too vigorous CPR) and/or the physical examination (jugular venous distention, muffled heart sounds), pericardiocentesis should be performed. Withdrawing as little as 50 ml of fluid under these circumstances may be lifesaving.

Emergency pericardiocentesis is best performed through a subxiphoid approach with insertion of the needle at a 20° to 30° angle with the frontal plane. The needle should be directed toward the tip of the left shoulder, and aspiration should be continuous. Entry into the pericardium usually produces a distinct "giving" sensation that should be followed by the appearance of nonclotting blood in the syringe. If the blood clots, it most likely has been removed from the right ventricle.

Finally, EMD that occurs with **trauma** should prompt the emergency care provider to actively consider an alternative set of causes. The mechanism of injury may be enlightening. Learning that a victim's automobile was demolished in a high-speed freeway accident in which the patient's chest deformed the steering wheel before his head crashed through the windshield should suggest at least four possible etiologies to explain EMD including:

—acute blood loss (internal hemorrhage from abdominal injury, pelvic fracture, etc.)
—cardiogenic shock from myocardial contusion (the result of the steering wheel injury)
—neurogenic shock from cervical spine injury
—pericardial tamponade, bilateral pneumothorax, or tension pneumothorax from trauma to the chest wall.

REFERENCES

Ewy GA: Defining electromechanical dissociation. Ann Emerg Med **13:**830, 1984.

Niemann JT, Haynes KS, Garner D, Rennie CJ, Jagels G, Stormo O: Postcountershock pulseless rhythms: Response to CPR, artificial cardiac pacing, and adrenergic agonists. Ann Emerg Med **15:**112, 1986.

CHAPTER 5

FINDING THE ERROR: MORE PRACTICE FOR MEGA CODE

This chapter has been added to provide a final practice for MEGA CODE. Six code vignettes are presented. One or more flagrant errors in treatment have been made. You are asked to review the sequence of events and to "find the error."

The points brought out by these scenarios should once again reinforce the principles that are essential to master in order to effectively run a cardiac arrest. Recognition of these errors and understanding why the treatment given was not the most appropriate are important preparatory exercises for MEGA CODE.

EXERCISE A

Preceding Scenario

A middle-aged man of average ($\approx$70 kg) size is admitted to the coronary care unit (CCU) with chest pain to rule out acute myocardial infarction. He is on oxygen and has received some morphine but no other medications. Shortly thereafter the rhythm shown in **Figure 5A-1** is noted on telemetry.

Present Scenario

Clinical: The patient is complaining of mild chest discomfort. He appears to be relatively comfortable.

Hemodynamic status: BP = 90 palpable.

Sequential treatment given for present scenario:

1) Lidocaine—75 mg IV bolus
2) Bretylium—mix 500 mg in 50 cc of D5W and infuse over 10 minutes. Then start constant infusion at 1–2 mg/min.
3) Epinephrine—1 mg IV
4) Defibrillate with 200 joules

Your Impressions:

Your Interpretation of Figure 5A-1

Agree with Treatment Given? What Might You Do Differently?

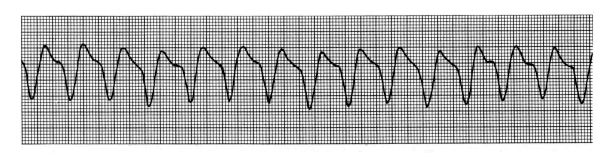

Figure 5A-1

Analysis

RHYTHM INTERPRETATION

A regular, wide QRS complex tachycardia is present at a rate of about 115 beats/min. One must assume this to be *ventricular tachycardia* until proved otherwise.

TREATMENT ANALYSIS

While the rate of the VT is not extremely rapid, this patient has been admitted with suspected acute myocardial infarction, and he has mild chest discomfort with a borderline blood pressure—all causes for concern. Treatment is therefore definitely indicated.

Because the patient is conscious, appears relatively comfortable, and is maintaining a blood pressure of 90 mm Hg, a *brief* trial of medical therapy is reasonable. Were hemodynamic decompensation to occur at any time during such therapy, immediate *synchronized* cardioversion would be indicated.

Alternatively, some emergency care providers might argue that cardioversion should be performed initially, given the patient's borderline hemodynamic status. This approach would also be reasonable. Were this the path you chose, you would have time to sedate the patient, call anesthesia to the bedside, and select a relatively low energy level (50 joules) for the initial cardioversion attempt.

If you preferred to begin with medical therapy, lidocaine would definitely be the drug of choice. The initial bolus prescribed (75 mg) is an appropriate amount for a patient this size. How-ever, a constant infusion of the drug should have been started at the time the bolus was given.

Administration of bretylium is *not* the next step. Although bretylium is an effective *antifibrillatory* agent, it is recommended only as a *third-line* drug for treatment of ventricular tachycardia. Lidocaine *and* procainamide in therapeutic doses should generally be tried before turning to bretylium. In this particular case, if the initial 75 mg IV bolus of lidocaine didn't work, the next step would be to rebolus with one or more additional 50–75 mg doses of lidocaine before moving on to procainamide.

Administration of epinephrine is obviously wrong. This potent chronotropic and inotropic agent would serve only to make the arrhythmia worse. Epinephrine is the drug of choice for *ventricular fibrillation,* but it is contraindicated with ventricular tachycardia. Finally, the patient should not have been defibrillated with an unsynchronized countershock. If electrical therapy were needed, energy delivery should be by *synchronized* cardioversion for ventricular tachycardia with a pulse so as to minimize the chance of the shock falling on the T wave (the vulnerable period) and precipitating ventricular fibrillation.

EXERCISE B

Preceding Scenario

An EMS unit is called to the scene of a cardiac arrest. The victim is an elderly woman who has

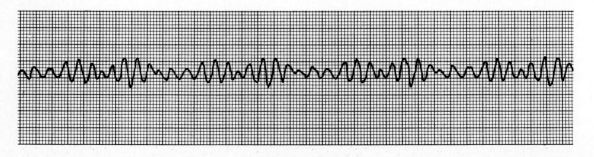

Figure 5B-1

been down for an estimated "5 minutes" before arrival. CPR was performed by a witness at the scene. The paramedics have intubated the patient and secured a peripheral IV line. The rhythm observed on quick-look paddles is shown in **Figure 5B-1.**

Present Scenario

Clinical: The patient is unresponsive.

Hemodynamic status: No pulse. No blood pressure.

Sequential treatment given for present scenario:

1) Epinephrine—1mg by IV or ET
2) Sodium bicarbonate—2 ampules IV
3) Defibrillate with 300 joules
4) Defibrillate with 360 joules
5) Bretylium—500 mg IV

Your Impressions:

Your Interpretation of Figure 5B-1

Agree with Treatment Given? What Would You Do Differently?

Analysis

RHYTHM INTERPRETATION

This is *ventricular fibrillation.*

TREATMENT ANALYSIS

The key to treating ventricular fibrillation is defibrillation of the patient *as soon as possible.* Although quick-look paddles were used on the scene here to identify the initial rhythm of the arrest, defibrillation was unnecessarily delayed! Clearly the patient should have been defibrillated *before* being intubated, having an IV

started, and receiving epinephrine and sodium bicarbonate.

The recommended energy level for initial defibrillation is 200 joules—not the 300 joules that were administered in this scenario. The lower energy level is equally effective yet less likely to produce asystole or other conduction disturbance. If initial defibrillation is unsuccessful, a second countershock attempt with increased energy (300 joules) should be tried, to be followed in rapid succession by a *third* attempt with maximal energy (360 joules). Only two attempts at defibrillation were made in this case.

If countershock is unsuccessful in converting ventricular fibrillation, epinephrine is the drug of choice. It was correctly given here in the appropriate dose. However, it may not yet have been time for sodium bicarbonate. The acidosis that develops during the early minutes of cardiac arrest is primarily respiratory in nature. A significant metabolic component usually does not develop for *at least* 5–10 min after patient collapse. Sodium bicarbonate probably should not be ordered before this time has elapsed unless evidence of a preexisting metabolic acidosis is present or ventricular fibrillation remains refractory to other therapy. Even in the setting of a severe metabolic acidosis, some investigators now question the utility of sodium bicarbonate and refrain from its use due to the potential deleterious effects of this drug (i.e., production of a paradoxical intracellular acidosis).

Bretylium has become a *second-line* agent for refractory ventricular fibrillation. It is recommended that a bolus of lidocaine be tried first. If this is unsuccessful, one then has the option of either repeating the lidocaine or changing to bretylium.

Because of the markedly decreased clearance of lidocaine in the arrested heart, it is not essential to start an infusion of this drug as long as ventricular fibrillation persists. Once converted out of ventricular fibrillation, however, the patient should be rebolused with lidocaine, and an infusion begun.

The final point to emphasize about antifibrillatory therapy (with lidocaine or bretylium) is that by itself the drug rarely results in spontaneous conversion of ventricular fibrillation. Instead, CPR must be performed for 1–2 min following administration in order to circulate the drug, and only then should defibrillation be repeated.

EXERCISE C

Preceding Scenario

An elderly man is admitted to the CCU for chest pain which is relieved by small doses of

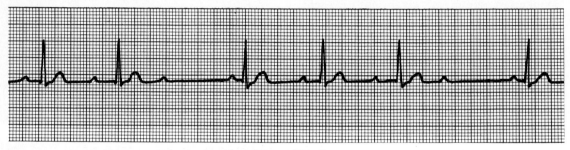

Figure 5C-1

morphine and nitroglycerin. ECG shows sinus rhythm and acute inferior myocardial infarction. Shortly thereafter the rhythm shown in **Figure 5C-1** is noted.

Present Scenario

Clinical: The patient is comfortable and is not having any more chest pain.

Hemodynamic status: Blood pressure is 110/70 mm Hg.

Sequential treatment given for present scenario:
1) Atropine—1 mg IV
2) Consult cardiology for transvenous pacemaker insertion
3) While waiting, repeat the 1 mg dose of atropine

Your Impressions:

Your Interpretation of Figure 5C-1

Agree with Treatment Given? What Would You Do Differently?

Analysis

RHYTHM INTERPRETATION

Although the ventricular response is not regular, the atrial rate for the most part is. Each QRS complex is preceded by a P wave, and the PR interval gradually increases until a beat is dropped. This is *2° AV block Mobitz type I (Wenckebach)*.

TREATMENT ANALYSIS

Mobitz I 2° AV block occurs much more commonly than does the Mobitz II variety of 2° AV block. This is fortunate because, in general, prognosis for Mobitz I is much better than it is for Mobitz II.

Mobitz I is frequently seen in the setting of acute inferior myocardial infarction. Patients usually are hemodynamically stable and do *not* require treatment. The conduction disturbance most often resolves spontaneously, and pacemaker insertion is *rarely* needed. Such is the case in this example.

In contrast, Mobitz II more often occurs in association with acute anterior myocardial infarction. The block is usually lower down in the conduction system. Consequently, the QRS complex is almost always wide (whereas it is most often narrow with Mobitz I), and the ventricular response is slower and less reliable. Pacemaker insertion is essential.

Atropine should not be given for either conduction disturbance unless there are clear signs of hemodynamic compromise. It is important to emphasize that this drug is *not* a benign medication. Activity of *both* sympathetic and parasympathetic components of the autonomic nervous system is often increased with acute myocardial infarction. With inferior infarction, parasympathetic tone usually predominates, which is why one commonly sees associated bradycardia and hypotension. Administration of vagolytic doses of atropine blocks this parasympathetic tone. If underlying sympathetic hyperactivity was also present, however, it may now be unopposed. Giving atropine may thus result in tachycardia, increased oxygen consumption, and potentially serious tachyarrhythmias. Because of this, atropine should be administered with caution to patients with myocardial infarction, with the dose being limited to 0.5 mg at a time if the patient shows only signs of "mild" hemodynamic compromise. In contrast, when heart rate is markedly decreased (40 beats/min or less) and blood pressure is extremely low (60 mm Hg systolic or less), administration of 1 mg increments of atropine is reasonable. In this patient, the blood pressure was normal and he was asymptomatic, so *no atropine at all was indicated.*

EXERCISE D

Preceding Scenario

An elderly woman arrests in the outpatient clinic. She is immediately attended to by the staff, who utilize the clinic crash cart at the scene. An initial rhythm of ventricular fibrillation responds to the first 200 joule countershock attempt and converts to the rhythm shown in **Figure 5D-1.** An IV of D5W has been started.

Present Scenario

Clinical: The patient is unresponsive and is not spontaneously breathing.

Hemodynamic status: No pulse. No blood pressure.

Sequential treatment given for present scenario:
1) Intubate the patient
2) Atropine—1 mg IV. Repeat another 1 mg in short order if no response
3) Sodium bicarbonate—2 ampules
4) Isoproterenol—mix 1 g in 250 cc of D5W and begin the drip at 30 drops/min.
5) Calcium chloride—500 mg ($\frac{1}{2}$ ampule) IV

Your Impressions:

Your Interpretation of Figure 5D-1

Agree with Treatment Given? What Would You Do Differently?

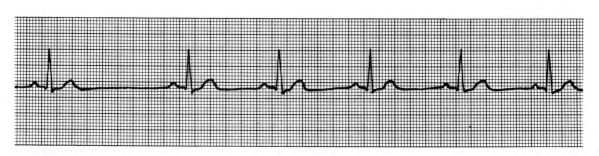

Figure 5D-1

Analysis

RHYTHM INTERPRETATION

The mechanism of the rhythm is sinus, as each QRS complex is preceded by a P wave with a fixed PR interval. A pause follows the first beat, after which the rhythm becomes regular at 52 beats/min. It is hard to be sure of the reason for the pause with only this short rhythm strip available. However, this becomes academic when one considers that the patient is pulseless and unresponsive. She is therefore in *electrical-mechanical dissociation (EMD)*.

TREATMENT ANALYSIS

Intubation of the patient is appropriate. However, none of the medications shown above should have been given. Lack of a pulse in this case is not due to the slow heart rate. Giving atropine is therefore not the solution. As discussed in Section B, sodium bicarbonate is not routinely indicated for at least the first 10 minutes of cardiac arrest unless evidence of a preexisting metabolic acidosis is present. Such is not the case here. Isoproterenol is contraindicated in asystole and EMD. The pure beta-adrenergic action of this drug results in peripheral vasodilation which lowers aortic diastolic blood pressure and minimizes blood flow to the arrested heart. [Note that the dose of isoproterenol ordered for mixing the drip was wrong by a factor of 1000! One milligram (*not* one gram) should be diluted in 250 cc of D5W when preparing an IV infusion of this drug.] Similarly, calcium chloride has been removed from the recommended treatment protocols for asystole and EMD because its efficacy has never been proved in this situation, and the drug appears to adversely affect survival.

By definition, EMD is a nonperfusing rhythm. Therefore, the first priority *must* be to resume CPR. Epinephrine is the pharmacologic agent of choice because it is the one drug that favors blood flow to the heart and brain. Realistically, however, the chances for survival with this disorder are usually minimal unless one is able to identify and correct an underlying cause.

EXERCISE E

Preceding Scenario

A middle-aged man complaining of chest pain presents to the emergency department. An IV is started and he is hooked up to a monitor. As the rhythm shown in **Figure 5E-1** is recorded, the patient becomes unresponsive.

Present Scenario

Clinical: Unresponsive. Not breathing spontaneously

Hemodynamic status: No pulse

Sequential treatment given for present scenario:
1) Lidocaine—100 mg IV bolus. Begin infusion at 2 mg/min.

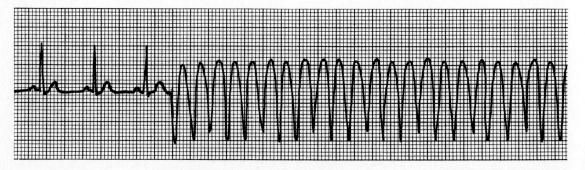

Figure 5E-1

2) Rebolus with 75 mg IV <u>lidocaine</u> and increase drip to 3 mg/min.
3) <u>Synchronized cardioversion</u> with 200 joules

Your Impressions:

Your Interpretation of Figure 5E-1

Agree with Treatment Given? What Would You Do Differently?

Analysis

RHYTHM INTERPRETATION

Sinus rhythm is present for the first three beats of this strip. This is interrupted by a run of sustained *ventricular tachycardia* with an extremely rapid ventricular response.

TREATMENT ANALYSIS

Treatment of ventricular tachycardia depends on the patient's hemodynamic status. The first priority when hemodynamic compromise sets in must be to restore perfusion. In the case of *pulseless* ventricular tachycardia (as occurs here), this should be done by immediate delivery of <u>unsynchronized countershock</u>. A <u>precordial thump</u> may be tried in this case (witnessed onset of pulseless ventricular tachycardia) while someone is getting the defibrillator and charging it. However, there is no justification for delaying therapy to administer lidocaine when the patient is pulseless. [In contrast, if a pulse and acceptable blood pressure are present with ventricular tachycardia (as was the case in Exercise A), a trial of medical therapy with lidocaine would be appropriate.]

The reason unsynchronized countershock is usually preferred over synchronized cardiover-

sion for pulseless ventricular tachycardia is that the former can usually be applied faster with at least equal success. The extremely rapid rates of ventricular tachycardia that usually accompany the pulseless state frequently preclude accurate synchronization by the defibrillator. Distinction between the QRS complex and the T wave may become difficult, and/or the T wave itself may be sensed instead of the QRS if it is tall in amplitude. Using unsynchronized countershock in this situation obviates this problem.

Lidocaine should be started *after* countershock.

EXERCISE F

Preceding Scenario

A cardiac arrest has been in progress. The patient was initially in ventricular fibrillation which converted to a supraventricular tachycardia after a third countershock with maximal energy. Lidocaine was administered, but despite this, ventricular fibrillation recurred, and the patient was shocked again with 360 joules. The rhythm shown in **Figure 5F-1** is the response to this treatment. The patient has been intubated, a large bore peripheral IV has been started, and CPR is being performed.

Present Scenario

Clinical: The patient is unresponsive. No spontaneous respirations.

Hemodynamic status: No pulse. No blood pressure.

Sequential treatment given for present scenario:

1) <u>Sodium bicarbonate</u>—2 ampules IV
2) <u>Atropine</u>—5 mg IV. Repeat in 5 minutes.
3) <u>Dopamine</u>—mix 200 mg in 250 cc of D5W and begin drip at 30 drops/min.
4) <u>Transvenous pacemaker</u> insertion
5) <u>Calcium chloride</u>—500 mg IV
6) <u>Epinephrine</u>—0.5 mg IV

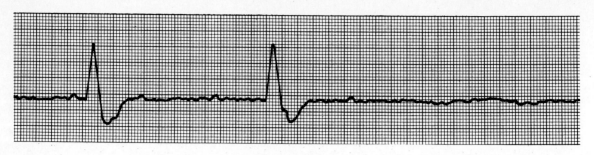

Figure 5F-1

Your Impressions:

Your Interpretation of Figure 5F-1

Agree with Treatment Given? What Would You Do Differently?

Analysis

RHYTHM INTERPRETATION

Two idioventricular complexes are seen, and then asystole results. This is an *agonal rhythm*.

TREATMENT ANALYSIS

The sequential treatment administered in this scenario is less than ideal. Sodium bicarbonate should not be routinely given during the early minutes of cardiac arrest. Atropine is occasionally effective for asystole and is definitely worth a try. However, the dose for this indication is 1 mg (not the 0.5 mg that was given here). It should be repeated in short order (in *less* than 5 min) if there is no response. Low-dose dopamine as was ordered here will not exert a potent enough alpha-adrenergic (vasoconstrictor) effect to favor myocardial blood flow. Pacemaker insertion may be tried, but its effectiveness with asystole is usually inversely proportional to the amount of time that has passed until this can be accomplished. (Application of an external pacer may be more expeditious.) Calcium chloride is contraindicated.

The treatment of choice for asystole or agonal rhythm is to resume CPR and administer epinephrine. In this particular case, it seems as if this drug was given as an afterthought when other medications and modalities had failed. Instead, early administration of epinephrine is essential. Increments of 1 mg (rather than 0.5 mg) probably should be used and repeated liberally every few minutes.

CHAPTER 6

SELF-ASSESSMENT: PRACTICE FOR THE WRITTEN TEST

This section provides an opportunity for self-assessment and preparation for the written test in the ACLS Course. Select the best answer(s) to the following questions.

1) Steps in the assessment and management of the unconscious victim include:

  i) Calling for help
  ii) Establishing unresponsiveness
  iii) Positioning the victim
  iv) Applying the ABCs of CPR

Which of the following indicates the correct order in which these steps should be performed?

  A) i, ii, iii, iv
  B) i, iii, ii, iv
  C) ii, i, iii, iv
  D) ii, iii, iv, i
  E) iv, i, ii, iii

2) Treatment for asystole includes which of the following?

  A) Epinephrine
  B) Atropine
  C) Calcium chloride
  D) Pacemaker insertion
  E) Isoproterenol

3) The single most common cause of airway obstruction in the unconscious victim is:

  A) A foreign body
  B) Food
  C) Dentures
  D) The tongue
  E) Edema from epiglottitis or tracheobronchitis

4) For external chest compression to be effective in an adult, the sternum must be depressed:

  A) $\frac{1}{2}$ to $\frac{3}{4}$ inch
  B) 1 inch
  C) $1\frac{1}{2}$ to 2 inches
  D) $2\frac{1}{2}$ inches
  E) 3 to 4 inches

5) Which of the following measures may be useful in the treatment of paroxysmal supraventricular tachycardia?

  A) Sedation
  B) Verapamil
  C) Carotid sinus massage
  D) Infusion of isoproterenol
  E) Digitalization

6) Which of the following factors are important in determining survival from out-of-hospital ventricular fibrillation?

  A) Prompt recognition of cardiac arrest by the lay public and early activation of emergency medical services.
  B) Initiation of CPR by a bystander within 4 min.
  C) Initiation of ACLS within 8 min.
  D) The mechanism of the arrest.
  E) All of the above.

7) Regarding the diagnosis of acute myocardial infarction, which one of the following is the *most* important factor to consider in deciding to admit a patient with chest pain?

  A) Initial ECG
  B) Chest x-ray film

C) Cardiac enzymes

D) Technetium pyrophosphate scan

E) History

8) Which of the following statements is/are true regarding supraventricular bradyarrhythmias with acute myocardial infarction?

A) They are particularly common during the first hour following the onset of symptoms.

B) They are most often associated with anterior infarction.

C) They usually reflect increased parasympathetic tone.

D) They should be routinely treated with atropine.

E) All of the above

9) Which of the following statements is/are true regarding current recommendations for the performance of 2-rescuer CPR in the unintubated patient?

A) At least 80 compressions should be performed each minute.

B) There should be a 15:2 ventilation to compression ratio.

C) Each compression should be sustained for 40% of the cycle.

D) CPR may be stopped for up to 45 seconds at a time when needed for endotracheal intubation or moving a patient.

E) The cardiac output produced by properly performed external chest compression may be 60% of normal output.

10) One establishes pulselessness in an infant by checking for the presence of:

A) Carotid pulse

B) Brachial pulse

C) Radial pulse

D) Precordial activity

E) Femoral pulse

11) The most common mechanism of sudden cardiac death is:

A) Ventricular tachycardia/fibrillation

B) Asystole

C) Electromechanical dissociation

D) Long QT syndrome

E) Idioventricular rhythm

12) In an unmonitored arrest situation, which of the following should be done first after the diagnosis of a ventricular fibrillation has been established?

A) Apply countershock with 200 joules of delivered energy.

B) Apply countershock with 360 joules of delivered energy.

C) Administer epinephrine IV or by intratracheal instillation.

D) Administer sodium bicarbonate.

E) Administer lidocaine.

13) Which of the following statements about sodium bicarbonate is/are true?

A) The drug should be routinely given as soon as possible in cardiac arrest.

B) The initial dose for a patient in cardiac arrest is 0.5 mEq/kg.

C) Indiscriminate use may result in a paradoxical intracellular acidosis.

D) The drug is probably unnecessary if the period of cardiac arrest is only a few minutes in duration.

E) Each ampule of sodium bicarbonate contains 25 mEq of drug.

14) The recommended dose of epinephrine for IV administration is:

A) 0.05 to 0.10 mg of a 1:10,000 solution

B) 0.5 to 1.0 mg of a 1:10,000 solution

C) 5 to 10 mg of a 1:10,000 solution

D) 0.5 mg to 1.0 mg of a 1:1000 solution

E) 5 to 10 mg of a 1:1000 solution

15) Clinical indications of lidocaine toxicity include which of the following?

A) Disorientation

B) Paresthesias

C) Diarrhea

D) Agitation

E) Seizures

16) What would you expect the pH to be for a patient with a pure respiratory acidosis if the $PaCO_2$ is 55 torr?

A) 7.36
B) 7.32
C) 7.28
D) 7.24
E) 7.20

17) Which of the following statements about procainamide is/are true?

A) The drug may be administered in 100 mg increments IV every minute until a loading dose of 1 g has been given.
B) Its use is indicated for venticular arrhythmias that are resistant to lidocaine.
C) Its use may widen the QRS complex.
D) It rarely causes hypotension when given IV.
E) The drug may lengthen the QT interval.

18) Which of the following statements about dopamine is/are true?

A) The drug is a chemical precursor of norepinephrine.
B) At doses above 20 $\mu g/kg/min$ it dilates renal and mesenteric blood vessels.
C) It primarily exerts an alpha-receptor stimulating action at low doses.
D) It is indicated for treatment of cardiogenic shock and hemodynamically significant hypotension.
E) It comes in 1 ml ampules that contain 500 mg of drug.

19) Cannulation of the internal jugular vein by the central approach is performed by introducing the needle:

A) 1 cm below the junction of the middle and medial thirds of the clavicle
B) At the midpoint of the anterior border of the sternomastoid muscle
C) At the junction of the lower and middle thirds of the anterior border of the sternomastoid muscle

D) At the apex of the triangle formed by the two heads of the sternomastoid muscle and the clavicle
E) Under the sternomastoid muscle near the junction of the middle and lower thirds of the lateral border of this muscle

20) Which of the following statements about airway obstruction is/are true?

A) Dentures and an elevated blood alcohol level are frequently associated with choking on food.
B) Foreign body obstruction of the airway accounts for nearly as many cases of cardiopulmonary arrest as does coronary heart disease.
C) Back blows and manual thrusts should be applied in the management of both partial and total airway obstruction.
D) Foreign body obstruction of the airway rarely occurs during eating.
E) The abdominal thrust to relieve airway obstruction cannot be applied by the victim on himself/herself.

21) Which of the following statements is/are true regarding the performance of basic life support in infants and children?

A) Only two fingers are needed to perform adequate external chest compression in the infant.
B) The proper area of compression in the infant is the midsternum.
C) The sternum should be depressed $\frac{1}{4}$ to $\frac{1}{2}$ inch with external chest compression in the infant.
D) The compression to ventilation ratio is 5:1 for one and two rescuers.
E) The compression rate in infants is at least 80/min.

22) What is the recommended initial energy dose for the defibrillation of a 20 kg child?

A) 10 joules
B) 20 joules
C) 40 joules

D) 60 joules
E) 80 joules

23) Which of the following statements about the esophageal obturator airway (EOA) is/are true?

A) It should be used only in unconscious patients.
B) It may be used in children over the age of 10 years.
C) It should not be used when esophageal disease is suspected.
D) Endotracheal intubation cannot be accomplished while the EOA is in place.
E) Inflation of the EOA cuff requires as much air as inflation of the cuff of an endotracheal tube.

24) The most common cause of sudden cardiac death is:

A) Mitral valve prolapse
B) Coronary heart disease
C) Acute myocardial infarction
D) Hypertrophic cardiomyopathy
E) Massive pulmonary thromboembolism

25) Which of the following statements about Mobitz I 2° AV block is/are true?

A) This form of block usually occurs below the level of the AV node.
B) The conduction defect is usually transient.
C) The block may be the result of the increased parasympathetic tone that is commonly associated with acute inferior infarction.
D) Group beating is commonly seen.
E) The block may be caused by digitalis toxicity.

26) Which of the following statements about atrial flutter in adults is/are true?

A) The atrial rate is usually ≈ 200–240 beats/min.
B) The ventricular response is usually ≈ 100–120 beats/min.
C) The rhythm is a common manifestation of digitalis toxicity.

D) The rhythm can usually be converted to sinus rhythm with low energy cardioversion.
E) Application of carotid sinus massage may be helpful in confirming the diagnosis.

27) Which of the following factors would suggest that an abnormal QRS complex is an aberrantly conducted PAC rather than a PVC?

A) The finding of a premature P wave in front of the abnormal complex
B) The presence of a full compensatory pause
C) A QRS complex width of greater than 0.14 second for the abnormal complex
D) A right bundle branch block pattern of the abnormal complex in a right-sided monitoring lead
E) The presence of atrial fibrillation

28) Treatment of ventricular tachycardia may include which of the following?

A) Cardioversion
B) Lidocaine
C) Procainamide
D) Verapamil
E) Bretylium

29) Treatment for 3° AV block may include which of the following?

A) Verapamil
B) Isoproterenol
C) Insertion of a pacemaker
D) Calcium chloride
E) Atropine

30) Insertion of a subclavian or internal jugular line is preferable on the right side because of which of the following reasons?

A) The dome of the right lung and pleura is lower than that of the left side.
B) Both veins are larger on the right side.
C) There is more or less a straight line to the atrium.
D) The landmarks are easier to recognize on the right side.
E) The large thoracic duct is not endangered.

31) The esophageal obturator airway (EOA):

A) Requires visualization of the airway for insertion

B) When removed is frequently followed by immediate regurgitation

C) Should be removed before endotracheal intubation is performed

D) Presents some potential for damage to the esophagus

E) Is a superior technique to endotracheal intubation

32) Endotracheal intubation:

A) Should always be performed as a first step in CPR

B) Should be preceded by oxygenation of the lungs by other methods of ventilation

C) Allows adequate lung inflation without causing gastric distention

D) Is always necessary for adequate lung ventilation

E) Provides a route for administration of medication

33) Oxygen-powered mechanical breathing devices for use during CPR:

A) Are satisfactory only if pressure cycled

B) Are satisfactory only if manually triggered

C) Must provide flow rates of at least 100 liters/min

D) Are not capable of delivering high concentrations of oxygen to the patient

E) Can be used in patients of all ages and sizes

34) Epinephrine:

A) Increases peripheral vascular resistance

B) Can restore electrical activity in asystole

C) Can facilitate defibrillation of ventricular fibrillation

D) Increases myocardial contractility

E) Is contraindicated in electromechanical dissociation

35) Atropine sulfate:

A) Is of no value in ventricular tachycardia

B) Is always required if the heart rate is less than 50 beats/min

C) Is usually given in 0.1 mg boluses up to a total of 0.5 mg

D) May be of value in symptomatic bradyarrhythmias

E) Is a benign treatment

36) Lidocaine:

A) May facilitate defibrillation of ventricular fibrillation

B) Has no significant effect on myocardial contractility

C) May be useful in treating multiform PVCs

D) Is not indicated in ventricular tachycardia

E) May cause seizures

37) Which of the following ECG rhythms may mimic ventricular tachycardia?

A) Paroxysmal supraventricular tachycardia (PSVT) with aberration

B) PSVT with left bundle branch block (LBBB)

C) Atrial tachycardia with block

D) Very rapid atrial fibrillation with LBBB

E) PSVT with right bundle branch block (RBBB)

38) Which of the following drugs may be useful in preparing the heart for electrical conversion from ventricular fibrillation to an effective rhythm?

A) Oxygen

B) Calcium chloride

C) Epinephrine

D) Morphine

E) Verapamil

39) Isoproterenol:

A) Increases myocardial irritability

B) Results in alpha-adrenergic stimulation

C) Lowers peripheral vascular resistance

D) Speeds the heart rate

E) Increases myocardial oxygen consumption

40) Which of the following drugs used in therapeutic doses do not directly depress the pumping function of the heart muscle?

A) Atropine
B) Lidocaine
C) Propranolol
D) Isoproterenol
E) Verapamil

41) Arterial blood gas values of pH $= 7.30$,
$pCO_2 = 60$ torr; $HCO_3 = 30$ mEq/L suggest
which of the following:

A) Metabolic acidosis
B) Metabolic alkalosis
C) Respiratory acidosis
D) Respiratory alkalosis
E) A mixed acid-base disorder

42) Risk factors of coronary heart disease
include:

A) Hypertension
B) Smoking
C) Level of fitness
D) Male sex
E) Type A personality

43) Which of the following drugs may be useful
in treating asystole after an unwitnessed cardiac
arrest?

A) Lidocaine, epinephrine, and sodium bicar-
bonate
B) Epinephrine, sodium bicarbonate, atro-
pine
C) Verapamil, atropine, and calcium chloride
D) Isoproterenol, dopamine, and atropine
E) Epinephrine, bretylium, calcium chloride

44) Which of the following statements regarding
IV lines in the setting of cardiac arrest is/are
true?

A) A large bore IV is preferable.
B) A femoral line is undesirable for adminis-
tering drugs.
C) Sterile technique must always be used.
D) The first thing to do in an arrest is to start
an IV.

E) Drug delivery may be improved by following drug administration with a 50 ml bolus
of fluid and elevating the arm.

45) Cardiac arrest in children is usually due to:

A) Myocardial infarction
B) Cardiac arrhythmias
C) Hypoxia secondary to respiratory arrest
D) SIDS (sudden infant death syndrome)
E) Valvular heart disease

46) Nitroglycerin:

A) May be effective in treating angina
pectoris
B) Reduces preload in patients with congestive heart failure
C) Relieves bronchospasm
D) Is useful in treating the chest pain of acute
myocardial infarction
E) May lower blood pressure in patients with
acute myocardial infarction

47) How much pressure should be exerted on
each electrode paddle during adult defibrillation?

A) 5 lbs
B) 10 lbs
C) 15 lbs
D) 20 lbs
E) 25 lbs

48) Which of the following are considered end
points during the administration of IV
procainamide?

A) QRS widening of 100% of its pretreatment
width
B) Hypotension
C) A loading dose of 2 g
D) Control of the arrhythmia
E) Hypertension

49) During the course of synchronized cardioversion, a patient suddenly develops ventricular
fibrillation. Which of the following steps should
be taken?

A) Begin external chest compression immediately.

B) Administer 50–100 mg lidocaine IV.

C) Immediately repeat synchronized cardioversion with the same energy.

D) Immediately turn off the synchronizer switch and proceed with unsynchronized countershock.

E) Administer epinephrine.

50) Reasons sodium bicarbonate has been deemphasized in the treatment of cardiac arrest are that:

A) It may shift the oxyhemoglobin dissociation curve to the right (thus resulting in easier release of oxygen to the tissues).

B) It may cause a paradoxical intracellular acidosis.

C) It may cause hypoosmolality.

D) Its use may result in production of iatrogenic metabolic alkalosis.

E) Hyperventilation is the preferred way to correct the acidosis that is associated with the initial minutes of the arrest.

True/False Questions

51) In the "sniffing" position, the neck is extended backward as the head is flexed forward.

52) To intubate a patient with a curved blade, the tip is inserted into the vallecula, and traction is exerted upward and forward to displace the epiglottis anteriorly and expose the glottis.

53) The tidal volumes generated with a bag-valve-mask device are much greater than those delivered by the mouth-to-mouth technique.

54) A Venturi mask is advantageous for use in patients with chronic obstructive pulmonary disease because of it ability to deliver a controlled oxygen concentration.

55) The femoral vein lies medial to the artery in the femoral sheath.

56) The most common adverse reaction to a bretylium infusion is hypertension.

57) Nitroglycerin is contraindicated in the management of acute myocardial infarction, since there is the risk of it causing hypotension.

58) Ventricular fibrillation is up to 10 times more common during the first 2 hours after the onset of symptoms of an acute myocardial infarction than during the subsequent 24 hours.

59) The Killip classification for patients with acute myocardial infarction can reliably predict which patients will have elevated pulmonary capillary wedge pressures with hemodynamic monitoring.

60) Induction of diuresis is the treatment of choice for right-sided heart failure associated with pure right ventricular infarction.

61) Insertion of a pacemaker significantly reduces mortality in patients who develop complete right bundle branch block with acute myocardial infarction.

62) Mobitz I 2° AV block is slightly more common than Mobitz II with acute myocardial infarction.

63) The dose of lidocaine should be reduced in the presence of congestive heart failure.

64) For a malpractice claim to be successful, the plaintiff must establish only that a patient-physician relationship existed and that the physician was negligent in the care rendered to the patient.

65) A "do not resuscitate" (DNR) order cannot be written unless the patient or the family is competent and willing.

66) The dose of atropine for a 15 kg infant is 0.75 mg IV.

67) Acute epiglottitis is most commonly seen in patients who are more than 2 years of age.

68) The pediatric response to hypoxemia is tachycardia.

69) A 3° AV block that occurs at the level of the AV node (with an escape rhythm that has a narrow QRS complex) and is associated with acute inferior myocardial infarction is usually transient and frequently has a good prognosis.

70) The esophageal obturator airway (EOA) is inserted with the patient's head in the sniffing position.

71) The presence of "warning arrhythmias" reliably predicts those patients most likely to develop ventricular fibrillation with acute myocardial infarction.

72) A patient initially has ventricular tachycardia. He is unresponsive, has only a weak pulse, and no blood pressure is obtainable. Lidocaine is the treatment of choice.

73) The diagnosis of acute myocardial infarction should be based primarily on the initial ECG and cardiac enzymes.

74) In general, thrombus formation occurs as a result of acute myocardial infarction and is not the cause of it.

75) It is unsafe to perform cardiac catheterization or angioplasty in acute myocardial infarction.

Answers to Self-Assessment: Practice for the Written Test

1) The correct order of steps in assessment and management of the unconscious victim is **establishing unresponsiveness (ii), calling for help (i), positioning the victim (iii), and applying the ABCs of CPR (iv)- (Choice C).**

(See Chapter 10.)

2) Treatment for asystole includes **epinephrine (A), atropine (B), and pacemaker insertion (D).**

Calcium chloride is no longer recommended for treatment of asystole. Data proving its efficacy are lacking, and some studies suggest mortality to be increased with the use of this agent. Similarly, isoproterenol is no longer recommended for treatment of asystole. The vasodilatory effect of this agent lowers aortic diastolic blood pressure, resulting in reduced myocardial blood flow. (See Chapter 1.)

3) The single most common cause of airway obstruction in the unconscious victim is **the tongue (D).**

The tongue has been dubbed "the enemy of the airway" because in the unconscious victim the musculature that normally supports this structure relaxes, allowing the tongue to fall back and obstruct the airway. (See Chapter 7.)

4) For external chest compression to be effective in an adult, the sternum must be depressed **1.5 to 2 inches (C).**

For chest compression to be effective, the sternum must be depressed at least 0.5 to 1 inch for infants, 1 to 1.5 inches for children between 1 and 8 years old, and 1.5 to 2 inches for children older than 8 and adults. (See Chapter 17.)

5) Measures that may be useful in treatment of paroxysmal supraventricular tachycardia include **sedation (A), verapamil (B), carotid sinus massage (C), and digitalization (E).**

Although verapamil has become the drug of choice for treatment of PSVT in adults, digoxin may also be effective. Vagal maneuvers (such as carotid massage) may occasionally be effective even without medication. Not generally appreciated is the fact that sedation may also be helpful. In addition to relieving the anxiety that so often accompanies this tachyarrhythmia, sedation lowers sympathetic tone. Enhanced sympathetic tone appears to play a role in perpetuating PSVT because it shortens the refractory period of AV nodal tissue and speeds conduction through the area. (See Chapters 1 and 16.)

6) Factors important in determining survival from out-of-hospital ventricular fibrillation include **prompt recognition of cardiac arrest by the lay public and early activation of emergency medical services, initiation of CPR by a bystander within 4 minutes, initiation of ACLS**

within 8 minutes, and the mechanism of the arrest (all of the above = **Choice E**).

(See Chapter 11.)

7) The *most* important factor to consider in deciding whether to admit a patient with chest pain to the hospital is **the history (E).**

The initial ECG may remain normal for the first few hours of acute infarction. Occasionally it *never* shows changes. Cardiac enzymes should *not* be used to decide whether to admit the patient. If the history is at all suggestive, the patient should be admitted. (See Chapter 12.)

8) Supraventricular bradyarrhythmias with acute myocardial infarction **are particularly common during the first hour following the onset of symptoms (A) and usually reflect increased parasympathetic tone (C).**

Supraventricular bradyarrhythmias are most commonly associated with acute *inferior* infarctions. Treatment with atropine should be administered only if the patient is symptomatic (hypotensive, or having chest pain, dyspnea, mental status changes, or ventricular ectopy) as a result of the bradycardia. (See Chapters 3, 12, and 16.)

9) According to current recommendations for performance of 2-rescuer CPR in the unintubated patient, **at least 80 compressions should be performed each minute (A).**

The new recommendations advocate a 5:1 compression:ventilation ratio for performance of 2-rescuer CPR in which compressions are delivered at a rate of 80–100 per minute, and a 1–1.5 second pause for slow ventilation is inserted after each 5 compressions. The 15:2 compression:ventilation ratio is still recommended for performance of 1-rescuer CPR, whereas ventilations and compressions in the intubated patient may be asynchronous. (See Chapter 10.)

10) Pulselessness in an infant is established by checking for the presence of a **brachial pulse (B).**

Because of the short, chubby neck of infants, location of the carotid pulse is extremely difficult in this age group (infants simply "don't have necks"). After 1 year of age, either the carotid or brachial

pulse may be used. In the past, the femoral pulse had been selected as an alternative site for palpating the pulse; however, the femoral *vein* rather than the artery is sometimes palpated when this method is used! (See Chapter 17.)

11) **Ventricular tachycardia/fibrillation (A)** is the most common mechanism of sudden cardiac death.

In the past, ventricular fibrillation had always been cited as the most common mechanism of sudden cardiac death. Recently it has become evident that a period of ventricular tachycardia probably precedes development of ventricular fibrillation in most cases of cardiac arrest. (See Chapter 11.)

12) In an unmonitored arrest situation, once the diagnosis of ventricular fibrillation has been established one should **apply countershock with 200 joules of delivered energy (A).**

Prior to countershock, a precordial thump may be delivered. (See Chapter 1.)

13) Regarding sodium bicarbonate, **indiscriminate use may result in a paradoxical intracellular acidosis (C), and the drug is probably unnecessary if the period of cardiac arrest is only a few minutes in duration (D).**

Each ampule of sodium bicarbonate contains 50 mEq of drug. More important than a patient's weight in determining the dose to administer is the clinical circumstance of the arrest. In the absence of a preexisting metabolic acidosis, sodium bicarbonate is definitely not indicated if the period of arrest is brief. (See Chapter 2.)

14) The recommended dose of epinephrine for IV administration is **0.5 to 1.0 mg of a 1:10,000 solution (B).**

(See Chapter 2.)

15) Clinical indications of lidocaine toxicity include **disorientation (A), paresthesias (B), agitation (D), and seizures (E).**

(See Chapter 13.)

16) For a patient with a pure respiratory acidosis in which the $PaCO_2$ is 55 torr, one would expect the pH to be **7.28 (C).**

In the acute setting, a change in $PaCO_2$ (either up or down) of 10 torr is associated with an approximate increase or decrease in pH of 0.08 units. Therefore, since the $PaCO_2$ in this example was increased by 15 (over the usual $PaCO_2$ of 40 torr), the pH would be expected to decrease by 0.12 units. (Golden Rule #1 from the 1984 ACLS Textbook.)

17) Procainamide **is indicated for ventricular arrhythmias that are resistant to lidocaine (B), may widen the QRS complex (C), and may lengthen the QT interval (E).**

Procainamide should not be given more rapidly than 20 mg/min, or hypotension is likely to occur. (See Chapter 14.)

18) Dopamine is **a chemical precursor of norepinephrine (A) and is indicated for treatment of cardiogenic shock and hemodynamically significant hypotension (D).**

The drug is usually dispensed in ampules of 200 mg. The dopaminergic effect (dilatation of renal and mesenteric blood vessels) prevails at low infusion rates (1–2 μg/kg/min), while alpha-receptor stimulating effects predominate at high infusion rates (>10 μg/kg/min). At intermediate infusion rates (2–10 μg/kg/min), beta-receptor stimulating effects predominate. (See Chapter 2.)

19) Cannulation of the internal jugular vein by the central approach is performed by introducing the needle **at the apex of the triangle formed by the two heads of the sternomastoid muscle and the clavicle (D).**

(See Chapter 8.)

20) Regarding airway obstruction, **dentures and an elevated blood alcohol level are frequently associated with choking on food (A).**

Foreign body airway obstruction frequently occurs during eating, especially in patients with dentures who have consumed too much alcohol. Although back blows are no longer recommended by the AHA for relief of complete airway obstruction in the adult, there are still some advocates of its use. However, *neither* back blows nor abdominal thrusts should be delivered to the patient manifesting only *partial* airway obstruction! (See Chapter 17.)

21) Regarding the performance of basic life support in infants and children, **only 2 fingers are needed to perform adequate external chest compression in the infant (A), and the compression to ventilation ratio is 5:1 for one and two rescuers (D).**

The sternum must be depressed at least 0.5 to 1 inch for infants, and the compression rate should be at least 100 times per minute. The recommended hand position for infants is no longer over the midsternum (parallel to the nipple line) but instead should be 1 fingerbreadth *below* the nipple line. (See Chapter 17.)

22) The recommended initial energy dose for the defibrillation of a 20 kg child is **40 joules (C).**

The energy recommended for the initial countershock attempt in children is 2 joules per kilogram. If unsuccessful, this energy level should be doubled (to 4 joules per kilogram) for repeat defibrillation. (See Chapter 17).

23) Regarding the esophageal obturator airway (EOA), **it should be used only in unconscious patients (A), and it should not be used when esophageal disease is suspected (C).**

The EOA should not be used in children less than 16 years of age. Endotracheal intubation can easily be achieved while the EOA is in place, and the EOA should not be removed until endotracheal intubation has been performed. Inflation of the EOA cuff requires approximately 30 ml or air, which is much more than the 5–10 cc of air required with endotracheal intubation. Inadvertent endotracheal intubation by an EOA with inflation of the cuff to the full 30 ml of air may result in disastrous consequences. (See Chapter 7.)

24) The most common cause of sudden cardiac death is **coronary heart disease (B).**

The overwhelming majority of victims of out-of-hospital cardiac arrest have underlying coronary artery disease. Surprisingly, only about $\frac{1}{3}$ of such individuals have an acute myocardial infarction at the time of their episode. (See Chapter 11.)

25) Regarding Mobitz I 2° AV block, **the conduction defect is usually transient (B), the block may be the result of the increased para-**

sympathetic tone that is commonly associated with acute inferior infarction (C), group beating is commonly seen (D), and the block may be caused by digitalis toxicity (E).

(See Chapter 3.)

26) Regarding atrial flutter in adults, **the rhythm can usually be converted to sinus rhythm with low energy cardioversion (D), and application of carotid sinus massage may be helpful in confirming the diagnosis (E).**

The usual atrial rate of flutter in adults is 250–350 beats/min, providing that the patient is not being treated with a medication (such as quinidine or procainamide) that might slow the atrial response. Most commonly there is a 2:1 AV conduction, so that the usual ventricular response is between 125 and 175 beats/min. Although digitalis toxicity may produce almost any arrhythmia, it rarely produces atrial flutter. (See Chapter 3.)

27) Factors suggesting that an abnormal QRS complex is aberrantly conducted include **the finding of a *premature* P wave in front of the abnormal complex (A) and a right bundle branch block pattern (with a taller right rabbit ear) in a right-sided monitoring lead (D).**

The finding of a full compensatory pause and a QRS complex width of greater than 0.14 second are factors in favor of ventricular ectopy. (See Chapter 15.)

28) Treatment of ventricular tachycardia may include **cardioversion (A), lidocaine (B), procainamide (C), and bretylium (E).**

Verapamil is contraindicated for the treatment of ventricular tachycardia because its cardiac depressant and vasodilatory effects not infrequently result in deterioration of the rhythm to ventricular fibrillation. For this reason verapamil should *not* be given as a therapeutic trial to patients with a regular wide complex tachycardia when the possibility exists that the rhythm may be ventricular tachycardia. (See Chapters 1 and 2.)

29) Treatment for a 3° AV block may include **isoproterenol (B), insertion of a pacemaker (C), and atropine (E).**

(See Chapter 1.)

30) Insertion of a subclavian or internal jugular line is preferable on the right side because **the dome of the right lung and pleura is lower than the dome on the left side (A), there is more or less a straight line to the atrium (C), and the large thoracic duct is not endangered (E).**

(See Chapter 8.)

31) The esophageal obturator airway (EOA) **when removed is frequently followed by immediate regurgitation (B) and presents some potential for damage to the esophagus (D).**

An EOA provides a means of controlling the airway when operators skilled in endotracheal intubation are not available. An advantage of the EOA is that it can be inserted without the need for visualization of the airway. To minimize the chance of regurgitation, the EOA should *not* be removed until after the endotracheal intubation has been performed. (See Chapter 7.)

32) Endotracheal intubation **should be preceded by oxygenation of the lungs by other methods of ventilation (B), allows adequate lung inflation without causing gastric distention (C), and provides an alternative route for administration of medication (E).**

Endotracheal intubation need *not* be performed as the first step in CPR. Adequate ventilation can often be maintained by proper use of respiratory adjuncts. (See Chapter 8.)

33) Oxygen-powered mechanical breathing devices for use during CPR **are satisfactory only if manually triggered (B) and must provide flow rates of at least 100 liters/minute (C).**

Oxygen-powered mechanical breathing devices have come under increasing scrutiny in recent years. Although capable of delivering high concentrations of oxygen, they are especially prone to producing gastric insufflation when used in the patient with an unprotected airway. They should not be used in children. (See Chapter 7.)

34) Epinephrine **increases peripheral vascular resistance (A), can restore electrical activity in asystole (B), can facilitate defibrillation of ven-**

tricular fibrillation, and increases myocardial contractility (D).

(See Chapter 2.)

35) Atropine sulfate **is of no value in ventricular tachycardia (A) and may be of value in symptomatic bradyarrhythmias (D).**

Atropine is usually administered in 0.5–1.0 mg boluses up to a total of 2 mg. Because of its potential to produce supraventricular or ventricular tachyarrhythmias, the drug should *not* be used to treat bradycardia unless the patient is symptomatic. (See Chapter 2.)

36) Lidocaine **may facilitate defibrillation of ventricular fibrillation (A), has no significant effect on myocardial contractility (B), may be useful in treating multiform PVCs (C), and may cause seizures (E).**

(See Chapters 2 and 13.)

37) ECG rhythms that may mimic ventricular tachycardia include **paroxysmal supraventricular tachycardia (PSVT) with aberration (A), PSVT with LBBB (B), very rapid atrial fibrillation with LBBB (D), and PSVT with RBBB (E).**

Although one should always assume that a wide complex tachycardia is ventricular tachycardia until proved otherwise, the possibility of a supraventricular tachycardia with either preexisting bundle branch block or aberrancy should also be kept in mind. Because rapid atrial fibrillation often appears as a fairly regular rhythm, it may also mimic ventricular tachycardia if there is preexisting bundle branch block. (See Chapters 3 and 15.)

38) Drugs that may be useful in preparing the heart for electrical conversion from ventricular fibrillation to an effective rhythm include **oxygen (A) and epinephrine (C).**

(See Chapter 1.)

39) Isoproterenol **increases myocardial irritability (A), lowers peripheral vascular resistance (C), speeds the heart rate (D), and increases myocardial oxygen consumption (E).**

Because of the above effects of isoproterenol, use of the drug has been deemphasized in recent years. It is best reserved as a temporizing measure for treatment of hemodynamically significant bradyarrhythmias that have not responded to atropine. (See Chapter 2.)

40) Drugs that do not directly depress the pumping function of the heart when used in therapeutic doses include **atropine (A), lidocaine (B), and isoproterenol (D).**

Both propranolol and verapamil may decrease cardiac contractility, so that use of these agents must proceed with extreme caution (if at all) in patients with a history of congestive heart failure. (See Chapters 2 and 14.)

41) Arterial blood gas values of pH = 7.30, pCO_2 = 60 torr; HCO_3 = 30 mEq/L suggest **a mixed acid-base disorder (E).**

The acid-base abnormality in this example is *mixed*, since both pCO_2 and the HCO_3 values are abnormal. The pCO_2 is increased by 20 torr over the normal value of 40 (respiratory *acidosis*), while HCO_3 is increased by 6 mEq/L over the normal value of 25 (metabolic *alkalosis*). Since the body usually does not overcorrect the pH and an acidosis is present, one can assume that this is the *primary* abnormality.

In the acute setting, a change in $PaCO_2$ (either up or down) of 10 torr is associated with an approximate increase or decrease in pH of 0.08 units. Thus one would have expected the pH to drop by 0.16 units (to a pH = 7.24) if one were simply dealing with an acute respiratory acidosis. The fact that the pH is higher than this, and that HCO_3 has also been increased suggests adaptation by the body in an attempt to compensate for the primary acid-base disorder. Thus this example illustrates a primary respiratory acidosis with partial metabolic compensation.

42) Risk factors of coronary heart disease include **hypertension (A), smoking (B), level of fitness (C), male sex (D), and type A personality (E).**

The five most important risk factors for coronary heart disease are smoking, hypertension, positive family history, hypercholesterolemia, and level of fitness. Lesser risk factors include male sex, age, obesity, diabetes mellitus, and type A personality. Although family history, sex, and age cannot be changed, the other risk factors may all be modified to at least some extent by a motivated patient.

43) Drugs that may be useful in treating asystole after an unwitnessed cardiac arrest include **epinephrine, sodium bicarbonate, and atropine (B).**

(See Chapters 1 and 2.)

44) Regarding the use of IV lines in the setting of cardiac arrest, **a large bore IV is preferable (A), a femoral line is undesirable for administering drugs (B), and drug delivery may be improved by following drug administration with a 50 ml bolus of fluid and elevating the arm (E).**

Circulation of drugs in the arrested heart is most effectively accomplished when administered into a *central* vein such as the internal jugular or subclavian. However, achieving access at these sites requires the presence of a provider skilled in their insertion and may still be attended by complications such as pneumothorax. The femoral vein is no longer recommended as a site for drug delivery during cardiac arrest because blood flow during CPR is significantly diminished below the diaphragm. Drug delivery may be optimized when administered from a peripheral IV line if a proximal site (such as the antecubital fossa) is chosen, a large bore needle is used, a 50–100 ml bolus of fluid "flushes" the medication in, and the arm is elevated (See Chapter 8.)

45) Cardiac arrest in children usually is due to **hypoxia secondary to respiratory arrest (C).**

(See Chapter 17.)

46) Nitroglycerin **may be effective in treating angina pectoris (A), reduces preload in patients with congestive heart failure (B), is useful in treating the chest pain of acute myocardial infarction (D), and may lower blood pressure in patients with acute myocardial infarction (E).**

(See Chapters 12 and 14.)

47) The amount of pressure that should be exerted on each electrode paddle during adult defibrillation is **25 lbs (E).**

Among the factors that decrease transthoracic resistance (TTR) during defibrillation are the pressure of the electrode paddles against the chest wall and the phase of ventilation of the patient. Exerting firm pressure (of 25 pounds) on each paddle may lower TTR by up to 25%. It also helps assure forced expiration of the victim, decreasing the distance between paddle electrodes and the heart and thus further lowering TTR. (See Chapter 2.)

48) End points during the administration of procainamide include **hypotension (B) and control of the arrhythmia (D).**

Other end points for the IV administration of procainamide include QRS widening by 50% of the pretreatment width and infusion of the full 1 g loading dose. (See Chapter 14.)

49) If during the course of synchronized cardioversion a patient suddenly develops ventricular fibrillation, one should **immediately turn off the synchronizer switch and proceed with unsynchronized countershock (D).**

Immediately defibrillating the patient minimizes the time that ventricular fibrillation is present and maximizes the chance for successful conversion. A precordial thump may be delivered prior to countershock. (See Chapter 1.)

50) Reasons sodium bicarbonate has been deemphasized in the treatment of cardiac arrest are that it **may cause a paradoxical intracellular acidosis (B), its use may result in production of iatrogenic metabolic alkalosis (D), and hyperventilation is the preferred way to correct the acidosis that is associated with the initial minutes of the arrest (E).**

Significant metabolic acidosis may not develop in cardiopulmonary arrest for at least some time (5–15 minutes?) after patient collapse. Since the primary abnormality in the initial minutes is hypoventilation (respiratory acidosis), it would therefore seem far more appropriate to correct the acidosis of cardiac arrest by improving ventilation (by hyperventilating the patient) than by administering sodium bicarbonate.

Sodium bicarbonate therapy is *not* benign. Adverse effects of excessive administration of this agent include extreme alkalosis, hyperosmolality, hypokalemia, sodium overload, shifting of the oxyhemoglobin dissociation curve leftward with consequent impaired oxygen release to the tissues, and precipitation of convulsions and/or arrhythmias. Moreover, unless adequate ventilation is achieved, carbon dioxide (CO_2) will tend to accumulate. Since CO_2 is freely diffusible across cellular and organ membranes, it readily enters the brain and heart where it may further depress function by producing a *paradoxical intracellular acidosis*. Giving sodium bicarbonate only aggravates this acidosis. (See Chapter 2.)

True/False Questions

51) **False.**

The "sniffing" position is achieved in children by sliding a small rolled washcloth (or your hand) under the patient's shoulders. This allows the head to slightly tilt back on its axis until the jaw forms a 90° angle to the long axis of the body. (See Chapter 17.)

52) **True.**

(See Chapter 7.)

53) **False.**

The most difficult part about using a bag-valve-mask device is that one rescuer must simultaneously perform three tasks. A patent airway and tight face seal must be maintained with one hand while the other hand is used to ventilate the patient. The tidal volume generated by squeezing the reservoir bag with one hand is much less than that delivered by the mouth-to-mouth technique. (See Chapter 7.)

54) **True.**

(See Chapter 7.)

55) **True.**

The mnemonic *VAN*, may help recall that the femoral vein lies medial to the artery, and the artery lies medial to the nerve.

56) **False.**

Bretylium has a complex mechanism of action including adrenergic stimulation that results in an initial release of norepinephrine, followed several minutes later by adrenergic blockade in which uptake of norepinephrine and epinephrine into postganglionic adrenergic nerve endings is prevented.

This latter effect becomes the predominant one and accounts for the fact that, following an initial increase in blood pressure, *hypotension* commonly occurs and is the most common adverse reaction to bretylium infusion. (See Chapter 2.)

57) **False.**

Although in the past nitroglycerin was not used in acute myocardial infarction for fear of causing hypotension, the drug is now commonly recommended in this setting as an agent of choice for treatment of chest pain, ischemia, or hypertension. If administered cautiously to patients with systolic blood pressure readings of at least 100 mm Hg, hypotension usually does not pose a problem. (See Chapters 12 and 14.)

58) **True.**

(See Chapter 11.)

59) **False.**

The Killip classification of patients with acute myocardial infarction was first proposed in 1967 and is still in use today. It consists of four classes:

  i) Class I—uncomplicated myocardial infarction (no rales or S3)
  ii) Class II—mild ventricular failure (rales in the lower lung field and an S3)
  iii) Class III—severe ventricular failure (pulmonary edema)
  iv) Class IV—cardiogenic shock (systolic blood pressure of less than 90 mm Hg, oliguria, mental obtundation)

The problem with this classification is that it is based on bedside assessment of the patient's circulatory status. Differentiation of patients with mild-to-moderate failure from those with severe failure is sometimes difficult to do on clinical grounds alone. (See Chapter 12.)

60) **False.**

Diuresis is an important component of the therapy of patients with acute myocardial infarction and left ventricular failure. In contrast, *volume expansion* (rather than diuretic therapy) is the initial treatment of choice for hemodynamically significant right ventricular infarction. The goal is to increase right ventricular contractility by the Frank-Starling principle. Decreasing preload (with diuretics) would be counterproductive. (See Chapter 12.)

61) **False.**

Development of intraventricular conduction defects with acute myocardial infarction is thought to reflect extensive myocardial damage. Mortality most often results from power failure rather than from progression of the conduction disturbance to complete AV block. Consequently, prophylactic pacing usually will not increase survival, although on rare occasions it may benefit patients with bundle branch block and high-degree AV block in the absence of significant heart failure. (See Chapter 12.)

62) **False.**

Mobitz I 2° AV block is *much* more common than Mobitz II in the setting of acute myocardial infarction. In general the former conduction disturbance is most often associated with acute inferior infarction, while the latter is seen with acute anterior infarction. The importance of distinguishing between Mobitz I and Mobitz II AV block is that the former is usually a benign, transient disturbance, while the latter requires pacemaker insertion. (See Chapter 3.)

63) **True.**

Lidocaine is eliminated from the body by hepatic metabolism. The half-life of this elimination phase is proportional to hepatic blood flow and under normal circumstances takes between 1 and 2 hours. Patients in shock or congestive heart failure in whom hepatic blood flow may be greatly diminished would be expected to have a prolonged elimination phase half-life and be more susceptible to accumulation of drug and lidocaine toxicity. Other groups at high risk of developing lidocaine toxicity include patients with liver disease, those taking drugs such as propranolol or cimetidine that decrease hepatic clearance of lidocaine, the elderly in whom cardiac output is less, and patients with low body weight. (See Chapter 13.)

64) **False.**

For a malpractice claim to be successful, four conditions must be satisfied:

i) A relationship must have been established between the patient and health care provider.
ii) Negligence on the part of the health care provider must have occurred.
iii) The patient must have suffered an injury.
iv) A direct *cause-and-effect* relationship must be proved to exist between the negligence and the injury that resulted. (See Chapter 18.)

65) **False.**

"Do not resuscitate" (DNR) orders may be written if the patient is competent and willing, if the patient was competent in the past and made out a valid advance directive, or if the legal guardian and/or proxy decision-maker of an incompetent patient agrees with the physician that a DNR order is in the best interests of the patient. (See Chapter 18.)

66) **False.**

The recommended dose of atropine for infants and children is 0.02 mg/kg. Therefore the appropriate dose for a 15 kg infant is 0.3 mg. (See Chapter 17.)

67) **True.**

Acute epiglottitis is a bacterial infection that usually occurs in children between 2 and 7 years of age. In contrast, the viral form of croup (laryngotracheobronchitis) tends to be seen in younger individuals between 3 months and 3 years old. (See Chapter 17.)

68) **False.**

The pediatric heart responds to hypoxemia by *slowing* its rate. As a result, bradycardia and asystole are by far the most common arrhythmias associated with cardiopulmonary arrest in children. (See Chapter 17.)

69) **True.**

Pacemaker insertion is routinely performed in patients who develop 3° AV block as the result of acute *anterior* infarction. The escape pacemaker tends to be idioventricular (wide QRS complex) and is often associated with a slow heart rate and signs of hemodynamic compromise. On the other hand, 3° AV block that develops with acute *inferior* infarction may occur with a stable junctional escape rhythm (narrow QRS complex) that is able to maintain the patient's hemodynamic status. The mechanism of AV block in this setting may simply reflect increased parasympathetic tone and/or ischemia of the AV node rather than irreversible myocardial damage. The conduction defect usually is transient. If the heart rate remains close to 60 beats/min, no treatment at all may be indicated. With slower heart rates, atropine may effectively accelerate the ventricular response and/or improve AV conduction. Pacemaker insertion is often not needed. (See Chapter 3.)

70) **False.**

The EOA is not inserted with the patient's head in the sniffing position. Instead, the head is gently flexed *forward* to assist in directing the tube into the esophagus. (See Chapter 7.)

71) **False.**

In the past it was thought that "warning arrhythmias" ($\geq$ 5PVCs per minute, $\geq$ 2PVCs in a row, multiform PVCs, and the "R-on-T" phenomenon) regularly preceded development of primary ventricular fibrillation in patients with acute myocardial infarction. Consequently, one would wait for the occurrence of such arrhythmias before initiating antiarrhythmic treatment in patients admitted with acute chest pain.

Today we know that ventricular fibrillation frequently occurs in acute myocardial infarction without being preceded by warning arrhythmias. Even when warning arrhythmias do occur, they do not reliably predict which patients will subsequently develop ventricular fibrillation. (See Chapters 12 and 14.)

72) **False.**

The treatment of choice for hemodynamically significant ventricular tachycardia is immediate cardioversion. Time should not be lost instituting medical treatment. Lidocaine should be started after cardioversion or in patients with ventricular tachycardia in whom an adequate blood pressure is maintained. (See Chapter 1.)

73) **False.**

The diagnosis of acute myocardial infarction is based on history, ECG changes, and cardiac enzyme abnormalities. Although the ECG is most helpful when suggestive changes are present, a normal tracing does not rule out acute infarction. In general, cardiac enzymes play little (or no) role in determining whether a patient with new-onset chest pain should be admitted to the hospital. This leaves *history* as an essential factor in diagnosing acute myocardial infarction. (See Chapter 12.)

74) **False.**

Although in the past it was thought that thrombus formation occurred secondary to acute myocardial infarction, we now know that acute thrombotic occlusion is the cause (not the result) in the vast majority of cases. (See Chapter 12.)

75) **False.**

Although in the past it was taboo to perform cardiac catheterization and angioplasty in the setting of acute myocardial infarction, these procedures have been shown to be remarkably safe in most instances. Consequently, cardiac catheterization is performed almost routinely with acute myocardial infarction in many centers, and angioplasty is frequently utilized as the method of choice for reperfusion therapy. (See Chapter 12.)

PART II:

ESSENTIALS OF THE AIRWAY AND IV ACCESS

CHAPTER 7

MANAGEMENT OF AIRWAY AND VENTILATION

Dan Cavallaro, NREMT
Ken Grauer, MD

The importance of controlling the airway in patients presenting with cardiac and/or respiratory emergencies cannot be overemphasized. For outcome to be favorable, spontaneously breathing patients should be provided with supplemental oxygen, those who are not adequately ventilating must be assisted, and patients in respiratory arrest must be intubated and oxygenated. This chapter discusses the modalities and techniques used to accomplish these tasks.

OPENING THE AIRWAY

The first priority in managing the patient with respiratory difficulty is to assure patency of the airway. The two maneuvers recommended for doing this are the chin lift and jaw thrust.

In the unconscious supine patient, the musculature that normally supports the tongue and epiglottis relaxes. As a result, one or both of these structures may fall back and occlude the airway (**Figure 7-1**). This accounts for the fact that the most common cause of airway obstruction in the unconscious patient is soft tissue in origin.

The degree of airway obstruction may be aggravated in the patient who is making spontaneous attempts to breathe. Inspiratory efforts create a negative pressure that frequently draws the tongue and epiglottis back even more into the throat, further compromising the airway. Because the tongue and epiglottis are attached to the lower jaw, procedures aimed at displacing the mandible forward will lift these structures off the posterior pharynx and open the airway.

This is the way in which the chin lift and jaw thrust maneuvers work.

The Head-Tilt/Chin-Lift

The new guidelines recommended the *head-tilt/chin-lift* maneuver because it is easier to learn and more effective than the jaw thrust (Clinton and Ruiz, 1985). The technique is performed by placing the palm of one hand on the patient's forehead and the fingers of the other hand under the patient's chin. The fingers are positioned on the bony structure of the chin so as to avoid compression of soft tissues which might compromise the airway. With the hand on the forehead acting as a stabilizing force, the head is tilted backward by gently pushing the chin in a cephalad direction (**Figure 7-2**).

As the head is tilted back, the mouth will almost always open. When this occurs, resist the urge to force the mouth closed. Instead, concentrate on using the fingers under the chin to assist in supporting the head-tilt position.

The Jaw Thrust

Although slightly more difficult to perform than is the head-tilt/chin-lift maneuver, the *jaw thrust* is the procedure of choice when the possibility of cervical spine injury exists. This maneuver allows the rescuer to support the head and open the airway without flexing or extending the cervical spine. One hand is placed on each side of the patient's head and the index and/or middle fingers are used to displace the mandible anteriorly. This lifts the tongue off the hypopharynx (**Figure 7-3**).

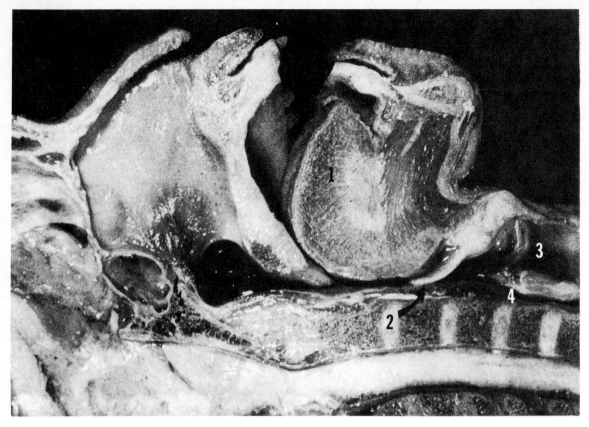

Figure 7-1. Cross-section of the head demonstrating the tongue and epiglottis occluding the airway. 1) tongue; 2) epiglottis; 3) trachea; 4) esophagus. (Reproduced with permission from Yokochi, C., Rohen, J. W.: *Photographic Anatomy of the Human Body,* University Park Press, Baltimore, 1978.)

The Head-Tilt/Neck-Lift

Although the *head-tilt/neck-lift* technique used to be the most commonly taught method for opening the airway, it is no longer recommended. Tilting the head back and lifting the neck is an indirect method of opening the airway and is much less effective than procedures which displace the mandible forward. It also poses the greatest risk when cervical spine injury is a possibility.

ASSESSING THE ADEQUACY OF VENTILATION

In order to determine optimal airway management, the emergency care provider must assess the adequacy of ventilation. The parameters to monitor include color, breath sounds, tidal volume, respiratory rate, and the work of breathing.

Evaluating the patient's *color* is perhaps the easiest way to determine hypoxia. Cyanosis is an obvious indicator of inadequate oxygenation. Pallor and/or an ashen appearance suggests in addition diminished cardiac output.

All lung fields should be auscultated for *breath sounds*. The finding of good, symmetric breath sounds indicates that the airway is patent and that air movement is adequate. On the other hand, asymmetric or abnormal breath sounds suggest a problem in the airway. This may be due to obstruction (from foreign body, soft tissue, mucous plugging), cardiopulmonary disease (bronchospasm, pneumonia, congestive heart failure), or improper tube placement

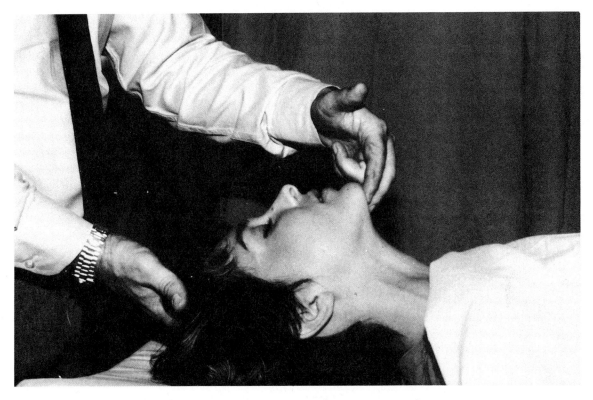

Figure 7-2. Head-tilt/chin-lift.

(right mainstem intubation, tracheal intubation with the esophageal obturator).

The next two parameters to monitor are *tidal volume* and *respiratory rate*. The product of these two make up the *minute ventilation*. Most adults breathe in about 500 ml of air an average of 12 times each minute. This results in a minute ventilation of 6 L (500 × 12 = 6000). Because of the inverse relationship between tidal volume and respiratory rate, alterations in one of these parameters may be at least partially compensated by corrective alterations in the other. For example, minute ventilation may remain adequate despite a decrease in tidal volume provided respiratory rate increases proportionately.

Accurate assessment of tidal volume requires the use of a spirometer. Without such equipment or in an emergency setting, one may surmise that the tidal volume is probably adequate if breath sounds are full and equal in the presence of good, symmetric chest excursion.

Respiratory rate should be counted. It is extremely easy to overestimate or underestimate the frequency of respiration by casual inspection. A conscious effort must also be made on the part of the observer to assess the *work of breathing*. Tachypnea and the use of accessory muscles are common signs of ventilatory insufficiency.

> The above parameters should be frequently assessed while caring for the patient in cardiac and/or respiratory distress. Without so doing, subtle changes in hemodynamic or ventilatory status may go unnoticed.

ADJUNCTS FOR IMPROVING OXYGENATION

In the conscious, spontaneously breathing patient, one of the main priorities is to provide

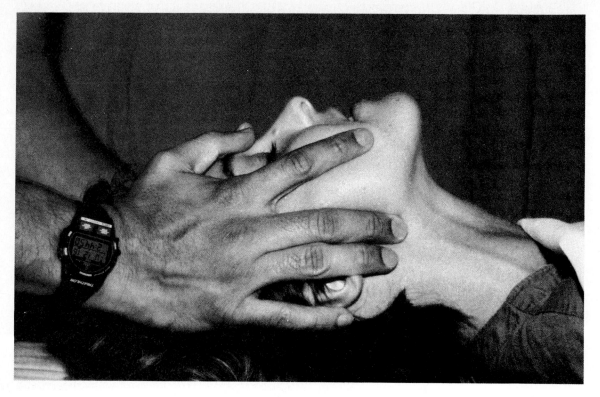

Figure 7-3.   Jaw thrust.

supplemental oxygen. Although many devices are available for accomplishing this, we will address only the four most commonly used modalities.

The Nasal Cannula

The *nasal cannula* is a piece of tubing with two ports designed to deliver supplemental oxygen through the nares. It is easily applied by slipping the tubing over the ears and sliding the prongs into the nares (**Figure 7-4**). Two to 6 L of oxygen may be administered per minute, providing the patient with inspired oxygen concentrations (F_iO_2) of 24–40%.

The advantage of this device is that it is well tolerated by most individuals. The nasal cannula is particularly valuable in patients with chronic obstructive pulmonary disease for whom low concentrations of oxygen (24–28%) are desira-

ble. However, when higher concentrations of oxygen are needed, the non-rebreathing oxygen mask and Venturi mask are preferable provided they can be tolerated by the patient.

In normal persons, respiratory drive depends on arterial carbon dioxide concentration. In contrast, hypercarbia loses its value as a stimulus for respiration in many patients with chronic obstructive pulmonary disease (COPD). Such individuals come to depend on hypoxemia for their respiratory drive. Administration of high concentrations of oxygen to such patients is potentially dangerous because it may correct hypoxemia and suppress ventilation to the point of respiratory arrest. The F_iO_2 of supplemental oxygen should therefore be kept at low levels for patients at risk of carbon dioxide retention.

The problem with the nasal cannula is that the actual amount of inspired oxygen varies greatly and depends on both tidal volume and whether the patient predominantly breathes through the nose or mouth.

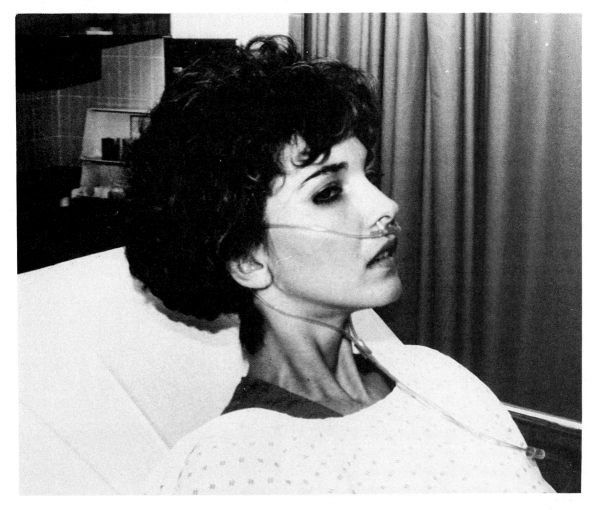

Figure 7-4.   Nasal cannula.

The Oxygen Mask

The *oxygen mask* is a plastic device with a number of small vents on each side which allow for inspiration and expiration of ambient air. There is also a port for delivery of supplemental oxygen on the lower portion of the mask. Five to 10 L of oxygen may be administered, providing an F_iO_2 of up to 50%.

The principal drawback of this device is the tremendous variability in actual inspired oxygen concentration. This is because the amount of air entrained from the outside (that mixes with the supplemental oxygen) is dependent on the pa-

tient's inspiratory flow rate. Because of the variability in delivered F_iO_2 with the oxygen mask, a non-rebreather or Venturi mask may be preferable when high concentrations of oxygen are required.

The Non-Rebreathing Oxygen Mask

The *non-rebreathing oxygen mask* is far superior to the basic plastic oxygen mask described above. It is the adjunct of choice when high con-

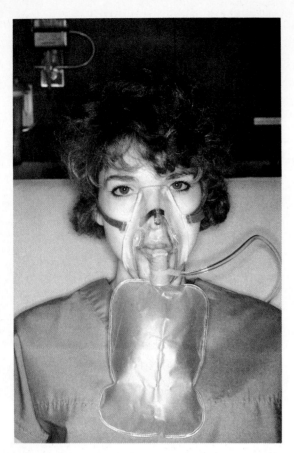

Figure 7-5.   Non-rebreathing oxygen mask.

is much less than 100% because supplemental oxygen has mixed with ambient air.

Special Considerations

The reservoir bag should remain completely filled when using the non-rebreathing oxygen mask so that ample supplemental oxygen is available for each breath. In order to assure that this occurs, high flow rates (10–15 L/min) must be used. In addition, the mask must fit snugly on the face to prevent ambient air from mixing with oxygen inhaled from the reservoir bag.

The Venturi Mask

The *Venturi mask* is similar in concept to the basic oxygen mask with an important modification that allows relatively fixed concentrations of supplemental oxygen to be inspired. Oxygen concentrations of 24%, 28%, 35%, and 40% can be delivered, using either 4 or 8 L/min flow rates. The advantage of this mask is much greater control of the oxygen concentration administered to the patient. Consistent oxygen de-

centrations of oxygen are needed, because it can consistently deliver an F_iO_2 of up to 90%.

Several modifications account for the superiority of this device. The first is that a flutter (one-way) valve has been added to each side of the non-rebreather mask. This allows exhaled air to escape but prevents ambient air from being inspired. In contrast, the air holes on the sides of the basic mask allow passage of both inspired and expired air. The other major difference between these two devices is that the basic mask directs the supplemental oxygen into the mask, while the *non-rebreathing* mask directs it into a *reservoir* bag (**Figure 7.5**). A one-way valve prevents exhaled air from entering this reservoir, so that the patient entrains 100% oxygen from the reservoir on inhalation. In contrast, the concentration of inspired oxygen from the basic mask

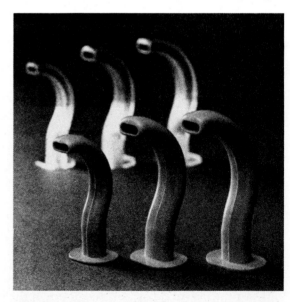

Figure 7-6.   Examples of oral pharyngeal airways. (Reproduced with permission of Ambu, Inc. from Lotz, P., Ahnefeld, F. W., Hirlinger, W. D., *A Systematic Guide to Intubation:* Atelier Flad, Eckental, West Germany.)

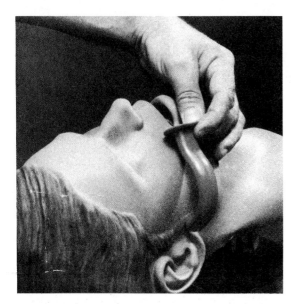

Figure 7-7. Sizing the oral pharyngeal airway. (Reproduced with permission of Ambu, Inc. from Lotz, P., Ahnefeld, F. W., Hirlinger, W. K.: *A Systematic Guide to Intubation*, Atelier Flad, Eckental, West Germany.)

livery has made the Venturi mask the favored device for providing precise F_iO_2 rates to patients with COPD.

AIRWAY ADJUNCTS

In the semiconscious or unconscious patient, invasive measures may be needed to maintain patency of the airway for ventilation. The two devices used are the oral and the nasopharyngeal airway.

The Oral Pharyngeal Airway

The *oral pharyngeal airway* is a semicurved, tubular device that is placed on top of the tongue (**Figure 7-6**). When properly positioned, the distal tip lies between the base of the tongue and the back of the throat. This prevents the tongue from occluding the airway and allows ventilation to occur through the lumen of the tube.

Appropriate sizing of the device may be estimated at the bedside or in the field by aligning

the tube on the side of the patient's face and choosing an airway that extends from the tragus to the corner of the mouth (**Figure 7-7**).

Technique for Insertion

There are two ways to position the airway. The quickest method is to insert the device upside down into the mouth (**Figure 7-8A**). As soon as the distal end reaches the hard palate, the airway is gently rotated 180° and slipped behind the tongue into the posterior phayrnx (**Figures 7-8B and 7-8c**).

The second technique requires a tongue blade. The tongue is depressed and the airway is inserted right side up into the oral pharynx. With either technique, the flange of the tube should sit comfortably on the lips if the device has been properly inserted (**Figure 7-9**).

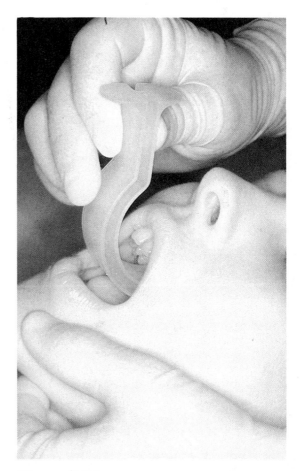

Figure 7-8A. Insertion of the oral pharyngeal airway. The device is inserted upside down into the mouth.

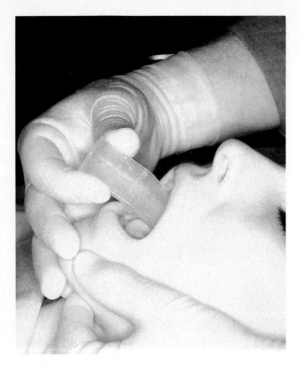

Figure 7-8B.   Rotation of the airway.

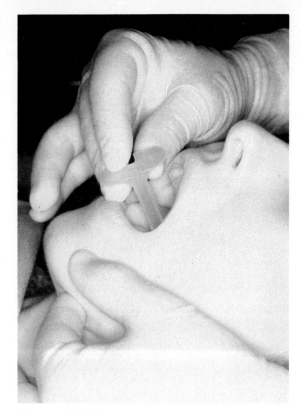

Figure 7-8C.   Final position of the oral pharyngeal airway.

Special Considerations

i) If the tube repeatedly comes out of the mouth, it may be improperly seated and compressing the tongue into the posterior pharynx. This may further obstruct the airway. Remove the tube and reinsert it.

ii) Although the lumen of the tube is adequate for ventilating the patient, it should *not* be used for suctioning. The suction catheter is inserted adjacent to the airway. Suction is then performed in the usual way.

iii) The oral pharyngeal airway should be used only in unconscious patients. Insertion of this device in a conscious or semiconscious patient may activate the gag reflex (when the back of the tongue or posterior pharyngeal wall are touched) and precipitate vomiting.

The Nasopharyngeal Airway (Nasal Trumpet)

The *nasopharyngeal airway* is an extremely compliant rubber tube approximately 15 cm in length (**Figure 7-10**). The tube is designed so that its distal tip sits in the posterior pharynx while the proximal tip rests on the external nares. The lumen of this device permits the passage of air into the lower respiratory tract.

The principal advantage of the nasal pharyngeal airway is that it is usually well tolerated in the patient who retains a sensitive gag reflex. This makes it the device of choice for the conscious or semiconscious patient with respiratory difficulty.

Technique for Insertion

The tube should be lubricated with 2% lidocaine gel prior to insertion. The purpose of the lidocaine is twofold. It anesthetizes the nasal mucosa in the posterior pharynx (so as to minimize sensitivity of the gag reflex) and lubricates the tube to facilitate insertion.

The nasopharyngeal airway is then advanced into the nares by placing the bevel against the septum of

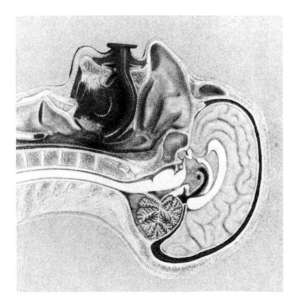

Figure 7-9. Correct position of oral pharyngeal airway after insertion. (Reproduced with permission of Ambu, Inc. from Lotz, P., Ahnefeld, F. W., Hirlinger, W. K.: *A Systematic Guide to Intubation*, Atelier Flad, Eckental, West Germany.)

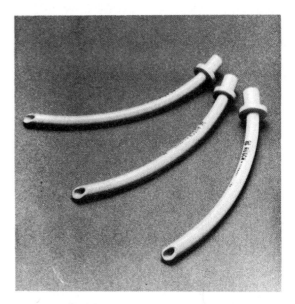

Figure 7-10. Examples of nasopharyngeal airways. (Reproduced with permission of Ambu, Inc. from Lotz, P., Ahnefeld, F. W., Hirlinger, W. K.: *A Systematic Guide to Intubation*, Atelier Flad, Eckental, West Germany.)

the nose (**Figure 7-11A**) and gently sliding the tube backward in line with the base of the ears (**Figure 7-11B**). In this way the tube passes parallel to the floor of the nasal cavity (**Figure 7-12**). When completely inserted the distal end is seated in the posterior pharynx (**Figure 7-13**).

Special Considerations

i) Although in most cases proper insertion of the nasal trumpet will result in correct position of the distal end in the posterior pharynx, on occasion the tube may be too short or too long. When this happens, adequate ventilation may not be achieved.

ii) While most conscious or semiconscious patients are able to tolerate this device, the gag reflex of certain particularly sensitive individuals may still be activated.

iii) Forceful introduction of the airway into the nasal passage should be avoided, since this may cause abrasions or lacerate the nasal mucosa and produce significant bleeding.

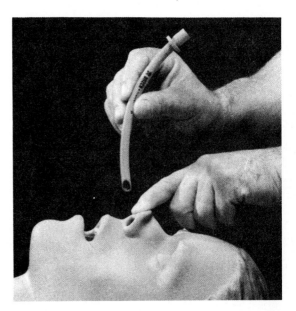

Figure 7-11A. Proper bevel position of the nasopharyngeal airway during insertion. (Reproduced with permission of Ambu, Inc. from Lotz, P., Ahnefeld, F. W., Hirlinger, W. K.: *A Systematic Guide to Intubation*, Atelier Flad, Eckental, West Germany.)

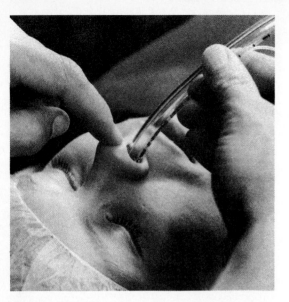

Figure 7-11B. Careful sliding of the naso-pharyngeal tube into the nasal cavity. (Reproduced with permission of Ambu, Inc. from Lotz, P., Ahnefeld, F. W., Hirlinger, W. K.: *A Systematic Guide to Intubation,* Atelier Flad, Eckental, West Germany.)

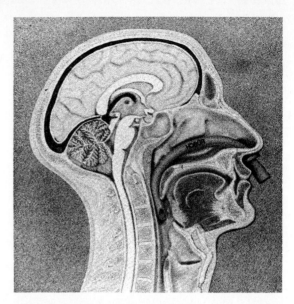

Figure 7-13. Correct position of nasopharyngeal airway after insertion. (Reproduced with permission of Ambu, Inc. from Lotz, P., Ahnefeld, F. W., Higlinger, W. K.: *A Systematic Guide to Intubation,* Atelier Flad, Eckental, West Germany.)

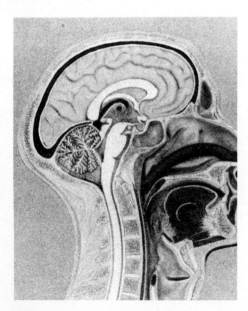

Figure 7-12. Passage of the nasopharyngeal airway parallel to the floor of the nasal cavity. (Reproduced with permission of Ambu, Inc. from Lotz, P., Ahnefeld, F. W., Hirlinger, W. K.: *A Systematic Guide to Intubation,* Atelier Flad, Eckental, West Germany.)

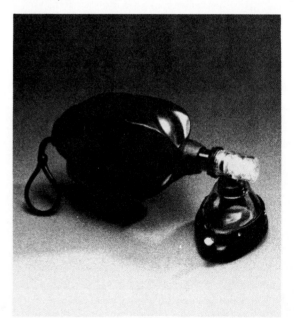

Figure 7-14. Example of a self-inflating resuscitation (Ambu) bag. (Reproduced with permission of Ambu, Inc. from Lotz, P., Ahnefeld, F. W., Hirlinger, W. K.: *A Systematic Guide to Intubation,* Atelier Flad, Eckental, West Germany.)

Suction

Immediate accessibility to properly functioning *suction* equipment is equally important as availability of other airway adjuncts. Such equipment is needed to remove secretions and particulate matter that might otherwise be aspirated or compromise the airway. Suction units should be portable, durable, and capable of generating at least 300 mm Hg of negative pressure. When suctioning the oral pharynx, a large bore catheter *and* tube should be used in order to assure that all large particulate matter will be evacuated. Smaller catheters are generally adequate for nasopharyngeal and/or endotracheal suction.

Suction Technique

Prior to suctioning, the patient should always be hyperventilated. The suction procedure itself should *never* be carried out for more than 15 seconds at a time to minimize the chance of hypoxemia.

Suction of the oral pharynx is performed by inserting the catheter in the patient's mouth and intermittently applying negative pressure. The trick to endotracheal suctioning is not to apply negative pressure during insertion of the catheter down the endotracheal tube. Instead, intermittent suction should only be applied while slowly withdrawing the catheter.

VENTILATORY ADJUNCTS

The devices described below are used to assist ventilation of patients in respiratory distress or to provide mandatory ventilation for those who are not breathing at all.

Self-Inflating Reservoir Bags

The *self-inflating resuscitation bag (bag-valve mask or BVM)* is a unit consisting of a bag and an adapter that can be attached to a mask or endotracheal tube (**Figure 7-14**).

The ideal BVM unit should have the following characteristics:
   i) A clear mask
   ii) A self-inflating, easy-to-grip bag
   iii) A system for delivery of supplemental oxygen
   iv) No pop-off valve

The reason for the *clear mask* is that it allows the emergency care provider to see if regurgitation has occurred. The bags of most BVM units are made of smooth rubber that becomes especially slippery when wet. An *easy-to-grip bag* would facilitate handling the unit when ventilating the patient.

A *system* for delivery of *supplemental oxygen* is important. An F_iO_2 of up to 40% may be provided by attaching a high-flow source of supplemental oxygen to the bag. With the additional attachment of an *oxygen reservoir* and a flow rate of 10–15 L/min, an F_iO_2 of up to 90% may be delivered.

Pop-off valves are not desirable for BVM units used to manage the airway of the patient in cardiac arrest because of the dramatic decrease in lung compliance that occurs in this setting. In order to ventilate such patients, much higher than usual airway pressures are often needed. Pop-off valves could be self-defeating, as they might prevent generation of sufficient peak airway pressure to overcome this increase in airway resistance.

BVM units are the most commonly employed ventilatory adjunct in emergency situations. Nevertheless, significant drawbacks are associated with their use. These include fluctuations in peak airway pressures, tidal volumes, and ventilatory rates; variability in delivered oxygen concentrations when a reservoir is not used; and face mask leaks.

Contrary to popular belief, tidal volumes generated with BVM units in the unprotected airway are far less than those generated by mouth-to-mouth or mouth-to-mask ventilation. This is not true for intubated patients, since leakage of air through the face mask is no longer a problem and both of the rescuer's hands are now free to squeeze the bag.

Technique for Use

The most difficult part of using a BVM unit is that one rescuer must simultaneously perform three tasks. A patent airway and tight face seal must be maintained with one hand while the other hand is used to ventilate the patient. Unless each of these tasks is performed correctly, inadequate ventilation is likely to result.

Insertion of an oral or nasopharyngeal tube may assist in maintaining patency of the airway. The mask of the BVM unit is then applied to the patient's face and secured by positioning the index finger on the portion that covers the chin while the thumb holds the upper part of the mask firmly against the bridge of the nose. The remaining three fingers are placed on the base of the mandible to support the head in the tilt position. The other hand is used to squeeze the bag.

To prevent high peak airway pressures and decrease the likelihood of gastric distention in the patient with an unprotected airway, the bag must be squeezed *slowly*. Use of a second rescuer is ex-

tremely helpful in this regard since it allows one rescuer to concentrate on securing a good face seal, while the other may use both hands to squeeze the bag. When proper ventilation is being administered, the chest will be observed to rise and fall with each insufflation of the bag. (An advantage of the BVM unit is that it provides the rescuer with a sense of the compliance of the patient's lungs.)

Flow-inflation Reservoir Bag

The *flow-inflation reservoir (anesthesia) bag (Mapelson-D bag)* requires much more skill to operate than does a BVM. It consists of an anesthesia bag, a piece of plastic tubing (that is approximately 1 foot long), an exhaust valve, and a standard endotracheal tube connector (**Figure 7-15**). The latter is usually attached to the oxygen source and an endotracheal tube. Advantages of this bag over the standard BVM are that you can

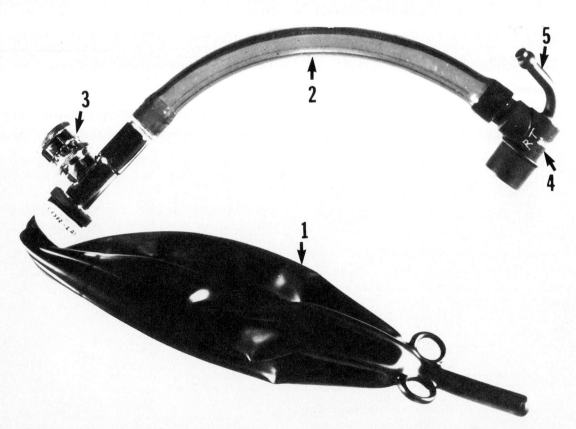

Figure 7-15.   Flow-inflation reservoir bag. 1) anesthesia bag; 2) plastic tubing; 3) exhaust valve; 4) standard ET tube connector; 5) connector for manometer (used to measure airway pressures).

apply CPAP (continuous positive airway pressure) and PEEP (positive end-expiratory pressure). In addition, ventilation with 100% oxygen is guaranteed. In contrast, one is never entirely sure of the concentration of oxygen delivered with the BVM because the amount of entrained room air is highly variable.

It should be emphasized that the Mapelson-D bag should be operated only by individuals highly trained in its use. In the hands of an inexperienced provider, the risk of barotrauma (and tension pneumothorax) is great.

Oxygen-Powered Breathing Devices (O₂PBD)

The *oxygen-powered breathing device* has been used to ventilate the victim in respiratory arrest

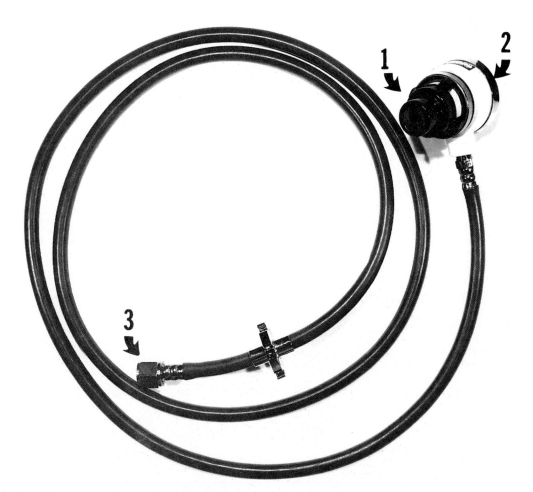

Figure 7-16. Oxygen-powered breathing device. 1) 15/22mm connector for attaching endotracheal tube; 2) flow regulator; 3) oxygen source connector.

and provide supplemental oxygen to spontaneously breathing patients. When used in the former setting, the O_2PBD functions as a manually cycled, pressure-limited ventilator (**Figure 7-16**). Activation of the unit by the rescuer provides spontaneous flow rates of up to 120 L/min. Ventilation is terminated either by release of the activation button or when peak airway pressure attains 40 mm Hg (54 cm H_2O).

> In recent years, this device has come under increasing scrutiny because of the high inspiratory flow rates it generates when manually operated and the potential for producing gastric insufflation in the patient with an unprotected airway. Consequently, the device is *not* recommended for use in patients unless they are intubated.
>
> The O_2PBD should not be used in children because of the risk of barotrauma.

In contrast, the O_2PBD may be much more useful when employed as a demand valve for spontaneously breathing patients. In this capacity, generation of as little as 1 cm H_2O negative airway pressure activates a flutter valve within the unit that allows the patient to inhale 100% oxygen. This aspect of the device is extremely

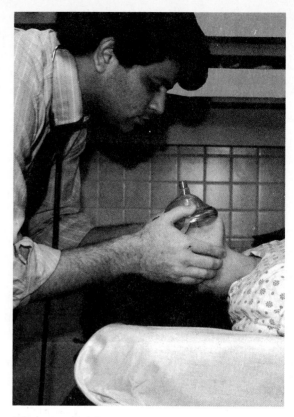

Figure 7-18. Proper positioning of the pocket mask.

advantageous in providing spontaneously breathing patients supplemental oxygen without requiring large volumes of stored oxygen.

The Pocket Mask (Mouth-to-mask)

The *pocket mask* is very similar to the mask used in conjunction with the bag-valve devices (**Figure 7-17**). The major difference is that the mouth-to-mask unit has an additional port where supplemental oxygen can be administered, providing inspired oxygen concentrations of 50% with a flow rate of 10 L/min. The port used for attachment of the reservoir bag with the bag-valve device is the port through which the rescuer ventilates the patient with the pocket mask.

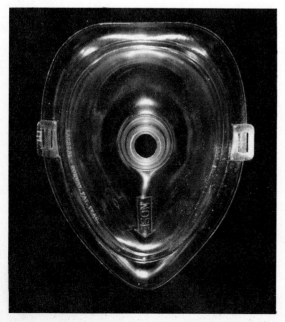

Figure 7-17. Pocket mask.

The most attractive feature of the pocket mask is that it allows the rescuer to perform mouth-to-mouth ventilation without the need for direct contact with the mouth of the victim.

Use of the Device

When using the pocket mask, the rescuer position himself/herself above the head of the patient. The mask is placed on the patient's face and secured through a coordinated interplay of the fingers of both hands. The thumbs stabilize the mask over the bridge of the nose, while the index fingers hold the mask in place over the chin. The three remaining fingers of each hand are positioned under the chin and act in concert to maintain the head tilt (**Figure 7-18**).

INTUBATION

Intubation is the definitive method of managing the airway of patients who are not breathing or who are unresponsive with an unprotected airway. The advantages of intubation are:

 i) Prevention of aspiration
 ii) Lower risk of gastric insufflation
 iii) Allows for administration of high inspired oxygen concentrations and positive pressure ventilations
 iv) Provides access for drug administration (with endotracheal intubation)

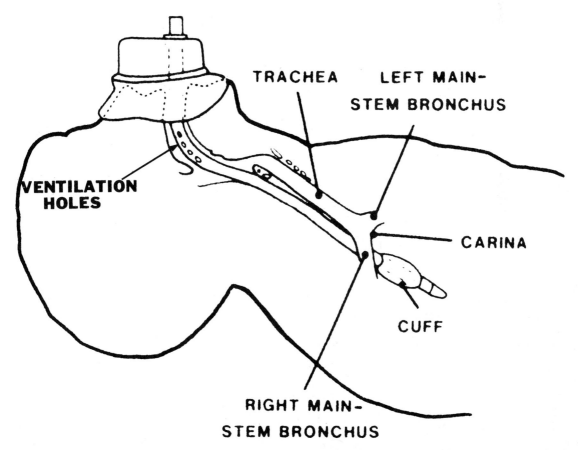

Figure 7-19.   Correct positioning of esophageal obturator airway (EOA) after insertion. (Reproduced with permission from McIntyre, K. M., Lewis, J. A. (editors): *Textbook of Advanced Cardiac Life Support,* American Heart Association, Dallas, 1981.)

v) Provides access for suctioning of the tracheobronchial tree (with endotracheal or nasotracheal intubation)

We will discuss the techniques and relative merits of each of the three available methods of intubation.

Esophageal Obturator Airways

The principal of the *esophageal obturator* is to occlude the esophagus so that gastric insufflation is prevented and the ventilatory efforts of the rescuer are directed into the trachea. Two types of obturators are currently available: the *esophageal obturator airway (EOA)* and the *esophageal gastric tube airway (EGTA)*. Although similar in appearance, important differences exist between the two types of obturators in the method of ventilation.

The EOA is the original esophageal obturator airway. This device was first described in 1968. It consists of a tube approximately 37 cm in length with a blind tip on its distal end. Inflation of a cuff just above this tip occludes the esophagus. When properly inserted, the cuff should lie slightly below the level of the carina of the trachea.

The proximal end of the tube is open and fits snugly into a specially designed face mask. Small ventilation holes are present in the uppper third of the tube. When the EOA is correctly positioned, the holes lie at the level of the posterior pharynx (**Figure 7-19**). It is through these small holes that ventilation occurs.

The EGTA was developed in 1977. It improved on the design of the EOA by adding a route for decompression of the stomach (**Figure 7-20A**). This lessens the chance of regurgitation and aspiration. Instead of having a blind tip on the distal end of the obturator tube, an opening was made through which a nasogastric tube could be passed into the stomach. The small holes which had previously been used for ventilation with the EOA are no longer present with the EGTA tube. Instead, a second port has been added to the mask through which ventilation oc-

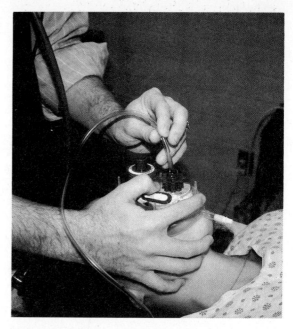

Figure 7-20A.   Inserting a nasogastric tube through the lumen of the EGTA tube to decompress stomach.

curs in a similar fashion as with the bag-valve mask (**Figure 7-20B**).

Technique of Insertion

The principle for insertion of the EOA and the EGTA is the same. The patient's head is gently flexed forward to assist in directing the tube into the esophagus (**Figure 7-21A and 7-21B**). The EOA/EGTA is inserted into the oral pharynx and *blindly* advanced. It should follow the natural curvature of the pharynx and enter into the esophagus (**Figure 7-21C**). At this point the mask should be seated on the face (**Figure 7-21D**).

Never force advancement of the tube. If resistance is encountered along the way, simply withdraw the tube slightly, reposition the patient's head if needed, and try again to advance the tube.

Confirming proper position of the tube is critical. If the trachea is inadvertently intubated and the cuff of the tube inflated with 30 ml of air, significant damage may occur to this structure. Several positive pressure ventilations should be delivered to test for tube position. Even though some of this air will enter the esophagus, enough should go

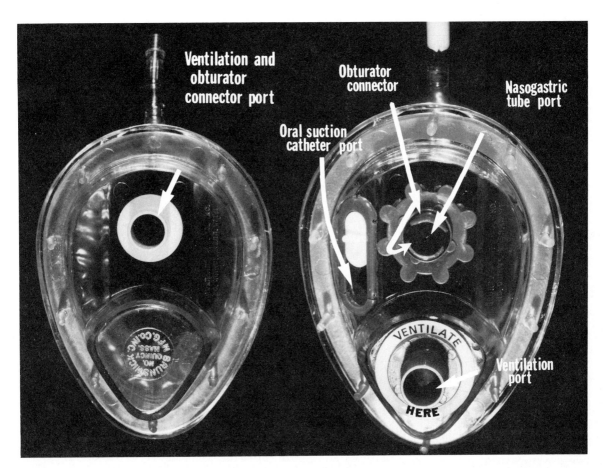

Figure 7-20B.   Comparison of EOA and EGTA (esophageal gastric tube airway) face mask.

into the trachea to produce a rise and fall of the chest wall if the tube is properly situated in the esophagus. The cuff may now be inflated with 30 ml of air. Further confirmation of proper tube placement can be obtained by auscultating over the apices and lateral lung fields for good bilateral breath sounds and observing for symmetric chest excursion.

Special Considerations

Although distinctly uncommon, esophageal rupture may complicate EOA placement. As a result,

Clinton and Ruiz (1985) suggest that inflation of the EOA cuff be limited to 20 ml of air instead of the customary 30 ml. In their experience, doing so has not resulted in leakage around the cuff and has virtually eliminated the risk of esophageal rupture.

The EOA/EGTA was initially advocated as an alternative method of endotracheal intubation. It has been most useful in the prehospital setting where operators skilled in endotracheal intubation are not always available. Advantages of the EOA are that insertion may be accomplished

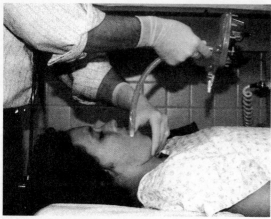

Figure 7-21A.   Position of the head while inserting the obturator airway.

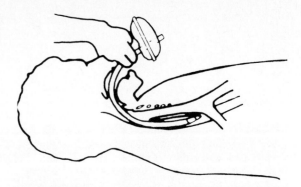

Figure 7-21C.   Advancing the obturator airway. (Reproduced with permission from McIntyre, K. M., Lewis, J. A. (editors): *Textbook of Advanced Cardiac Life Support,* American Heart Association. Dallas, 1981.)

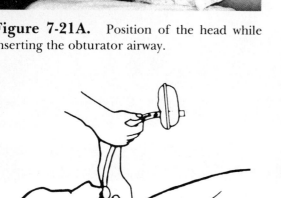

Figure 7-21B.   Schematic representation of Figure 7-21A. (Reproduced with permission from McIntyre, K. M., Lewis, J. A. (editors): *Textbook of Advanced Cardiac Life Support,* American Heart Association, Dallas, 1981.)

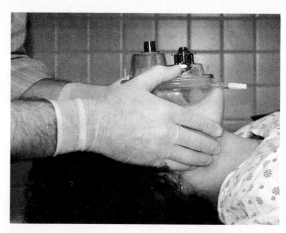

Figure 7-21D.   Final position of the obturator airway mask.

rapidly (in less than 10 seconds) by trained individuals (Clinton and Ruiz, 1985) and that neck extension is not needed for the procedure. However, significant problems have been associated with its use. These include:

i) Inadequate tidal volumes due to face mask leak

ii) Inadvertent endotracheal intubation

iii) Esophageal laceration and rupture

iv) High incidence of gastric regurgitation on removal of the tube

Because of these problems, endotracheal intubation is universally acknowledged as the procedure of choice for managing the unprotected airway.

Use of the EOA/EGTA is contraindicted if:

i) The victim is conscious.

ii) There is suspicion of caustic ingestion.

iii) The victim is less than 16 years of age.

iv) There is known esophageal disease.

Additional Considerations

Most emergency care providers will probably never have the opportunity to insert an EOA/EGTA. However, they may be involved with the removal of this device, particularly if they work in an emergency facility. It is therefore essential to gain familiarity with the technique for *removal* of the tube.

If the patient is still not breathing spontaneously on arrival in the emergency department, endotracheal intubation must be performed *before* the esophageal obturator is withdrawn. Because of the extremely high incidence of gastric regurgitation with removal of the EOA/EGTA, suction must be readily available. Hyperventilate the patient prior to any manipulation. The face mask of the obturator is then detached by squeezing the connector on the proximal end of the tube that protrudes through the mask (**Figure 7-22**). To make room for the laryngoscope, the tube is pushed to the left side of the mouth with the rescuer's index finger. Intubation can now be performed in the usual fashion. Due to the fact that the EOA/EGTA is still in place in the esophagus, the rescuer may be less likely to mistakenly intubate this structure.

Once correct placement of the endotracheal tube has been confirmed, the EOA/EGTA may be removed. This should be done by deflating the balloon, turning the patient on the side, and vigorously suctioning the oral pharynx at the same time that the tube is withdrawn.

Endotracheal Intubation

The most definitive means of managing the airway for the nonbreathing, unresponsive pa-

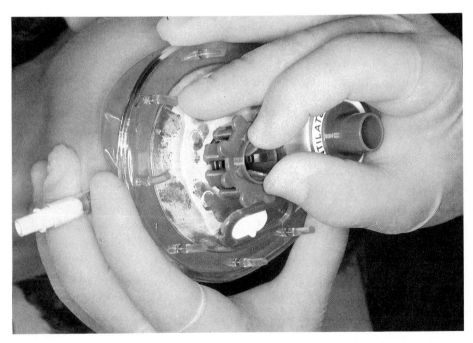

Figure 7-22. Releasing the EGTA mask.

tient is with *endotracheal intubation.* Two types of laryngoscope blades may be used to perform this procedure: the *Miller (straight) blade* and the *MacIntosh (curved) blade.*

The technique for visualization of the vocal cords is similar regardless of which blade is used. The only difference in the procedure is in the placement of the tip. When using the curved blade, the tip should be inserted into the vallecula. The soft tissue is then lifted and the laryngeal opening is visualized (**Figure 7-23**). In contrast when the straight blade is used, the epiglottis itself is lifted to provide visualization (**Figure 7-24**). *It matters little which blade is chosen for intubation.* Far more important for the emergency care provider is to decide on his/her preference and to become comfortable in the use of that *one* type of blade.

The size of the endotracheal tube most commonly used to intubate adults is 7.5–8.0 mm in diameter for females and 8.0–8.5 mm for males.

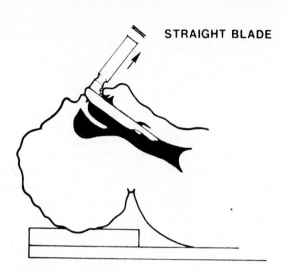

STRAIGHT BLADE

Figure 7-24. Proper placement of straight blade. (Reproduced with permission from McIntyre, K. M., Lewis, J. A. (editors): *Textbook of Advanced Cardiac Life Support,* American Heart Association, Dallas, 1981.)

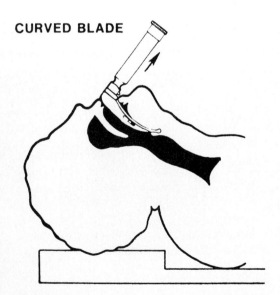

CURVED BLADE

Figure 7-23. Proper placement of curved blade. (Reproduced with permission from McIntyre, K. M., Lewis, J. A. (editors): *Textbook of Advanced Cardiac Life Support,* American Heart Association, Dallas, 1981.)

Prior to Intubation

All equipment must be routinely checked at frequent intervals. The time to find out that a laryngoscope bulb has burned out is not *after* the blade has been inserted into the pharynx. Similarly, the time to find out that the cuff is defective is not *after* the patient has been intubated.

Hyperventilation should always be performed prior to attempting intubation. At no time should a patient remain unventilated for more than 15–20 seconds. If intubation is not successful within this time frame, withdraw the tube, reventilate the patient, and try again.

Positioning the Patient

It is commonly assumed that hyperextension of the head and neck will facilitate endotracheal intubation. In reality, hyperextension produces the opposite effect because it causes the axes of the oropharynx and trachea to become misaligned (**Figure 7-25**). One technique that may make intubation easier is to place a small pillow or towel under the patient's occiput so as to lift the head slightly without extending it. This posture is known as the *sniffing* position (**Figure 7-26A**). As can be seen from **Figure 7-26B,** a much more direct line for visualization of the vocal cords (due to alignment of the axes of the oropharynx and trachea) is now evident.

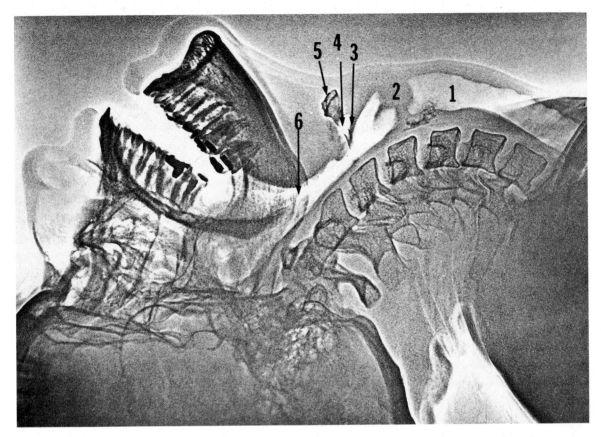

Figure 7-25. Hyperextension of the neck causes the axes at the oropharynx and trachea to become misaligned, thus making endotracheal intubation more difficult. 1) trachea; 2) vocal cords; 3) epiglottis; 4) vallecula; 5) hyoid cartilage; 6) oropharynx. (Reproduced with permission from Applebaum, E. L., Bruce, D. L.: *Tracheal Intubation*, W. B. Saunders Co., Philadelphia, 1976.)

Technique for Intubation

The key priorities for endotracheal intubation are speed of insertion and proper technique. The two are equally important. In the long run, attention to proper technique will improve speed by decreasing the need for repetitive intubation attempts.

A common mistake is to rapidly insert the full length of the laryngoscope blade. This frequently places the tip of the blade *beyond* the epiglottis and vallecula, making it extremely difficult for the rescuer to identify the anatomy. The rescuer is then forced to search for key structures on withdrawal of the blade. *It is far simpler and more effective to insert the blade in a more controlled manner.* This allows

one to visualize structures in their natural sequence as the blade is advanced through the airway.

The laryngoscope blade is carefully inserted into the patient's mouth, following the natural curvature of the tongue. The hard palate and uvula are visualized as one tracks through the oral pharynx. On arrival at the posterior pharynx, the tip of the blade is lifted. In most cases the epiglottis will now become readily visible. If using the straight blade, the epiglottis is lifted to visualize the cords. If the curved blade is used, the blade tip is inserted into the vallecula and then lifted a little higher to visualize the cords. Remember that the vallecula lies at the base of the tongue and is not nearly as deep in the throat as is commonly believed. Thus it is *not* necessary to insert the entire length of the laryn-

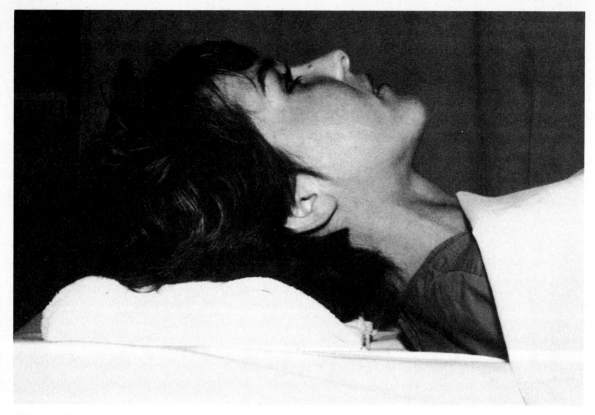

Figure 7-26A.   Sniffing position.

goscope blade into the patient's mouth for successful intubation.

   The teeth must not be used as a fulcrum to pry the mandible up when attempting to visualize the cords. Doing so makes it likely that a tooth will be fractured. Instead, the rescuer should concentrate on lifting the laryngoscope handle *forward* and *anteriorly* as if reaching to touch where the ceiling and wall meet (**Figure 7-27**).

   Once the epiglottis has been lifted and the laryngeal opening is in view, the following structures should be seen:
   i) The arytenoid cartilages
   ii) The vocal cords
   iii) The glottic opening

   The *arytenoid cartilages* lie at the bottom of the rescuer's field of vision. Behind them are found the white, glossy *vocal cords* which are separated by the dark glottic opening (**Figure 7-28**). It is through this opening that the endotracheal tube is inserted. The rescuer should watch the tube *as it passes*

through the opening until the cuff just disappears from sight (approximately 2 cm beyond the cords) (**Figure 7-29**).

   Once the tube is properly seated in the trachea, it is held in position with the rescuer's right hand as the laryngoscope is removed with the left hand. Care must be taken not to dislodge the endotracheal tube or fracture any teeth while removing the laryngoscope.

   The cuff is now inflated with 5–10 cc of air. Correct position of the tube can then be confirmed by auscultating the lung fields and epigastric area as several ventilations are administered. One listens for the presence of good bilateral breath sounds and looks for symmetric chest excursion. Absent or diminished breath sounds on the left side of the chest suggests intubation of the right mainstem bronchus. This can usually be rectified by withdrawing the tube a short distance until breath sounds become equal. Should gurgling sounds be heard over the epigastrium, the tube is in the stomach. Immediately deflate the balloon and remove the tube. Final confirmation of correct tube placement is demonstrated radiographically.

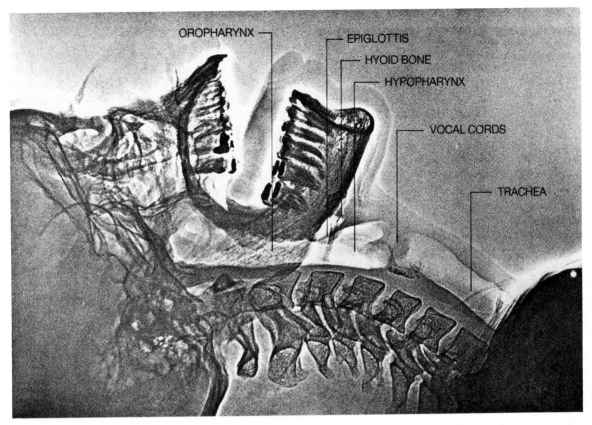

Figure 7-26B. X-ray demonstrating the sniffing position. (Reproduced with permission from Applebaum, E. L., Bruce, D. L.: *Tracheal Intubation*, W. B. Saunders Co., Philadelphia, 1976.)

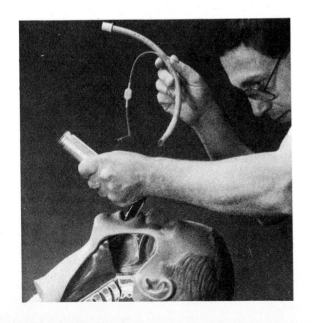

Figure 7-27. Correct technique for insertion of endotracheal tube, lifting laryngoscope handle forward and anteriorly. (Reproduced with permission of Ambu, Inc. from Lotz, P., Ahnefeld, F. W., Hirlinger, W. K.: *A Systematic Guide to Intubation*, Atelier Flad, Eckental, West Germany.)

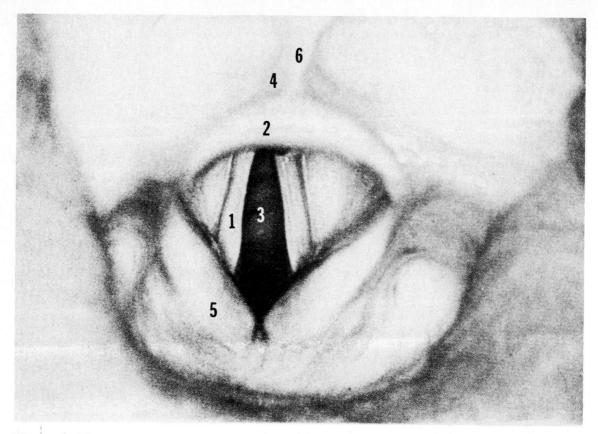

Figure 7-28.   Anatomy of the area around the entrance to the trachea. 1) vocal cords; 2) epiglottis; 3) aperture of the cords; 4) vallecula; 5) arytenoid cartilage; 6) tongue. (Reproduced with permission from Yokochi, C., Rohen, J. W.: *Photographic Anatomy of the Human Body*, University Park Press, Baltimore, 1978.)

Special Considerations

Insertion of an endotracheal tube may sometimes be aided by the use of a *stylet*. This malleable, firm wire is inserted into the endotracheal tube, with the distal end of the stylet lying at least 1 cm proximal to the distal end of the endotracheal tube. The reason for recessing the distal end of the stylet is to avoid traumatizing the airway. Molding the stylet so that the distal end of the endotracheal tube takes on a "hockey stick" appearance, and then guiding this curvature in an anterior direction often facilitates entry through the cords.

Another technique that may greatly assist the operator during endotracheal intubation is application of cricoid pressure (The *Sellick* maneuver).

This technique may serve the dual function of allowing visualization of the glottis and preventing regurgitation of gastric contents until intubation can be completed.

To perform the Sellick maneuver, one must first identify the cricoid cartilage. This is done by walking one's hands down in the midline from the thyroid cartilage (Adam's apple) into the depression below (the cricothyroid membrane) and onto the next lying structure. This is the cricoid cartilage. Apply firm, downward pressure on the anterolateral aspects of this cartilage with the thumb and index finger of either hand (**Figure 7-30**). Be sure to maintain downward pressure until *after* the endotracheal tube has been inserted and the cuff is inflated!

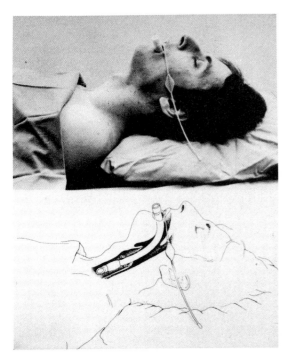

Figure 7-29. Correct position of the endo-tracheal tube after insertion. (Reproduced with permission from Applebaum, E. L., Bruce, D. L.: *Tracheal Intubation*, W. B. Saunders Co., Philadelphia, 1976.)

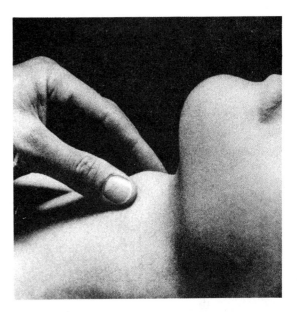

Figure 7-30. Application of the Sellick maneuver. (Reproduced with permission of Ambu, Inc. from Lotz, P., Ahnefeld, F. W., Hirlinger, W. K.: *A Systematic Guide to Intubation*, Atelier Flad, Eckental, West Germany.)

Blind Nasotracheal Intubation

The advantage of *nasotracheal intubation* is that it provides an alternative method for achieving definitive control of the airway in the spontaneously breathing patient who exhibits teeth clenching and/or who retains a sensitive gag reflex.

A slightly smaller (6.5–7.5 mm in diameter) endotracheal tube is recommended for this procedure than for endotracheal intubation.

Technique for Insertion

The technique for insertion is initially the same as that described for placement of a nasopharyngeal airway. The nasotracheal tube is lubricated with 2% lidocaine gel. It is inserted into the nares and advanced by placing the bevel against the sep-

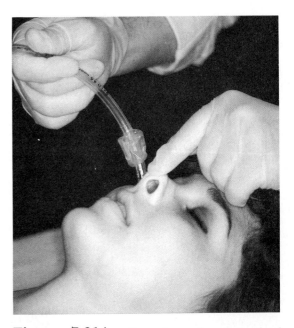

Figure 7-31A. Insertion of nasotracheal tube into the right nares.

tum of the nose and gently sliding the tube backward in line with the base of the ears (**Figure 7-31A**). In this way the tube passes parallel to the floor of the nasal cavity.

In passing from the nasopharynx to the posterior pharynx, the tube must take a downward turn. Occasionally it may get hung up trying to negotiate this turn and abut against the posterior pharyngeal wall. Clinically, this should be suspected if resistance to further advancement is encountered or there is loss of air movement through the tube. Should this happen, immediately withdraw the tube a short distance, reposition (slightly extend) the patient's head, and reattempt to advance the tube. Do *not* try to force the tube forward as this may result in mucosal injury and bleeding or even in retropharyngeal perforation!

The rescuer now directs his/her attention to listening (or feeling) for air movement through the tube (**Figure 7-31B**). As the distal end of the tube gets closer and closer to the laryngeal opening, the sound of air movement should become increasingly louder (**Figure 7-31C**). Continue to gently guide the tube toward the glottis. If at any time air movement ceases, withdraw the tube slightly, reposition the patient's head if needed, and resume the process. When air movement sounds are at their loudest, the rescuer should hold the tube still. At this point, anticipate the next inspiratory effort of the patient, and the moment this effort begins attempt to advance the tube into the trachea. This often

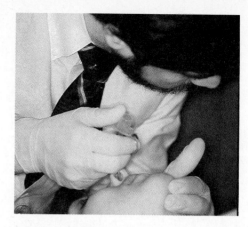

Figure 7-31C.   As the final position of the nasotracheal tube is approached, manipulation of the trigger may facilitate tracheal intubation.

stimulates the patient's cough reflex. If the attempt is successful, inspiratory and expiratory air flow will be heard through the tube. If not, the esophagus may have been intubated. The tube should be immediately withdrawn, and another attempt made.

Final tube placement should be confirmed in the same manner as for endotracheal intubation.

Special Considerations

Recently a device has been made available that greatly facilitates blind nasotracheal intubation (*Endotrol*, National Catheter Corporation, Brunswick, New York). By means of a trigger mechanism at the proximal end of the tube, controlled flexion of the distal end is now possible (**Fig. 7-32**). This allows the rescuer to direct the distal tip anteriorly in the direction of the laryngeal opening at the moment the tube is inserted into the trachea.

Finally, since accurate placement with blind nasotracheal intubation is predicated on hearing (or feeling) movement of air in the tube, it should be apparent that the procedure cannot be performed in the apneic patient.

ALGORITHM FOR MANAGEMENT OF THE ADULT AIRWAY

To help conceptualize the material covered in this chapter we have developed an Algorithm for Management of the Adult Airway (**Fig. 7-33**). The management sequence begins with the res-

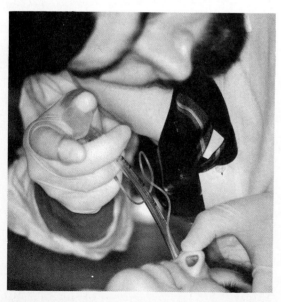

Figure 7-31B.   Listening for air movement as the tube is advanced.

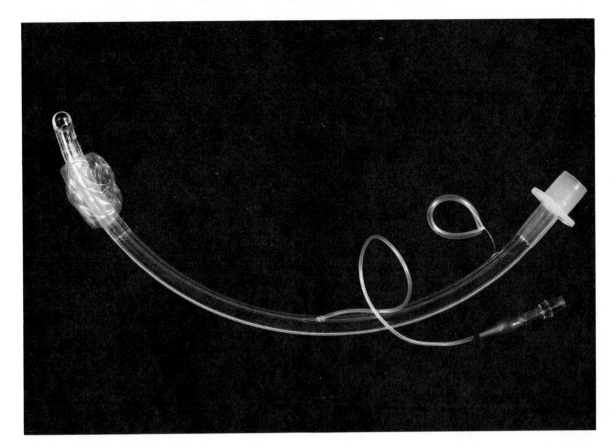

Figure 7-32.   Endotrol tube.

cuer simultaneously assessing ventilation and the level of consciousness (**1**).

> Many definitions exist for the terms *conscious, semiconscious,* and *unconscious.* For the purpose of determining optimal managment of the airway, we have defined these terms in the following manner:
>
> **Conscious**—a patient who is alert, awake, and responding appropriately.
> **Semiconscious**—a less alert patient who may not be awake and only responds to verbal or painful stimuli. The gag reflex may still be intact.
> **Unconscious**—a patient who cannot be aroused and does not respond to either verbal or painful stimuli. The gag reflex is absent.

If a patient is *conscious* or *semiconscious* and spontaneously breathing in a normal manner, all that may be needed is supplemental oxygen (**1-2-4**). The rescuer should then evaluate the adequacy of oxygenation (**5**). This may be done by physical examination (as described earlier in this chapter) and/or by arterial blood gas sampling (if indicated). If this evaluation suggests that oxygenation is inadequate, more definitive management of the airway (either by insertion of a nasopharyngeal airway or endotracheal intubation) is needed.

Unconscious patients, even if they are breathing normally, require definitive airway management with endotracheal intubation (**1-3-7**).

For patients who are breathing abnormally (and for those who are not breathing at all), appropriate management of the airway is the same regardless of the state of consciousness (**1-2-6**) or (**1-3-6**). In either case, the airway should be manually opened by either the chin lift or jaw

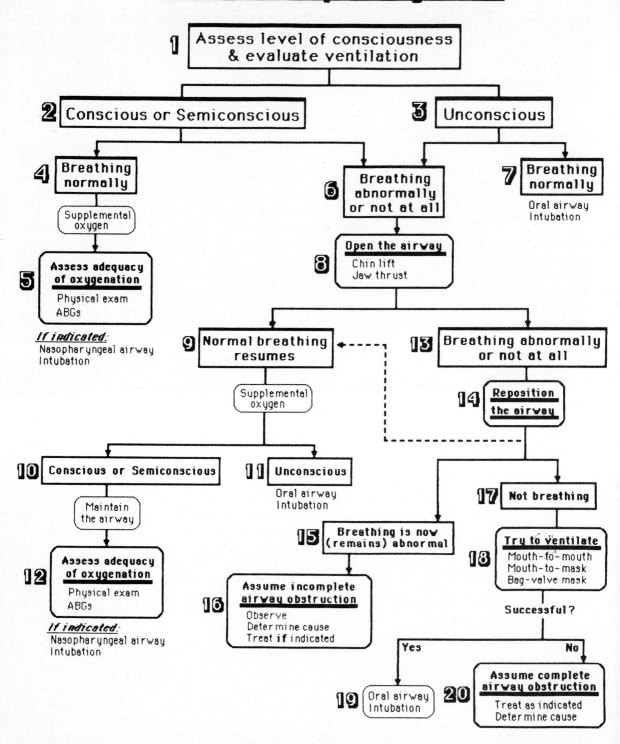

Figure 7-33. Algorithm for Management of the Adult Airway.

thrust maneuver **(8)**. If this results in resumption of normal breathing **(9)**, supplemental oxygen should be administered. For the *unconscious* patient, definitive airway management with endotracheal intubation is again the treatment of choice **(6-8-9-11)**. On the other hand, if the patient is *conscious* or *semiconscious* **(10)**, less definitive therapy may be needed. Manually maintain the airway. Further management will then hinge on assessment of the adequacy of oxygenation **(6-8-9-10-12)**.

If after initially opening the airway, the patient continues to breathe abnormally (or is still not breathing at all), the rescuer should reposition the airway **(6-8-13-14)**. If this results in resumption of normal breathing, management should follow the course described above **(8-9-10-12)** or **(8-9-11)**. On the other hand, if breathing is still abnormal after repositioning the airway **(15)**, the rescuer should assume *incomplete airway obstruction* is present and treat accordingly **(6-8-13-14-15-16)**.

If the patient remains in respiratory arrest even after repositioning the airway, an attempt should be made to ventilate the patient **(14-17-18)**. If successful, definitive airway management with endotracheal intubation should be performed **(19)**. If unsuccessful, the rescuer should assume *complete airway obstruction* and treat accordingly **(20)**.

REFERENCES

Auerbach PS, Geehr EC: *Inadequate oxygenation and ventilation using the esophageal gastric tube airway in the prehospital setting.* JAMA 250:3067–3071, 1983.

Clinton JE, Ruiz E: *Emergency airway management procedures.* In Roberts JR, Hedges JR (Eds): Clinical Procedures in Emergency Medicine. W.B. Saunders, Philadelphia, 1985, pp 2–45.

Harrison RR, Maull KI, Keenan RL, Boyan CP: *Mouth-to-mask ventilation: A superior method of rescue breathing.* Ann Emerg Med 11:74–76, 1982.

Hochbaum SR: *Emergency airway management.* In Kobernick MS, Burney RE (Eds): Emergency Medicine Clinics of North America. W.B. Saunders, Philadelphia, Vol 4, 1986, pp 441–425.

Montgomery WH: *Ventilation during cardiopulmonary resuscitation.* In Harwood AL (Ed): Cardiopulmonary Resuscitation. Williams & Wilkins, Baltimore, 1982, pp. 4–33.

White RD: *Controversies in out-of-hospital emergency airway control: Esophageal obstruction or endotracheal intubation?* Ann Emerg Med 13:778–781, 1984.

CHAPTER 8

INTRAVENOUS ACCESS

Dan Cavallaro, NREMT   Larry Kravitz, MD   Jerry Diehr, MD
Ken Grauer, MD   Harry Sernaker, MD   Paul Augereau, MD

Along with management of the airway and defibrillation, establishing intravenous (IV) access is one of the major priorities of cardiopulmonary resuscitation. Many techniques exist for accomplishing this goal, each with its own relative merits and drawbacks. The skill of the operator and individual preferences tempered by personal experience all play a large role in determining which technique is chosen for any given situation and how the technique is performed. *The best technique is the one that works for you.* We limit our discussion here to a brief overview of the standard methods for obtaining intravenous access, with commentary on techniques that have been helpful in our experience.

INITIAL PRIORITIES

Circulation of drugs in the arrested heart is most effectively accomplished when administered into a *central* vein such as the internal jugular or subclavian. These veins offer the advantage of having a fairly constant location with respect to easily identifiable anatomic landmarks. This usually allows rapid cannulation, even in a state of cardiovascular collapse (when peripheral veins may be exceedingly difficult to visualize.) However, achieving access at these sites is not without problems such as:

i) The need for an operator skilled in the technique
ii) The need to stop CPR
iii) Significant risk of pneumothorax, hemothorax

Selection of the femoral vein as the site for central venous access avoids the latter two problems but raises an additional concern. Recent studies suggest that blood flow during CPR is significantly diminished below the diaphragm (Dalsey et al., 1983; Neimann et al., 1981). Thus drugs administered through this route during cardiopulmonary resuscitation may not adequately reach the central circulation.

Practically speaking, the most commonly chosen site for intravenous access during cardiopulmonary resuscitation is a *peripheral* line. This is particularly true when operators skilled in the insertion of central lines are not on the scene. One should remember that the smaller the catheter and the more distal the site, the less likely there will be adequate drug delivery to the central circulation. Four suggestions may be helpful to optimize drug delivery by this route:

i) Select a proximal site (antecubital fossa) if possible, as this is superior to using a vein on the dorsum of the wrist
ii) Use a *large* bore needle (ideally 16 gauge or larger, although this may not always be possible)
iii) Elevate the arm after administering the medication (to favor venous return)
iv) Follow administration of the medication with a 50–100 cc bolus of fluid (to help "flush" the medication toward the central circulation)

Finally, one should not forget the *endotracheal* route. Three of the most commonly used drugs in cardiopulmonary resuscitation (epinephrine, lidocaine, and atropine) are effectively given in this manner. Although the pharmacokinetics of these drugs is probably more favorable when they are administered through a central venous route, one should not hesitate to give drugs endotracheally if this is the only route available.

Technique for Endotracheal Drug Administration

Three techniques have been proposed for endotracheal drug administration (Ward, 1985). In each, the drug should be diluted to a volume of at least 10 ml. The first method is the simplest and probably the most commonly used. Drug is drawn up in a 10–20 ml syringe with an 18 gauge needle firmly attached to the end of the syringe. The drug is then rapidly injected down the lumen of the ET tube, followed by several forceful insufflations of the Ambu bag. This promotes more distal delivery of drug into the tracheobronchial tree. Should the patient cough during the procedure, the ET tube opening should be covered to prevent expulsion of the medication. External chest compressions should be stopped momentarily while the drug is injected, since this too may result in expulsion of the medication.

In the second method of endotracheal drug administration, instead of injecting the drug down the opening of the ET tube the 18 gauge needle is inserted *into* the ET tube itself. An advantage of this method is that the ventilatory device need not be disconnected from the ET tube opening in order to administer the drug. Medication is injected through the side of the ET tube during the inspiratory phase of ventilation, in this manner being forcefully delivered to the distal tracheobronchial tree.

In the final method of endotracheal drug administration, a CVP catheter is attached to the syringe instead of the 18 gauge needle. The catheter is inserted down the lumen of the ET tube. In this way, drug may be injected directly into the distal trachea and bronchi, without loss of solution onto the lumen walls of the ET tube.

Although data demonstrating the superiority of one method over another are lacking, intuitive advantages of the latter two techniques are that they probably deliver drug more directly to the distal tracheobronchial tree.

Our Suggestion for Obtaining IV Access

If on your arrival at the scene of a cardiac arrest the patient is already intubated or has a large bore proximal IV in place, medications should initially be administered by one (or both) of these routes. If the patient does not respond (or if neither of these routes has been established), it is certainly reasonable to stop CPR momentarily to attempt insertion of an internal jugular or subclavian vein provided you are adept with these techniques.

INTRAVENOUS ACCESS SYSTEMS: GENERAL CONSIDERATIONS

In general, three types of cannulas are used to achieve intravenous access: 1) catheter-*over*-the-needle units; 2) catheter-*through*-the-needle units; and 3) catheters inserted over a guidewire which was previously introduced through a needle (*Seldinger technique*) (**Figure 8-1**). Catheter-over-the-needle units are the kind used for obtaining peripheral venous access, while the other two types of catheters are used for central venous insertion.

With the catheter-*over*-the needle system, the catheter must necessarily be larger in diameter than the needle. After cannulation of the vein with the needle, the catheter must then be advanced over the needle and in through the puncture site of the vessel wall. Because the diameter of the catheter is a little larger than the diameter of the puncture site, the catheter may sometimes fail to enter the vein. This is a marked disadvantage of the system.

The chances of threading the catheter into the vein are much greater with the second system, because the catheter is advanced *through* the needle. However, this system is marked by several disadvantages. Catheter size is limited by (and must be slightly smaller than) the diameter of the needle. If in the midst of an arrest situation the operator becomes momentarily distracted and *withdraws* the catheter back through the needle, a portion of the catheter may be sheared off and embolize distally in the vessel. Finally, because the catheter lumen is slightly smaller than the lumen of the needle, it will also be smaller than the diameter of the puncture site. Extravasation of fluid may therefore occur at the site where the catheter enters the vein.

In the past, the catheter-through-the-needle system was a favored technique for achieving rapid access into the central circulation during an emergency situation. Because of the above disadvantages of the system, it is now being replaced by the Seldinger technique.

The *Seldinger technique* is the ideal system for obtaining intravenous access. It not difficult to

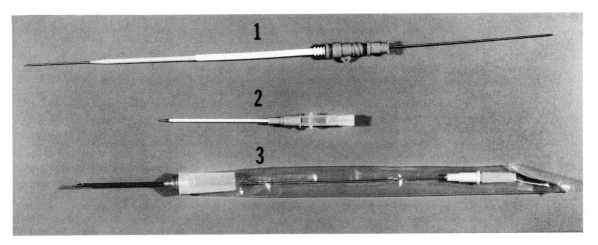

Figure 8-1. The three types of cannulas used to achieve intravenous access. 1) guide wire and sheath dilator unit; 2) catheter over-the-needle cannula; 3) catheter through-the-needle cannula.

learn and provides rapid access (with a large bore catheter) to the central circulation with a minimum of complications. Initially the vein is cannulated with a relatively small bore introducing needle. The diameter of this needle may be small (18 gauge)—*it only has to be large enough to accommodate the guide wire.* Because initial intravenous access is accomplished with a small bore needle, the chances of successfully cannulating a vein in a state of cardiovascular collapse (when the lumen of the vein is small and hard to enter) are increased, while the potential for damaging surrounding structures by errant needle puncture is minimized. Once the guidewire is threaded through the introducing needle, the dilator and large bore (8.0–8.5 French) catheter sheath may be inserted over the guide wire. The dilator and wire can then be removed, and access for rapid administration of medication, fluids, blood, or passage of a temporary transvenous pacemaker or Swan-Ganz catheter is secured. (We describe the Seldinger technique in more detail at the end of this chapter.)

Another advantage of the Seldinger technique is that in a matter of moments an existing IV (such as an 18 gauge peripheral line placed by paramedics in the field) may be converted into a large bore site of intravenous access. All one has to do is slip the guide wire through the existing peripheral catheter, remove the catheter, and then proceed as above to insert the dilator/catheter sheath unit over the wire.

Rate of Fluid Administration

The rate of fluid administration depends on the diameter and *length* of the particular catheter and IV tubing used. As an example of how dramatically these parameters affect the rate of fluid administration, consider the following:

Flow rate through a 18 gauge × 4.3 cm catheter ≈ 55 ml/min
Flow rate through a 16 gauge × 20 cm catheter ≈ 25 ml/min
Flow rate through a 16 gauge × 13.3 cm catheter ≈ 57 ml/min
Flow rate through a 16 gauge ×5.7 cm catheter ≈ 83 ml/min
Flow rate through a 14 gauge ×5.7 catheter ≈ 94 ml/min
Flow rate through a 8.5 French × 12 cm catheter ≈ 108 ml/min

(Sacchetti, 1985)

Thus the larger the bore and the shorter the catheter, the greater the flow rate. Although this statement may seem intuitively obvious, it is surprising how common the principle is overlooked in practice. For example, a 16 gauge, 20 cm long catheter-through-the-needle unit (as is commonly used for central venous cannulation) provides *less than one third the flow* as a 16 gauge, 5.7 cm long unit (as is commonly used for securing peripheral venous access). Clearly, cannulation of a central vein with a catheter-through-the-needle does not provide ideal access for rapid administration of large amounts of fluid.

Complications of IV Access Systems

Certain complications are common to all IV access systems. These include local complications (infiltration with resultant hematoma formation, infection, and thrombosis) and systemic complications (sepsis, pulmonary embolism, air embolism, and catheter fragment embolism). Technique-specific complications (pneumothorax, hemothorax) are addressed below.

Although strict aseptic technique is often not feasible during an emergency situation, one must remember to change contaminated IV lines as soon as possible in patients who have been successfully resuscitated.

PERIPHERAL LINES

Veins in the Upper Extremity

Most readers are thoroughly familiar with the techniques for insertion of a peripheral line in the upper extremity. Therefore we will limit our comments to a few selected points.

     i) If unable to visualize a suitable vein for cannulation, apply a tourniquet, hang the arm off the bed, *and go to the other side.* If after 2 additional minutes you are unable to cannulate a vein on the other side, return to the original side (with the tourniquet). A vein may now be distended.

     ii) A trick for establishing a large bore IV in a proximal upper extremity vein is to first establish distal access on the dorsum of the wrist with a 22 gauge butterfly. Then infuse 10–15 ml of fluid into this vein with a syringe. Frequently this will distend a larger more proximal vein that can then be cannulated directly.

     iii) Perhaps the best method for facilitating insertion of a peripheral IV line is to apply a warm towel to the arm for several minutes.

Alternatively, nitroglycerin ointment may be applied to the skin. The underlying veins will usually distend. Unfortunately the time involved with these techniques may preclude their use in an emergency situation.

External Jugular Vein

The external jugular vein lies superficially along the lateral aspect of the neck. It extends from the angle of the mandible and runs downward until it enters the thorax at a point corresponding to the middle of the clavicle. Shortly thereafter it terminates in the subclavian vein (**Figure 8-2**).

Under normal circumstances, the external jugular vein is surprisingly easy to cannulate. Its advantage is that despite being a peripheral vein, it provides rapid access into the central circulation. The problem is that during a code situation, the external jugular is often not readily accessible, especially if rescuers are actively working on controlling the airway. Other drawbacks are that the vein tends to be very mobile and tortuous. Consequently, intravenous access may be tenuous (easy to dislodge) and positional (with flow sometimes varying greatly with even slight movement of the head).

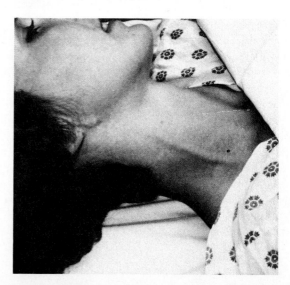

Figure 8-2. Anatomical location of the external jugular vein.

Technique for Insertion

With the patient in the supine, head-down position, rotate the head to the opposite side. Applying digital pressure to the vein distally (just above the clavicle) will often assist in distending the vein. Insert the needle in the middle of the vein (**Figure 8-3**). Cannulation is then performed by essentially the same technique that is used with other peripheral veins.

Veins in the Lower Extremity

As noted above, the lower extremity is not a preferred site for intravenous cannulation, since it appears that blood flow from below the diaphragm is significantly decreased during CPR.

CENTRAL LINES

Internal Jugular Vein

The internal jugular vein runs from the base of the skull downward along the carotid artery until it enters the chest to meet with the subclavian vein behind the clavicle (**Figure 8-4**). For those skilled in the technique, it is a favored site for obtaining intravenous access.

The right side of the neck is preferred for three reasons: 1) the dome of the lung and pleura are lower on the right side; 2) insertion of a cannula on this side follows a direct line to the right atrium; 3) the thoracic duct empties on the left side.

A major advantage of selecting the internal

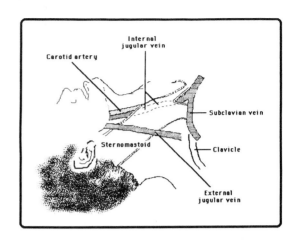

Figure 8-4. Anatomical location of the internal jugular vein.

jugular instead of the subclavian vein is the significantly lower risk of pneumothorax. Unfortunately during a code situation, this site may not be readily accessible, especially if rescuers are actively working on controlling the airway.

Special Considerations

One complication unique to internal jugular cannulation is *neck hematoma*. This may be due to extravasation from either the vein or inadvertent puncture of the artery. Fortunately in either case, local pressure will usually be sufficient to control the bleeding (although 10–20 minutes of firm pressure may be needed to control hemorrhage with arterial puncture). Should one suspect arterial puncture, *the operator must not attempt cannulation of the internal jugular vein on the other side*, since bilateral hemorrhage (with compression of the trachea) could occur. Instead, subsequent attempts at central venous cannulation should preferably be on the subclavian vein of the *same* side (to avoid the possibility of producing an iatrogenic bilateral complication).

Carotid artery disease is a relative contraindication to internal jugular cannulation for two reasons: 1) inadvertent arterial puncture may dislodge a plaque and 2) should neck hematoma complicate the procedure, application of firm pressure to control the hemorrhage might further compromise carotid artery flow.

Body habitus may play a role in determining the likelihood of success with this technique. Cannulation is most difficult in patients with short, stubby necks. Finally in conscious patients, one should bear in mind that internal jugular cannulation is

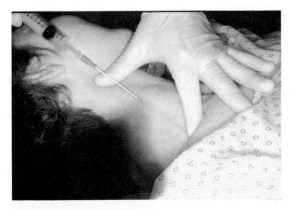

Figure 8-3. Cannulation of the external jugular vein.

more uncomfortable than subclavian cannulation, due to the restriction it places on neck movement.

Techniques for Insertion

There are three techniques for insertion of an internal jugular central line. *For each of them,* the patient is supine and in slight (15°–30°) Trendelenburg position with the head turned to the contralateral side. Additional maneuvers that may be helpful in distending the vein include asking the conscious patient to bear down (Valsalva) and having an assistant apply pressure to the abdomen of the unconscious patient.

Posterior Approach

The needle is inserted at the junction of the middle and lower thirds of the lateral border of the sternomastoid muscle. It is then advanced *under* this muscle, aiming toward the suprasternal notch (**Figure 8-5**).

Most providers do not use this approach. It appears to be more difficult for the novice to master, is associated with potentially significant complications, and entails insertion of the needle a long way (5–7 cm) before the vein is entered.

Anterior Approach

The index and middle fingers are placed on the carotid artery and retract it medially away from the anterior border of the sternocleidomastoid muscle. The needle is then inserted at the midpoint of the medial aspect of the sternocleidomastoid muscle at a 30° to 45° angle with the frontal plane, aiming for the ipsilateral nipple (**Figure 8-6**).

Most providers do not use this approach either. The major problem is the close proximity of the carotid artery. Because the carotid sheath is fairly well fixed to underlying structures, even the most diligent efforts to retract it medially are often less than successful. In the hands of the novice, the risk of arterial puncture appears to be significant.

Central (Middle) Approach

The patient is supine and in slight Trendelenberg position, with the head rotated to the contralateral side. The needle is inserted at the apex of the triangle formed by the two heads of the sternocleidomastoid muscle and directed slightly lateral in the direction of the ipsilateral nipple. Although many texts suggest to enter the skin at a 30° angle to the frontal plane, increasing the angle of entry

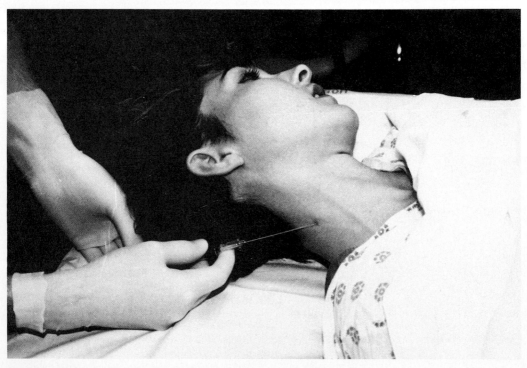

Figure 8-5. Posterior approach to the internal jugular vein.

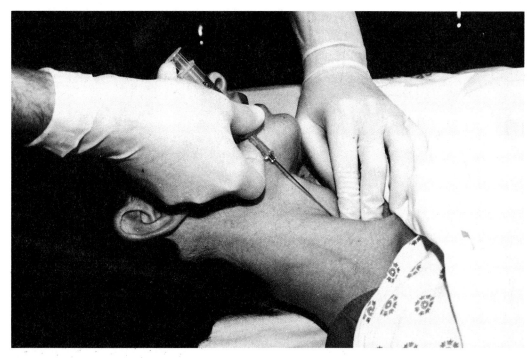

Figure 8-6. Anterior approach to the internal jugular vein.

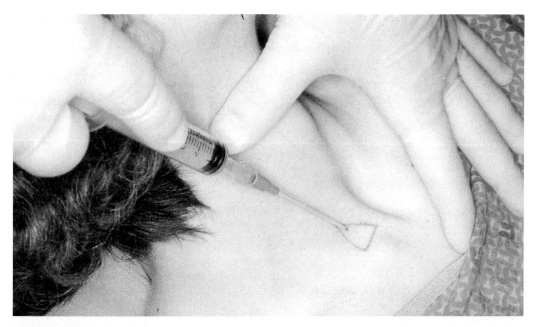

Figure 8-7. Central approach to the internal jugular vein. The needle is inserted at the apex of the triangle formed by the two heads of the sternocleidomastoid muscle (here marked in ink).

to between 45° and 60° may be more effective (**Figure 8-7**). The vein is usually entered within 1–3 cm. If unsuccessful, withdraw the needle and redirect it in a slightly more medial orientation on the next attempt.

This is the preferred approach of most emergency care providers who choose the internal jugular site, and the one we suggest. Anatomic landmarks (the two heads of the sternocleidomastoid muscle) are easy to identify on virtually all subjects, and the risk of carotid artery puncture is much less than with the anterior approach (since at this level of the neck the jugular vein lies lateral [and away from] the common carotid artery).

Subclavian Vein

The subclavian vein is the continuation of the axillary vein, beginning at the point where this vessel passes over the first rib and under the medial third of the clavicle. It then meets with the internal jugular vein to form the brachiocephalic (innominate) vein (**Figure 8-8**).

The subclavian vein is the central venous access site preferred by many providers because:

i) It may have been the only method taught during their training.

ii) It may be more accessible than the internal jugular vein during cardiopulmonary resuscitation.

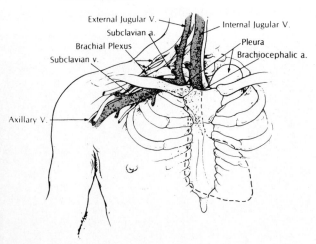

Figure 8-8. Anatomical location of the subclavian vein. (Reproduced with permission from Roberts, J. R. and Hedges, J. R. (editors): *Clinical Procedures in Emergency Medicine*, W. B. Saunders Co., Philadelphia, 1985.)

iii) It may be easier for the novice to master than the internal jugular technique.

A significant drawback is the substantial risk of pneumothorax and other complications (hemothorax, subclavian artery puncture).

Additional contraindications to subclavian cannulation include anticoagulation and coagulopathy. Unlike the case for internal jugular cannulation, there is no way to locally tamponade bleeding should either venous extravasation or inadvertent arterial puncture occur.

Special Considerations

As for the internal jugular vein, selecting the right side for the initial attempt at cannulation is favored, since this lowers the risk of pneumothorax (lower dome of the pleura on the right) and eliminates the possibility of thoracic duct puncture. Many clinicians feel these considerations outweigh the potential benefit offered by the smoother trajectory of the catheter when it is inserted from the left side.

Ideally, one should not make multiple attempts at cannulating the subclavian vein. Doing so only increases the risk of causing a pneumothorax. If unsuccessful on one side, instead of attempting subclavian cannulation on the opposite side (which invites the possibility of producing a bilateral iatrogenic complication), *it may be preferable to attempt internal jugular cannulation on the same side.*

Technique for Insertion

Again, the patient ideally is supine and in slight Trendelenberg position, with the head rotated to the contralateral side. Optimal positioning for subclavian cannulation may be further facilitated by placing a pillow or rolled towel between the scapulae; however, allowing the shoulders to fall too far back may be counterproductive by narrowing the space between the clavicle and the first rib. Make sure the arms are at the side of patient and not hanging off the bed. (Having an assistant exert gentle downward traction on the ipsilateral arm [pulling toward the feet] sometimes helps maintain optimum positioning.)

Insert the needle at the junction of the middle and medial thirds of the clavicle. Then "walk" the needle down under the clavicle and advance it *parallel to the frontal plane.* Do not direct the needle downward, as this greatly increases the risk of pneumothorax. Position the index fingertip of the free hand in the suprasternal notch and use this as a reference point. The advancing needle should be aimed just above and posterior to this fingertip (**Figure 8-9A**). Aspirate on the syringe until a blood flash is obtained (**Figure 8-9B**). Then remove the

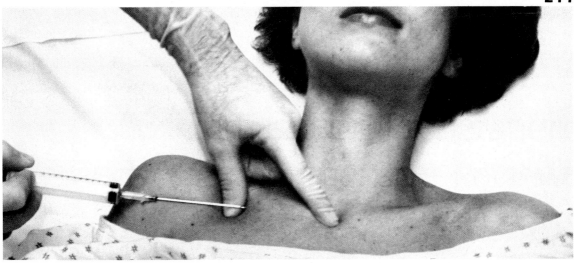

Figure 8-9A. Cannulation of the subclavian vein.

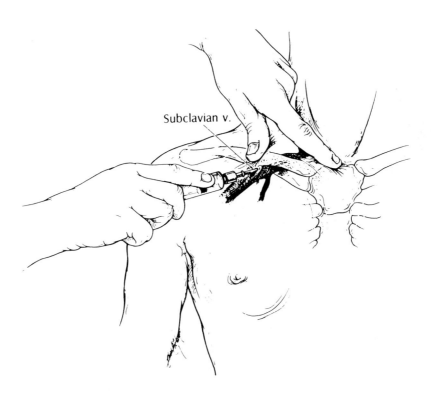

Subclavian v.

Figure 8-9B. Schematic representation of subclavian vein cannulation. Aspirate until blood flash is obtained. (Reproduced with permission from Roberts, J. R. and Hedges, J. R. (editors): *Clinical Procedures in Emergency Medicine,* W. B. Saunders Co., Philadelphia, 1985.)

syringe and feed in the catheter. *At no time expose the catheter hub to free air,* as this greatly increases the risk of air embolus.

In order to facilitate the catheter in making the downward turn into the brachiocephalic vein (instead of traveling up the neck), the bevel of the needle should be direcrted downward as soon as the lumen of the vein is entered. Aligning the bevel of the needle with the numerical markings on the syringe *before* beginning the procedure is a handy trick for knowing which way the needle will have to be rotated.

The catheter should thread easily. If it doesn't, it may have kinked, encountered an obstruction, or passed out of the vessel lumen. *Never force the catheter and above all do not withdraw it through the needle if it does not thread.*

Femoral Vein

As noted above, the femoral vein is no longer a favored site for central venous access during cardiac arrest.

The Seldinger Technique

In recent years the Seldinger technique has become an increasingly popular method for central venous cannulation. As discussed in our introduction, the advantages of this technique are

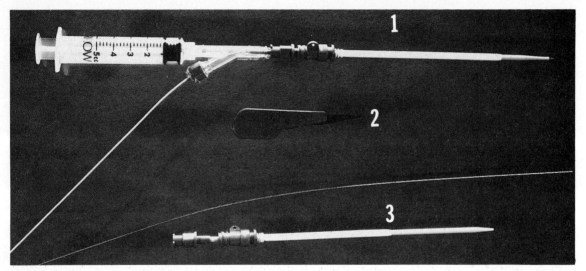

Figure 8-10.   Pre-packaged kits* for performing the Seldinger technique. 1) combined kit containing syringe, needle, guide wire, dilator, and sheath; 2) small #11 blade for nicking the skin; 3) guide wire and dilator/sheath devices as separate units.

*Manufactured by Arrow International, Inc., Reading, Pennsylvania.

Figure 8-11.   Overview of the Seldinger technique.

Procedure for placement of Seldinger-type guide wire catheter. A) The selected vessel is cannulated. B) The guide wire is threaded through the vessel with the flexible end first into the lumen of the vessel. C) The needle is removed so that only the wire now exits from the vessel. D) The skin entry site is enlarged with a #11 scalpel. E) The catheter sheath and the dilator are threaded over the wire and advanced to the skin. The wire must be visible through the back of the device. F) If the proximal wire is not visible, it is pulled from the skin through the catheter until it appears at the back of the catheter. G) The sheath and the dilator are advanced as a unit into the skin with a twisting motion. It is best to grasp the unit at the junction of the sheath and the dilator to prevent bunching up of the sheath. H) Once the sheath and the dilator are well within the vessel, the wire guide and the dilator are removed.

(Reproduced with permission from Roberts, J. R. and Hedges, J. R. (editors): *Clinical Procedures in Emergency Medicine,* W. B. Saunders Co., Philadelphia, 1985.)

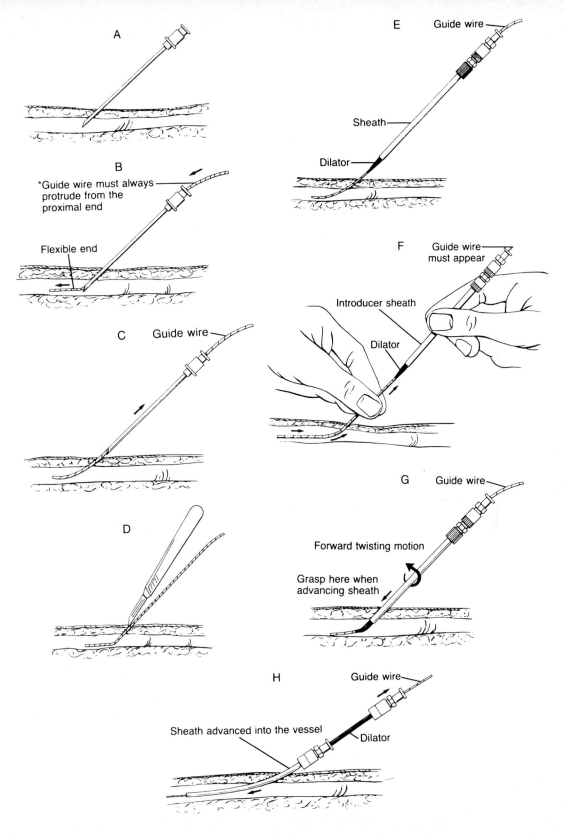

A

B

*Guide wire must always protrude from the proximal end

Flexible end

C

Guide wire

D

E

Guide wire

Sheath

Dilator

F

Guide wire must appear

Introducer sheath

Dilator

G

Guide wire

Forward twisting motion

Grasp here when advancing sheath

H

Guide wire

Sheath advanced into the vessel

Dilator

that it provides rapid access with a large bore catheter to a central vein with minimal complications.

A variety of prepackaged kits are commercially available. Some come complete with introducing needle, syringe, guide wire, dilator, and catheter sheath. Other kits do not contain the needle and syringe (**Figure 8-10**). In either case, the technique for insertion is the same.

> Having the necessary equipment readily available in a prepackaged kit is most welcome in a code situation, as it avoids having to find and assemble material piecemeal during the haste of an emergency.

Guide wires may be straight or J-shaped. The purpose of the latter is to help negotiate vessel tortuosity if it is encountered. In general, straight guide wires are more than adequate for cannulation of the internal jugular or subclavian veins.

> As is the case for threading an intravenous catheter, guide wires should never be forced. Doing so only increases the chance that the wire may unwind, bend, or break (and possibly cause wire embolization). If gentle rotation of the wire does not facilitate easy advancement, remove the wire and try to confirm correct intravascular placement.

The *dilator* and *catheter sheath* function as a unit, with the 8.0–8.5 French catheter fitting over the dilator. The lumen through the dilator allows the unit to be threaded over the guide wire.

Technique for Insertion

> **Figure 8-11** provides an overview of the entire procedure. The introducing needle with attached syringe is inserted into the vein in the standard fashion (Figure 8-11). Once the vein is cannulated, remove the syringe and insert the *soft* tip of the guide wire through the needle and into the vein (**Figure 8-12**). The guide wire should be inserted 5–10 cm making sure that a substantial portion of it still exposed. The needle is now removed.
>
> A small nick should be made in the skin with a no. 11 scalpel blade (**Figure 8-13**). This nick must be deep enough to penetrate both the dermis and epidermis, since it must allow passage of the dilator through the skin. The dilator/catheter sheath unit is now slipped *over* the guidewire and into the incised area of skin (**Figure 8-14**). A twisting motion may facilitate skin penetration and subsequent

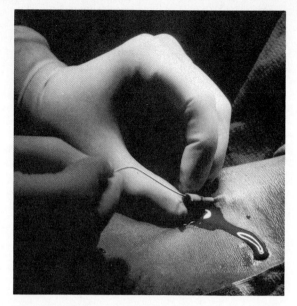

Figure 8-12.   Insertion of guide wire into the IV catheter.

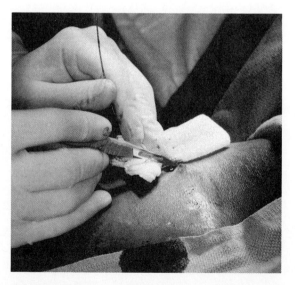

Figure 8-13.   Nicking the skin with a #11 scapel blade.

entry into the vein (**Figure 8-15**). *The proximal tip of the guide wire should always protrude out of the distal end of the dilator/catheter sheath unit.* Advancing the unit without checking for the protruding wire tip may result in distal migration of the guide wire with embolization into the vessel.

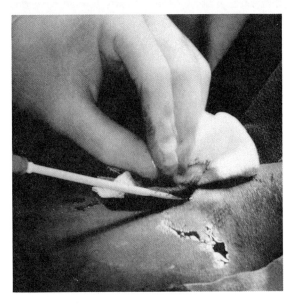

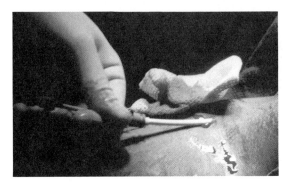

Figure 8-15. Advancing the unit with a twisting motion.

Figure 8-14. Slipping the dilator/sheath catheter unit over the guide wire into the vein.

After the dilator/catheter sheath unit is well into the vein, the wire and dilator are sequentially removed from the catheter. This leaves the large bore catheter sheath in place in the vein, ready to be used as needed for administration of drugs, fluid, blood, or for passage of a transvenous pacemaker or Swan-Ganz catheter (**Figure 8-16**).

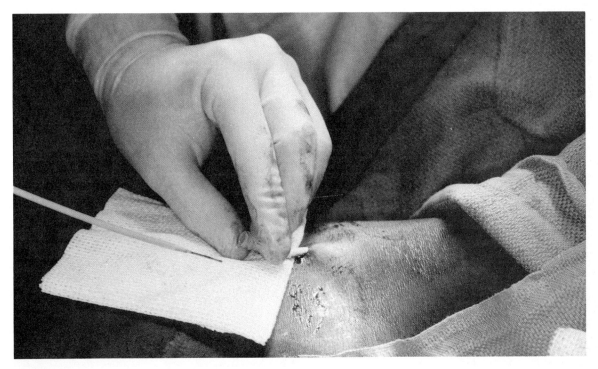

Figure 8-16. Final position of the sheath in the vein.

Catheter Confirmation

One should always confirm correct placement of any central venous catheter. At the bedside this is done by immediately aspirating for blood after cannulation or by lowering the IV bag below bed level to look for blood return.

> One should be aware that in addition to suggesting arterial placement of the catheter, a *pulsating* flashback of blood may be due to ventricular tachycardia (if there is retrograde conduction to the atria), atrial fibrillation (when the right atrium contracts against the closed tricuspid valve), or tricuspid regurgitation (Wyte and Barker, 1985).

Ultimate confirmation of correct central line placement in the superior vena cava (and reassurance that neither pneumothorax nor hemothorax was produced) should be by chest x-ray at the first convenient moment.

REFERENCES

Becker A: *Central venous catheter placement and care.* In Rippe JM, Csete ME (Eds): Manual of Intensive Care Medicine. Little, Brown and Company, Boston, 1983, pp 9–15.

Dalsey WC, Barsan WG, Joyce SM, Hedges JR, Lukes SJ, Doan LA: *Comparison of superior vena cava vs inferior vena cave access for delivery of drugs using a radioisotope technique during normal perfusion and CPR (Abstract).* Ann Emerg Med 12:247–248, 1983.

Dronen SC: *Subclavian venipuncture.* In Roberts JR, Hedges JR (Eds): Clinical Procedures in Emergency Medicine. W.B. Saunders, Philadelphia, 1985, pp 304–321.

Hollinshead WH: *Textbook of Anatomy.* Harper & Row Publishers, New York, 1969, pp 758–789.

Kaye W: *Intravenous Techniques.* In McIntyre KM, Lewis AJ (Eds): Textbook of Advanced Cardiac Life Support. American Heart Association, Texas, 1983, pp. 151–162.

Neimann JT, Rosborough J, Hausknecht M, Ung S, Criley JM: *Blood flow without cardiac compression during closed chest CPR.* Crit Care Med 9:380–381, 1981.

Rosen P, Sternbach G: *Atlas of Emergency Medicine.* Williams & Wilkins, Baltimore, 1979, pp 51–58.

Sacchetti A: *Large-bore infusion catheters (Seldinger technique) of vascular access.* In Roberts JR, Hedges JR (Eds): Clinical Procedures in Emergency Medicine. W.B. Saunders, Philadelphia, 1985, pp 286–293.

Ward JT: *Endotracheal drug administration.* In Roberts JR, Hedges JR (Eds): Clinical Procedures in Emergency Medicine. W.B. Saunders, Philadelphia, 1985, pp 343–351.

Wyte SR, Brker WJ: *Central venous catheterization: Internal jugular approach and alternatives.* In Roberts JR, Hedges JR (Eds): Clinical Procedures in Emergency Medicine. W.B. Saunders, Philadelphia, 1985, pp 321–332.

PART III:

PITFALLS IN THE MANAGEMENT OF CARDIAC ARREST

CHAPTER 9

PITFALLS IN THE MANAGEMENT OF CARDIAC ARREST

The techniques of basic and advanced cardiac life support have been taught to thousands of medical and paramedical personnel across the country. Yet despite this widespread dispersion of knowledge, certain fundamental mistakes in the application of these techniques continue to be made on a frequent basis. The purpose of this chapter is to draw attention to some of these pitfalls in the management of cardiac arrest in the hope of increasing awareness of such problems and improving delivery of emergency cardiac care.

Listed below are a number of common problems encountered in management of various aspects of cardiac arrest:

General Management of Cardiac Arrest

1) Failure of Someone to Assume Command of the Resuscitation Effort. This does not necessarily have to be a physician but may be the first qualified emergency care provider on the scene. Whether this role is subsequently passed on to more knowledgeable authorities as they arrive is not nearly as important as having a *single* person clearly defined as the one responsible for making decisions.

Some of the many roles of the **code director** are to:

a) Oversee and coordinate the overall resuscitative effort.
b) Clear the room of unnecessary personnel.
c) Verify that CPR is being done correctly and that a pulse is produced by external chest compressions.
d) Make sure that the patient is adequately

ventilated at all times (by bag-valve mask, pocket mask, mouth-to-mouth ventilation, or an endotracheal tube).
e) Following endotracheal intubation, make sure equal bilateral breath sounds are present.
f) Make sure that a pulse is checked for whenever the cardiac rhythm changes. If there is a pulse, check for a blood pressure.
g) Have the patient hooked up to a monitor and make sure someone is constantly checking the patient's rhythm.
h) Order administration of drugs in the appropriate dosage and by the appropriate route.
i) Delegate an experienced specific individual to inquire about the patient's history, his/her overall health status, and the events leading up to the arrest. Resuscitation of a person with diabetes in ketoacidosis is vastly different from resuscitation of a patient who has overdosed or who is uremic. Moreover, how aggressively one proceeds with the resuscitative effort may be strongly influenced by factors in the patient's history, such as whether or not he/she has a terminal disease.
j) Order appropriate radiographic and laboratory tests as they are needed. Blood for determining arterial blood gases (ABGs) should be drawn to guide respiratory therapy and assist in the decision of whether to administer sodium bicarbonate. Once a stable rhythm is established, a chest x-ray film should be done to verify correct positioning of the endotracheal tube, central lines, and/or pacemaker wires and to rule out pneumothorax. A 12-lead ECG should be obtained to look for infarction. Finally, serum electrolyte concentrations and other

blood work may be needed to help determine the etiology of the arrest and the need for corrective therapy.

k) Consult with the patient's primary physician at the earliest opportunity.

l) Talk to the patient's family.

m) Decide when the resuscitation effort should be terminated.

n) Talk to your colleagues. Let them know why various actions are being taken ("the patient is in ventricular tachycardia with a pulse—let's cardiovert with 200 joules"). State all orders clearly (and loudly) so that there is no misunderstanding of your intentions. Insist that team members do the same and announce all completed tasks ("one ampule of epinephrine given by the ET route"). Proceeding in this manner enables everyone present to follow the course of the resuscitation effort in a meaningful way, allows anticipation of future actions that will need to be taken, and prevents duplication of effort.

o) Acknowledge the efforts of those who helped.

p) Do not forget to write a progress note after the code.

2) Failure to Record the Sequence of Events as They Unfold During the Arrest.

The **code sheet** should reflect the following information:

a) The various cardiac rhythms that occurred during the code and whether or not they were associated with a pulse and blood pressure.

b) The time of administration, dose, route, site, and indication for all medications given during the code.

c) The number of countershock attempts and the energies used.

d) The performance of any procedures such as endotracheal intubation, pericardiocentesis, and insertion of a pacemaker or of central IV lines. Indicate who did the procedure, the time, and any complications.

e) The names of the emergency care providers in attendance.

f) The time the arrest began and the time and reason the resuscitation effort was terminated.

Keeping track of this information during the code is particularly important with regard to administration of drugs that are frequently given on a *timed* basis (ie, atropine, epinephrine, and boluses of lidocaine and bretylium). If sodium bicarbonate is used, correlation of the time of administration with respect to the timing of endotracheal intubation and drawing of ABGs is critical.

Medicolegally, the code sheet provides documentation. However, for this documentation to be accurate, it is essential that events be recorded *as they happen*. It is difficult enough to keep track of all that happens *during* a code even when someone is specifically assigned to accomplish nothing but this function. *After the code*, accurate reconstruction of the sequence of events becomes virtually impossible.

3) Failure to Review the Resuscitation Effort.
The importance of this undertaking cannot be overemphasized. Review should be done both immediately and at a later date.

The last thing most emergency care providers want to do immediately following a code is to reflect on the process. This is especially true if the patient died. Yet going back over the code sequence and reviewing events (and/or the actual ECG recordings) and *thinking about how things may have gone better* may provide invaluable feedback. Discussing the case with a trusted colleague who was present may likewise be immensely insightful.

Periodic review of code sheets by ICU personnel or a code committee is another helpful mechanism of assuring regular feedback with the intent of improving future resuscitation efforts. It is also a way of verifying that adequate documentation of code events is being obtained.

4) Not Regularly Checking to See That All Crash Cart Drugs Are Restocked and All Emergency Equipment Is In Working Order.
Laryngoscope bulbs, Ambu bags, defibrillator gel or pads, and suction equipment all have a disturbing tendency to "disappear" at

the moment they are needed for a call of cardiac arrest. Similarly, essential drugs such as epinephrine, dopamine, and bretylium may not be available when needed, and defibrillator function (and/or batteries) may be impaired unless provisions for regularly scheduled crash cart maintenance checks have been made.

5) Failure to Consider "Do Not Resuscitate" (DNR) Orders Before the Cardiac Arrest Occurs.

A routine practice should be made when admitting any patient to the hospital of assessing whether or not resuscitation efforts should be initiated in the event of a cardiopulmonary arrest. This decision should be arrived at jointly by the physicians caring for the patient, the patient's family, and the patient himself/herself if he/she is competent to participate in the decision-making process. If the patient's condition subsequently changes during the course of hospitalization, the decision regarding whether or not to initiate resuscitation may need to be reconsidered. If it is felt to be in the patient's best interests not to initiate cardiopulmonary resuscitation (CPR) because of a terminal illness, this decision *must* be adequately documented on the chart and made clear to all hospital personnel involved in the care of the patient.

6) Failure to Inquire About a Living Will When Appropriate.

Advance directives in the form of a **Living Will** have become legal in many states. All that is required is for the patient to be competent at the time he/she fills out this document. Specific aspects of resuscitation may be defined by the patient. For example, he/she may indicate a desire to be made as comfortable as possible with analgesics and a willingness to allow chemical and electrical resuscitation but may firmly refuse to be intubated.

While it may be awkward and inappropriate to routinely ask each patient at the time of admission to the hospital whether he/she has filled out a Living Will, awareness of the existence of such documents (if they are legal in the state where you practice) and sensitivity to the issues encompassed by them will go a long way in helping the emergency care provider elicit such information

at an opportune moment. Available family that are close to the patient may occasionally assist if they know of the patient's desires or of advance directives that have already been filled out.

Provision of Basic Life Support

1) Delay in Making the Diagnosis of Cardiopulmonary Arrest.

As soon as unresponsiveness has been verified, it is imperative to call for help while checking for the adequacy of spontaneous ventilation and circulation. Basic life support *must* be started promptly for pulselessness and/or apnea. If the patient is not breathing and a bag-valve mask is not readily available (and will be delayed more than momentarily), mouth-to-mouth resuscitation should be started. (*Ready availability of pocket masks at the bedside would alleviate concern of disease transmission*—see section "On Mouth-to-Mouth" in Chapter 10).

2) Delay in Securing an Airway.

The resuscitation is doomed to failure unless an airway can be established and maintained. CPR should not be repeatedly interrupted by inexpert attempts at intubation, since ventilation with a properly positioned mask usually is sufficient to maintain adequate oxygenation until personnel experienced in intubation arrive.

3) Failure to Place a Bed Board Under the Patient.

Cardiac massage is not effective when performed on a mattress.

4) Unnecessarily Interrupting CPR.

CPR should not be stopped for more than 5 seconds except for intubating or moving the patient. No more than a 15–20-second interruption should be permitted for these maneuvers.

5) Improper Application of External Chest Compression.

The rescuer should be correctly positioned over the patient's sternum with arms extended. Pressure is then applied to the lower sternum with the heels of both hands, displacing it downward by 1.5 to 2 inches toward the spine. Standing on a stool may optimize body mechanics. The rescuer should not remove his/her hands from the sternum between compressions but must release pressure completely. Fingers should not rest on the patient's chest, and jerking or bouncing movements must be avoided. Instead, external chest compression should be as smooth and regular as possible and *occupy at least 50% of the cycle* to assure maximum blood flow during CPR.

In the past, too much emphasis was placed on compressing exactly at a specified rate. The new guidelines reflect this by now allowing a *range* of compressions (ie, 80–100/min) instead of demanding that a certain number be performed each minute. Aiming for the higher side of this range will probably result in optimal blood flow. (See the Addendum at the end of Chapter 10.)

6) Ignoring Gastric Distention.   Even when performed correctly, CPR frequently results in gastric distention. This can compromise left ventricular filling and predispose the patient to regurgitation of stomach contents. Increasing gastric distention during CPR should be recognized and relieved by early insertion of a nasogastric tube after protecting the airway by endotracheal intubation.

The new guidelines have taken several steps toward rectifying this problem. The most important of these is to slow delivery of ventilation. It is now recommended that rescue breathing be performed over a period of 1–1.5 seconds so as to allow delivery of a *full* ventilation. This significantly reduces airway inflation pressures and minimizes the amount of air that enters the esophagus.

7) Forgetting About the Sellick Maneuver.   Application of backward pressure on the cricoid cartilage against the cervical vertebra minimizes the chance of regurgitation during performance of CPR. The technique is not difficult to learn, but it does require an assistant.

Administration of Drugs

1) Unnecessary Concern with Sterile Techniques During Resuscitation.   Although ideally all procedures should be performed with as sterile a technique as possible, the primary concern during cardiac arrest obviously must be to *save* the patient. Sterile technique may have to take a back seat role to this.

2) Forgetting About the Intra(endo)tracheal Route.   The onset of action of intratracheally administered epinephrine in patients with cardiovascular collapse is comparable to that when the drug is given intravenously (Parmley et al., 1982; Redding, 1979). Thus in the event that a patient is intubated but an IV line cannot be started, one should not hesitate to give epinephrine through the endotracheal tube.

Atropine and lidocaine may also be administered by this route, although the pharmacokinetics of these agents appear to be more favorable when they are given intravenously (McDonald, 1985; Greenberg et al., 1982). The mnemonic **ALE** (**a**tropine, **l**idocaine, **e**pinephrine) may help recall that these three drugs can be given by the ET route.

[Other medications that can be given by the endotracheal route include Narcan and Valium (Greenberg, 1984). Expansion of the mnemonic to *NAVEL* {**N**arcan, **a**tropine, **V**alium, **e**pinephrine, **l**idocaine} may help remember these five drugs.]

3) Preoccupation with Inserting a Central Line.   During closed chest compression, circulation of drugs by a central IV line is preferable to using a peripheral IV (Kuhn et al., 1981). Administration through a central IV allows immediate access into the central circulation and accommodates a larger volume than does a peripheral IV. However, insertion of an internal jugular or subclavian line requires cessation of CPR and exposes the patient to a sig-

nificant risk of pneumothorax. Although these disadvantages do not apply to the insertion of a femoral line, blood flow during CPR is diminished below the diaphragm (Dalsey et al., 1983; Niemann et al., 1981), making this an undesirable route for administration of medications during a code.

As noted above, three of the most commonly used medications during cardiac arrest may be effectively given by the endotracheal route. Although circulation of drugs administered through IV lines inserted at a *distal* peripheral site (that is, dorsum of the wrist, hand, or lower leg) is less reliable in the arrested heart, establishment of a peripheral IV in a more *proximal* site (such as the antecubital fossa) is more likely to provide adequate access for blood flow to the central circulation (JAMA Suppl, 1986). Thus, if an operator skilled in the insertion of central lines is not available, administration of medications through either the antecubital vein or the endotracheal route will probably be both sufficient and preferable to inexpert attempts at cannulation of a central vein.

4) Failure to Optimize Drug Delivery Through a Peripheral IV.

As noted above, the more distal the site for a peripheral IV, the less likely it is that there will be adequate delivery of drugs to the central circulation. Thus a tiny "butterfly" IV in the dorsum of the wrist may not provide much better access for delivering drugs during cardiac arrest than no access at all!

There are four simple things one may do to improve drug delivery from a peripheral IV:

i) *Choose an appropriate site.* This should ideally be from an upper extremity vein in the antecubital fossa or a more proximal site.

ii) *Use a short length and large bore catheter for the IV.* According to the Laws of Poiseuille and Hagen, flow of fluid is proportional to the *fourth* power of the diameter of the catheter and *inversely* proportional to its length. Therefore, a small increase in IV lumen diameter may make a substantial difference in the rate of fluid administration!

Optimal flow will be obtained when large bore catheters of *short* length are used.

iii) *Elevate the patient's arm after administering the medication.* This favors venous return.

iv) *Follow administration of the medication with a bolus of fluid.* This helps "flush" the medication toward the central circulation.

5) Failure to Flush the IV Line After the Administration of Sodium Bicarbonate.

Catecholamines (epinephrine, dopamine, isoproterenol) and calcium salts are inactivated when mixed with sodium bicarbonate. For this reason the IV line must be especially well flushed after giving sodium bicarbonate before additional drugs can be infused.

6) Inappropriate Administration of Medication by Intracardiac Injection.

This route of drug administration should be reserved as a last resort because of the unjustifiably high incidence of complications associated with its use. These include induction of intractable ventricular fibrillation, laceration of a coronary artery, pneumothorax, and hemopericardium with tamponade.

7) Dosing Atropine Inappropriately.

The recommendation for the use of atropine in treating hemodynamically significant bradyarrhythmias is to administer 0.5 mg IV every 5 minutes until a total of 2 mg has been given. Errors occur in both underdosing and overdosing of this drug. Atropine is *not* a benign medication. When given in a high dose (ie, 1 mg at a time) to a patient with only minimal hemodynamic compromise, the drug may unmask underlying sympathetic hyperactivity and result in tachycardia, increased myocardial oxygen consumption, and even ventricular tachycardia or fibrillation.

In contrast, giving only 0.5 mg every 5 minutes for a patient with a heart rate in the 30s and a barely palpable blood pressure would require no less than 15 minutes to administer the whole 2 mg. A happy medium for dosing atropine must be struck which is based on the clinical significance of the bradyarrhythmia.

8) Forgetting That Drug Administration During (or Preceding) Cardiac Arrest

May Alter Pupil Size and Responsiveness.   Thus resuscitation should not be terminated because of pupillary unresponsiveness if atropine was administered during the code since pupillary dilatation may last for hours. Other drugs that may alter pupillary responsiveness include narcotics, amphetamines, cocaine, and tricyclic antidepressants. Overdose from any of these agents can precipitate cardiac arrest.

9) Reflexively Administering Sodium Bicarbonate.   Sodium bicarbonate has been liberally administered during cardiac arrest in the past. The new guidelines have strongly deemphasized the use of this agent. We now know that the acidosis that occurs during arrest is primarily respiratory for at least the first 5 to 15 minutes following patient collapse (Sanders et al., 1984; Weil et al., 1984), and that administration of sodium bicarbonate is potentially deleterious (because it may exacerbate *intra*cellular acidosis). Unless a preexisting metabolic acidosis was present before the arrest, sodium bicarbonate should probably not be given. Even then its use is questionable. (See section on Sodium Bicarbonate.)

10) Using Calcium Chloride for Asystole or EMD.   The new guidelines no longer recommend calcium chloride for use in asystole or EMD. The reason for this is the absence of clinical data supporting efficacy of the agent and increasing reports of adverse outcome associated with its use (Stueven et al., 1983 and 1984). The *only* remaining indications for calcium chloride are hypocalcemia, hyperkalemia, and asystole that follows the use of a calcium channel blocking agent.

11) Using Isoproterenol in the Arrested Heart.   The new guidelines no longer recommend isoproterenol for use in the arrested heart. The reason is that the pure beta-adrenergic stimulating action of this drug produces vasodilatation. This results in a lowering of aortic diastolic pressure and minimizes coronary perfusion while CPR is being performed. Epinephrine is the pharmacologic treatment of choice for asystole and ventricular fibrillation, since its alpha-adrenergic (vasoconstrictor) effect increases aortic diastolic pressure and favors blood flow to the heart.

12) Indiscriminately Using Verapamil as a Diagnostic and Therapeutic Trial with Wide QRS Complex Tachyarrhythmias.   Regular, wide QRS complex tachyarrhythmias must always be assumed to be ventricular tachycardia until proved otherwise. The common practice of administering verapamil as a diagnostic and therapeutic trial to help distinguish between a supraventricular and ventricular etiology for the arrhythmia is potentially dangerous since a large percentage of patients in ventricular tachycardia will hemodynamically deteriorate if given verapamil (Stewart et al., 1986). Instead, other means (such as scrutiny of QRS morphology in different leads, looking for P waves) should be used to assist in differentiating supraventricular from ventricular tachyarrhythmias.

13) Withholding Oxygen for Fear of Causing Carbon Dioxide Retention.   Carbon dioxide retention in an acutely ill patient who is being intensively monitored is of relatively little concern. In general, such patients are not left alone long enough for this to happen. High flow oxygen in this setting is safe (and often essential) and may be administered until ABG studies and/or clinical evaluation indicate otherwise.

14) Not Optimally Monitoring Patients on Potent Cardioactive Agents. Blood pressure cuff readings on patients in shock often do not truly reflect intraarterial pressure. An *arterial line* may be needed to obtain accurate readings. Similarly, clinical assessment of hemodynamic status for patients with acute myocardial infarction, shock, or just after resuscitation from cardiopulmonary arrest is notoriously inaccurate. Invasive hemodynamic monitoring with a *Swan-Ganz catheter* is often essential.

15) Inappropriate Use of Bretylium for Refractory Ventricular Fibrillation.   Although bretylium is an effective agent for refractory ventricular fibrillation, the new guidelines have made it a second-line drug to lidocaine for this purpose. If lidocaine is not effective and one chooses to use bretylium, it is important to keep several points in mind:

More than one dose of the drug may be needed. If the first 5 mg/kg bolus does not work, give a second dose of 10 mg/kg. This may be repeated if needed up to a total of 30 mg/kg.

Bretylium usually does not convert ventricular fibrillation on its own. Remember to circulate the drug with CPR for about 2 minutes following each dose, and then to defibrillate the patient.

Although the antifibrillatory effect of bretylium usually works within a few minutes, it is sometimes delayed for 10–15 minutes. Continued CPR may be needed for this time in order to allow the drug adequate opportunity to work.

Lidocaine and procainamide are preferable to bretylium for treating PVCs and ventricular tachycardia.

16) Forgetting to Administer Lidocaine Prophylactically Following Successful Conversion of Ventricular Fibrillation.
Because of the altered pharmacokinetics of lidocaine in the arrested heart, only bolus therapy is needed as long as the patient remains in ventricular fibrillation (McDonald, 1985). As soon as the patient is converted out of ventricular fibrillation, however, it is important to rebolus with lidocaine and initiate a maintenance infusion. Failure to do this significantly increases the risk of recurrent ventricular fibrillation.

17) Failure to Use the Lowest Possible Dose of a Pressor Agent.
Use of pressor agents such as dopamine, isoproterenol, and epinephrine is often essential for supporting the circulation during cardiac resuscitation. It is essential, however, to use the *lowest possible dose* of these agents. As soon as spontaneous circulation is restored, efforts should be made to down titrate the rate of infusion. Failure to do so may result in tachyarrhythmias that could precipitate a recurrence of the arrest.

Defibrillation

1) Forgetting to Clear the Area Before Defibrillation.
Although seemingly obvious, careless application of countershock without first verifying that no one is in direct (or indirect) contact with the patient still results in accidental defibrillation of hospital personnel. Standing in spilled IV fluids and "the hanging stethoscope" are two nemeses that may catch the unaware rescuer who is holding the paddles.

2) Failure to Apply 25 Pounds of Firm Pressure to Each Paddle When Defibrillating.
Application of firm pressure to the chest wall reduces transthoracic resistance and increases the efficacy of defibrillation.

3) Unfamiliarity with the Defibrillation Equipment.
The time to learn about the specifics of your defibrillator/cardioverter is *not* during a cardiac arrest.

4) Failure to Use the Quick-Look Paddles.
Most defibrillators are equipped to provide a quick look at the cardiac rhythm on contact of the paddles to the patient's chest. This saves the time of applying monitoring leads and in the case of ventricular fibrillation allows for more rapid initial defibrillation.

5) Delay in Defibrillation.
The chance for successful conversion of ventricular fibrillation is inversely proportional to the time from the onset of this rhythm until countershock is applied. One should defibrillate the patient immediately on confirming the diagnosis of ventricular fibrillation rather than losing time trying to first intubate or secure an IV line.

6) Use of Excessive Energy with the Initial Defibrillation Attempt.
Weaver et al. (1982) have shown that initial defibrillation with 175 joules of delivered energy is as effective in converting ventricular fibrillation as countershock with 320 joules yet is associated with a lower incidence of advanced atrioventricular (AV) block after defibrillation. Consequently,

the delivered energy of the initial countershock attempt should be limited to 200 joules.

7) Forgetting to Immediately Deliver a Second Countershock if the Initial Attempt at Defibrillation is Unsuccessful.

Successive countershocks reduce transthoracic resistance, increasing the amount of *current* that will flow through the heart with the second attempt. If the patient remains in ventricular fibrillation after the second countershock, the new guidelines recommend that a third attempt at defibrillation be made with maximal energy (360 joules).

8) Failure to Use Synchronized Cardioversion When Indicated.

Synchronized cardioversion is indicated for the treatment of patients with supraventricular tachycardias or ventricular tachycardia if they demonstrate hemodynamic compromise. By delivering the electrical impulse during that portion of the cardiac cycle when the ventricles are most refractory, synchronized cardioversion is less likely to cause ventricular fibrillation than is unsynchronized countershock.

Miscellaneous

1) Misuse of the Precordial Thump.

Although the precordial thump may restore sinus rhythm if delivered soon after the onset of ventricular tachycardia or ventricular fibrillation, it may also cause ventricular tachycardia to go into ventricular fibrillation or may result in a pulseless idioventricular rhythm or asystole. Consequently, the precordial thump should *not* be routinely administered for ventricular tachycardia when a pulse is present. Indications for use of this maneuver may be best remembered if one views the thump as a "no-lose" procedure. Thus it is reasonable to use it at the onset of ventricular fibrillation or *pulseless* ventricular tachycardia. If a defibrillator is readily available, this mode of therapy (using either synchronized cardioversion or unsynchronized countershock) is preferable to the random delivery of 2–5 joules at an unpredictable point in the cardiac cycle that the thump provides.

2) Failure to Actively Seek Out an Underlying Cause of Electromechanical Dissociation (EMD).

(See Case Study D and Table 4D-1 for a review of the causes of EMD.)

3) Delay in Arranging for Emergency Pacing.

A patient with a hemodynamically significant bradyarrhythmia who has not responded to atropine is in need of cardiac pacing. The use of pressor agents should be employed only as a stopgap measure to support the patient until the pacemaker has been inserted. (See the algorithm for treatment of bradyarrhythmias in Section D, Chapter 1 and the specific indications for cardiac pacemakers in Section D, Chapter 2.)

REFERENCES

American Heart Association Subcommittee on Emergency Cardiac Care: Standards and guidelines for cardiopulmonary resuscitation (CPR) and emergency cardiac care (ECC). JAMA 255:2905–2992, 1986.

Dalsey WC, Barsan WG, Joyce SM, Hedges JR, Lukes SJ, Doan LA: Comparison of superior vena cava vs inferior vena cava access for delivery of drugs using a radioisotope technique during normal perfusion and CPR (abstract). Ann Emerg Med 12:247–248, 1983.

Doan LA: Peripheral versus central venous delivery of medications during CPR. Ann Emerg Med 13:784–786, 1984.

Greenberg MI: Endotracheal drugs: State of the art. Ann Emerg Med 13:789–790, 1984.

Greenberg MI, Mayeda DY, Chrzanowski R, Brumwell D, Baskin SI, Roberts JR: Endotracheal administration of atropine sulfate. Ann Emerg Med 11:546–548, 1982.

Grundler W, Weil MH, Rackow EC, Falk JL, Bisera J, Miller JM, Michaels S: Selective acidosis in venous blood during human cardiopulmonary resuscitation: A preliminary report. Crit Care Med 13:886–887, 1985.

Kuhn GJ, White BC, Swetnam RE, Mumey JF, Rydesky MF, Tintinalli JE, Krome RL, Hoehner PJ: Peripheral vs central circulation times during CPR: A pilot study. Ann Emerg Med 10:417–419, 1981.

McDonald JL: Serum lidocaine levels during cardiopulmonary resuscitation after intravenous and endotracheal administration. Crit Care Med 13:914, 915, 1985.

Niemann JT, Rosborough J, Hausknecht M, Ung S, Criley JM: Blood flow without cardiac compression during closed chest CPR. Crit Care Med 9:380–381, 1981.

Parmley WW, Hatcher CR, Ewy GA, Furman S, Redding J, Weisfeldt ML: Task Force V: Physical interventions and adjunctive therapy. Thirteenth Bethesda Conference on Emergency Cardiac Care. Am J Cardiol 50:409–420, 1982.

Redding JS: Cardiopulmonary resuscitation: An algorithm and some common pitfalls. Am Heart J 98:788–797, 1979.

Sanders AB, Ewy GA, Taft TV: Resuscitation and arterial blood gas abnormalities during prolonged cardiopulmonary resuscitation. Ann Emerg Med 13:676–679, 1984.

Stewart RB, Bardy GH, Greene HL: Wide complex tachycardia: Misdiagnosis and outcome after emergent therapy. Ann Intern Med 104:766–771, 1986.

Stueven H, Thompson BM, Aprahamian C, Darin JC: Use of calcium in prehospital cardiac arrest. Ann Emerg Med 12:136–139, 1983.

Stueven HA: Calcium chloride: Reassessment of use in asystole. Ann Emerg Med 13:820–822, 1984.

Weaver WD, Cobb LA, Compass MK, Hallstrom AP: Ventricular defibrillation—A comparative trial using 175-J and 320-J shocks. N Engl J Med 307:1101–1106, 1982.

PART IV:

TOPICS OF GENERAL INTEREST IN EMERGENCY CARDIAC CARE

CHAPTER 10

NEW DEVELOPMENTS IN CPR

CPR (cardiopulmonary resuscitation) is one of the most important treatment modalities for the victim of cardiopulmonary arrest. Its impact is immense. In addition to being the first line of therapy for cardiopulmonary arrest, CPR plays a major role in educating the public about primary prevention (risk factor modification) and recognition of coronary artery disease, acute myocardial infarction, and sudden cardiac death. Awareness of CPR in this country has mushroomed; almost 90% of adult Americans have heard of the technique, and 40 million individuals have already received formal training.

In this chapter we will take a close look at the benefits of CPR. How effective is this technique? What changes in CPR have been recommended by the new guidelines? What is the rationale for these changes? And how has our new understanding of the mechanism for blood flow with CPR influenced our utilization of this procedure?

THE NEW GUIDELINES: RECOMMENDATIONS FOR BASIC LIFE SUPPORT (BLS)

THE SEQUENCE OF BLS: ONE-RESCUER CPR

Performance of basic life support (BLS) is predicated on the ABCs (**A**irway, **B**reathing, and **C**irculation). In addition to **a**irway, the **A** should recall that **a**ssessment is the initial step of each phase. The recommended sequence for one-rescuer CPR is as follows:

Airway
1) **Assessment**—Determine unresponsiveness ("Are you OK?").

2) Call for help.
3) Position the victim (so he/she is supine on a flat firm surface).
4) Open the airway. (Use the head-tilt/chin-lift or jaw-thrust maneuver.)

Breathing
1) **Assessment**—Determine breathlessness. (*Look, listen,* and *feel* for air movement.)
2) If the victim is not breathing, *begin rescue breathing.* (Give two *slow* breaths over 2–3 seconds.)

If the victim is breathing, maintain an open airway while waiting for help to arrive.

If the victim is not breathing and you are unable to give two breaths, reposition the victim's head and attempt to ventilate again. If still unable to ventilate, initiate treatment for **foreign-body airway obstruction** with the Heimlich maneuver (subdiaphragmatic abdominal thrusts or chest thrusts). Follow this with a finger sweep to dislodge and/or remove the foreign body obstruction. Reposition the victim's head and attempt to ventilate again. If unsuccessful, repeat this sequence.

Circulation
1) **Assessment**—Determine pulselessness. (Spend a good 5–10 seconds feeling for a carotid pulse.)
2) If there is no pulse, *begin external chest compressions.* (Compress at a rate of 80–100/min.)

If a pulse is present, maintain an open airway and continue rescue breathing (at a rate of 12/min) while waiting for help to arrive.

3) Perform 15 chest compressions and then stop to deliver two *slow* breaths (1–1.5 seconds per breath). Perform four complete cycles of this 15:2 compression/ventilation ratio and then reassess the patient. If the patient is still breathless and pulseless, resume CPR and continue until help arrives.

TWO-RESCUER CPR

<u>A</u>irway—Same as for One-Rescuer CPR
<u>B</u>reathing—Same as for One-Rescuer CPR
<u>C</u>irculation—Same as for One-Rescuer CPR except that one rescuer ventilates the patient while the other performs chest compressions. After completing 5 compressions (given at a rate of 80–100/min), the first rescuer *pauses* for 1–1.5 seconds while the second rescuer delivers a *slow* ventilation. The first rescuer then resumes compressions. The 5:1 compression/ventilation ratio is continued.

TWO-RESCUER CPR IN THE INTUBATED PATIENT

<u>A</u>irway—Same as for Two-Rescuer CPR
<u>B</u>reathing—Same as for Two-Rescuer CPR
<u>C</u>irculation—Same as for Two-Rescuer CPR except ventilation and compression are *asynchronous*. One rescuer performs 80–100 compressions per minute while the other independently delivers 12–15 ventilations per minute.

Rationale for Changes in the New Guidelines

SLOWER VENTILATION

"Staircase" breathing is no longer recommended to initiate CPR. This phenomenon is an artifact of Resusci Annie that can be produced only because the mannikin has an exhalation valve. It is impossible to achieve in human subjects, since air is expired almost as rapidly as it is taken in (Melker et al., 1981). Even if one could staircase breaths in humans, this would not be desirable. The gastroesophageal sphincter of most patients opens as soon as pressure in the unprotected airway exceeds 25 cm H_2O. Were one to deliver 2 liters of air within 1 second as required by the staircase effect, pressures much higher than this would have to be generated. Gastric insufflation would certainly result,

leading to ineffective CPR and eventual regurgitation of gastric contents with aspiration (Melker and Banner, 1985).

To prevent this sequence of events, it is now recommended that ventilation be delivered *slowly* over 1–1.5 seconds. In addition, when two-rescuer CPR is administered to a victim with an unprotected airway, one should *pause* at the end of each five compressions to allow ample time for delivery of a slow, complete ventilation.

Once the patient is intubated, however, the pause is no longer needed. In the past, the recommendation was to *interpose* ventilations between the upstroke of the fifth compression and the downstroke of the first compression for the subsequent cycle. The time allotted to complete each ventilation by this method was necessarily short. As a result, there was a tendency to prematurely terminate ventilations so as to be sure to finish before the first compression of the next cycle. Because of our improved understanding of how blood flows with CPR, we now know that this is no longer necessary (Melker and Cavallaro, 1983). Rescuers need not concern themselves with the timing of ventilation and compression in the intubated patient. The increased intrathoracic pressure that may result if ventilation and compression occur simultaneously does not impair blood flow with CPR. On the contrary, it actually *increases* blood flow, as we will see momentarily.

MORE RAPID RATE OF COMPRESSION

The second major change recommended by the new guidelines is an increase in the *rate* of compressions to 80–100/min for both one- and two-rescuer CPR. There are two reasons for this change. First, insertion of the 1- to 1.5-second pause for each ventilation reduces the total time allotted for compressions. A faster rate of compressions is needed to make up for this.

Equally important is the fact that an increased rate improves the *efficacy* of chest compression. Traditionally, a rate of 60 compressions per minute had been recommended for two-rescuer CPR, with each compression ideally lasting for 50% of the compression-relaxation cycle. In practice, more attention was usually directed to complying with the rate criterion. Rescuers would often meticulously count off one per second cardiac compressions but pay little attention to whether each compression was maintained for the proper amount of time.

It has been shown that rate of compression per se is a relatively *unimportant* determinant of blood flow with CPR (Luce et al., 1980). In contrast, the *force* and *duration of compression* are extremely important (Taylor et al., 1977; Maier et al., 1984). Carotid blood flow increases directly with increases in compression duration, and maximal antegrade flow is achieved when compression duration is extended to occupy 60–70% of the compression-relaxation cycle (Luce et al., 1980; Parmley et al., 1982).

The problem is that sustaining each compression for at least 50% of the cycle is hard to accomplish at slow compression rates. However, with faster compression rates, the total time for each cycle is less. As a result, the *percentage* of time devoted to compression becomes proportionately greater. In addition, rescuers tend to apply greater *force* with each compression when working at a faster rate (*high-impulse CPR*). Thus efficiency of CPR is improved by increasing the rate of compressions. (See the Addendum at the end of this chapter.)

How Does Blood Flow with CPR?

THE CARDIAC PUMP THEORY

How does blood flow with CPR? Although in the past, direct compression of the heart between the sternum and vertebral column was thought to provide the main impetus for blood flow (*cardiac pump theory*), recent evidence suggests otherwise. While the cardiac pump theory may explain what occurs in infants, young children, and other individuals with compliant chest walls, direct cardiac compression is probably *not* the major mechanism for generating blood flow during CPR in the majority of adults (Niemann et al., 1981; Weisfeldt et al., 1981; Rogers, 1983).

A number of observations led researchers to believe that other mechanisms might be operative. If blood flow were simply the result of direct cardiac compression, one would expect pressure in the left ventricle to dramatically increase as blood was "squeezed" out of this chamber. The mitral valve would then close in response to the high pressure gradient produced between the left ventricle and the left atrium, and heart size would decrease as blood was ejected from the aorta. Similar events should occur on the right side of the heart as blood was ejected into the pulmonary bed (**Fig. 10-1**). However, cardiac chamber size does not change significantly during CPR, pressures remain equal in all cardiac chambers and intrathoracic vessels, and heart valves remain open throughout the entire cardiac cycle (Luce et al., 1980; Bircher, 1982). Rather than acting as a pump, the heart is a *passive conduit* for blood flow during CPR. No pressure gradient is produced anywhere within the thorax, and the increase in intrathoracic pressure that occurs with external chest compression is generalized.

Further evidence against the cardiac pump theory is provided by observations on blood flow during CPR performed on patients with emphysema and flail sternum. If the heart functioned as a pump, blood flow with CPR should be minimal in the former, since one would expect direct cardiac compression to be much more difficult to accomplish in "barrel-chested" individuals. In contrast, blood flow should be maximal in traumatized patients with flail sternum. What better opportunity for direct cardiac compression could there be than when the sternum is unrestricted by its costal attachments? In fact, neither of these expectations are realized. Blood flow in emphysematous individuals is comparable to blood flow in individuals with normal chest wall configurations. Traumatized victims with flail sternum demonstrate minimal blood flow with CPR *unless* the thorax is bound and stabilized to allow for a generalized increase in intrathoracic pressure.

Final evidence against the cardiac pump theory was provided by Criley et al. (1976) with the introduction of a new technique known as *cough*

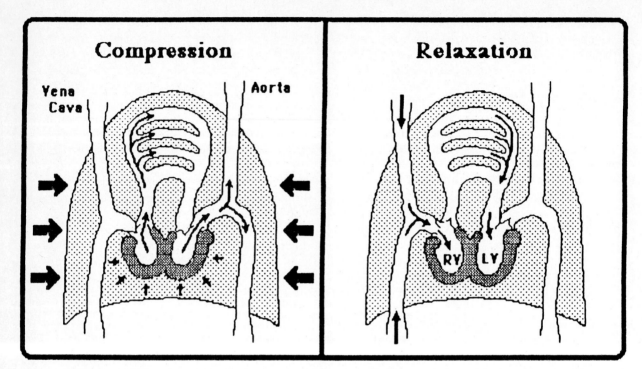

Figure 10-1   Sequence of events during the compression and relaxation phases of CPR according to the **cardiac pump** theory. Compression produces an increase in intraventricular pressure. This generates a pressure gradient that causes the mitral and tricuspid valves to close while blood is simultaneously ejected from the aorta and pulmonary artery. With relaxation, pressure in the ventricles drops significantly, and blood is returned to the thorax.

CPR. With this self-administered form of CPR, a number of subjects were able to sustain consciousness during ventricular fibrillation for periods of up to 90 seconds simply by forceful repetitive coughing. Such coughing generated high intrathoracic pressures (of up to 140 mm Hg!) that somehow resulted in adequate blood flow despite the presence of a nonperfusing rhythm (ventricular fibrillation). *How could the cardiac pump theory be operative when coughing alone* (without any chest compression) *was enough to maintain consciousness?*

THE THORACIC PUMP THEORY

To try and answer this question, the *thoracic pump theory* was proposed. Rather than saying that a pressure gradient is generated between cardiac and vascular structures *within* the thorax, this theory suggests that the pressure gradient develops *outside* the thorax. The intrathoracic-extrathoracic pressure differential produced provides the impetus for forward (antegrade) flow of blood out of the aorta (**Fig. 10-2**).

Three factors allow unidirectional flow of blood to occur with sternal compression. They are:

i) Functional venous closure at the thoracic inlet
ii) Preserved patency of the carotid artery
iii) Greater *capacitance* of the extrathoracic venous bed

(Because veins have greater capacitance than arteries, lower pressures are generated in the venous system for an equal volume of blood.)

Researchers have postulated that a valve exists in the jugular vein at the thoracic inlet. Com-

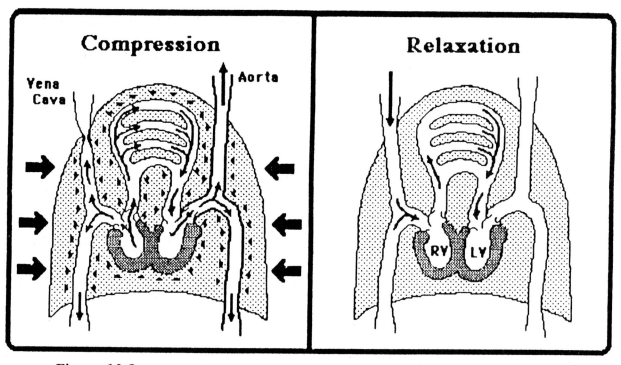

Figure 10-2 Sequence of events during the compression and relaxation phases of CPR according to the **thoracic pump theory.** The impetus for blood flow results from generation of an *intra*thoracic- *extra*thoracic pressure gradient. The increase in intrathoracic pressure with compression is generalized. Undirectional forward flow is made possible by functional venous closure at the thoracic inlet, preserved patency of the thick-walled carotid artery, and greater capacitance of the extrathoracic venous bed. The drop in intrathoracic pressure with relaxation allows blood return to the thorax. Blood flow below the diaphragm is minimal due to the lack of valves in the inferior vena cava.

petence of this valve would explain why retrograde flow does not occur out of the thoracic cavity with chest compression. That valves exist elsewhere in the jugular vein is evidenced by the fact that blood does not flow up the neck during a Valsalva maneuver. However, whether or not a valve is present precisely at the thoracic inlet is still the subject of controversy. In any event the lack of retrograde flow out of the thoracic cavity can be explained by a *functional* closure that occurs when the thin-walled jugular vein is collapsed by the increase in intrathoracic pressure generated by external chest compression.

In contrast, the thick-walled carotid artery resists compression and remains patent throughout CPR. By doing so it allows transmission of intrathoracic pressure to the extrathoracic arterial bed. This increase in pressure is also transmitted to the extrathoracic venous bed but, because of the greater *capacitance* of venous structures, pressures do not rise to nearly the same degree as they do on the arterial side. An *intrathoracic-extrathoracic* pressure gradient is thus established, and blood flows out of the thorax (Luce et al., 1980; Niemann et al., 1981). Blood returns during the relaxation phase of CPR. With release of chest compression, pressure within the thorax drops to virtually zero. The residual pressure in the extrathoracic venous bed now exceeds pressure within the thorax, and blood flows back into the chest.

The presence of venous valves is essential in producing and maintaining a pressure difference between the carotid artery and the internal jugular vein. Without this valving mechanism, blood would not flow during CPR. No such valving mechanism is present in the inferior vena cava. As a result, pressures in the arteries and veins of the abdomen and lower extremities are nearly equal during external chest compression, and circulation to the lower extremities is significantly less than that to the thorax and head (Niemann et al., 1981). Clinically this is important in explaining why the femoral vein is no longer a favored route for drug administration during CPR.

Acceptance of the thoracic pump theory led researchers to explore whether cardiac output during CPR might not be enhanced even more by further increasing intrathoracic pressure. As opposed to the situation with traditional CPR in which ventilations are interposed after every fifth cardiac compression, coordination of external chest compressions to occur *simultaneously* with ventilation (simultaneous compression-ventilation, or SCV-CPR) would maximize intrathoracic pressure. Experimentally, the result is a dramatic increase in peripheral and common carotid blood flow (Chandra et al., 1980).

The New CPR

Researchers came up with other ways to enhance blood flow during CPR. In addition to high pressure ventilations with SCV-CPR, the following were proposed:

—Abdominal binding
—Reduction in the rate of compression to 40/min
—Prolongation of compression duration to 60% of the compression-relaxation cycle

Taken together, these modifications made up the *"New CPR"* (Bircher, 1982). Abdominal binding was added to increase intrathoracic pressure. This is probably accomplished by limiting passive movement of the diaphragm during CPR (Niemann et al., 1982). The result is an increase in common carotid blood flow. Aortic afterload also increases, and presumably leads to preferential redistribution of blood to the coronary and cerebral vascular beds. Other investigators have suggested that application of mili-

tary antishock trousers (MAST suit) might result in a similar favorable redistribution of carotid blood flow during CPR (Lilja et al., 1981).

It should be emphasized that the New CPR is a research tool that is *not* recommended for clinical application by either the lay public or trained health care personnel. It cannot be, for a number of reasons. First, the high pressure ventilation of the New CPR requires endotracheal intubation. This alone prevents its use by the lay public. With the New CPR, one ventilation is delivered with each chest compression (SCV-CPR). At a rate of 40 compressions per minute, this means that 40 ventilations must be delivered each minute—a rate far too rapid for use in the field. Finally, coordinating ventilation so that it occurs simultaneously with compression and extending compression duration to occupy at least 60% of the cardiac cycle are both difficult objectives to consistently achieve by human endeavor. Laboratory use of a mechanical compression device (thumper) is needed.

Despite these limitations, the New CPR has been instrumental in providing us with a wealth of information on the mechanism of blood flow during cardiopulmonary resuscitation. Application of this knowledge has led to our realization that duration of compression is a far more important determinant of cardiac output during CPR than rate. Awareness that an increase in intrathoracic pressure is probably the major mechanism for blood flow has resulted in elimination of the previous recommendation to interpose ventilations with compression and has led to adoption of the asynchronous mode of CPR for the intubated patient.

Is CPR Effective?

ARE THE VITAL ORGANS PERFUSED?

Two final questions remain:

1) Does the increase in carotid blood flow produced by the New CPR result in improved cerebral perfusion?
2) Does it improve coronary blood flow?

Although one might logically assume that increases in common carotid blood flow result in improved cerebral perfusion, this is not necessarily the case (Luce et al., 1980; Rogers, 1983; Sanders et al., 1984). The common carotid artery divides into two branches: the external and internal carotid arteries. The tongue, face, scalp, and neck are supplied by the former, while the internal branch supplies the brain. When CPR is performed in the absence of pharmacologic therapy, blood is preferentially shunted to the external carotid artery. Thus, even though common carotid blood flow may more than double with SCV-CPR, cerebral perfusion remains minimal.

Although the use of adjuncts such as abdominal binding has been advocated, such measures are of questionable benefit and may even be deleterious. Blood flow to the brain is determined by cerebral perfusion pressure. This is equal to mean arterial pressure minus resting intracranial pressure (ICP). Abdominal binding increases intrathoracic pressure. Because of free communication between veins in the intrathoracic and intracerebral compartments, increases in intrathoracic pressure lead to increases in resting ICP. Such increases in ICP reduce blood flow to the brain (Rogers, 1983; Ewy, 1984; Michael et al., 1984).

What about coronary perfusion? Although external chest compression may generate systolic blood pressure peaks of more than 100 mm Hg, diastolic blood pressure is extremely low in the absence of pharmacologic therapy. The coronary arteries are perfused during diastole. Thus, increasing systolic blood pressure by external chest compression without also increasing diastolic blood pressure should have little effect on coronary blood flow (Luce et al., 1980; Niemann et al., 1982; Sanders et al., 1984; Martin et al., 1986).

Once again, abdominal binding and/or application of the MAST suit have been advocated in the hope of favorably redistributing blood flow to the coronary circulation during CPR. However, these techniques are cumbersome to employ during cardiac resuscitation, and their use cannot be recommended at the present time.

Moreover, to encourage use of the MAST suit or abdominal binding while CPR is being performed on patients in ventricular fibrillation might divert attention and delay treatment (defibrillation) of the primary disorder.

Another intervention that had been recommended in the past for increasing common carotid blood flow is *volume loading*. Application of the MAST suit hoped to take advantage of this concept by *autotransfusion* of lower extremity circulating volume to the intravascular compartment above the diaphragm. Although volume loading does increase common carotid flow, overall perfusion of vital organs (the heart and brain) is paradoxically decreased by this technique (Ditchey and Lindenfeld, 1984). Volume loading cannot be recommended for the normovolemic victim in cardiac arrest.

Open-Chest CPR

The problem of perfusing vital organs by closed-chest cardiac massage (CCCM) can be resolved by thoracotomy, cross-clamping the aorta, and direct manual cardiac compression (*open-chest CPR*). This technique was first described in the early 1900s and was the most commonly accepted method of cardiac resuscitation until the introduction of CCCM in 1970. Survival with open-chest CPR varied greatly, but success rates of up to 50% were reported in selected cases when open-chest CPR was performed in the operating room. Unlike CCCM, the limitations of blood flow to vital organs imposed by the heart being contained within the intrathoracic cavity (compartment) are obviated by opening the chest (thoracotomy). Direct cardiac compression more than triples cardiac output, and blood flow to the heart and brain are favored (Bircher and Safar, 1984; Sanders et al., 1984; Sanders et al., 1985). The technique may be lifesaving when patients fail to respond to CCCM. However, if it is to be effective, open-chest CPR must be started early (Sanders et al., 1985). Because of the risks of the procedure, its restriction to centers with readily accessible trained personnel comfortable with the procedure, and a lack of convincing evidence of its superiority over CCCM, the impact of open-chest CPR has not been appreciable.

Epinephrine

Short of opening the chest, how can one increase blood flow to the vital organs (the heart and brain) during CPR? The answer is with pharmacologic therapy. Alpha-adrenergic agents such as *epinephrine* favor blood flow to the heart by increasing peripheral vascular resistance and aortic diastolic blood pressure (Otto et al., 1981; Parmley et al., 1982; Redding, 1979). In addition, the drug *stiffens* the carotid artery, allowing intrathoracic pressure to be transmitted intact to the extrathoracic arterial bed. This is a prerequisite for circulation of blood by the thoracic pump theory. Finally, by increasing extracranial arterial resistance, epinephrine preferentially shunts blood from the external to the internal carotid artery, leading to increased cerebral perfusion (Rogers, 1983).

IS CPR EFFECTIVE?

Much controversy has centered around the question of whether CPR initiated by a lay bystander is important in saving lives of patients with out-of-hospital cardiac arrest. This is understandable considering our previous discussion of how blood flow to the heart and brain is minimal when CPR is performed without pharmacologic therapy. Determining the true value of CPR is made all the more difficult because of the virtually impossible task of separating out bystander-initiated CPR from the host of other variables that influence survival from cardiac arrest. Response time from patient collapse until arrival of EMS units capable of providing ACLS is especially hard to control for. Lay person perception of time under the stress of witnessing a cardiac arrest (especially if it is on a loved one) is notoriously inaccurate. Although one may clock in the time that a witness notifies EMS and accurately calculate response time from that moment, there is no way to verify how long it really took the witness to recognize the arrest in the first place. Nor is there any way to determine how long it actually took the witness to make the emergency phone call after recognizing the arrest.

This is the problem with most of the studies to date. Cummins and Eisenberg (1985) suggest that lay bystander CPR is effective in their comprehensive review of the literature on survival from prehospital cardiac arrest. However, the studies they quote did not control for the variables of witnessed arrest or paramedic response time, and only a few of them controlled for the variable of presenting rhythm. Uncontrolled studies that demonstrate improved survival with bystander-initiated CPR may be misleading because they are more likely to select cases in which the arrest was witnessed, where the initial rhythm was ventricular fibrillation, and for whom the call for help was put in sooner.

Stueven et al. (1986) reached a different conclusion about the efficacy of CPR in a retrospective review of 1500 prehospital cardiac arrests that occurred over a 10-year period. Their results suggest that when the variables of witnessed arrest, paramedic response times, and presenting rhythm are controlled for, performance of CPR by lay bystanders is *not* of benefit in improving ultimate survival from ventricular fibrillation, ventricular tachycardia, or asystole.

What then is the value of CPR? As we will discuss in Chapter 11 on Sudden Cardiac Death, the most important treatment of out-of-hospital cardiac arrest is defibrillation. The sooner patients with ventricular fibrillation or pulseless ventricular tachycardia can be countershocked, the better the chances for survival. While CPR per se is no substitute for definitive therapy, it may buy time until the defibrillator arrives (Niemann, 1985). In cases of pure respiratory arrest (as may occur with victims of near-drowning, lightning strikes, drug overdoses), the *rescue breathing* component of CPR alone may be curative. Perhaps the greatest impact CPR has on cardiopulmonary resuscitation is to teach the lay public to promptly recognize cardiac arrest and mobilize EMS personnel early (Eisenberg et al., 1979; Thompson et al., 1985).

COMPLICATIONS FROM CPR

CPR is not benign. In addition to the almost universal subjective complaint of sore chest reported by CPR survivors, serious complications may occur in up to 25% of all recipients (Nagel et al., 1984; Kern et al., 1986). Rib and sternal fractures are exceedingly common. These may lead to pneumothorax, pericardial tamponade, and flail chest. Other complications that may directly result from CPR include aspiration, aortic laceration, myocardial contusion, gastric mucosal tears with hemorrhage, gastric rupture, liver laceration, pulmonary edema, and lung herniation (Bjork et al., 1982; McDonnel et al., 1984; Nagel et al., 1984; Batra, 1986). This is *not* to say that CPR should not be promptly initiated by witnesses at the scene of a cardiac arrest but rather to point out that potential complications associated with its use are surprisingly common. Awareness that such complications may be caused by CPR becomes particularly important in the postresuscitation management of survivors of cardiac arrest.

CPR Training and the Lay Public

LAYPERSON CPR: ARE WE TRAINING THE RIGHT PEOPLE?

CPR then is our link with the community in the treatment and prevention of cardiopulmonary arrest. Yet, are we training the right people? In a study by Goldberg et al. (1984) of family members of patients with coronary artery disease, CPR training was felt to be important by the overwhelming majority. However, only 22% of these family members had ever taken a CPR course, and only 9% had done so within the past 3 years!

One might expect doctors to feel at least equally positive about the importance of CPR as the lay public. Yet a large Massachusetts survey revealed only 6% of physicians in that area routinely provided information about CPR training to family members of their patients with coronary artery disease (Goldberg et al., 1984). In these days of preventive medicine when health maintenance procedures such as mammography, testing for occult blood, and sigmoidoscopy are in vogue, instruction in CPR should probably command at least equal priority.

The Usual Scenario

What is the usual scenario of out-of-hospital cardiac arrest? Most such arrests occur in the home. Frequently, only one other person (the spouse) is around. Since the most common victims are men over 40, women over 40 (spouses) form the most likely group to witness a cardiac arrest. Yet the people who seek instruction in CPR tend to be in their 20s and 30s, and men seek training more commonly than do women (Goldberg et al., 1984; Mandel and Cobb, 1985). Even after the episode, most spouses of the victim still do not learn CPR. *Are we training the right people?*

Layperson CPR: How Quickly They Forget

One of the problems involved in teaching CPR to the lay public is the rapidity with which cognitive and psychomotor skills are forgotten. A study by Weaver et al. (1979) showed that while immediate retention of skills following a 4 hour BLS course was excellent, less than 15% of lay individuals were able to correctly perform one-person CPR according to AHA standards when retested 6 months later. Although disappointing, this result should not be unexpected when one considers how infrequently lay individuals are called on to perform CPR in a real situation.

Simplification of CPR for the Lay Public

In an attempt to improve retention of skills by the lay public, the new guidelines have simplified the standards for performance of CPR. No longer need lay individuals concern themselves with compressing at precisely 60 times per minute. A range of between 80 and 100 per minute is the new standard. Similarly, lay persons will no longer be taught two-person CPR. As noted above, it is extremely uncommon for out-of-hospital cardiac arrest to occur in the presence of two or more lay individuals who are trained in CPR. The two-rescuer sequence adds complexity to the task and may detract from performance of one-rescuer CPR. The victim would probably best be served if the most knowledgeable person on the scene initiated one-rescuer CPR while any additional witnesses promptly summoned an EMS unit. Trained professionals capable of taking over BLS (and hopefully of instituting ACLS) should then arrive shortly thereafter.

ON MOUTH-TO-MOUTH RESUSCITATION*

The setting is all too familiar. A cardiac arrest is called in the far reaches of your hospital. You run to the bedside and find yourself among the first to arrive. Neither respiratory therapy nor the code team (or crash cart) are yet on the scene. Health care providers are feverishly putting on monitor leads, obtaining IV access, getting a bedboard under the patient, and performing external chest compressions . . . and no one is breathing for the patient. And the patient is blue. Knowing looks pass back and forth from those in attendance . . . and no one is breathing for the patient. As precious seconds (which seem like hours) pass by, you reflect on your options. You could:

1) Perform mouth-to-mouth resuscitation.
2) Wait a little longer and hope that help (in the form of someone with a bag-valve mask) arrives.
3) Perform mouth-to-mouth resuscitation.
4) Yell at a nurse.
5) Look for a medical student and have him/ her perform mouth-to-mouth resuscitation.
6) Busy yourself with the ECG monitor.
7) Wait a little longer.
8) Let the patient die.
9) Perform mouth-to-mouth resuscitation.

In 1987, the act of performing mouth-to-mouth resuscitation in a medical environment is

*Reproduced with permission from Grauer K, Kravitz L: On Mouth-to-Mouth. Journal of American Board of Family Practice, Lexington KY, to be published in Vol. 1;1, winter, 1987.

at risk of becoming an extinct art (Lawrence, 1985). Fear of AIDS has overcome all reason. Even elderly ladies and gentlemen who haven't ventured out of nursing homes for years are not receiving rescue breathing because of the possibility that they somehow contracted *the* disease.

Ironically, reluctance to perform mouth-to-mouth resuscitation seems to be less of a problem with prehospital cardiac arrest. Most events that occur outside the hospital take place in the home. Lay person witnesses in this setting most often know the victim well and are frequently aware of their medical history. If lay person witnesses know CPR, they usually administer it promptly.

Delay in providing respiratory support is also less of a problem in hospital emergency departments and intensive care units. While reluctance to perform mouth-to-mouth resuscitation among health care providers is still prevalent in these areas, the crash cart is usually nearby and the personnel in attendance so familiar with emergency cardiopulmonary care that the time for control of the airway is frequently minimal. In contrast, the problem of achieving airway control in other medical environments (on regular wards, in waiting rooms, out-patient clinics, and medical offices) is significant. Reluctance to perform mouth-to-mouth resuscitation in these settings has reached epidemic proportions. Considering that respiratory equipment (and the crash cart) is often just too many minutes away, prompt administration of rescue breathing must be looked on as the essential first step in the life-saving process.

The facts are these:

1) Although the HIV AIDS virus is present in saliva, no transmission of infection during mouth-to-mouth resuscitation has ever been documented (MMWR, 1985; FDA Drug Bulletin, 1985; JAMA Suppl, 1986).

2) The epidemiology of HIV infection is similar to that of hepatitis B virus infection. The risk of hepatitis B virus transmission in health care settings far exceeds that for HIV virus transmission. While experience with AIDS is still fairly limited, more than 15 years of experience in management has been accumulated

with hepatitis B virus infection. No transmission of infection during mouth-to-mouth resuscitation has ever been documented for hepatitis B (MMWR, 1985).

3) Although final answers are not yet in, the potential risk of transmission of AIDS by mouth-to-mouth resuscitation appears to be extremely small.

We suggest the following:

1) If a patient arrests outside the hospital and you don't do CPR, the chances are good that no one else will. If the cause of the arrest is purely respiratory (such as drowning or drug overdose), prompt administration of rescue breathing could be lifesaving. *Breathe* for the patient.

2) If a patient arrests in a hospital setting and you know help (and a bag-valve mask) is on the way, it may be reasonable to wait a few moments for their arrival. Ventricular tachycardia/fibrillation is the most common cause of cardiopulmonary arrest in this setting. Defibrillation is the treatment of choice. Putting off management of the airway for a few moments (although less than ideal) probably will not adversely affect outcome in most instances. However, if help in the hospital is late in arriving and the patient is not being ventilated, *breathe* for the patient.

3) If nothing in the available history of the patient even remotely suggests that he might have AIDS, hepatitis B, herpes, active tuberculosis, or meningococcal meningitis, do not even wait the few moments. If the patient is not being ventilated and a bag-valve mask unit is not available at the bedside, *breathe* for the patient.

4) Consider more widespread use of the *pocket mask*. This underutilized, inexpensive device has been shown to be far superior to bag-valve mask systems in ventilating the patient in respiratory arrest (Harrison et al., 1982; Elling and Politis, 1983). Because the mask eliminates direct contact between rescuer and victim, the risk of disease transmission is dramatically lessened. The device may be made even safer by adding a *one-way valve* to the mask (so that air expired by the victim is directed away from the rescuer). Greater availability of this inexpensive airway adjunct in medical settings where cardiac arrest may occur (for example, nursing stations on all

floors, waiting rooms, medical offices) would go a long way to alleviating the problem.

5) Anticipate. Consider keeping a pocket mask (preferably with a one-way valve) or bag-valve mask unit at the bedside of those patients at particularly high risk of coding.

6) Do not let the patient die of hypoxemia.

ADDENDUM:

As a footnote to this chapter, one should appreciate that the thoracic pump model has not been unquestionably accepted by all investigators in the field as the principal mechanism for blood flow in adults during CPR. Advocates of *high impulse CPR* assert that direct cardiac compression is an important mechanism in many adults, and that maximal cardiac output will only be obtained when manual massage is performed at a rapid rate with brief compressions of moderate force (Maier et al., 1984). Although all of the data are not yet in, the "true" explanation for blood flow during CPR is probably best thought of as part of a spectrum. Direct cardiac compression doubtlessly plays a major role in infants, young children, and individuals with thin and compliant chest walls. At the other end of the spectrum, in many adults (especially those with emphysema) the thoracic pump model provides a more rational explanation for blood flow. In between these two extremes, a combination of the cardiac and thoracic pump models is probably operative.

Until more definitive data are obtained, our feeling is that both mechanisms for blood flow be taken into account in making recommendations for compression rate during CPR. Thus, although a range of between 80–100 compressions per minute has been recommended by the American Heart Association for both one and two-rescuer CPR, we suggest that one err on the higher side of this range. Compressing at the more rapid rate should lead to increased blood flow regardless of whether the cardiac or thoracic pump model is the predominant mechanism for a particular individual.

REFERENCES

American Heart Association Subcommittee on Emergency Cardiac Care: Standards and guidelines for cardiopulmonary resuscitation (CPR) and emergency cardiac care (ECC). JAMA 255:2905–2992, 1986.

Batra AK: Lung herniation after CPR. Crit Care Med 14:595–596, 1986.

Bircher N: New concepts in cardiopulmonary resuscitation. ER Reports 3:45–48, 1982.

Bircher N, Safar P: Manual open-chest cardiopulmonary resuscitation. Ann Emerg Med 13:770–773, 1984.

Bjork RJ, Snyder BD, Campion BC, Loewenson RB: Medical complications of cardiopulmonary arrest. Arch Intern Med 142:500–503, 1982.

Chandra N, Rudikoff M, Weisfeldt ML: Simultaneous chest compression and ventilation at high airway pressure during cardiopulmonary resuscitation. Lancet 1:175–178, 1980.

Criley JM, Blaufuss AH, Kissel GL: Cough-induced cardiac compression: Self-administered form of cardiopulmonary resuscitation. JAMA 236:1246–1250, 1976.

Cummins RO, Eisenberg MS: Prehospital cardiopulmonary resuscitation: Is it effective? JAMA 253:2408–2412, 1985.

Ditchey RV, Lindenfeld J: Potential adverse effects of volume loading on perfusion of vital organs during closed chest resuscitation. Circulation 69:181–189, 1984.

Eisenberg MS, Bergner L, Hallstrom A: Cardiac resuscitation in the community: Importance of rapid provision and implications for program planning. JAMA 241:1905–1907, 1979.

Elling R, Politis J: An evaluation of emergency medical technicians' ability to use manual ventilation devices. Ann Emerg Med 12:765–768, 1983.

Ewy GA: Current status of cardiopulmonary resuscitation. Mod Conc Cardiovasc Dis 53:43–45, 1984.

FDA Drug Bulletin: Progress on AIDS. 15:26–32, 1985.

Goldberg RJ, Gore JM, Love DG, Ockene JK, Dalen JE: Layperson CPR—Are we training the right people? Ann Emerg Med 13:701–704, 1984.

Harrison RR, Maull KL, Keenan RL, Boyan CP: Mouth-to-mask ventilation: A superior method of rescue breathing. Ann Emerg Med 11:74–76, 1982.

Kern KB, Carter AB, Showen RL, Voorhees WD, Babbs CF, Tacker WA, Ewy GA: CPR-induced trauma: Comparison of three manual methods in an experimental model. Ann Emerg Med 15:674–679, 1986.

Kowalski R, Thompson BM, Horwitz L, Stueven H, Aprahamian C, Darin JC: Bystander CPR in prehospital coarse ventricular fibrillation. Ann Emerg Med 13:1016–1020, 1984.

Lawrence PJ: Ventilation during cardiopulmonary resuscitation: Which method? Med J Aust 143:443–447, 1985.

Lilja GP, Long RS, Ruiz E: Augmentation of systolic blood pressure during external cardiac compression by use of the MAST suit. Ann Emerg Med 10:182–184, 1981.

Luce JM, Cary JM, Ross BK, Culver BH, Butler J: New developments in cardiopulmonary resuscitation. JAMA 244:1366–1370, 1980.

Maier GW, Tyson GI, Olsen CO, Kernstein KJ, Davis JW, Cohn EH, Sabiston DC, Rankin JS: The physiology of external cardiac massage: high-impulse cardiopulmonary resuscitation. Circulation 70:86–101, 1984.

Mandel LP, Cobb LA: CPR training in the community. Ann Emerg Med 14:669–671, 1985.

Martin GB, Carden DL, Nowak RM, Lewinter JR, Johnston W, Tomlanovich MC: Aortic and right atrial pressures during standard and simultaneous compression and ventilation CPR in human beings. Ann Emerg Med 15:125–130, 1986.

McDonnell PJ, Hutchins GM, Hruban RH, Brown CG: Hemorrhage from gastric mucosal tears complicating cardiopulmonary resuscitation. Ann Emerg Med 13:230–233, 1984.

McIntyre KM, Parisi AF, Benfari R, Goldberg AH, Dalen JE: Pathophysiologic syndromes of cardiopulmonary resuscitation. Arch Intern Med 138:1130–1133, 1978.

Melker RJ, Banner MJ: Ventilation during CPR: Two-rescuer standards reappraised. Ann Emerg Med 14:397–402, 1985.

Melker R, Cavallaro D, Krischer J: One-rescuer CPR: A reappraisal of present recommendation for ventilation. Crit Care Med 9:423, 1981.

Melker RJ, Cavallaro DL: Cardiopulmonary resuscitation during synchronous and asynchronous ventilation (abstract). Ann Emerg Med 12:142, 1983.

Michael JR, Guerci AD, Koehler RC, Shi AY, Tsitlik J, Chandra N, Niedermeyer E, Rogers MC, Traystman RJ, Weisfeldt ML: Mechanisms by which epinephrine augments cerebral and myocardial perfusion during cardiopulmonary resuscitation in dogs. Circulation 69:822–835, 1984.

Nagel EL, Fine EG, Krischer JP, Davis JH: Complications of CPR. Crit Care Med 9:424, 1981.

Niemann JT: Artificial perfusion techniques during cardiac

arrest: Questions of experimental focus versus clinical need. Ann Emerg Med 14:761–768, 1985.

Niemann JT, Rosborough J, Hausknecht M, Ung S, Criley JM: Blood flow without cardiac compression during closed chest CPR. Crit Care Med 9:380–381, 1981.

Niemann JT, Rosborough JP, Ung S, Criley JM: Coronary perfusion pressure during experimental cardiopulmonary resuscitation. Ann Emerg Med 11:127–131, 1982.

Otto CW, Yakaitis RW, Blitt CD: Mechanism of action of epinephrine in resuscitation from asphyxial arrest. Crit Care Med 9:321–324, 1981.

Parmley WW, Hatcher CR, Ewy GA, Furman S, Redding J, Weisfeldt ML: Task Force V: Physical interventions and adjunctive therapy. Thirteenth Bethesda Conference on Emergency Cardiac Care. Am J Cardiol 50:409–420, 1982.

Recommendations for Preventing Transmission of Infection with Human T-Lymphotropic Virus Type III/Lymphadenopathy-Associated Virus in the Workplace. MMWR 34:681–696, 1985.

Redding JS: Cardiopulmonary resuscitation: An algorithm and some common pitfalls. Am Heart J 98:788–797, 1979.

Redding JS: Commentary on the proceedings: Second Wolf Creek Conference on CPR. Crit Care Med 9:432–435, 1981.

Rogers MC: New development in cardiopulmonary resuscitation. Pediatrics 71:655–658, 1983.

Rosborough JP, Hausknecht M, Niemann JT, Criley JM: Cough supported circulation. Crit Care Med 9:371–372, 1981.

Safar P: Cardiopulmonary Cerebral Resuscitation. Asmund S. Laerdal, Stavanger, Norway, 1981.

Sanders AB, Kern KB, Ewy GA: Time limitations for open-chest cardiopulmonary resuscitation from cardiac arrest. Crit Care Med 13:897–898, 1985.

Sanders AB, Kern KB, Ewy GA, Atlas M, Bailey L: Improved resuscitation from cardiac arrest with open-chest massage. Ann Emerg Med 13:672–675, 1984.

Sanders AB, Meislin HW, Ewy GA: The physiology of cardiopulmonary resuscitation: An update. JAMA 252:3283–3286, 1984.

Stueven H, Troiano P, Thompson B, Mateer JR, Kastenson EH, Tonsfeldt D, Hargarten K, Kowalski R, Aprahamian C, Darin J: Bystander/first responder CPR: Ten years experience in a paramedic system. Ann Emerg Med 15:707–710, 1986.

Taylor GJ, Tucker WM, Greene HL, Rudikoff MT, Weisfeldt ML: Importance of prolonged compression during cardiopulmonary resuscitation in man. N Engl J Med 296:1515–1518, 1977.

Thompson BM, Stueven HA, Mateer JR, Aprahamian CC, Tucker JF, Darin JC: Comparison of clinical CPR studies in Milwaukee and elsewhere in the United States. Ann Emerg Med 14:750–754, 1985.

Weaver FJ, Ramirez AG, Dorfman SB, Raizner AE: Trainees' retention of cardiopulmonary resuscitation: How quickly they forget. JAMA 241:901–903, 1979.

Weisfeldt ML, Chandra N, Tsitlik J: Increased intrathoracic pressure—not direct heart compression—causes the rise in intrathoracic vascular pressures during CPR in dogs and pigs. Crit Care Med 9:377–378, 1981.

White BC, Gadzinski DS, Hoehner PJ, Krome C, Hoehner T, White SD, Trombley JH: Effect of flunarizine on canine cerebral cortical blood flow and vascular resistance post cardiac arrest. Ann Emerg Med 11:119–126, 1982.

CHAPTER 11

SUDDEN CARDIAC DEATH

OUT-OF-HOSPITAL CARDIAC ARREST

Sudden cardiac death (SCD) has been defined as unexpected death of cardiac etiology occurring either immediately or within 1 hour of the onset of symptoms (Eisenberg et al., 1981). It claims the lives of almost half a million individuals in the United States each year. Although most of these victims have significant coronary artery disease, in many the disease is silent and sudden death is the first manifestation in an otherwise healthy adult.

In a sense, the very term "sudden cardiac death" has become almost obsolete. Initially the designation was applied synonymously with the occurrence of out-of-hospital ventricular fibrillation, as the latter event was almost uniformly fatal—hence, sudden "death." Today this is no longer the case. Overall outcome for patients with out-of-hospital cardiac arrest has improved tremendously. In many communities where advanced emergency medical service (EMS) systems exist, the rate of successful resuscitation and ultimate discharge home has more than doubled during the past decade. In Seattle, Washington, for example, response time from dispatch until arrival of a basic life support team averages less than 3 minutes, and a paramedic unit capable of administering ACLS arrives 4 minutes later. As a result, up to 60% of cases of ventricular fibrillation are successfully resuscitated on the scene, and 25% survive to leave the hospital (Cobb and Werner, 1982). In addition to their advanced EMS system, more than a third of the population now know CPR (compared to only 5% a decade ago). Thus, Seattle has become the prototype community for delivery of BLS and ACLS, and being victim to an out-of-hospital cardiac arrest there is no longer synonymous with mortality. The same holds true in other areas of the country where community interest in CPR is high and advanced EMS systems exist.

The ACLS Score

What determines the likelihood of survival from out-of-hospital cardiac arrest? One factor which is unalterable is the underlying disease process. A patient who develops ventricular fibrillation secondary to a massive pulmonary embolus or rupture of a ventricular aneurysm may be unsalvageable regardless of how sophisticated resuscitation techniques are. Beyond the underlying disease process, *four* factors appear to be most important in determining survival. They have been incorporated by Eisenberg into a mnemonic known as the **"A-C-L-S"** Score:

A —Was the **A**rrest witnessed?
C—What was the initial **C**ardiac rhythm documented by the paramedics on arrival?
L—Was **L**ay bystander CPR performed?
S—How long did it take for help to arrive (ie, **S**peed of paramedic response time)?

Eisenberg et al. (1981) examined the importance of each of these factors in a review of 611 cases of out-of-hospital cardiac arrest (defined as a pulseless condition confirmed by paramedics) during a 3-year period from 1976–1979. For arrests that were witnessed **(A),** 28% of 380 patients were ultimately discharged from the hospital. In contrast, only 3% of 231 victims of unwitnessed cardiac arrest survived. When the mechanism of the arrest (the initial **C**ardiac rhythm) was ventricular tachycardia or fibrillation, 28% of 389 patients survived, compared to a dismal 3% survival in the 222 patients for whom the initial documented rhythm was asystole. In those 168 patients for whom a lay bystander performed CPR **(L),** a 32% survival rate was seen. When CPR was delayed until arrival of the EMTs, that figure dropped to 14%. Finally, when paramedics were able to respond with ACLS in less than 4 minutes (**S**peed), 56% of patients were saved. Survival decreased to 35% when response time was between 4 and 8 minutes, and to only 17% if response time exceeded 8 minutes.

Mechanisms of Out-of-Hospital Cardiac Arrest

From the above, it can be seen that the initial mechanism of an arrest is an extremely important determinant of survival. Statistically, about two thirds of patients arresting outside the hospital are initially found in ventricular fibrillation. An additional 5–10% are in ventricular tachycardia when the rescue team arrives, and the remainder are in a bradyarrhythmia (including asystole). Prognosis is by far best for those patients found in ventricular tachycardia. The large majority of these individuals can be successfully resuscitated on the scene, and up to two thirds of them will be ultimately discharged from the hospital (Myerburg et al., 1982). In contrast, patients initially found in a bradyarrhythmia or asystole have a dismal prognosis with a minuscule ultimate survival rate. Outcome of patients initially found in ventricular fibrillation is intermediate between these two groups. The data collected by Myerburg et al. from Miami during the 3-year period from 1975–1978 demonstrated a 23% long-term survival rate for 220 such patients with out-of-hospital ventricular fibrillation. Slightly higher figures have been obtained from Seattle.

> In discussing the mechanism of out-of-hospital cardiac arrest, the obvious question to raise is how can one be sure that the initial cardiac rhythm documented by the EMS unit on the scene is truly the *precipitating* mechanism of the arrest. The answer is that one cannot. In the Miami experience, this was assumed to be the case because data were included only from episodes in which the onset of cardiac arrest was witnessed, EMS personnel were summoned without delay, and arrival on the scene was documented to have occurred within 4 minutes of summons. Nevertheless it is still quite possible that at least some of the bradyarrhythmias represented a *secondary* rather than primary mechanism of arrest in which asystole or EMD succeeded ventricular fibrillation as time from patient collapse until arrival of the EMS unit elapsed.
> Similarly, ventricular tachycardia could have preceded development of ventricular fibrillation. That this probably occurs much more commonly than is generally appreciated is suggested by several obser-

vations. SCD survivors who have a second cardiac arrest while being monitored in the hospital often demonstrate ventricular tachycardia as the initial rhythm of their recurrence (Josephson et al., 1980). In addition, patients sustaining cardiac arrest during Holter monitoring frequently demonstrate ventricular tachycardia of variable duration as the precipitating mechanism of arrest (Pratt et al., 1983; Kempf and Josephson, 1984; Milner et al., 1985). *Ventricular tachycardia* (rather than ventricular fibrillation) may well be the primary (precipitating) mechanism of many *(if not most)* cardiac arrests (Buxton, 1986).

The significance of this finding lies with the much better chance for successful resuscitation if ventricular tachycardia is the initial rhythm found on arrival of the EMS unit. The reason this rhythm has been documented so infrequently in previous studies of out-of-hospital cardiac arrest may be due to the time it takes for help to arrive. During these critical minutes, ventricular tachycardia probably deteriorates to ventricular fibrillation in many cases. Were it possible for emergency care providers to get to the scene sooner (when ventricular tachycardia is still present), survival from out-of-hospital cardiac arrest would doubtlessly improve.

The Immediate Postresuscitation Rhythm

The poor prognostic implications of bradyarrhythmias carry over to the *immediate postresuscitation rhythm* (ie, the *first* rhythm seen *after* conversion out of ventricular fibrillation). For patients initially discovered in ventricular fibrillation, conversion to a supraventricular rhythm with a heart rate greater than 100 beats/min is associated with greater than 40% long-term survival (Nagel et al., 1975). In contrast, long-term survival is only 5% when the initial postresuscitation rhythm is bradycardia. Patients in whom the heart rate immediately following conversion from ventricular fibrillation is between 60 and 100 beats/min have an intermediate prognosis.

Clinical Implications

Awareness of the primary mechanism for out-of-hospital cardiac arrest may provide the rescue team with important prognostic information regarding the chances for successful resuscitation and ultimate survival. This is *not* to say that little attempt should be made to resuscitate a patient who suffers an unwitnessed arrest and is found in a bradyarrhythmia such as asystole or EMD. On the contrary, rescuers are always obligated to initiate and continue basic and advanced life support measures until it becomes evident that effective cardiovascular function cannot be restored. Nonetheless, knowledge of the clinical context in which an arrest occurs and appreciation of what the cardiac rhythm was *at the time of arrival* of the EMS unit may be extremely helpful to the emergency care provider in determining how aggressively resuscitation efforts should be pursued.

It should be evident from the discussion so far that time is critical in cardiac resuscitation. If a patient is still in ventricular tachycardia at the time help (the defibrillator) arrives, the chances of successful resuscitation are extremely good. If the patient is in ventricular fibrillation, a 20–30% chance for long-term survival still remains. The longer the patient remains in ventricular fibrillation, the less likely it becomes that defibrillation will be successful (Weaver et al., 1984; Eisenberg et al., 1985). By the time ventricular fibrillation has deteriorated to bradycardia (or in those instances when a bradyarrhythmia itself is the primary mechanism of arrest), prognosis is dismal.

For practical purposes then, potentially treatable mechanisms of out-of-hospital cardiac arrest are ventricular tachycardia and ventricular fibrillation. Early defibrillation (or synchronized cardioversion for ventricular tachycardia with a pulse) is the treatment of choice. Institution of lay bystander CPR is *not* a substitute for this definitive therapy. CPR by itself (without adjunctive use of drugs such as epinephrine) will not result in adequate perfusion of vital organs such as the heart and brain (Michael et al., 1984; Sanders et al., 1984). At most, performance of CPR buys a small amount of time until definitive care can be provided (Cummins et al., 1985; Stueven et al., 1986). CPR does *not* prevent ventricular tachycardia or ventricular fibrillation from deteriorating to asystole (Enns et al, 1983). What CPR does do, however, is teach the lay public to recognize cardiac arrest sooner. This is vitally important because it leads to earlier activation of EMS personnel and more rapid initiation of definitive therapy.

Historically, efforts to transport the victim of cardiac arrest to a defibrillator have not been successful (Eisenberg et al., 1980; Stults et al., 1984). It simply takes too long to get the patient to the hospital. As a result, emphasis has switched to transporting the defibrillator to the scene. This idea first gained support in the 1960s with the advent of mobile coronary care units that carried defibrillators. Initially, physicians were used to staff these units. By the 1970s, a number of communities had begun to use specially trained lay personnel (paramedics) instead of physicians for this purpose. With paramedics providing initial emergency care at the scene, both prompter and wider dispersion of medical services was possible. Earlier countershock could be delivered to patients with ventricular fibrillation, and survival rates from out-of-hospital cardiac arrest more than doubled (Eisenberg et al., 1980).

In succeeding years, lay personnel with much less extensive training were used to provide emergency care and on-the-scene defibrillation. In communities without paramedics, this meant firemen, policemen, and ambulance drivers received training to become emergency medical technicians (EMTs). With as little as 10 hours of formal instruction, it was shown that such providers could be taught to identify ventricular fibrillation and defibrillate effectively (Eisenberg et al., 1980). Even when such personnel were not allowed to do anything other than defibrillate victims of out-of-hospital cardiac arrest (ie, no intubation and no administration of medication), lives were saved (Stults et al., 1984; Eisenberg et al., 1984).

Automatic External Defibrillators

As an extension of the idea that providing prompter defibrillation for victims of out-of-hospital cardiac arrest improved survival, the *automatic external defibrillator (AED)* was developed. Designed for both the lay public and EMS personnel, this device is now commercially available.

The AED is relatively easy to use, although frequent retraining is essential to ensure retention of skills (Cummins et al., 1985). Most lay people can be taught to effectively operate it in as little as 3 hours (Eisenberg et al., 1985). All that is required is to insert an oral airway and apply a pregelled adhesive pad to the anterior chest of the victim. The machine does the rest. Electrodes attached to the oral airway and chest pad sense the cardiac rhythm, analyze it, and deliver 200 to 335 joules of electrical energy if ventricular fibrillation is present.

> In earlier models, a breath detector was incorporated into the oral airway to verify the absence of respiration, thus serving as a double check that the victim was truly in cardiopulmonary arrest. However, due to the recently appreciated fact that agonal respirations may persist despite the presence of ventricular fibrillation, the breath detector has proved to be a double-edged sword. It has been removed from newer models to avoid the potential situation where the AED might not shock a patient with gasping respirations who was nevertheless in ventricular fibrillation.

Preliminary results (Cummins et al., 1984) with the AED show a sensitivity of 81% for detection of ventricular fibrillation and a specificity of 100% (no inappropriate countershocks of patients who are not in ventricular fibrillation). Prospective trials are underway to obtain more data and to evaluate the efficacy of the AED when used by family members of patients at high risk of sudden cardiac death.

In an attempt to increase the ability of EMTs to deliver definitive care in the field, a move has been made to allow such individuals to operate the AED at the scene of cardiac arrest. This is particularly important for rural communities where funding usually is inadequate to provide paramedic programs. Because volunteerism for ambulance services is often high in such areas, while the incidence of out-of-hospital cardiac arrest is quite low, most EMTs who work in communities with populations under 25,000 will not have an opportunity to test their defibrillation skills in a real situation more often than once

every year (Stults et al., 1984; Ornato et al., 1984). The obvious advantage of the AED is that it minimizes the need for the constant retraining that would be necessary to maintain the skills of individuals who are called on to defibrillate so infrequently.

Currently, prospective, randomized, controlled studies of automatic defibrillation by EMTs are in progress in Seattle, Washington. Preliminary results are encouraging. They suggest that communities lacking the resources necessary for more extensive EMT training and supervision may improve survival from out-of-hospital cardiac arrest by implementing automatic defibrillation programs by EMS personnel (Cummins et al., 1985). Considering the extremely poor prognosis of persons suffering cardiac arrest in rural communities (Bachman et al., 1986), instituting some mechanism for expediting emergency defibrillation would seem to offer the only realistic chance for improving survival in such areas of the country.

FOLLOW-UP TREATMENT OF SURVIVORS OF OUT-OF-HOSPITAL CARDIAC ARREST

The overwhelming majority of victims of out-of-hospital cardiac arrest have underlying coronary artery disease (CAD). In at least 20% of these individuals, cardiac arrest is the first (and last) manifestation of CAD (Cobb et al., 1980; Kannel et al, 1975). Surprisingly, acute myocardial infarction is the actual cause of the cardiac arrest in less than one third of cases (Myerburg et al., 1982). Subsequent mortality depends on whether acute infarction is the inciting mechanism. This is because ventricular electrical instability is common during the early hours of myocardial infarction. Consequently, most deaths from acute infarction result from primary ventricular fibrillation that develops within the first few hours of the onset of symptoms. Electrical instability associated with acute infarction is usually a transient phenomenon that resolves as the patient recovers. The occurrence of ventricular fibrillation during the early hours of acute infarction does not seem to affect long-term survival. Patients who have an otherwise uncomplicated course demonstrate an equally good prognosis as those with uncomplicated myocardial infarction who never had ventricular fibrillation (Bigger and Coromilas, 1983).

In contrast, patients who develop out-of-hospital cardiac arrest without associated infarction do not have any obvious inciting cause. When Holter monitoring is performed on these patients after their episode, extremely frequent and complex ventricular ectopy with runs of ventricular tachycardia is the rule (Myerburg et al., 1982).

Treatment of such individuals poses a true dilemma. Left alone, the rate of recurrence for a second episode of cardiac arrest approaches 30% during the year following the initial episode and 50% by the second year (Bigger, 1984). Although total elimination of PVCs might seem to be the ideal end point of therapy, this goal is an unrealistic (if not impossible) one to achieve. Moreover, even if PVCs could be completely eliminated, current knowledge suggests that this does *not* guarantee such patients will be at less risk of developing a lethal arrhythmia such as sustained ventricular tachycardia or ventricular fibrillation (Ruskin et al., 1983).

Programmed Electrophysiologic Stimulation (PES) Studies

Several potential end points of therapy for survivors of out-of-hospital cardiac arrest have been proposed. Ideally such individuals should probably be studied with *programmed electrophysiologic stimulation (PES) studies*. An intravenous electrode catheter is fluoroscopically guided into the right ventricle, and one or more ventricular extrastimuli are introduced at various points in the cardiac cycle in an attempt to induce ventricular tachycardia. Ability to induce this arrhythmia in the laboratory appears to be

an excellent indicator of which patients are at greatest risk of its spontaneous occurrence. For those patients in whom induction of sustained ventricular tachycardia is no longer possible following administration of an antiarrhythmic agent, recurrence of the arrhythmia becomes much less likely when the drug is continued on a long-term basis (Horowitz et al., 1980; Akhtar, 1982; Swerdlow et al., 1983). Unfortunately, PES studies are invasive, time-consuming, expensive, and not universally available. In addition, they are successful in finding an effective drug in only about one third of cases (Bigger, 1984).

Surgery for Refractory Ventricular Arrhythmias

Surgery has taken on an increasingly important role in the treatment of survivors of out-of-hospital cardiac arrest. Given that coronary artery disease is so common in these individuals, coronary artery bypass grafting (CABG) may control arrhythmias in some of these patients simply by treating the underlying ischemic disease.

In other patients, a ventricular aneurysm or endocardial scarring may be the anatomic substrate for recurrent episodes of ventricular tachycardia. Utilization of intraoperative electrophysiologic mapping may allow precise localization of an arrhythmogenic focus. If such a focus is found, surgical ablation by endocardial resection and/or cryothermia may control the arrhythmias in up to 85% of cases, frequently without the need for additional antiarrhythmic therapy (Cox, 1985; Lawrie et al., 1985; Wetstein et al., 1985).

Automatic Implantable Defibrillator

An exciting new modality for treatment of patients with lethal ventricular arrhythmias is the *automatic implantable defibrillator (AID)*. The current device consists of a pulse generator that is the size of a package of cigarettes. This is implanted in the abdomen. Two defibrillating electrodes that also serve as sensors are positioned in the superior vena cava and over the apex of the heart. Newer models also include a bipolar right ventricular electrode that allows R-wave synchronization and cardioversion.

Conceptually, the AID functions essentially as a pacemaker. Instead of sensing bradyarrhythmias and pacing, it senses tachyarrhythmias and cardioverts or defibrillates, depending on the rhythm detected.

Survival rates for patients who have received implantable defibrillators have been truly remarkable. One-year mortality from sudden death is reduced to well below 10%, compared to the 30% expected mortality for patients left untreated (Mirowski et al., 1983; Echt et al., 1985; Mirowski, 1985). Over 400 individuals in more than 40 centers across the country have already received this device. Its use will probably become even more widespread within the very near future.

Empiric Therapy for Survivors of Out-of-Hospital Cardiac Arrest

Use of PES studies, endocardial electrophysiologic mapping, and implantation of the automatic defibrillator are all excellent modalities for treatment of patients with lethal ventricular arrhythmias. They clearly are more sensitive than Holter monitoring for determining the population at highest risk of recurrence from sudden cardiac death. They are also decidedly more effective than empiric antiarrhythmic therapy in preventing such recurrences (Skale et al., 1986). Unfortunately, these procedures are costly, invasive, and require specialized centers with highly skilled personnel for their implementation. They are not currently accessible to many survivors of out-of-hospital cardiac arrest.

When these modalities are not available, empiric therapy may be a reasonable (necessary) alternative. Myerburg et al. (1982) followed a number of survivors of out-of-hospital cardiac

arrest with this approach over a 2-year period. Patients were treated with antiarrhythmic agents (quinidine and procainamide) and closely monitored with antiarrhythmic blood levels. Significant reduction in PVC frequency could not be achieved even among those patients who were able to consistently maintain therapeutic antiarrhythmic blood levels. Virtually all patients continued to demonstrate greater than 100 PVCs per hour! However, mortality was significantly decreased in the group for whom therapeutic serum levels of antiarrhythmic drugs were maintained. Although the number of patients studied was small, the data suggest that a more practical and realistic end point to aim for when sophisticated modalities are unavailable is partial (rather than complete) reduction in PVC frequency with elimination of worrisome forms (long runs of ventricular tachycardia) and maintenance of therapeutic antiarrhythmic drug levels.

IN-HOSPITAL CARDIAC ARREST

Most individuals who suffer cardiac arrest outside the hospital have underlying coronary artery disease. In contrast, in-hospital cardiac arrest is frequently the common terminal event for a variety of end-stage disease processes. Cardiac arrests occur in 1–2% of all patients admitted to the hospital (Lowenstein et al., 1986). Among those who die, cardiopulmonary resuscitation is attempted about one third of the time (Bedell et al., 1983). Overall survival for in-hospital cardiac arrest is somewhat poorer than for arrest that occurs outside the hospital. This has been attributed to the fact that hospitalized patients are usually sicker and carry a poorer prearrest prognosis than ambulatory individuals. Across the board, half of the patients who arrest in the hospital are initially resuscitated, one third are still alive the next day, and about 15% survive to leave the hospital (Bedell et al., 1983; Scaff et al., 1984).

Factors Influencing Survival

Success rates for in-hospital resuscitation do *not* appear to be significantly influenced by *where* in the hospital the arrest occurs. Instead, *time until discovery* is a much more critical factor in determining whether the resuscitation effort will be successful (Bedell et al., 1983). Although patients who arrest in the emergency department and intensive care unit often do better than those arresting on a general ward, this is probably because such patients are more often monitored and discovered sooner after collapse. For the same reason, the *time of day* that an arrest occurs is not thought to be important except for the fact that arrests occurring during early morning hours are more likely to go a longer period of time until discovery (Gulati et al., 1983; Scaff et al., 1984). Were there some way to monitor a greater number of patients (or better predict who was going to have an arrest), survival from resuscitation during early morning hours on general wards would doubtlessly improve.

An important factor in predicting outcome from in-hospital cardiac arrest is *duration* of the code. Among 241 patients in the study by Bedell (1983) for whom cardiac arrest lasted longer than 15 minutes, 95% died. No one survived when the arrest lasted longer than 30 minutes. In contrast, 56% of patients survived to leave the hospital when resuscitation took less than 15 minutes.

Equally poor statistics have been seen by others for survival after prolonged resuscitation (Scaff et al., 1984). Although some patients are brought back initially, ultimate survival is extremely rare. Thus, it may be reasonable for the emergency care provider to consider terminating resuscitation efforts in *adults* as code duration approaches 30 minutes, especially if there have been no signs that a patient is responding. (A notable exception to this generality is the arrested patient who is *hypothermic,* for whom a code should never be called until adequate core rewarming has been achieved.)

The likelihood of survival for patients who arrest more than once during a given hospital stay is extremely small (Debard, 1981; Scaff et al., 1984). Careful thought must be given to whether a patient should be recoded a second or third time if an initial resuscitation is unsuccessful.

Surprisingly, *age* has absolutely no effect on survival from in-hospital cardiac arrest (Bedell et al., 1983; Gulati et al., 1983; Scaff et al., 1984). Although one commonly perceives "quality" of life to be less for older individuals, this is not necessarily the case. Even though other underlying disease processes are usually present, survival rates after resuscitation are equally as good for the elderly as they are for younger patients. Thus, *age* per se should *not* be a determining factor in deciding who should be resuscitated.

Finally, with respect to personnel directing the code, whether housestaff or attending physicians are in charge is not nearly as important as whether emergency care providers are trained in ACLS (Scaff et al., 1984). In a study by Lowenstein et al. (1986), survival from in-hospital cardiac arrest nearly doubled following such training.

Precipitating Mechanisms of In-Hospital Cardiac Arrest

As is the case for out-of-hospital events, ventricular fibrillation is thought to be an extremely common precipitating mechanism of in-hospital cardiac arrest. This is especially true for patients seen during the first few hours of acute myocardial infarction when ventricular fibrillation is most likely to arise. As alluded to earlier, in noninfarcting patients, ventricular tachycardia probably precedes many *(if not most)* episodes of ventricular fibrillation. The importance of acute care monitoring is that potentially lethal arrhythmias such as ventricular tachycardia may be detected *before* deterioration to ventricular fibrillation occurs.

Next to ventricular tachycardia/fibrillation, *primary respiratory arrest* may be the most common precipitating mechanism of in-hospital cardiac arrest (Debard, 1981; Bedell et al., 1983). This is important because discovery of the patient at the time of respiratory arrest *before cardiac arrest has occurred* is an easily treatable problem in a hospital setting. Management of the airway by rescue breathing, ventilation with airway adjuncts, and/or intubation is usually all that is needed. In contrast, by the time the EMS unit arrives on the scene of a respiratory arrest that occurred outside the hospital, the rhythm has usually deteriorated to ventricular fibrillation or asystole.

Special mention should be made of *asystole* as a mechanism of in-hospital cardiac arrest. While prognosis for asystole is never good, the outlook for the patient may not be quite as bleak when asystole is seen in a hospital setting as when it occurs on the outside. Again, this may be due to the shorter time until discovery of the arrest. In addition, the pathogenesis of asystole may differ for the two conditions. Asystole occurring on the outside is most often a preterminal event that develops following prolonged cardiopulmonary arrest and deterioration from ventricular fibrillation. Structural damage is frequently present, which renders the myocardium unresponsive to therapy (Coon et al., 1981; Niemann et al., 1985). In contrast, asystole occurring with in-hospital cardiac arrest may sometimes result from massive parasympathetic discharge. As such, it is less likely to be asociated with irreversible structural damage and may on occasion respond to atropine (Coon et al., 1981).

PRE- AND POST-ARREST VARIABLES PREDICTIVE OF PROGNOSIS

Five *pre-arrest* variables have been found to be predictive of prognosis from in-hospital cardiac arrest (Bedell et al., 1983). These include:

   i) Pneumonia
   ii) Hypotension (systolic blood pressure of less than 100 mm Hg for at least 1 day before the arrest)
   iii) Renal failure

   iv) Cancer (excluding skin cancer)
   v) Homebound life-style *before* hospitalization

In Bedell's study of 294 patients who suffered in-hospital cardiac arrest, long-term survival after the arrest was *only* 5% if any of the above five factors were present beforehand. In contrast, long-term survival was 66% when none of these factors were present prior to the arrest.

While it may not be surprising that patients with hypotension, renal failure, and cancer fare poorly following cardiac arrest, the finding that none of the 58 patients who had pneumonia before the arrest survived was indeed unexpected. It is also insightful to learn that preadmission ambulatory status is a predictive factor of survival.

Important prognostic information regarding the likelihood of ultimate survival from in-hospital cardiac arrest is also provided by the patient's clinical condition on the day following the arrest. Patients who are alert and off pressor agents by 24 hours after CPR is performed have a greater than 90% chance of living to be discharged from the hospital. In contrast, long-term survival is less than 20% for patients who are still comatose or on pressor drugs the day after. Only 1 of the 52 patients in Bedell's study who were still in coma at this time lived to leave the hospital, and that patient remained lethargic until succumbing 2 months later.

Patient Recollection of the Arrest

Most survivors of cardiac arrest do not recall anything of the event itself. A few in Bedell's study remembered receiving a "hard bang on the chest." All had a sore chest the next day. Some recalled the "look of terror in the eyes of the doctors and nurses" who worked to revive them. Only one described a "near-death" experience. For him the arrest "was peaceful, beautiful, and accompanied by angels over my head. It would have been an easy death."

HOW WELL ARE THE SURVIVORS?

A prevalent fear among hospitalized patients is that they will be successfully resuscitated only to lead a long-lingering life in a vegetative state. Although this may occur, it appears to be the exception rather than the rule. Thirty-eight of the 41 patients in Bedell's study who survived to leave the hospital had an intact mental status at the time of discharge. Two of the survivors were demented but had been so before the arrest. Only one survivor developed a grossly impaired mental status as a direct result of the arrest. Thus by and large, most persons who survive in-hospital cardiac arrest are mentally intact. Those who become comatose or mentally impaired following resuscitation usually die within the next few days, and few live to leave the hospital.

Psychologically, most of the survivors in Bedell's study were depressed at the time of discharge. Yet within 6 months, this depression had almost uniformly lifted. Physically, all of the survivors reported a decrease in functional capacity. For some this simply meant that although they could still pursue the same activities as before their arrest, they had to do them slower. However, of the 38 mentally intact survivors, 5 of 9 who were previously employed retired, 10 became newly homebound, and 5 required new institutionalization. In many cases the investigators felt the degree of impairment to be out of proportion to the extent of organic disease. More than half of the survivors seemed to limit their physical activities because of fear. The message is clear. Survivors of cardiopulmonary resuscitation need continued encouragement and support from health care providers in order to maximize functional recovery.

DECIDING ABOUT DNR STATUS

A final take-home message from Bedell's study comes from the survey she conducted on the 38 mentally competent survivors. These individuals were asked if they would want to be resuscitated again in the event of a second cardiac arrest. Initially 21 of the 38 patients answered affirmatively, 16 preferred to be made DNR (*Do Not Resuscitate*), and 1 patient was ambivalent. Six months later, over 90% of these patients held firm to their initial request. This suggests

that competent patients have often thought about cardiopulmonary resuscitation and that many (if not most) of these individuals have definite feelings about what they would like to be done should they arrest.

Unfortunately, all too often the patient is *not* involved in such decisions. In a follow-up study by Bedell et al. (1986), discussion with the patient regarding resuscitation status was undertaken *before* DNR orders were written in only 22% of 389 cases. A major reason given for this was that 76% of the patients in Bedell's study were mentally incompetent and therefore unable to participate in the decision-making process at the time DNR status was determined. However, when one considers that an average of 7 days passed before resuscitation status was addressed and that the overwhelming majority of patients (89%) were mentally competent at the time of admission, the need for health care providers to routinely inquire about a patient's wishes for resuscitation *early* in the hospitalization is evident.

(More detailed discussion on deciding about DNR status is presented in Chapter 18 on Medicolegal Aspects.)

REFERENCES

Akhtar M: Management of ventricular tachyarrhythmias (I and II). JAMA 247:671–674, 1982.

Bachman JW, McDonald GS, O'Brien PC: A study of out-of-hospital cardiac arrests in Northeastern Minnesota. JAMA 256:477–483, 1986.

Bedell SE, Delbanco TL, Cook EF, Epstein FH: Survival after cardiopulmonary resuscitation in the hospital. N Engl J Med 309:569–576, 1983.

Bedell SE, Pelle D, Maher PL, Cleary PD: Do-not-resuscitate orders for critically ill patients in the hospital: How are they used and what is their impact? JAMA 256:233–237, 1986.

Bigger JT: Antiarrhythmic treatment: An overview. Am J Cardiol 53:8B–16B, 1984.

Bigger JT, Coromilas J: Identification of patients at risk for arrhythmic death: Role of Holter ECG recording. In Josephson ME (Ed): Sudden Cardiac Death, Cardiovascular Clinics. FA Davis, Philadelphia, Vol 15, No. 3, 1983, pp 131–143.

Buxton FE: Sudden cardiac death—1986 (editorial). Ann Intern Med 104:716–718, 1986.

Cobb LA, Werner JA: Predictors and prevention of sudden cardiac death. In Hurst JW (Ed): The Heart. McGraw-Hill, New York, 1982, pp 599–610.

Cobb LA, Werner JA, Trobaugh GB: Sudden cardiac death. Mod Conc Cardiovasc Dis 49:31–36, 1980.

Coon GA, Clinton JE, Ruiz E: Use of atropine for brady-asystolic prehospital cardiac arrest. Ann Emerg Med 10:462–467, 1981.

Cox JL: The status of surgery for cardiac arrhythmias. Circulation 71:413–417, 1985.

Cummins RO, Eisenberg MS: Prehospital cardiopulmonary resuscitation: Is it effective? JAMA 253:2408–2412, 1985.

Cummins RO, Eisenberg MS, Bergner L, Hallstrom A, Hearne T, Murray JA: Automatic external defibrillation: Evaluations of its role in the home and in emergency medical services. Ann Emerg Med 13:798–801, 1984.

Cummins RO, Eisenberg MS, Graves JR, Hearne TR, Litwin PE, Hallstrom AP, Pierce J: Automatic external defibrillators used by emergency medical technicians: A controlled clinical trial (abstract). Crit Care Med 13:945–946, 1985.

Cummins RO, Eisenberg MS, Litwin PE, Hallstrom AP: Survival benefit of prehospital cardiopulmonary resuscitation for cardiac arrest (abstract). Crit Care Med 13:944–945, 1985.

Cummins RO, Eisenberg MS, Moore JE, Hearne TR, Andresen E, Wendt R, Litwin PE, Graves JR, Hallstrom AP, Pierce J: Automatic external defibrillators: Clinical, training, psychological, and public health issues. Ann Emerg Med 14:755–760, 1985.

Debard ML: Cardiopulmonary resuscitation: Analysis of six years experience and review of the literature. Ann Emerg Med 10:408–416, 1981.

Echt DS, Armstrong K, Schmidt P, Oyer PE, Stinson EB, Winkle RA: Clinical experience, complications, and survival in 70 patients with the automatic implantable cardioverter/defibrillator. Circulation 71:289–296, 1985.

Eisenberg MS, Bergner L, Hallstrom A: Out-of-hospital cardiac arrest: Improved survival with paramedic services. Lancet 1:812–815, 1980.

Eisenberg MS, Copass MK, Hallstrom AP, Blake B, Bergner L, Short FA, Cobb LA: Treatment of out-of-hospital cardiac arrest with rapid defibrillation by emergency medical technicians. N Engl J Med 302:1379–1393, 1980.

Eisenberg MS, Cummins RO, Hallstrom AP, Hearne T: Defibrillation by emergency medical technicians. Crit Care Med 13:921–922, 1985.

Eisenberg MS, Cummins RO, Moore J, Hallstrom AP, Hearne T, Litwin P: Use of automatic external defibrillators in the home (abstract). Crit Care Med 13:946–947, 1985.

Eisenberg M, Hallstrom A, Bergner L: The ACLS Score—Predicting survival from out-of-hospital cardiac arrest. JAMA 246:50–52, 1981.

Enns J, Tween WA, Donen N: Prehospital cardiac rhythm deterioration in a system providing only basic life support. Ann Emerg Med 12:478–481, 1983.

Grauer K: Sudden cardiac death. Cont Ed 17:82–86, 1983.

Grauer K, Gums J: Pitfalls in the evaluation and management of ventricular arrhythmias. JABFP (in press)

Gulati RS, Bhan GL, Horan MA: Cardiopulmonary resuscitation of old people. Lancet 2:267–269, 1983.

Hershey CO, Fisher L: Why outcome of cardiopulmonary resuscitation in general wards is poor. Lancet 1:31–34, 1982.

Horowitz LN, Josephson ME, Kastor JA: Intracardiac electrophysiologic studies as a method for the optimization of drug therapy in chronic ventricular arrhythmia. Prog Cardiovasc Dis 23:81–98, 1980.

Josephson ME, Horowitz LN, Spielman SR, Greenspan AM: Electrophysiologic and hemodynamic studies in patients resuscitated from cardiac arrest. Am J Cardiol 46:948–955, 1980.

Kannel WB, Doyle JT, McNamara PM, Quickenton P, Gordon T: Precursors of sudden coronary death: Factors related to incidence of sudden death. Circulation 51:606–613, 1975.

Kempf FC, Josephson ME: Cardiac arrest recorded on ambulatory electrocardiograms. Am J Cardiol 53:1577–1582, 1984.

Lawrie GM, Wyndham CRC, Krafcheck J, Luck JC, Roberts R, DeBakey ME: Progress in the surgical treatment of cardiac arrhythmias: Initial experience of 90 patients. JAMA 254:1464–1468, 1985.

Lowenstein SR, Sabyan EM, Lassen CF, Kern DC: Benefits of training physicians in advanced cardiac life support. Chest 89:512–516, 1986.

Michael JR, Guerci AD, Koehler RC, Shi AY, Tsitlik J, Chandra N, Niedermeyer E, Rogers MC, Traystman RJ, Weisfeldt ML: Mechanisms by which epinephrine augments cerebral and myocardial perfusion during cardiopulmonary resuscitation in dogs. Circulation 69:822–835, 1984.

Milner PG, Platia EY, Reid PR, Griffith LSC: Ambulatory electrocardiographic recordings at the time of fatal cardiac arrest. Am J Cardiol 56:588–592, 1985.

Mirowski M: The automatic implantable cardioverter-defibrillator: An overview. J Am Coll Cardiol 6:461–466, 1985.

Mirowski M, Reid PR, Winkle RA, Mower MM, Watkins L, Stinson EB, Griffith LSC, Kallman CH, Weisfeldt ML: Mortality in patients with implanted automatic defibrillators. Ann Med Intern 98:585–588, 1983.

Myerburg RJ, Kessler KM, Zaman L, Conde CA, Castellanos A: Survivors of prehospital cardiac arrest. JAMA 247:1485–1490, 1982.

Nagel EL, Liberthson RR, Hirshman JC, Nussenfeld SR: Emergency care. In Prineas JR, Blackburn H (Eds): Sudden Coronary Death Outside Hospital. Circulation 52 (suppl 3):216–218, 1975.

Niemann JT, Adomien GE, Garner D, Rosborough JP: Endocardial and transcutaneous cardiac pacing, calcium chloride, and epinephrine in postcountershock asystole and bradycardias. Crit Care Med 13:599–604, 1985.

Ornato JP, McNeill SE, Craren EJ, Nelson NM: Limitation on effectiveness of rapid defibrillation by emergency medical technicians in a rural setting. Ann Emerg Med 13:1097–1099, 1984.

Pratt CM, Francis MJ, Luck JC, Wyndham CR, Miller RR, Quinones MA: Analysis of ambulatory electrocardiograms in 15 patients during spontaneous ventricular fibrillation with special reference to preceding arrhythmic events. J Am Coll Cardiol 2:789–797, 1983.

Ruskin JN, McGovern B, Garan H, DiMarco JP, Kelly E: Antiarrhythmic drugs: A possible cause of out-of-hospital cardiac arrest. N Engl J Med 308:1302–1306, 1983.

Sanders AB, Meislin HW, Ewy GA: The physiology of cardiopulmonary resuscitation: An update. JAMA 252:3283–3286, 1984.

Scaff B, Munson R, Hastings DF: Cardiopulmonary resuscitation at a community hospital with a family practice residency. J Fam Pract 18:561–565, 1984.

Skale BT, Miles WM, Hegar JJ, Zipes DP, Prystowsky EN: Survivors of cardiac arrest: Prevention of recurrence by drug therapy as predicted by electrophysiologic testing or electrocardiographic monitoring. Am J Cardiol 57:113–119, 1986.

Stueven H, Troiano P, Thompson B, Mateer JR, Kastenson EH, Tonsfeldt D, Hargarten K, Kowalski R, Aprahamian C, Darin J: Bystander/first responder CPR: Ten years experience in a paramedic system. Ann Emerg Med 15:707–710, 1986.

Stults KR, Brown DD, Schug VL, Bean JA: Prehospital defibrillation performed by emergency medical technicians in rural communities. N Engl J Med 310:219–223, 1984.

Swerdlow CD, Winkle RA, Mason JW: Determinants of survival in patients with ventricular tachyarrhythmias. N Engl J Med 308:1436–1442, 1983.

Weaver WD, Copass MK, Bufi D, Ray R, Hallstrom AP, Cobb LA: Improved neurologic recovery and survival after early defibrillation. Circulation 69:943–948, 1984.

Wetstein L, Engel TR, Kowey PR, Kelliher GJ: Surgical management and mapping of cardiac arrhythmias. In Dreifus LS (Ed): Cardiac Arrhythmias: Electrophysiologic Techniques and Management. FA Davis, Philadelphia, Vol 16, No. 1, 1985, pp 151–166.

Witte KL: Variables present in patients who are either resuscitated or not resuscitated in a medical intensive care unit. Heart Lung 13:159–163, 1984.

CHAPTER 12

ACUTE MYOCARDIAL INFARCTION

Acute myocardial infarction (AMI) occurs in well over a half million Americans each year. Although many patients have an uneventful hospital course and are discharged within 7–14 days, the ever-present threat of complications during the early phase of AMI demands constant vigilance and a readiness to intervene at any moment. Our purpose in this chapter is to discuss the role of the emergency care provider in the evaluation and management of these patients.

Until the past decade, the etiology of AMI was unclear. This was because autopsy studies performed the day after the event frequently failed to reveal acute thrombosis at the site of infarction. Cardiac catheterization during AMI was unheard of at the time due to the fear of precipitating a potentially lethal complication. In contrast, coronary angiography in the acute setting is performed almost routinely today in many centers and is a prerequisite procedure when considering most forms of reperfusion therapy. As a result, we have learned that sudden thrombotic occlusion of a major coronary artery is in fact the primary cause of AMI in the overwhelming majority of cases (DeWood et al., 1980).

Catheterization within the first 4 hours of infarction virtually always reveals total or near-total (>95%) occlusion. The reason previous investigators failed to detect this is that spontaneous lysis of clot begins almost immediately. By 12–24 hours following an infarct, total occlusion is present in only 65% of cases. Unfortunately, the process of myocardial necrosis is too well underway by this time for spontaneous lysis to have an appreciable effect on prognosis. However, improved understanding of the pathophysiology of acute infarction has provided the impetus for reperfusion therapy. Restoration of the coronary circulation within the first few hours of the acute insult may salvage myocardium that has not yet become irreversibly damaged. Results to date have been promising, but much work remains to determine which subsets of patients are most likely to benefit and what the time course for embarking on such interventions should be.

PROGNOSTIC DETERMINANTS OF AMI

Practically speaking, the two most important factors influencing acute and long-term prognosis of patients with myocardial infarction are the presence and severity of ventricular arrhythmias and the amount of myocardium damaged by the acute event. Arrhythmias are most important early in the course, with the incidence of *primary* ventricular fibrillation being several times greater during the first 2 hours of the infarction than during the rest of the hospital stay (Hancock, 1986). Yet even today, many individuals fail to seek emergency care as promptly as they should, and delays of several hours ("to see if the chest pain goes away") are all too common. As a result, primary ventricular fibrillation *prior* to the patient's arrival in the hospital remains the most common cause of death from AMI.

Once in the hospital, intensive care monitoring and antiarrhythmic therapy have largely eliminated mortality from ventricular arrhythmias. Extent of the infarct now assumes the most important role in determining survival. Simply stated, the greater the amount of myocardium affected, the less likely it is that adequate hemodynamic function can be maintained.

As the amount of myocardium involved approaches 35–40%, the chance of developing pump failure becomes substantial. Unfortunately, despite advances in virtually all other aspects of management, treatment of cardiogenic shock (once the full-blown syndrome has set in) remains unsatisfactory. Ventricular fibrillation may develop in these individuals, but in this setting the arrhythmia is the result of extensive myocardial damage (*secondary* ventricular fibrillation) rather than a primary event from electrical instability of the infarct itself. This secondary ventricular fibrillation (associated with cardiogenic shock) is rarely amenable to pharmacologic therapy.

In order to reduce mortality from AMI once the patient has reached the hospital, efforts must therefore be directed at limiting infarct size. Although standard measures such as pain control and adequate oxygenation are of some help in attaining this goal, reperfusion therapy (with streptokinase, angioplasty, or bypass surgery) offers the greatest potential for lessening the chance of developing pump failure. Patients who stand to benefit most from this form of treatment are those with anterior infarctions (since these infarctions tend to be larger) and those with a history of previous events (as the amount of myocardial damage needed to produce pump failure is cumulative).

Following recovery from AMI, the occurrence of ventricular arrhythmias and the amount of residual myocardial damage again become the principal factors determining mortality over the ensuing year. Interestingly, development of ventricular fibrillation during the early hours of AMI does not seem to affect long-term survival, and patients who have an otherwise uncomplicated course demonstrate an equally good prognosis as those with uncomplicated AMI who never had ventricular fibrillation (Stannard and Sloman, 1969; Bigger and Coromilas, 1983). It is only when ventricular arrhythmias persist into the late infarction period (beyond the first 3–5 days) that long-term survival is adversely affected (Bigger et al., 1982; Bigger and Coromilas, 1983). As a result, routine Holter monitoring is advocated by many prior to discharge after AMI (Bigger et al., 1982; Bigger, 1984), and an-

tiarrhythmic treatment is recommended if frequent and complex ventricular ectopy is found.

PITFALLS IN DIAGNOSIS OF AMI

Because of the high risk of potentially lethal ventricular arrhythmias during the early hours of infarction, accurate diagnosis with appropriate observation and treatment in a protective environment is the essential first step toward minimizing mortality. Several points merit special mention to the emergency care provider entrusted with making the diagnosis:

i) Presenting symptoms of AMI may be atypical or totally absent.
ii) The initial ECG may be entirely normal.
iii) Despite these drawbacks, history, physical examination, and the initial ECG remain *the* most important evaluative parameters in making the decision of whether to admit the patient with acute chest pain to the hospital.

Atypical (or Absent) Presenting Symptoms

There is little question that the previously healthy middle-aged individual with cardiac risk factors who complains of the sudden onset of severe substernal chest pain radiating up the neck and down the left arm needs immediate admission to the coronary care unit. All too often, however, the history is much less typical. Patients with inferior (diaphragmatic) infarction may present with only epigastric discomfort or signs of gastrointestinal upset. Not infrequently, these symptoms are partially or even totally relieved by belching or a "GI cocktail." In other instances, a purely referred pattern of pain may be noted. Thus the patient may describe pain down the left arm, in either shoulder blade, or in the neck and/or jaw without the slightest indication of chest discomfort. At least 20% of the time, AMI is entirely "silent" or at most accompanied by vague symptoms such as malaise or myalgias (Margolis et al., 1973; van der Does et al., 1980, Zarling et al., 1983). The absence of symptoms is particularly likely to occur in patients with diabetes mellitus (due to decreased pain sensation from neuropathy) and the elderly. In the latter group, a change in mental status (confusion, disorientation), an arrhythmia, dizziness, syncope, stroke, dyspnea, or the insidious development of congestive heart failure may be the only clue to AMI.

Drawbacks of the Initial ECG

It is important to appreciate that the initial ECG of a patient with AMI may fail to reveal findings suggestive of the diagnosis. There are several reasons for this (Grauer and Curry, 1986):

i) A lag time of hours (or even days) may exist before diagnostic electrocardiographic changes become evident.

ii) Changes may be subtle (nonspecific ST-T wave abnormalities, loss of R wave amplitude, development of "insignificant" q waves).

iii) The ECG may be one of *transition* (obtained at a time when ST segments have returned to the baseline just after the period of ST segment elevation and just before the period of T wave inversion).

iv) ECG changes of AMI may be obscured by a *competitive* condition (bundle branch block, left or right ventricular hypertrophy, pulmonary disease pattern, early repolarization, electrolyte disorders, Wolff-Parkinson-White syndrome) or by previous infarction.

v) A previous ECG may not be available for comparison.

vi) The infarction may be taking place in an "electrically silent" area of the heart (the apex, right ventricle, or posterobasal portion of the left ventricle)

The initial ECG is most helpful in diagnosis when it is clearly abnormal. The absence of diagnostic changes, however, in no way rules out the possibility of acute infarction. In such instances, history becomes the pivotal factor in deciding whether a patient should be admitted to a protective environment. Considering the potential for life-threatening arrhythmias during the early hours of infarction, it is usually wiser to err on the side of caution (admission to the hospital) if doubt remains.

It is of interest that the finding of an *unremarkable* initial ECG (either a normal tracing, one with only minor nonspecific ST-T wave abnormalities, or one without significant change from previous tracings) at the time of admission in patients with AMI is a strong predictor of a relatively benign hospital course (Brush et al., 1985; Lee et al., 1985). In contrast, the presence of acute ST segment changes (either ST segment elevation or depression), diagnostic Q waves, or an intraventricular conduction defect on the initial ECG is associated with a fairly high incidence of complications. Other factors predictive of a high-risk hospital course include ongoing chest pain at the time of admission, pulmonary rales, persistent sinus tachycardia, and/or PVCs on the initial 12-lead ECG (Fuchs and Scheidt, 1981; Crimm et al., 1984). Surveillance in a coronary care unit is usually preferable for individuals with any of these findings. In their absence and when the initial ECG is unremarkable, observation in a step-down (telemetry) unit is a reasonable course of action for those patients in whom the history dictates the need for hospital admission.

The Role of Cardiac Enzymes

The occurrence of AMI is characteristically accompanied by elevations in serum concentrations of cardiac enzymes. In general, the larger the infarct, the greater the rise in cardiac enzymes. The earliest change is usually noted with CK* (creatine kinase), which begins to rise within 3–6 hours of the onset of AMI, peaks at 10–18 hours, and returns to normal by 3–4 days. AST† (aspartate aminotransferase) increases by 8–12 hours, peaks in 18–36 hours, and returns to normal by 3–4 days. LD‡ (lactic dehydrogenase) is the last enzyme to rise. It usually increases by 24–48 hours, peaks in 3–6 days, and then gradually returns to normal over 8–14 days.

Unfortunately, CK elevations may be significantly delayed and not show any increase at the time of presentation. In addition, numerous other conditions may falsely elevate cardiac enzymes, including skeletal muscle injury from trauma or injection, primary liver disease, hepatic congestion from congestive heart failure, shock, seizures, myocarditis, pulmonary embolism, hypothyroidism, hemolysis, anemia, certain neoplasms, and electrical countershock. Differentiation of these conditions from AMI may usually be made reliably by obtaining cardiac isoenzyme studies. However, because such determinations generally require 1–2 days to be processed, they are of no assistance to the emergency care provider faced with making the "on-the-spot" decision of whether to admit the patient with chest pain to the hospital. Moreover, since the time course for elevation of cardiac isoenzymes is similar to that for the standard studies, falsely negative (normal) readings may be obtained if blood is sampled too early.

Our feeling is that standard cardiac enzyme studies (CK, AST, and LD) should play no role in making the decision of whether to admit the patient with chest pain to the hospital. Normal studies provide a false sense of security (since they in no way rule out infarction), while abnormal studies may be due to any of the causes in the above list. History, physical examination, and the initial ECG should be the principal parameters assessed in the emergency department

(Seager, 1980; Lee et al., 1985; Nowakowski, 1986). If these do not confidently exclude the possibility of an acute ischemic event (AMI, unstable angina), the patient should be admitted to the hospital (at least to a telemetry unit). It is at this point that cardiac enzymes (and isoenzymes) become invaluable in confirming AMI and in providing a rough estimation of infarct size.

Many of the topics covered in the rest of this chapter are discussed in detail elsewhere in the book. Consequently, we will limit our comments here and refer the reader to those sections where more material may be found.

CONVENTIONAL THERAPY

Treatment of AMI may be divided into standard measures that are generally accepted by all in the field (*conventional* therapy) and *innovative* therapy that is practiced by many but remains controversial.

OXYGEN THERAPY

Provision of supplemental oxygen by nasal cannula (at 2–4 L/min) is routinely recommended for patients suspected of AMI. While such treatment may have little effect on the arterial oxygen content of otherwise normal individuals, it significantly improves oxygenation of an ischemic myocardium in the patient with hypoxemia from pulmonary congestion.

PAIN RELIEF

A strong effort should be made to relieve the chest pain of acute ischemic heart disease. Failure to do so may result in tachycardia and further release of endogenous catecholamines. This in turn increases cardiac work and oxygen demand on an already ischemic myocardium. A faster heart rate causes the diastolic interval to shorten, compromising blood flow even more.

---

*CK was formerly designated CPK (creatine phosphokinase).
†AST was formerly designated SGOT (serum glutamic oxaloacetic transaminase).
‡LD was formerly designated LDH.

All these effects may be aggravated when chest pain is accompanied by a significant anxiety component.

Morphine sulfate is a potent analgesic agent that also allays anxiety and exerts beneficial hemodynamic effects in the patient with pulmonary congestion. By increasing venous capacitance and inducing mild arterial vasodilatation, the drug reduces both preload and afterload and thus improves cardiac performance.

Morphine should be administered in 2- to 5-mg IV increments every 5–30 minutes according to the patient's symptoms and clinical response. Although excessive use of the drug may result in bradycardia, hypotension, oversedation, nausea or respiratory depression, these undesirable effects can usually be avoided by cautious dosing. Respiratory depression can be reversed with 0.4 mg of naloxone (Narcan), while vagotonic actions are easily treated in most instances by placing the patient in Trendelenburg position, fluid infusion and/or 0.5–1.0 mg of IV atropine sulfate. (See Chapter 2.)

Nitroglycerin has resurfaced as an agent of choice for relief of the chest pain associated with AMI. While its predominant action is to increase venous capacitance (decrease preload), nitroglycerin also reduces afterload by arteriolar vasodilatation and improves coronary artery blood flow by a direct effect on these vessels. The drug can be administered in a number of ways, with the sublingual form usually being tried first (often by the patient) at the onset of symptoms. Although topical administration may be reasonable for treating patients who are only mildly symptomatic, persistence of severe chest pain beyond several minutes is an indication for initiating an IV infusion of the drug. This allows moment-to-moment titration and provides the best opportunity for pain relief and hemodynamic control. In general, the drug is safely given in the setting of AMI to patients who are normovolemic and closely monitored. (See Chapter 14.)

Finally, oral *diazepam* (Valium) or other anxiolytic agents should be considered as an adjunct to morphine when a marked anxiety component complicates the chest pain of AMI.

USE OF HEPARIN

The question of whether to routinely anticoagulate patients with AMI has long been the subject of controversy. Despite numerous trials, the data in favor of full anticoagulation remain inconclusive (Genton and Turpie, 1983). As a result, most authorities still reserve IV heparinization for specific indications such as prolonged immobilization, documented deep venous thrombosis, pulmonary embolism, mural thrombi, or as an adjunct to thrombolytic therapy (Hancock, 1986).

In contrast, many centers routinely employ low-dose subcutaneous heparin (5000 Units 2–3 times daily) to lower the incidence of deep venous thrombosis. Even though early mobilization is the most important factor in reducing this complication (Wray et al., 1973), subcutaneous heparin is both relatively benign and effective.

Mural thrombi occur more frequently than is generally appreciated. Autopsy data in patients with AMI suggest an incidence of between 20% and 60% (Genton and Turpie, 1983), with this complication being most common among individuals who had large anterior infarcts, ventricular hypertrophy, congestive heart failure, or ventricular aneurysm. It is only rarely associated with inferior infarction. While sensitivity of two-dimensional echocardiography for detecting mural thrombi is poor, the test is noninvasive, easily performed at the bedside, and of surprisingly good specificity. Patients who develop mural thrombi during the course of AMI face a particularly high risk of systemic embolization and should be fully anticoagulated with IV heparin and maintained on warfarin (Coumadin) for at least 6 months after the infarct (Weinreich et al., 1984; Ezekowitz, 1985; Spirito et al., 1986).

USE OF LIDOCAINE

In the past, lidocaine had only been recommended for patients demonstrating "warning arrhythmias" (≥5 PVCs/minute, ≥2 PVCs in a row, multiform PVCs, or the R-on-T phenomenon). It is now generally accepted that ventricular fibrillation commonly occurs without such premonitory arrhythmias and sometimes even without preexisting PVCs. In addition, many episodes of ventricular ectopy (including ventricular tachycardia) go undetected in even the best intensive care units. Withholding lidocaine until ventricular arrhythmias are observed on the monitor may thus resut in a potentially lethal delay for a significant number of patients. We have thus come to recommend *prophylactic* use of lidocaine for patients with acute ischemic chest pain in the following circumstances:

i) For patients in whom a high index of suspicion for AMI exists.

ii) When patients are seen within the first 24 hours of the onset of symptoms (since the incidence of primary ventricular fibrillation declines markedly after this period).

iii) For patients under 70 years of age (since the risk of primary ventricular fibrillation is much less in the elderly, while the chance of developing lidocaine toxicity becomes much greater).

One should distinguish between *prophylactic* and *therapeutic* use of lidocaine. The former category includes patients with new onset chest pain suggestive of acute ischemic heart disease in whom cardiac monitoring reveals only rare ventricular ectopy without complex forms or no PVCs at all. The rationale for prophylactically treating such individuals is that 5–10% of subjects with AMI develop primary ventricular fibrillation, and prophylactic treatment decreases this incidence. In contrast, treatment of frequent and/or complex ventricular ectopy in the setting of acute ischemic chest pain is a *therapeutic* use of the drug, since the arrhythmia is already manifest. In general, more vigorous treatment is in order. However, it is important to emphasize that *not* all PVCs need be eliminated for lidocaine to be protective. Attempting to do so enhances the risk of toxicity without necessarily increasing the drug's therapeutic effect. (See Chapter 13 for a more complete discussion on the use of lidocaine.)

Should therapeutic use of lidocaine prove ineffective (if frequent and complex PVCs persist despite optimal dosing), *procainamide* is the sec-

ond drug of choice. Increments of 100 mg may be administered IV over a 5-minute period, until either the arrhythmia is controlled, a total loading dose of 1 g has been given, or untoward side effects appear (hypotension or widening of the QRS complex). This may be followed by a continuous procainamide infusion of 2–4 mg/min (1–2 mg/min in patients with renal impairment). Alternatively, procainamide loading may be accomplished by infusing 500–1000 mg over a 30- to 60-minute period. (See Chapter 14.)

Autonomic Nervous System Dysfunction with AMI

Autonomic nervous system overactivity occurs in a majority of patients during the early minutes and hours of AMI. Parasympathetic overactivity is most often associated with acute inferior infarction, while sympathetic overactivity generally occurs with acute anterior infarction.

PARASYMPATHETIC OVERACTIVITY: USE OF ATROPINE

Patients with acute inferior infarction frequently demonstrate sinus bradycardia and hypotension (*parasympathetic* overactivity). Atropine sulfate effectively counteracts such increases in vagal tone, accelerating the rate of sinus node discharge and improving atrioventricular conduction. However, indiscriminate use of the drug may result in inappropriate acceleration of the sinus rate, hypertension, and induction of ventricular arrhythmias (including ventricular tachycardia or fibrillation). This may be due in part to an "unmasking" effect—the parasympatholytic action of atropine now leaves underlying sympathetic overactivity unopposed. Use of atropine should, therefore, not be taken lightly in the setting of AMI; the drug is indicated for bradycardic individuals only when they manifest signs of hemodynamic compromise (hypotension, PVCs, or chest pain as a direct result of the slow heart rate).

Atropine appears to be most effective at reversing sinus bradycardia and hypotension that occur within the first 6 hours of infarction.

After that time, factors other than vagal over-activity more frequently come into play. Increments of 0.5 mg may be repeated every 5 minutes as needed, with a maximum total dose of 2–3 mg. One should use as low a dose as possible in order to minimize the chance of an untoward response.

SYMPATHETIC OVERACTIVITY: BETA-BLOCKER USE WITH AMI

Patients with acute anterior infarction frequently demonstrate sinus tachycardia and hypertension (*sympathetic* overactivity). In addition, sympathetic overactivity during the early minutes to hours of an infarct may account for the high incidence of primary ventricular fibrillation during this period and at least partially explain the beneficial response to IV administration of beta-blockers. Whether to routinely recommend IV beta-blocker therapy during the acute phase of myocardial infarction is another matter.

Data have conclusively shown that beta-blockers decrease mortality, the incidence of nonfatal reinfarction, and sudden cardiac death in the 1- to 2-year period *after* AMI (Norwegian Multicenter Study Group, 1981; BHAT Research Group, 1982; Yusuf et al., 1985). However, the mechanism that accounts for these favorable results is still open to question. The effect is probably *multifactorial* and due to a combination of sympathetic blockade, decreased myocardial workload and oxygen consumption, antiarrhythmic activity, improved collateral blood flow, and decreased platelet aggregation (Lichstein, 1985; Campbell et al., 1986).

Beta-blockers also appear to lower mortality when administered *acutely* during the course of AMI (Hjalmarson et al., 1981; Hjalmarson, 1984). In the prospective, double-blind, placebo-controlled Göteborg trial, 1395 patients presenting with suspected or definite AMI received either IV metoprolol (3 IV injections totalling 15 mg) or placebo as soon as possible after admission to the hospital. Less than 7% of the patients who were given the drug were unable to tolerate it (Hjalmarson, 1984). Oral therapy (100 mg of metoprolol b.i.d.) was started in the others. Mortality was decreased by 36%

(compared to placebo-treated patients) after 90 days and remained low when treatment was continued over the first year after the infarct. In addition, chest pain (and the need for analgesic drugs), ventricular arrhythmias, infarct size, and hospital stay were all decreased in those given IV metoprolol acutely compared to the placebo group.

Thus it appears that early administration of IV beta-blockers (preferably within the first 12 hours of the onset of symptoms) may exert a favorable effect on the course of AMI. However, even though the incidence of adverse reactions to the therapy was only slightly increased compared to the placebo group, acute administration of IV beta-blockers carries the potential risk of hypotension, bradyarrhythmias, and myocardial depression. As a result, caution is urged if this intervention is contemplated. Fortunately, the half-life of IV metoprolol is less than 10 minutes, so that even if adverse effects occur they are usually short-lived.

IV metoprolol should not be given to patients with bronchospasm, significant bradycardia, hypotension, or pulmonary edema. However, the drug may be safely used in most cases even when bibasilar rales are present if other evidence of congestive heart failure is absent, a systolic blood pressure of greater than 100 mm Hg is maintained, and heart rate remains over 60 beats per minute. Initial dosing with small increments of the drug (1–2 mg IV) may further help to minimize untoward reactions to IV beta-blocker therapy. If patient tolerance is good, 3–5 mg IV boluses may be repeated q. 5–10 min until the 15 mg IV loading dose has been administered. Oral dosing may then be started (50 mg to be given 15 minutes after the last injection, followed by 50 mg orally q. 6h for 2 days, and then 100 mg orally q. 12h for at least 3 months).

Conduction System Disturbances

Atrioventricular (AV) block is a frequent complication of AMI. Prognosis and management vary greatly, depending on the degree of block, the location of the infarct, the ventricular response, and the patient's clinical status.

AV BLOCK

AV block most commonly occurs with acute inferior infarction, since the right coronary artery characteristically supplies the AV node. Treatment is generally not necessary for 1° AV block or 2° AV block Mobitz type I (Wenckebach), since blood pressure and heart rate usually remain adequate. Even with 3° (complete) AV block from acute *inferior* infarction, insertion of a transvenous pacemaker is often unnecessary, because such blocks tend to be transient, respond to atropine when treatment is needed, and are usually associated with a reliable AV junctional escape mechanism. Close observation with bedside availability of atropine (and ideally access to an external pacemaker) may be all that is needed.

In contrast, AV block with acute *anterior* infarction carries a much poorer prognosis. Anatomically, this type of block occurs lower in the conduction system (at the level of the His-Purkinje fibers) and is usually of the Mobitz II variety. The QRS complex is typically wider, and the escape mechanism is slower and less reliable. As a result, patients with Mobitz II AV block are much more likely to develop complete AV block (or ventricular standstill) than are those with the Mobitz I variety (Scheinman and Gonzalez, 1980). Transvenous pacemaker insertion is mandatory. Atropine may be tried if needed in the interim but will usually not be effective, since the block almost always occurs below the bundle of His. Pressor infusion (with isoproterenol, dopamine, or epinephrine) and/or placement of an external pacemaker may provide temporizing treatment until transvenous pacemaker insertion is accomplished.

BUNDLE BRANCH BLOCK

Bundle branch block is encountered more frequently with acute *anterior* infarction than with inferior infarction. This is because blood supply to the septum and the bundle branches contained therein is provided mainly by the left anterior descending artery, the vessel occluded in anterior myocardial infarction. Bundle branch block is estimated to develop in 10–15% of patients during the course of hospitalization for AMI. At times it may be difficult to discern whether the block is new and the *result* of infarction or whether it was present beforehand. In any event, mortality is significantly increased in patients with bundle branch block and AMI.

Development of intraventricular conduction defects with AMI is thought to reflect extensive myocardial damage. Mortality most often results from power failure rather than from progression of the conduction disturbance to complete AV block. Consequently, prophylactic pacing will not usually increase survival, although on rare occasions it may benefit patients with bundle branch block and high-degree AV block in the absence of significant heart failure (Hindman et al., 1978).

Controversy still exists regarding the need for pacemaker insertion with unifascicular block and AMI. There is general agreement, however, that new onset of bifascicular block or of 2° or 3° AV block in association with bundle branch block is a definite indication for prophylactic pacing.

Invasive Hemodynamic Monitoring

INDICATIONS

Most patients with AMI have either normal hemodynamic indices or pulmonary congestion with only mild to moderate left ventricular failure. More than 90% of such patients survive, and invasive hemodynamic monitoring is not generally needed in these cases.

The mortality rate from AMI rises with increasing degrees of left ventricular failure. Unfortunately, differentiating patients with mild-to-moderate failure from those with severe failure is often difficult to do on clinical grounds alone. Bedside assessment underestimates the degree of hemodynamic compromise at least 15% of the time (Genton and Jaffe, 1986). It is in these patients in whom there is uncertainty

TABLE 12-1   INDICATIONS FOR INVASIVE HEMODYNAMIC MONITORING IN AMI

Persistent chest pain
Persistent tachycardia
Hypertension
Hypotension
Significant left ventricular failure
Suspicion of hemodynamically significant right ventricular infarction
Use of intravenous inotropic or vasodilator agents for the management of any of the above
Development of a new systolic murmur (differentiation of ventricular septal defect from mitral regurgitation)

about the degree of left ventricular failure, as well as those in whom significant failure is obvious, that hemodynamic monitoring assumes its greatest importance.

Other indications for invasive hemodynamic monitoring in AMI are indicated in **Table 12-1.** For example, a patient may manifest tachycardia from persistent chest pain and/or anxiety, hypovolemia due to inappropriate peripheral vasodilation, sympathetic overactivity, or frank congestive failure. Because of dramatically differing therapeutic implications, determining which of these factors is predominant may be essential to effective management. This may not be possible without invasive monitoring.

MANAGEMENT ACCORDING TO HEMODYNAMIC SUBSETS

The management goal in patients with AMI is to improve ventricular performance while minimizing myocardial oxygen demand. The four most useful parameters to follow in achieving this goal are heart rate, arterial blood pressure (afterload), left ventricular filling pressure (which reflects preload), and cardiac output. Ideally, left ventricular filling pressure should be maintained between 15 and 18 mm Hg. At this level, cardiac output is optimized by the Starling mechanism. Values above this filling pressure increase the degree of pulmonary congestion, while reductions below this level (5–10 mm Hg) may result in substantially decreased cardiac output.

Classifying patients into clinical subsets according to hemodynamic indices has practical clinical applications, both for prognosis and for therapeutic decisions. These subsets consist of:

i) Patients who are normotensive and have adequate peripheral perfusion.
ii) Patients who have pulmonary congestion.
iii) Patients who have systolic hypertension.
iv) Patients who have peripheral hypoperfusion but no pulmonary congestion.
v) Patients who have both pulmonary congestion and peripheral hypoperfusion.

In patients with uncomplicated infarction who are normotensive and have signs of adequate peripheral perfusion (warm skin, sufficient urine output, and clear sensorium), no treatment other than observation is required.

Patients with pulmonary congestion, as manifested by an elevated left ventricular filling pressure, require diuretic therapy. However, diuretic therapy can be hazardous, since a number of patients considered to have pulmonary congestion clinically (basilar rales) are found to have a normal or even a low filling pressure on Swan-Ganz catheterization. Indiscriminate use of furosemide in such patients may result in unnecessary (and potentially dangerous) volume depletion.

In patients with systolic hypertension, the addition of vasodilators such as intravenous nitroglycerin or nitroprusside improves cardiac output by lowering the preload and afterload. Although *nitroprusside* has a more balanced effect on arteriolar resistance and venous capacitance vessels and may be a more effective antihypertensive agent, intravenous *nitroglycerin* with its predominant effect on veins reduces preload, selectively dilates coronary arteries, and offers at least a theoretical advantage in being less likely to produce "coronary steal." It is probably the drug of choice in the setting of persistent ischemic pain. However, patients with marked hypertension (diastolic blood pressure ≥110 mm Hg) will often require nitroprusside for blood pressure reduction. (See Chapter 14.)

In patients who have peripheral hypoperfusion without pulmonary congestion, volume infusion is the cornerstone of therapy. Left ventricular filling pressure should be increased to 15–18 mm Hg in an attempt to maximize contractility and cardiac output by the Starling mechanism. Once intravascular volume is restored, hypotension and tachycardia usually resolve.

CARDIOGENIC SHOCK

The final clinical subset comprises patients who have "power failure," with manifestations of both pulmonary congestion and peripheral hypoperfusion. The extreme form (systolic blood pressure under 90 mm Hg, oliguria, and mental confusion) represents the syndrome of *cardiogenic shock*. Clinically differentiating these patients from those with isolated peripheral hypoperfusion may be difficult. Patients in both groups present with tachycardia, hypotension, and a shock-like appearance. Invasive hemodynamic monitoring reveals left ventricular filling pressures of over 20 mm Hg and a markedly decreased cardiac output in patients with power failure.

Therapy is aimed at correcting these hemodynamic derangements with diuretics (to decrease preload), vasodilators (to decrease preload and afterload), and positive inotropic agents such as dopamine or dobutamine (to improve cardiac output).

Failure of these conventional measures is an indication for mechanical circulatory assist devices (such as intraaortic balloon counterpulsation) and consideration of cardiac catheterization to define the problem. A number of patients with heart failure may be saved by prompt surgical revascularization and/or repair of mechanical complications of myocardial infarction, such as ventricular septal defect, acute mitral regurgitation from papillary muscle rupture, or left ventricular aneurysm. Despite all these therapeutic interventions, hospital mortality for patients with power failure still exceeds 60%.

Right Ventricular Infarction

Due to the absence of a reliable method for diagnosing right ventricular infarction, little attention was paid to this entity in the past. However, development of myocardial scintigraphy, the increased use of two-dimensional echocardiography in the acute care setting, and more frequent application of right-sided electrocardiographic monitoring leads have resulted in more widespread recognition of acute right ventricular infarction. When one considers how much treatment of AMI may vary depending on whether significant right ventricular infarction is present, the clinical importance of making this distinction becomes obvious.

Isolated right ventricular infarction is rare. However, because the right coronary artery supplies both the right ventricle and the inferior wall of the left ventricle in most individuals, up to 40% of inferior infarctions will also demonstrate some degree of right ventricular involvement (Nixon, 1982; Kulbertus et al., 1985). While in most cases both clinical findings and prognosis are determined by the degree of left ventricular involvement, right ventricular manifestations can predominate on occasion. In such instances, one would expect to see jugular venous distention with hepatic tenderness and/or enlargement (suggesting right ventricular failure) in the absence of pulmonary congestion (left ventricular failure). A Kussmaul sign (distention of the jugular veins during inspiration) may also be present.

Diuresis is an important component of the treatment of patients with AMI and congestive failure from predominant left ventricular involvement. In contrast, *volume expansion* (rather than diuretic therapy) is the initial treatment of choice for hemodynamically significant right ventricular infarction. The goal is to increase right ventricular contractility by the Frank-Starling principle (see Chapter 2). Decreasing preload (with diuretics) would be counterproductive. In addition to cautious volume expansion, many of these individuals also require inotropic and/or vasodilator agents (Nixon, 1982; Shah et al., 1985; Genton and Jaffe, 1986).

Diagnosis of acute right ventricular infarction should be suspected when suggestive clinical signs (as described above) occur in the setting of acute inferior infarction. Utilization of right-sided monitoring leads (especially a V_{4R} lead) may provide further supportive evidence. The finding of a Q wave and ST segment elevation in lead V_{4R} that exceeds the degree of ST segment elevation in leads V_1–V_3 is both a sensitive and highly specific clue to the diagnosis (Lopez-Sendon et al., 1985). Invasive hemodynamic monitoring is helpful both in confirming the diagnosis and in assisting with optimal management. (Typically, right atrial pressure and right ventricular end diastolic pressure are elevated to an equal or greater extent than pulmonary capillary wedge pressure.)

Subendocardial (Non–Q–Wave Infarction)

In the past, distinction was made between *transmural* and *subendocardial* myocardial infarction depending on whether or not Q waves developed on the ECG. Since more of the myocardial wall was thought to be involved in the former, one expected prognosis to be correspondingly poorer with this type of infarct. Neither of these tenets necessarily holds true. Transmural infarctions do *not* always produce Q waves, while subendocardial infarctions may occasionally do so (Madias et al., 1974). Moreover, *long-term* prognosis for these two entities appears to be quite similar. Although initial mortality for transmural infarction may be somewhat greater, subendocardial infarction is a more unstable entity associated with a higher incidence of postinfarction angina and a higher recurrence rate of infarction during the first few months following hospital discharge (Madias and Gorlin, 1977). A reason this may occur is that such infarctions are more often "incomplete" (associated with subtotal occlusion of the infarct-related vessel) and therefore at greater risk of extension in the ensuing days and months (DeWood et al., 1986). Recently diltiazem (90 mg q. 6h started 1–3 days after the onset of infarction) has been shown to be effective in preventing early reinfarction and severe angina in patients with subendocardial infarction (Gibson et al., 1986).

Despite persistence in the literature of the potentially misleading terms *transmural* and *subendocardial,* the anatomically more accurate designations "*Q–wave*" and "*non–Q–wave producing*" are therefore preferable for describing the type of infarction.

Unstable (Preinfarction) Angina

The syndrome of *unstable angina* can be divided into three clinical subsets:

i) Patients with new onset angina.
ii) Patients in whom a previously "stable" pattern of angina is now superceded by progressively increasing severity, duration, and/or frequency of attacks despite appropriate medical therapy.
iii) Patients with continued anginal pain following recovery from AMI.

Because a significant number of individuals with this syndrome go on to develop AMI (hence the term, *preinfarction* angina), prompt recognition and aggressive treatment are essential (Rahimtoola, 1985).

Differentiation of unstable angina from AMI may be extremely difficult (if not impossible) at the time of presentation, especially if the admission ECG is inconclusive. Precipitating mechanisms (progression of atherosclerosis, acute coronary thrombosis, coronary artery spasm, and platelet aggregation) and the extent of underlying disease are similar for both entities (Rackley et al., 1982; Epstein and Palmeri, 1984). For the most part, initial treatment is also similar: patients are closely observed in a protective environment, and efforts are directed at relieving acute ischemic chest pain.

Nitrates provide the first line of therapy. Most patients will already have taken one or more sublingual nitroglycerin tablets by the time they arrive at the hospital. If pain is not promptly relieved, there should be little hesitation about starting an IV infusion of the drug (to allow more rapid titration to an effective dose).

Whereas morphine sulfate is the usual next choice for treatment of chest pain associated with AMI, use of a beta-blocker and/or calcium channel blocker is generally preferred when the diagnosis is more likely to be unstable angina (Flaherty, 1984; Epstein and Palmeri, 1984). In addition, *aspirin* should be started, since this drug has been shown to significantly reduce mortality and the incidence of AMI when given (in the dose of 325 mg a day) to patients with unstable angina (Lewis et al., 1983; Lewis and the VA Cooperative Study Group, 1985).

In most cases, the above measures will be effective in relieving acute ischemic chest pain. In the event that they are not, strong consideration should be given to cardiac catheterization (to define the problem) and to more aggressive forms of therapy (intracoronary nitroglycerin, thrombolytic therapy, percutaneous transluminal coronary angioplasty, and/or emergency coronary artery bypass grafting).

INNOVATIVE THERAPY

THROMBOLYTIC THERAPY

The idea of using thrombolytic therapy in AMI as a means of salvaging myocardium not yet irreversibly damaged is an extremely attractive one. Since an occlusive thrombus is associated with AMI more than 90% of the time, reestablishment of myocardial perfusion would

seem to be the ideal way to limit infarct size. However, despite its introduction as long ago as 1959, the use of thrombolytic therapy in AMI did not really gain popularity until 20 years later. At first only intracoronary (IC) *streptokinase* was tried. later, IV administration of the drug and the less allergenic (but much more expensive) *urokinase* were added. Most recently, *tissue plasminogen activator (TPA)* has been introduced.

Prompt institution of thrombolytic therapy in AMI reestablishes coronary perfusion a majority of the time. Successful reperfusion rates in major centers are achieved in 70–90% of cases with IC streptokinase (Laffel and Braunwald, 1984; Kennedy et al., 1985; Campbell et al., 1986). Although in the past lower reperfusion rates had been obtained with IV administration of the drug, earlier use of IV streptokinase (within 3 hours of the onset of infarction) has recently shown promise of offering almost comparable success rates as IC administration (Ganz et al., 1984; Taylor et al., 1984; Anderson et al., 1984). Because coronary angiography is not a prerequisite to giving IV streptokinase, this form of thrombolytic therapy avoids the expense, risk, and 1- to 2-hour delay involved with performing angiography. Thrombolytic therapy with IV streptokinase is thus more amenable to widespread use in areas of the country where emergency catheterization facilities and/or personnel are not readily available. Unfortunately, IV streptokinase induces a systemic lytic state that increases the risk of bleeding complications.

In the near future, TPA will probably become the thrombolytic agent of choice. Because TPA is highly "clot selective," it is hoped that this agent will induce fibrinolysis at the thrombus site *without* creating a systemic lytic state. Preliminary results following IV administration of the drug have been favorable and demonstrate rapid onset of action (within minutes), comparable efficacy to IV and IC streptokinase, and fewer complications (Van de Werf et al., 1984; the TIMI Study Group, 1985; the Health and Public Policy Committee, 1985). Although work still needs to be done to assure the safety of this agent (Sherry, 1985), the day may not be far off when paramedics in the field are given standing orders to administer TPA to all suspected victims of AMI.

By far the most important factor in determining whether thrombolytic therapy will be successful is the duration of time from the onset of symptoms until initiation of treatment. Ideally this interval should be less than 4 hours (Laffel and Braunwald, 1984; Health and Public Policy Committee, 1985). Significant improvement in myocardial function becomes much less likely once more than 6 hours have elapsed. In any event, even if coronary reperfusion is established, the question still remains as to whether such reperfusion will actually salvage jeopardized myocardium and result in improved left ventricular function (Rentrop et al., 1984). Preliminary evidence suggests that it will; however, a conclusive answer is not yet forthcoming from the literature due to spontaneous changes in left ventricular function that occur immediately after AMI (making it difficult to demonstrate objective improvement with thrombolytic therapy) and significant delays initiating streptokinase in many of the earlier studies (Laffel and Braunwald, 1984).

Signs of Reperfusion

Clinical evidence of acute reperfusion is occasionally dramatic and may be signaled by the sudden disappearance of chest pain and ST segment elevation. *Reperfusion arrhythmias* are common and most often consist of accelerated idioventricular rhythm (due to increased automaticity from reperfused areas of myocardium) and frequent PVCs. Fortunately, ventricular tachycardia and ventricular fibrillation are rare. Cardiac isoenzymes may become markedly elevated as a result of "CK washout" from reperfused areas.

Angioplasty and Emergency Cardiac Surgery

It is important to appreciate that acute thrombolytic therapy does little to reverse the under-lying processes (progressive atherosclerosis, coronary artery spasm, and/or platelet aggregation) responsible for infarction. Even after successful reperfusion, the risk of a recurrent ischemic event (silent reocclusion of the vessel, recurrent angina, reinfarction, or sudden death) is great (Urban et al., 1984; Meyer et al., 1985). Systemic anticoagulation (with heparin and then warfarin) is recommended after the procedure and may reduce this risk. In general, however, thrombolytic therapy is probably best viewed as a *temporizing* measure to reestablish flow and stabilize the patient until a more definitive procedure such as angioplasty or bypass surgery can be performed.

Percutaneous transluminal angioplasty (PTCA) and emergency coronary bypass surgery represent two alternative methods for restoring reperfusion during the initial phase of AMI. Both have been shown to be safe when performed by operators skilled in the technique. Whether to proceed with one of these procedures instead of attempting thrombolytic therapy depends on a number of factors, including the time from onset of symptoms until arrival at the hospital, the time for mobilization of the cardiac catheterization laboratory and/or the operating room, availability of skilled personnel for performing a particular technique, and the individual preferences of the patient and personnel involved. Streptokinase is most successful if administered within the first few hours of the onset of symptoms. It is of questionable benefit if delayed by more than 6 hours. On the other hand, PTCA may improve left ventricular function even after a more prolonged ischemic interval. Many centers now perform this technique either as the primary procedure or in the 25–40% of cases when thrombolytic therapy fails (Reeder and Vlieststra, 1986). Other institutions reserve PTCA as the secondary (more definitive) procedure to be performed in the days to weeks following successful reperfusion with thrombolytic therapy. Considering that the natural history of streptokinase-treated vessels is unknown, the degree of residual stenosis after thrombolytic therapy may *spontaneously* diminish in the weeks following the procedure, and the early reocclusion rate after emergency PTCA is as high as 20%, it is difficult to formulate general guidelines for optimal utilization and coordination of thrombolytic therapy and PTCA.

Coronary bypass surgery has also been performed on an emergency basis in patients with AMI. The procedure may prove to be lifesaving in selected patients with cardiogenic shock from AMI who have not responded to conventional medical therapy (Gray et al., 1983). Although certain centers have routinely performed emergency revascularization for acute evolving myocardial infarction, bypass surgery is perhaps best reserved for patients who demonstrate significant left main coronary artery disease at the time of emergency catheterization, cases of unstable angina refractory to medical therapy, patients who have received thrombolytic therapy but are unable to continue systemic anticoagulation, and as a backup procedure when emergency PTCA fails.

PRACTICAL CONSIDERATIONS FOR THE EMERGENCY CARE PROVIDER

Innovative therapy for AMI is a rapidly changing field with much potential for reducing infarct size and preserving myocardial function. Keeping abreast of all of the intricacies involved is a near impossible task for the nonspecialist. We offer the following practical suggestions:

i) Consider the possibility of an acute intervention *early* when evaluating patients who present with acute ischemic chest pain. In potential cases, consult your cardiologist *as soon as possible* in the process to review the case and determine which intervention (if any) may be suitable for the patient.

Surprisingly, the major cause of delay in performing emergency angiography (in preparation for IC streptokinase or PTCA) is not trying to mobilize the catheterization team but rather convincing the patient that 1) he/she is suffering an acute myocardial infarction, 2) a technique which is investigational offers hope of reducing the extent of the infarct, and 3) the decision of whether or not

not to proceed with the technique must be made immediately.

ii) Although subject to local variation, the following parameters serve to define potential candidates for acute thrombolytic therapy:
   —recent onset chest pain (of less than 4 hours, duration)
   —definite ST segment elevation that persists after treatment with nitroglycerin
   —no abnormal Q waves (that would suggest a completed infarction)
   —no contraindications to thrombolytic therapy (such as a history of a recent CVA, surgery, or GI bleeding; bleeding diathesis; marked hypertension; CPR; advanced age)

iii) Do *not* obtain arterial blood gas studies if acute thrombolytic therapy is being considered, since arterial puncture is a contraindication to this procedure.

iv) Don't forget about conventional therapy (pain relief, arrhythmia prophylaxis or control) while mobilizing personnel for an acute intervention.

REFERENCES

Alpert JS: Serum enzyme determination in patients with suspected myocardial infarction (editorial). Arch Intern Med 143:1522–1523, 1983.

Anderson JL, Marshall HW: A randomized trial of intravenous and intracoronary streptokinase in patients with acute myocardial infarction. Circulation 70:606–618, 1984.

Beta-Blocker Heart Attack Trial Research Group: A randomized trial of propranolol in patients with acute myocardial infarction: Mortality results. JAMA 247:1707–1714, 1982.

Bigger JT: Antiarrhythmic treatment: An overview. Am J Cardiol 53:8B–16B, 1984.

Bigger JT, Coromilas J: Identification of patients at risk for arrhythmic death: Role of Holter ECG recording. In Josephson ME (Ed): Sudden Cardiac Death, Cardiovascular Clinics. FA Davis, Philadelphia, Vol. 15, No. 3, 1983, pp 131–143.

Bigger JT, Weld FM, Rolnitzky LM: Which postinfarction ventricular arrhythmias should be treated? Am Heart J 103:660–666, 1982.

Brush JE, Brand DA, Acampora D, Chalmer B, Wackers FJ: Use of the initial electrocardiogram to predict in-hospital complications of acute myocardial infarction. N Engl J Med 312:1137–1141, 1985.

Campbell CA, Przyklenk K, Kloner RA: Infarct size reduction: A review of the clinical trials. J Clin Pharmacol 26:317–329, 1986.

Crimm A, Severance HW, Coffey K, McKinnis R, Wagner GS, Califf RM: Prognostic significance of isolated sinus tachycardia during first three days of acute myocardial infarction. Am J Med 76:983–988, 1984.

Dell'Italia LJ, Starling MR, O'Rourke RA: Physical examination for exclusion of hemodynamically important right ventricular infarction. Ann Intern Med 99:608–611, 1983.

DeWood MA, Spores J, Notske R, Mouser LT, Burroughs R, Golden MS, Lang LT: Prevalence of total coronary occlusion during the early hours of transmural myocardial infarction. N Engl J Med 303:897–902, 1980.

DeWood MA, Stifter WF, Simpson CS, et al.: Coronary arteriographic findings soon after non-Q-wave myocardial infarction. N Engl J Med 315:417–423, 1986.

Epstein SE, Palmeri ST: Mechanisms contributing to precipitation of unstable angina and acute myocardial infarction: Implications regarding therapy. Am J Cardiol 54:1245–1252, 1984.

Ezekowitz MD: Acute infarction, left ventricular thrombus and systemic embolization: An approach to management. J Am Coll Cardiol 5:1281–1282, 1985.

Fisher ML, Kelemen MH, Collins D, Morris F, Moran GW, Carliner NH, Plotnick D: Routine serum enzyme tests in the diagnosis of acute myocardial infarction: Cost-effectiveness. Arch Intern Med 143:1541–1543, 1983.

Flaherty JT: Unstable angina: Rational approach to management. Am J Med 76:52–57, 1984.

Forrester JS, Diamond G, Chatterjee K, Swan HJC: Medical therapy of acute myocardial infarction by application of hemodynamic subsets. N Engl J Med 295:1356–1362; 1404–1413, 1976.

Fuchs R, Scheidt S: Improved criteria for admission to cardiac care units. JAMA 246:2037–2041, 1981.

Ganz W, Geft I, Shah PK, Lew AS, Rodriguiz L, Weiss T, Maddahi J, Beman OS, Charuzi Y, Swan HJC: Intravenous streptokinase in evolving acute myocardial infarction. Am J Cardiol 53:1209–1216, 1984.

Genton E, Turpie AGG: Anticoagulant therapy following acute myocardial infarction. Mod Conc Cardiovasc Dis 52:45–48, 1983.

Genton R, Jaffe AS: Management of congestive heart failure in patients with acute myocardial infarction. JAMA 256:2556–2560, 1986.

Gibson RS, Boden WE, Theroux P, et al.: Diltiazem and reinfarction in patients with non-Q-wave myocardial infarction. N Engl J Med 315:423–429, 1986.

Grauer K: Early management of myocardial infarction. Am Fam Physician 28:162–170, 1983.

Grauer K, Curry RW: Clinical electrocardiography: A primary care approach. Medical Economics, Oradell, NJ, 1986, pp 237–311.

Gray RJ, Sethna D, Matloff JM: The role of cardiac surgery in acute myocardial infarction. II. Without mechanical complications. Am Heart J 106:728–735, 1983.

Hancock EW: Ischemic heart disease: Acute myocardial infarction. In Rubenstein E, Federman DD (Eds): Scientific American Medicine. New York, Scientific American, 1986, Section I, Chapter X, pp 1–23.

Health and Public Policy Committee, American College of Physicians: Thrombolysis for evolving myocardial infarction. Ann Intern Med 103:463–649, 1985.

Hindman MC, Wagner GS, JaRo M, et al.: The clinical significance of bundle branch block complicating acute myocardial infarction. Circulation 58:679–699, 1978.

Hjalmarson A, Elmfeldt D, Herlitz J, Holmberg S, Malek I, Nyberg G, Ryden L, Swedberg K, Vedin A, Waagstein F, Waldenstrom A, Waldenstrom J, Wedel H, Wilhelmsen L, Wilhelmsson C: Effect on mortality of metoprolol in acute myocardial infarction. Lancet 2:823–827, 1981.

Hjalmarson A: Early intervention with a beta-blocking drug after acute myocardial infarction. Am J Cardiol 54:11E–13E, 1984.

Johnston CC, Bolton EC: Cardiac enzymes. Ann Emerg Med 11:27–35, 1982.

Kennedy JW, Gensini GG, Timmis GC, Maynard C: Acute myocardial infarction treated with intracoronary streptokinase: A report of the Society for Cardiac Angioplasty. Am J Cardiol 55:871–877, 1985.

Kulbertus HE, Rigo P, Legrand Y: Right ventricular infarction: Pathophysiology, diagnosis, clinical course, and treatment. Mod Conc Cardiovasc Dis 54:1–5, 1985.

Laffel GL, Braunwald E: Thrombolytic therapy: A new strategy for the treatment of acute myocardial infarction. N Engl J Med 311:710–717, 770–776, 1984.

Lee TH, Cook F, Weisberg M, Sargent RK, Wilson C, Goldman L: Acute chest pain in the emergency room: Identification and examination of low-risk patients. Arch Intern Med 145:65–69, 1985.

Lewis HD, Davis JW, Archibald DG, Steinke WE, Smitherman TC, Doherty JE, Schnaper HW, LeWinter MM, Linares E, Pouget JM, Sabharwal SC, Chesler E, DeMots H: Protective effects of aspirin against acute myocardial infarction and death in men with unstable angina: Results of a Veterans Administration Cooperative Study. N Engl J Med 309:396–403, 1983.

Lewis HD, Veterans Administration Cooperative Study Group: Unstable angina: Status of aspirin and other forms of therapy. Circulation 72 (suppl V):V655–V160, 1985.

Lichstein E: Why do beta-receptor blockers decrease mortality after myocardial infarction? J Am Coll Cardiol 6:973–975, 1985.

Lopez-Sendon J, Coma-Canella I, Alcasena S, Sloane J, Gamallo C: Electrocardiographic findings in acute right ventricular infarction: Sensitivity and specificity of electrocardiographic alterations in right precordial leads V_4R, V_3R, V_1, V_2 and V_3. J Am Coll Cardiol 6:1273–1279, 1985.

Madias JE, Chahine RA, Gorlin R, Blacklow DJ: A comparison of transmural and nontransmural acute myocardial infarction. Circulation 49:498–507, 1974.

Madias JE, Gorlin R: The myth of acute "mild" myocardial infarction. Ann Intern Med 86:347–352, 1977.

Margolis JR, Kannel WS, Feinleib M, Dawbaer TR, McNamara PM: Clinical features of unrecognized myocardial infarction—silent and symptomatic: Eighteen year follow-up: The Framingham Study. Am J Cardiol 32:1–7, 1973.

Meyer J, Merx W: Sequential intervention procedures after intracoronary thrombolyis: Balloon dilatation, bypass surgery, and medical treatment. Int J Cardiol 7:281–293, 1985.

Nixon JV: Right ventricular myocardial infarction. Arch Intern Med 142:945–947, 1982.

Norris RM: β-Adrenoceptor blockers: An update on their role in acute myocardial infarction. Drugs 29:97–104, 1985.

Norwegian Multicenter Study Group: Timolol-induced reduction in mortality and reinfarction in patients surviving acute myocardial infarction. N Engl J Med 304:801–807, 1981.

Nowakowski JF: Use of cardiac enzymes in the evaluation of acute chest pain. Ann Emerg Med 15:354–360, 1986.

O'Neill WW: Interventions in acute myocardial infarction. In Kobernick MS, Burney RE (Eds): Emergency Medicine Clinics of North America. W. B. Saunders, Philadelphia, 1986, Vol 4, No. 3, pp. 467–486.

Rackley CE, Russel RO, Rogers WJ, Mantle JA, Papapietro SE: Unstable angina pectoris: Is it time to change our approach? Am Heart J 103:154–156, 1982.

Rahimtoola SH: Unstable angina: Current status. Mod Conc Cardiovasc Dis 54:19–23, 1985.

Reeder GS, Vlietstra RE: Coronary angioplasty: 1986. Mod Conc Cardiovasc Dis 55:49–53, 1986.

Rentrop KP, Feit F, Blanke H et al.: Effects of intracoronary streptokinase and intracoronary nitroglycerin infusion on coronary angiographic patterns and mortality in patients with acute myocardial infarction. N Engl J Med 311:1457–1463, 1984.

Scheinman MM, Gonzalez RP: Fascicular block and acute myocardial infarction. JAMA 244:2646–2649, 1980.

Seager SB: Cardiac enzymes in the evaluation of chest pain. Ann Emerg Med 9:346–349, 1980.

Shah PK, Maddahi J, Berman DS, Pichler M, Swan HJC: Scintigraphically detected predominant right ventricular dysfunction in acute myocardial infarction: Clinical and hemodynamic correlates and implications for therapy and prognosis. J Am Coll Cardiol 6:1264–1272, 1985.

Sherry S: Tissue plasminogen activator (t-PA): Will it fulfill its promise? N Engl J Med 333:1014–1017, 1985.

Spirito P, Bellotti P, Chiarella F, Domenicucci S, Sementa A, Vecchio C: Prognostic significance and natural history of left ventricular thrombi in patients with acute anterior myocardial infarction: A two-dimensional echocardiographic study. Circulation 72:774–780, 1985.

Stannard M, Sloman G: Ventricular fibrillation in acute myocardial infarction: Prognosis following successful resuscitation. Am Heart J 77:573, 1969.

Taylor GJ, Mikell FL: Intravenous versus intracoronary streptokinase therapy for acute myocardial infarction in community hospitals. Am J Cardiol 54:256–260, 1984.

The TIMI Study Group: Special report: The thrombolysis in myocardial infarction (TIMI) trial, Phase I findings. N Engl J Med 312:932–936, 1985.

Urban PL, Cowley M, et al.: Intracoronary thrombolysis in acute myocardial infarction: Clinical course following successful myocardial reperfusion. Am Heart J 108:873–878, 1984.

Van der Does E, Lubsen J, Pool J: Acute myocardial infarction: An easy diagnosis in general practice? J R Coll Gen Pract 30:405–409, 1980.

Van de Werf F, Ludbrook PA, Bergmann SR et al.: Coronary thrombolysis with tissue-type plasminogen activator in patients with evolving myocardial infarction. N Engl J Med 310:609–613, 1984.

Weinreich DJ, Burke JF, Pauletto FJ: Left ventricular mural thrombi complicating acute myocardial infarction: Long-term follow-up with serial echocardiography. Ann Intern Med 100:789–794, 1984.

Wray R, Maurer B, Shillingford J: Prophylactic anticoagulant therapy in the prevention of calf-vein thrombosis after myocardial infarction. N Engl J Med 288:815–817, 1973.

Yusuf S, Peto R, Lewis J, Collins R, Sleight P: Beta-blockade during and after myocardial infarction: An overview of the randomized trials. Prog Cardiovasc Dis 27:335–371, 1985.

Zarling EJ, Sexton H, Milnor P: Failure to diagnose acute myocardial infarction: The clinicopathologic experience at a large community hospital. JAMA 250:1177–1181, 1983.

CHAPTER 13

USE OF LIDOCAINE

Lidocaine is the most commonly used antiarrhythmic agent for the emergency treatment of ventricular arrhythmias. Despite its widespread use, opinions still vary about what constitutes an optimal protocol for administration of the drug. While virtually all therapeutic regimens employ an initial loading bolus, the need for one or more additional loading boluses remains open to question. Similarly, no general consensus exists regarding the ideal rate of infusion. Some authorities begin low (at an infusion rate of 1 mg/min) and adjust the infusion rate upward with each subsequent bolus. Others begin high (at an infusion rate of 4 mg/min) and adjust the infusion rate downward. A third group maintains a constant infusion rate of 2 mg/min regardless of whether additional boluses of drug are given.

With such an abundance of treatment protocols to choose from, it is not surprising that the emergency care provider may find it difficult to decide on the regimen best suited for a particular patient. This decision is further complicated by patient variables such as age, weight, use of concomitant drugs, and the presence of acute myocardial infarction, congestive heart failure, or liver disease, since each of these factors may affect lidocaine metabolism.

In addition to the divergence of opinions on lidocaine dosing is the lack of consensus on whether to routinely recommend the drug as a prophylactic agent for patients suspected of acute myocardial infarction. And finally, there is the question of whether lidocaine is an effective antifibrillatory agent.

The goal of this chapter is to clarify these points on the use of lidocaine. Basic pharmacokinetic principles of the drug are reviewed and applied in an attempt to demonstrate how to optimize therapy and minimize the risk of toxicity. Use of lidocaine prophylactically, therapeutically, and as an antifibrillatory agent is then discussed.

Lidocaine Pharmacokinetics

Lidocaine pharmacokinetics can best be understood by considering a two-compartment model **(Fig. 13-1).** The smaller *central compartment* includes the circulating blood volume and highly perfused organs such as the heart and brain. Because of rapid redistribution into the peripheral compartment, the half-life of lidocaine in the central compartment is less than 10 minutes. The larger *peripheral compartment* includes poorly perfused tissues such as skin, muscle, and most of the body fat stores. In healthy adults the half-life of lidocaine in this space is usually 1–2 hours.

> When a bolus of lidocaine is injected intravenously (into *blood*), it is administered directly into the central compartment. Since the *heart* is contained within this space, the antiarrhythmic effect of the drug begins almost immediately. Since the *brain* is also in this compartment, the size of the loading dose and the speed with which it is administered must be limited or central nervous system (CNS) toxicity may result.

Within 10 minutes, half of the initial loading bolus has already diffused into the peripheral compartment, and the level of drug in the bloodstream drops significantly. PVCs may recur at this time unless the serum drug concentration of lidocaine has been maintained within the therapeutic range (2–6 μg/ml) by additional loading boluses.

Lidocaine distribution from the central compartment to the peripheral compartment begins immediately following an IV bolus and continues until a state of equilibrium is established between these two compartments. By giving one or more loading boluses, therapeutic blood levels can be rapidly achieved so as to maintain an ad-

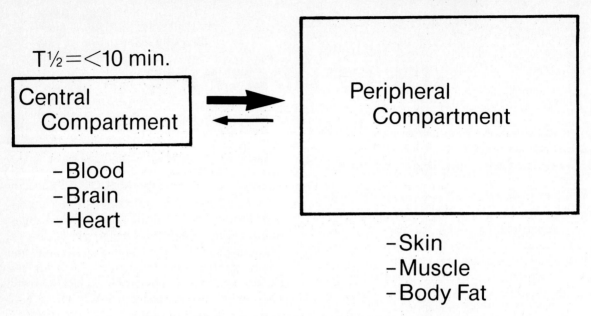

Figure 13-1   Pharmacokinetic model for lidocaine.

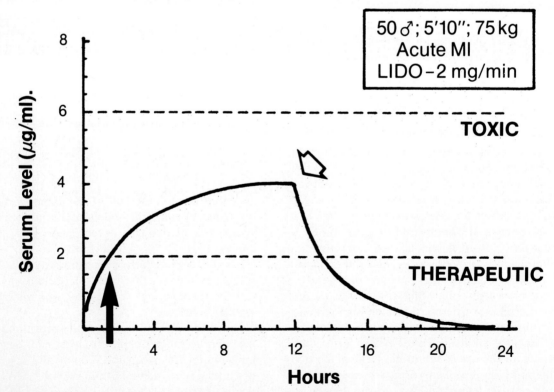

Figure 13-2   A 50-year-old man (5 feet 10 inches, 75 kg) with acute infarction is given an IV maintenance infusion of lidocaine at 2 mg/min. No loading dose is given. More than 1 hour passes before a therapeutic blood level is reached (arrow). The infusion is stopped after 12 hours (open arrowhead.) Therapeutic blood levels persist for at least 2 hours.

equate antiarrhythmic effect until the continuous intravenous infusion has had an opportunity to attain steady state. If instead one were to simply institute a maintenance infusion without first giving a loading dose, more than an hour would pass before serum drug levels would become therapeutic. This situation is illustrated in **Figure 13-2** in which a 75-kg man is started on a maintenance infusion of 2 mg/min.

If the same 75-kg man were to receive a 75-mg loading bolus of lidocaine (1 mg/kg) before starting the 2-mg/min maintenance infusion, therapeutic drug levels of lidocaine would be reached almost immediately **(Fig. 13-3)**. With the exception of a momentary dip below the therapeutic range (arrow in Fig. 13-3), adequate blood levels are maintained until steady state is established.

If one were to follow the initial 75-mg loading bolus with a second bolus given a short time later, even this transient "therapeutic hiatus" might be avoided **(Fig. 13-4)**.

The eventual steady state serum drug level (which in this case is just over 4 µg/ml) might be reached even sooner if a third and/or fourth loading bolus were administered **(Fig. 13-5)**. This type of aggressive loading protocol calls for an initial loading dose of 75-mg followed by 50-mg boluses every 5-10 minutes until a total loading dose of up to 225 mg has been given.

One may either keep the infusion rate constant at 2 mg/min (as in Fig. 13-5) or increase the infusion rate by 1 mg/min after each additional loading bolus is given, until a maximum rate of 4 mg/min is reached. The problem is that in an otherwise healthy 50-year-old man, the presence of any complicating factors that retard lidocaine metabolism (acute infarction, shock, congestive failure, or concomitant use of drugs such as propranolol or cimetidine) may be

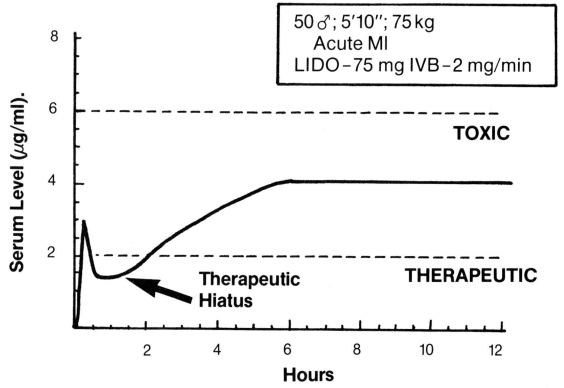

Figure 13-3   The same man described in Figure 13-2 is initially given a 75 mg bolus of lidocaine before starting an IV maintenance infusion at 2 mg/min. Therapeutic blood levels are reached almost immediately. They then transiently dip into the subtherapeutic range (arrow) until steady state is established.

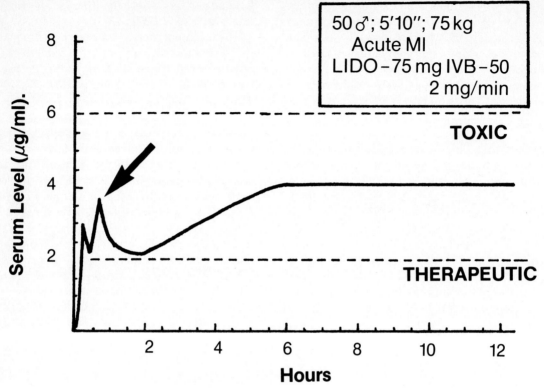

Figure 13-4   The second loading bolus of 50 mg (arrow) is given shortly after the initial 75 mg
loading dose. Blood levels never drop into the subtherapeutic range.

enough to cause the patient to become toxic when higher infusion rates are used **(Fig. 13-6)**.

> Pharmacokinetically, there is no need to increase the rate of infusion even if breakthrough PVCs occur during the initial hour of the loading period. This is because PVCs that recur during the 10–20 minutes following the loading bolus in Figure 13-3 probably are *not* due to the maintenance infusion being too slow but rather to the drop in the lidocaine blood level that occurs as the drug is redistributed from the central compartment to the peripheral compartment. This drop could be avoided by administering one or more additional loading boluses (Figs. 13-4 and 13-5).

One should note that the eventual steady state plasma concentration of lidocaine is *not* influenced by the manner in which the patient is loaded. As long as the rate of the maintenance infusion remains constant at 2 mg/min, the eventual level of lidocaine in the blood will be the same (a steady state level of just over 4 µg/

ml is ultimately reached in Figs. 13-3, 13-4, and 13-5). Only if a serum drug level of greater than 4 µg/ml is required for arrhythmia control would one have to increase the rate of the maintenance infusion above 2 mg/min.

Suggested Protocol for Lidocaine Administration

Considering the above, a reasonable protocol for administering lidocaine is to first give the patient a 50- to 100-mg IV bolus (1 mg/kg) while simultaneously beginning a maintenance infusion at 2 mg/min **(Fig. 13-7)**. Further administration of IV boluses should depend on the reason lidocaine is being given. If the drug is being used purely as a *prophylactic* measure to prevent ventricular fibrillation in a patient suspected of acute infarction but without ventricular ectopy, additional loading boluses are probably not es-

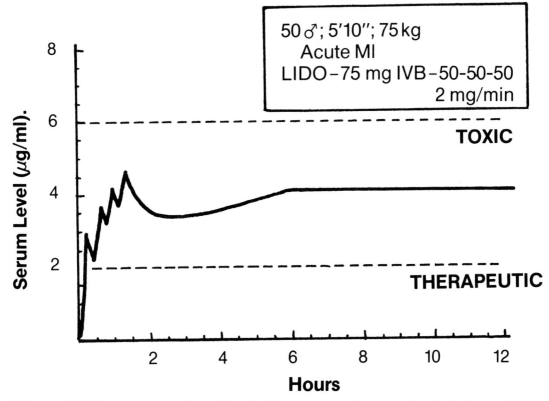

Figure 13-5 Loading regimen whereby the same man shown previously is given an initial loading dose of 75 mg followed by three additional 50 mg boluses. The maintenance infusion is set at 2 mg/min.

sential (Fig. 13-3). Alternatively, one might choose to administer a second loading bolus of 50- to 75-mg 5–10 minutes after the initial bolus (Fig. 13-4). More aggressive loading (Fig. 13-5) only increases the risk of toxicity and is probably not warranted when using lidocaine prophylactically.

On the other hand, if lidocaine is being used *therapeutically* to treat frequent and complex ventricular ectopy, it may be advisable to follow the initial loading dose with one or more additional 50- to 75-mg boluses spaced 5–10 minutes apart until a total loading dose of up to 225 mg has been given. If ventricular ectopy is controlled as this regimen is administered, the rate of the maintenance infusion need *not* be increased after each bolus.

Two points about this protocol are deserving of special mention. First, the short half-life of lidocaine in the central compartment makes it essential that adjustments in the rate of the IV infusion be enacted within 5–10 minutes of giving the IV bolus. Failure to do so will result in dissipation of the effect of the bolus. If one assumes that the half-life of lidocaine in the central compartment is 10 minutes and a 100-mg IV loading bolus is given, 10 minutes later only 50 mg will remain in the central compartment. Were one to delay initiating the maintenance infusion beyond this time, the effect of the bolus will have been lost.

The second point to emphasize is that *not every PVC must be treated for lidocaine to exert a protective effect*. The goal of both prophylactic and therapeutic administration of lidocaine is, after all, prevention of sustained ventricular tachycardia and ventricular fibrillation. Although in the past efforts were made to abolish all PVCs, recent evidence suggests this is probably not necessary. A more practical (and easily attainable) goal of lidocaine therapy might therefore be to decrease the overall frequency of ventricular ectopy and to markedly reduce the occurrence of repetitive forms (such as ventricular couplets and salvos) but not necessarily to eliminate all PVCs.

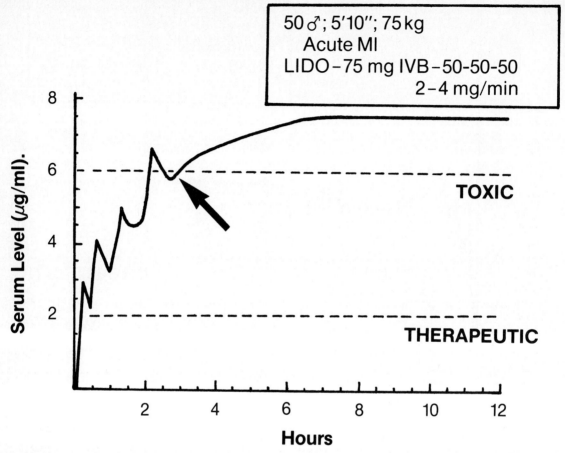

Figure 13-6   Patient in Figure 13-5 becomes toxic when the rate of infusion is increased following each of the loading boluses (arrow).

A number of questions on the usage of lidocaine may arise from the preceding discussion:

i) Why are loading doses of greater than 1 mg/kg not used?

ii) What are the clinical manifestations of lidocaine toxicity?

iii) Are there adverse cardiovascular effects that must be kept in mind when the drug is used?

iv) How is lidocaine eliminated from the body?

v) When administration of lidocaine is discontinued, can one abruptly stop the infusion or should it be tapered?

vi) What adjustments in administering the drug should be made for the elderly and/ or those with congestive heart failure, shock, or liver disease?

vii) When should lidocaine be used prophylactically? For how long should the infusion be maintained?

viii) Is there a role for lidocaine in the treatment of ventricular fibrillation?

Optimal Loading Dose of Lidocaine

The optimal initial loading dose of lidocaine is a 1-mg/kg bolus given intravenously. Despite common usage of the term *bolus,* this dose should not be injected as rapidly as possible. In-

Suggested Protocal for Lidocaine Administration

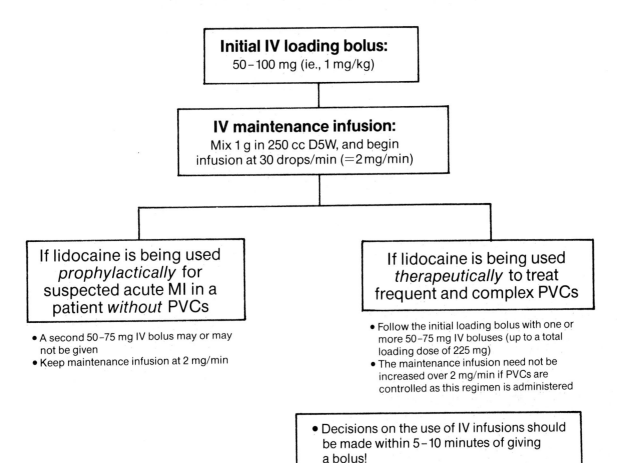

Initial IV loading bolus:
50–100 mg (ie., 1 mg/kg)

IV maintenance infusion:
Mix 1 g in 250 cc D5W, and begin
infusion at 30 drops/min (=2 mg/min)

If lidocaine is being used
prophylactically for
suspected acute MI in a
patient *without* PVCs

- A second 50–75 mg IV bolus may or may not be given
- Keep maintenance infusion at 2 mg/min

If lidocaine is being used
therapeutically to treat
frequent and complex PVCs

- Follow the initial loading bolus with one or more 50–75 mg IV boluses (up to a total loading dose of 225 mg)
- The maintenance infusion need not be increased over 2 mg/min if PVCs are controlled as this regimen is administered

- Decisions on the use of IV infusions should be made within 5–10 minutes of giving a bolus!
- It is not essential to eliminate every PVC for lidocaine to exert a protective effect!

Figure 13-7

stead it should be infused over a 1- to 2-minute period so as not to flood the central compartment with the drug. As mentioned previously, because the heart is contained within the central compartment, the antiarrhythmic effect of a loading dose of lidocaine begins almost immediately. However, since the brain is also contained within this central compartment, too rapid infusion of a loading bolus or administration of too large a dose may result in CNS tox-

icity. Consequently, while doses of more than 1 mg/kg of lidocaine may achieve steady state levels of drug more rapidly, because of the unwarranted risk of toxicity they are not recommended.

Manifestations of Toxicity

In general, lidocaine is an extremely well tolerated antiarrhythmic agent. When adverse effects do occur, they usually involve the central

TABLE 13-1   CLINICAL MANIFESTATIONS OF LIDOCAINE TOXICITY

↑	Respiratory arrest
	Seizures
	Muscle twitching
	Disorientation and confusion
Increasing Blood Level	Hearing impairment
	Dysarthria
	Mild agitation
	Euphoria
	Drowsiness
	Dizziness
	Feelings of dissociation
	Perioral paresthesias

nervous system. Clinical manifestations of CNS toxicity are listed in **Table 13-1.**

The therapeutic range of serum drug levels for lidocaine is between 2 and 6 μg/ml. Occasionally, mild signs of lidocaine toxicity (dizziness, feelings of dissociation, and perioral paresthesias) are seen at levels near 5 μg/ml, a serum drug concentration that overlaps with the upper limits of the therapeutic range. At other times these adverse reactions may follow infusion of a loading bolus, particularly if the drug was administered too rapidly. In the latter case, prompt resolution of adverse effects should follow discontinuation of the infusion. If, on the other hand, adverse effects are seen at a later stage during maintenance infusion of the drug, the picture is more suggestive of drug accumulation and impending toxicity. The drip should be stopped immediately. If possible, a blood level should be drawn to look for toxicity.

The problem with diagnosing lidocaine toxicity is that severe reactions such as seizures and respiratory arrest may occasionally occur without the milder premonitory symptoms. Thus, a patient convulsing during cardiac arrest may be hypoxic, hypotensive, alkalotic, or toxic from lidocaine. Unfortunately, clinical assessment without laboratory confirmation has not been shown to be accurate in differentiating among these possibilities (Deglin et al., 1980). Therefore, cautious dosing and a high index of suspicion are essential when treating patients at high risk of developing toxicity.

Adverse Cardiovascular Effects

Perhaps the most frequently observed adverse cardiovascular effect of lidocaine is hypotension. When this occurs, it is most often due to the too rapid administration of an IV bolus. Momentary placement of the patient in Trendelenburg and reducing the rate of infusion are usually all that is needed to resolve the problem.

Depression of left ventricular function and exacerbation of SA or AV conduction disturbances may occur but are distinctly uncommon. This is especially true for patients with intact interventricular conduction. In such individuals, lidocaine may be given almost with impunity. However, if SA or AV conduction is impaired (as it is in patients with sick sinus syndrome, bundle branch block, and second- or third-degree AV block), lidocaine may aggravate the conduction disturbance. In addition to slowing of the ventricular rate, case reports of asystole after lidocaine administration have been noted in such instances (Dunn et al., 1985; Hilleman et al., 1985). Although rare, the potential severity of these reactions warrants careful selection and monitoring of patients who are to receive the drug, particularly if they have preexisting conduction disturbances. Under such circumstances, availability of pacemaker insertion may be advisable before lidocaine infusion is begun.

A final but important cardiac effect that lidocaine may occasionally produce is acceleration of the ventricular response of supraventricular tachyarrhythmias (especially atrial flutter or atrial fibrillation). This results from a quinidine-like action of this drug that acts to decrease AV nodal refractoriness in certain patients. Consequently, lidocaine should *never* be given indiscriminately as a diagnostic measure to patients with wide complex tachyarrhythmias, since the drug may aggravate the condition (that is, accelerate the ventricular response) if the rhythm is supraventricular (Marriott and Bieza, 1972; Hilleman et al., 1985).

Lidocaine Elimination and Adjustments in Dosing

Lidocaine is eliminated from the body by hepatic metabolism. The half-life of this elimination phase is proportional to hepatic blood flow and under normal circumstances takes between 1 and 2 hours. Patients in shock or congestive heart failure in whom hepatic blood flow may be greatly diminished would be expected to have a prolonged elimination phase half-life and be more susceptible to accumulation of drug and lidocaine toxicity. Other groups at high risk of developing lidocaine toxicity include patients with liver disease, those taking drugs such as propranolol or cimetidine that decrease hepatic clearance of lidocaine, the elderly in whom cardiac output is less, and patients with low body weight **(Table 13-2).** In addition, the elimination phase half-life of lidocaine may increase in patients with acute infarction (due to altered protein-binding of lidocaine) and in those taking prolonged ($\geq$24 hour) infusions of the drug.

For this reason, one often decreases the rate of the maintenance infusion in patients on lidocaine for more than 24 hours.

Cimetidine inhibits the hepatic metabolism of a number of drugs, including lidocaine, warfarin, theophylline, and diazepam. The mechanism by which this occurs is thought to result from the drug's avid binding to the *cytochrome P-450 system* involved in drug elimination (Zimmerman and Schenker, 1985). When one considers the number of patients who are taking cimetidine and the fact that this drug is so commonly used as a prophylactic agent to prevent stress ulceration in patients admitted to intensive care units, *the importance of the interaction between cimetidine and lidocaine becomes obvious.* Failure to reduce the rate of lidocaine infusion for patients receiving both of these medications may precipitate lidocaine toxicity.

Although the other H-2 blocker that is currently in use *(ranitidine)* acts to reduce gastric acid production in much the same manner as cimetidine, it does not appear to bind to the cytochrome P-450 system to nearly the same degree (Zimmerman and Schenker, 1985). Significant clinical interactions between ranitidine and lidocaine have not been reported, and this drug may be preferable to cimetidine for stress ulceration prophylaxis in patients with ventricular arrhythmias.

Abruptly stopping an IV maintenance infusion of lidocaine will *not* immediately result in subtherapeutic blood levels. This point is well illustrated by Figure 13-2, in which serum drug levels do not fall into the subtherapeutic range for nearly 2 hours *after* the maintenance infusion is discontinued. Thus, *there would seem to be no pharmacokinetic rationale for tapering patients off lidocaine infusions!* The 1- to 2-hour elimination phase half-life of the drug automatically ensures a tapering effect.

TABLE 13-2   FACTORS IMPAIRING LIDOCAINE CLEARANCE

Congestive heart failure
Acute infarction
Shock
Liver disease
Drugs (ie, propranolol, cimetidine)
Older age
Low body weight
Prolonged infusion (ie, >24 hr)

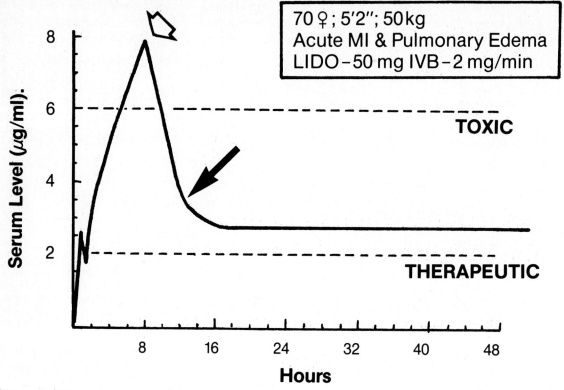

Figure 13-8   A 70-year-old woman (5 feet 2 inches, 50 kg) with acute infarction and pulmonary edema is given a 50 mg bolus and a maintenance infusion of 2 mg/min. The infusion is held after 8 hours (open arrowhead) when she becomes toxic, and then it is restarted at 12 hours (arrow) at the lower infusion rate of 0.5 mg/min.

What adjustments in dosing should be made for those patients at high risk of developing lidocine toxicity? Consider the case of a 50-kg elderly woman **(Fig. 13-8)** who is admitted with pulmonary edema from an acute myocardial infarction.

After receiving the standard 1-mg/kg loading dose (in this case 50 mg), the patient rapidly became toxic on a maintenance infusion of 2 mg/min. This rate is too high for an elderly subject of low body weight with acute infarction and significant congestive heart failure. After the infusion was held for 4 hours (open arrowhead), the drip was restarted (arrow) at a new infusion rate of 0.5 mg/min. In a patient such as this, an infusion rate of as low as 0.5 mg/min may be more than adequate to maintain therapeutic serum concentrations of the drug.

Let us assume that this same 50-kg elderly woman was admitted to the hospital with acute myocardial infarction but without congestive heart failure. In this case one might achieve and maintain adequate therapeutic blood levels by administering two 50 mg loading boluses and setting an IV infusion to run at 1 mg/min **(Fig. 13-9)**.

In summary, the initial loading dose of lidocaine is fairly independent of patient variables other than body weight. A dose of 1 mg/kg is the usual amount recommended for this first bolus. On the other hand, many factors impair lidocaine clearance and must be taken into account if subsequent boluses are given and when determining the rate of the maintenance infusion (Table 13-2). Failure to do so significantly increases the likelihood of lidocaine toxicity.

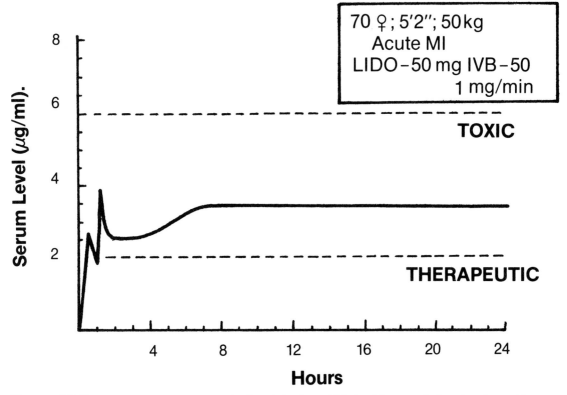

Figure 13-9 A 70-year-old woman (5 feet 2 inches, 50 kg) with acute infarction but without congestive heart failure is given two 50 mg loading boluses and then is maintained on an IV infusion at 1 mg/min.

Prophylactic Use of Lidocaine

In the past it was thought that "warning arrhythmias" (5 or more PVCs per minute, 2 or more PVCs in a row, multiform PVCs, and the "R-on-T" phenomenon) regularly preceded the development of primary ventricular fibrillation in patients with acute myocardial infarction. Consequently, one would wait for the occurrence of such arrhythmias before initiating antiarrhythmic treatment in patients admitted with acute chest pain.

Today the concept of warning arrhythmias has been conclusively disproved. Ventricular fibrillation frequently occurs in acute myocardial infarction without warning arrhythmias. Sometimes it even occurs without any prior ectopic activity. Moreover, when warning arrhythmias do occur, they do not reliably predict which patients will subsequently develop ventricular fibrillation.

In view of the fact that 5–10% of all patients with acute myocardial infarction develop primary ventricular fibrillation, it would seem prudent to consider the prophylactic use of antiarrhythmic therapy. Lidocaine has been the drug most commonly chosen for this purpose. It is easy to administer, is well tolerated by most patients, and effectively lowers the incidence of primary ventricular fibrillation associated with acute infarction. This drug should not be used indiscriminately, however, since its administration is associated with a 5–15% incidence of toxicity. The risk of lidocaine toxicity seems to be greatest for patients more than 70 years old

(Goldman and Batsford, 1979; Lie et al., 1974). Since the risk of developing primary ventricular fibrillation is significantly less in this age group, elderly patients could reasonably be excluded from consideration for lidocaine prophylaxis.

Patients who are most likely to benefit from lidocaine prophylaxis are those seen early during the course of their illness and in whom a high index of suspicion for acute infarction exists. This is because the greatest incidence of primary ventricular fibrillation associated with acute myocardial infarction occurs within the first few hours of the onset of symptoms. It is rare after 24 hours, and lidocaine prophylaxis is probably not warranted in patients who are first seen after this period.

The case for prophylactic use of lidocaine for patients with suspected myocardial infarction is not without controversy. A number of investigators maintain that, although the incidence of primary ventricular fibrillation may be lowered in treated patients, no study has ever demonstrated a decrease in mortality from the prophylactic use of this drug (Dunn et al., 1985; Carruth and Silverman, 1982). Therefore, they believe that lidocaine is not indicated in the absence of ventricular ectopy.

The caveat to beware of is the extremely small sample size and the low incidence of ventricular fibrillation in virtually all randomized trials on the prophylactic use of this drug. Such small trials may fail to show a statistically significant difference between controls and patients treated with lidocaine. In fact, when the data from these smaller studies are pooled, a significant benefit is observed in patients prophylactically treated with lidocaine (DeSilva et al., 1981).

In summary, lidocaine prophylaxis for the prevention of primary ventricular fibrillation is probably reasonable for the following patients who are admitted for suspected acute myocardial infarction:

   i) Patients less than 70 years of age
   ii) Those seen within the first 24 hours of the onset of symptoms
   iii) Those in whom a high index of suspicion for acute infarction exists

These patients should be given one or two IV loading boluses of lidocaine, and a continuous infusion of 1–2 mg/min should be started regardless of whether or not they are manifesting ventricular ectopic activity.

> In discussing the prophylactic use of lidocaine, it is important to differentiate between the primary and secondary forms of ventricular fibrillation. The former term refers to the acute electrical instability that develops as a direct consequence of the infarction. It is most often seen within the first few hours of infarction and is rare after 24 hours. In contrast, secondary ventricular fibrillation characteristically occurs several days after the onset of symptoms and is usually associated with the development of cardiogenic shock. As one might expect, the secondary form of ventricular fibrillation is notoriously resistant to any type of antiarrhythmic therapy.

Antifibrillatory Effect of Lidocaine

In the past, lidocaine was not recommended for treatment of ventricular fibrillation that was refractory to other measures. The fear was that administration of the drug in this setting might abolish the only ventricular activity that was present and lead to asystole. Recently this recommendation has changed, and lidocaine is now advocated as an antifibrillatory agent for treatment of ventricular fibrillation (White, 1984). Why should this be? How does lidocaine work to convert established ventricular fibrillation to a normal rhythm?

> To answer this question, we must first consider the mechanisms that sustain ventricular tachycardia and fibrillation. The substrate for the former is thought to be a fairly large reentry circuit that allows persistence of this tachyarrhythmia. In contrast, with ventricular fibrillation the wavefronts of depolarization are fragmented and follow circuitous paths. Seldom are such circuitous movements completed. Nevertheless, it appears that *reentry* is again the mechanism responsible for allowing the persistence of ventricular fibrillation.
>
> Lidocaine works by speeding conduction and prolonging refractoriness in ischemic zones. This may result in suppressing conduction along many of the fragmented wavefronts present with ventricular fibrillation. Subsequent electrical countershock might then facilitate removal of the remaining wavefronts sustaining ventricular fibrillation.

Lidocaine pharmacokinetics during cardiac arrest are somewhat unpredictable. Because of this, the new guidelines suggest that only bolus therapy be used in this setting. In addition, due to markedly decreased clearance of the drug, it appears that less frequent administration of loading boluses is needed during this low-flow state (McDonald, 1985). Thus, as little as one loading bolus (1 mg/kg) of lidocaine (or at most two boluses) is probably all that is required to maintain therapeutic levels of the drug during cardiac arrest.

> Once the patient has been converted out of ventricular fibrillation, clearance of the drug may markedly increase. Resumption of a normal dosing schedule (with rebolus and institution of a maintenance infusion) is then indicated.

REFERENCES

Adgey AAJ, Geddes JS, Webb SW, Allen JD, James RGG, Zaidi SA, Pantridge JF: Acute phase of myocardial infarction. Lancet 2:501–504, 1971.

Barnaby PF, Barrett PA, Lvoff R: Routine prophylactic lidocaine in acute myocardial infarction. Heart Lung 12:362–366, 1983.

Carruth JE, Silverman ME: Ventricular fibrillation complicating acute myocardial infarction: Reasons against the routine use of lidocaine. Am Heart J 104:545–550, 1982.

Church G, Biern RO: Intensive coronary care—A practical system for a small hospital without house staff. N Engl J Med 281:1155–1159, 1969.

Deglin SM, Deglin JM, Wurtzbacher J, Litton M, Rolfe C, McIntire C: Rapid serum lidocaine determination in the coronary care unit. JAMA 244:571–573, 1980.

DeSilva RA, Lown B, Hennekens CH, Casscells W: Lidocaine prophylaxis in acute myocardial infarction: An evaluation of randomized trials. Lancet 2:855–858, 1981.

Dunn HM, McComb JM, Kinney CD, Campbell NPS, Shanks RG, MacKenzie G, Adgey AAJ: Prophylactic lidocaine in the early phase of suspected myocardial infarction. Am Heart J 110:353–362, 1985.

El-Sherif N, Myerberg RJ, Scherlag BJ, Befeler B, Aranda JM, Castellanos A, Lazzara R: Electrocardiographic antecedents of primary ventricular fibrillation. Br Heart J 38:415–422, 1976.

Fuchs R, Schedit S: Improved criteria for admission to cardiac care units. JAMA 246:2037–2041, 1981.

Goldman L, Batsford WF: Risk-benefit stratification as a guide to lidocaine prophylaxis of primary ventricular fibrillation in acute myocardial infarction: An analytic review. Yale J Biol Med 52:455–466, 1979.

Grauer K: Should prophylactic lidocaine be routinely used in patients suspected of acute myocardial infarction? J Fla Med Assoc 69:377–379, 1982.

Harrison D: Should lidocaine be administered routinely to all patients after acute myocardial infarction? Circulation 58:581–584, 1978.

Hilleman DE, Mohiuddin SM, Destache CJ: Lidocaine-induced second-degree Mobitz II heart block. Drug Intell Clin Pharm 19:669–673, 1985.

Koster RW, Dunning AJ: Intramuscular lidocaine for prevention of lethal arrhythmias in the prehospitalization phase of acute myocardial infarction. N Engl J Med 313:1105–1110, 1985.

Lie KI, Wellens JH, van Capelle FJ, Durrer D: Lidocaine in prevention of primary ventricular fibrillation. N Engl J Med 291:1324–1326, 1974.

Lopez LM, Mehta JL, Robinson JD, Roberts RJ: Optimal lidocaine dosing in patients with myocardial infarction. Ther Drug Mon 4:271–276, 1982.

Marriott HJL, Bieza CF: Alarming ventricular acceleration after lidocaine administration. Chest 61:682–683, 1972.

McDonald JL: Serum lidocaine levels during cardiopulmonary resuscitation after intravenous and endotracheal administration. Crit Care Med 13:914–915, 1985.

Romhilt DW, Boomfield SS, Chou TC, Fowler NO: Unreliability of conventional electrocardiographic monitoring for arrhythmia detection in coronary care units. Am J Cardiol 31:457–461, 1973.

Stargel WW, Routledge PA: Lidocaine: Therapeutic use and serum concentration monitoring. In Taylor WJ, Finn AL (Eds): Individualizing Drug Therapy. Gross, Townsend, Frank, Inc., New York, 1981, pp 1–21.

White RD: Antifibrillatory drugs: The case for lidocaine and procainamide. Ann Emerg Med 13:802–804, 1984.

Wyman MG, Gore S: Lidocaine prophylaxis in myocardial infarction: A concept whose time has come. Heart Lung 12:358–361, 1983.

Wyman MG, Hammersmith L: Comprehensive treatment plan for prevention of primary ventricular fibrillation in acute myocardial infarction. Am J Cardiol 33:661–667, 1974.

Zimmerman TW, Schenker S: A comparative evaluation of cimetidine and ranitidine. Rational Drug Ther 19:1–7, 1985.

PART V:

BEYOND THE BASICS

CHAPTER 14

A COMPENDIUM OF ADDITIONAL DRUGS USED IN EMERGENCY CARDIAC CARE

AGENTS FOR SHOCK

DOBUTAMINE (DOBUTREX)
How Dispensed: 250 mg per 20-ml vial
Indication: Cardiogenic shock

Dose and Route of Administration

Mix 250 mg in 250 ml of D5W (1000 μg/ml) and begin drip at 10–15 drops/min. This will infuse $\approx$2.5 μg/kg/min for a 60- to 80-kg patient. Titrate according to clinical effect. Usual range of infusion = 2.5–10.0 μg/kg/min.

Comments

Dobutamine is a synthetic catecholamine with predominantly beta-1-adrenergic receptor stimulating effects. At usual doses (below 10 μg/kg/min), the drug improves myocardial contractility with only a minimal effect on heart rate and peripheral vascular resistance. It commonly produces reflex vasodilatation in response to this increased contractility and improved cardiac output. The drug is most useful for treatment of patients with cardiac failure who maintain a normal or near normal blood pressure, especially in the setting of acute myocardial infarction. However, for treatment of cardiac failure with hypotension, an agent such as dopamine (with its greater vasoconstrictor effect) is preferable.

The effects of dobutamine are frequently confused with those of dopamine. Dobutamine has no effect on dopaminergic receptors (in the renal or mesenteric vascular bed) and exerts a much lesser effect on the peripheral vasculature than does dopamine. It is in general less arrhythmogenic than

dopamine, and significant increases in heart rate usually are not seen unless high doses ($>$20 μg/kg/min) of the drug are used.

NOREPINEPHRINE (LEVOPHED)
How Dispensed: 1 mg/ml (4-ml vial)
Indications: Cardiogenic shock; hemodynamically significant hypotension (not due to hypovolemia)

Dose and Route of Administration

Mix 1 ampule (4 mg) in 250 ml of D5W (16 μg/ml) and begin drip at 10 drops/min ($\approx$2–3 μg/min). Titrate according to clinical effect and adjust the infusion to the lowest rate that maintains desired hemodynamic response.

Comments

Norepinephrine is an endogenous catecholamine with both alpha- and beta-receptor stimulating effects. It is an extremely potent vasoconstrictor that is used most often in the treatment of hypotension associated with reduced peripheral vascular resistance. (The drug should *not* be given to patients in shock from hypovolemia!)

The effects of norepinephrine on the heart are variable. Cardiac output may either increase or decrease, depending on circulating blood volume, peripheral vascular resistance, the state of the myocardium, and carotid baroreceptor reflex activity.

Significant drawbacks of norepinephrine are that the drug causes renal and mesenteric vasoconstriction and that skin sloughing may result if extravasation occurs from the IV site.

Because of the potential deleterious effects of norepinephrine, its use usually is reserved for patients in profound shock who have not responded to other vasoactive agents.

AMRINONE (INOCOR)

How Dispensed: 5 mg/ml (20-ml vial = 100 mg)

Indications: Short-term treatment of severe congestive heart failure refractory to conventional therapy

Dose and Route of Administration

An initial 0.75 mg/kg IV dose is administered over 2–3 minutes, followed by an IV infusion of 5–10 µg/kg/min. Titrate according to clinical effect.

> Note that amrinone should not be added directly to dextrose-containing solutions because the combination may result in a loss of the drug's activity (Medical Letter, 1984).

Comments

Amrinone is a nonglycoside, nonsympathomimetic (non-beta-agonist) positive inotropic agent. Although its precise mechanism of action is unclear, the drug enhances cardiac contractility (positive inotropic action) and is a potent vasodilator (of both arterial and venous vascular beds). Which of these effects predominate in any given individual appears to vary depending on the dose used and the patient's pretreatment condition.

IV administration of amrinone increases cardiac output and reduces systemic vascular resistance in selected patients with congestive heart failure (Colucci et al., 1986). At the usual dose prescribed, heart rate and blood pressure are not significantly affected in most individuals. In general the drug is well tolerated, and in 1984 the Food and Drug Administration (FDA) approved it for short-term use in treatment of patients with severe congestive heart failure refractory to conventional therapy. However, despite the fact that hemodynamic status may temporarily be improved, no evidence exists that the drug improves long-term survival (Medical Letter, 1984).

> Amrinone should be used with caution in the setting of acute myocardial infarction, particularly for

patients who are hypotensive and/or not in heart failure. In such individuals, the potent venodilator action of the drug may produce a hypotensive response.

> Adverse effects associated with IV administration include thrombocytopenia ($\approx$2%), arrhythmias ($\approx$ 3%), and hypotension ($\approx$1%).

Oral amrinone is not nearly as effective as the IV form of this drug. Due to an inordinately high incidence of side effects (gastrointestinal intolerance, headache, lightheadedness, thrombocytopenia, liver-function abnormalities, fever, and ventricular arrhythmias), oral amrinone is no longer being used in clinical trials. At present, related compounds (milrinone and others) are being studied for potential oral and parenteral use.

LEVODOPA (LARODOPA)

How Dispensed: 250- and 500-mg tablets and capsules

Indication: Congestive heart failure (experimental!)

Dose and Route of Administration

Begin at 250 mg, p.o., q.i.d., and gradually increase to 1.5–2.0 g, q.i.d.

Comments

Levodopa is a dopamine precursor with a positive inotropic effect. Although the drug has been used for years in the treatment of Parkinson's disease, it only recently has been studied for its potential application in patients with congestive heart failure. Its most attractive feature lies in the promise it holds as another orally active agent for the treatment of congestive heart failure.

Rajfer et al. (1984) showed that levodopa significantly improved cardiac output in selected patients with heart failure. However, the mechanism of action of the drug is unclear. Following oral ingestion, it is converted to dopamine. Its beneficial effect in congestive failure appears to be similar to that produced by low-dose dopamine and includes enhanced myocardial contractility (from beta-1-adrenergic stimulation) and peripheral vasodilatation (from dopaminergic receptor stimulation).

The major side effects of levodopa are nausea and vomiting, which are attentuated by beginning the drug at a low dose (250 mg, p.o., q.i.d.). Pyridoxine (50 mg/day) may also lessen these side effects, as well as assist in conversion of levodopa to dopamine.

More work definitely is needed before recommendations can be made regarding the use of this agent. It does not appear to have a role in emergency cardiac care at present.

AGENTS FOR HYPERTENSIVE CRISIS

NITROGLYCERIN
How Dispensed: Pharmacy dependent

Pharmacies vary greatly in the way they prepare IV nitroglycerin (dilutions may vary from 25–500 μg/ml) so that it is *essential* to become familiar with the concentrations employed at one's particular institution.

Indications: Acute ischemic chest pain (angina pectoris, coronary spasm, myocardial infarction); complications of acute myocardial infarction (hypertension, left ventricular failure)

Dose and Route of Administration
Mix 50 mg in 250 ml of D5W (200 μg/ml) and begin drip at 3 drops/min (10 μg/min). Carefully titrate according to clinical response.

Comments
The beneficial action of nitroglycerin in ischemic heart disease has been known for well over 100 years. Even today, the drug remains the first line of treatment for this disorder. Although multiple preparations of nitroglycerin are available, we have limited our comments to the intravenous form of administration.

The mechanism of action of nitroglycerin is multifactorial. The drug's most pronounced effect is to decrease venous tone. This produces a marked reduction in *preload*. Systemic vascular resistance is decreased (*afterload* reduction), although not nearly to the same extent as the reduction in preload. Ni-

troglycerin also increases coronary blood flow (by dilating epicardial coronary arteries) and dilates collateral vessels. Autoregulation of the normal vascular bed is preserved, however, so that shunting of blood flow away from ischemic areas of myocardium (*coronary "steal"*) tends not to occur (Frishman, 1985).

IV nitroglycerin is the drug of choice for treatment of severe chest pain and hypertension that complicate acute myocardial infarction. It is also extremely effective in treatment of congestive heart failure in this setting. Close observation (and frequent blood pressure checks) in an intensive care unit is essential, but invasive hemodynamic monitoring is not necessarily needed.

One should be particularly careful in using IV nitroglycerin when blood pressure is normal or slightly decreased and/or if left ventricular filling pressures are not elevated. Under such circumstances the drug's vasodilatory effect may actually lower stroke volume and cardiac output, resulting in hypotension and tachycardia. IV nitroglycerin appears to be most effective when used in patients with significantly impaired left ventricular function. In such individuals the drug exerts a greater afterload-lowering effect, resulting in an increase in stroke volume and cardiac output (Flaherty, 1984).

SODIUM NITROPRUSSIDE (NIPRIDE)
How Dispensed: 50 mg per 5-ml vial
Indications: Hypertensive crisis, treatment of complications of acute myocardial infarction (hypertension, left ventricular failure)

Dose and Route of Administration
Mix 50 mg in 250 ml of D5W (200 μg/ml) and begin drip at 3 drops/min (10 μg/min). This may be increased by 3 drops/min (10 μg/min) every 5 minutes.

Usual range of infusion = 0.5–8.0 μg/kg/min
Onset of action of the drug = within 1–2 minutes of starting the infusion; effects disappear within minutes of stopping the drip
Hemodynamic monitoring and minute-to-minute titration of dose is essential when nitroprusside is used.

Comments

Nitroprusside is an extremely potent peripheral vasodilator of both the arterial and venous vascular beds. It is the most effective agent currently available for treatment of hypertensive emergencies (Ferguson and Vlasses, 1986). It may also be useful in the treatment of congestive heart failure, due to its ability to lower preload and afterload.

> Compared to IV nitroglycerin, nitroprusside is a far more potent antihypertensive agent due to the greater arterial vasodilatation it produces. However, because nitroprusside is at least theoretically more likely to produce *coronary steal,* IV nitroglycerin is preferred by many for treating mild to moderate hypertension and congestive heart failure that complicate acute ischemic heart disease.

Problems associated with nitroprusside infusion include hypotension (from overaggressive use of the drug), headache, photodegradation of the solution (which is why the IV bottle should always be covered with aluminum foil), and *thiocyanate toxicity*. The earliest signs of the latter condition are weakening of the pulse, decreased intensity of heart sounds, shallow respiration, decreased or absent deep tendon reflexes, and development of a pinkish coloration. Later signs are tinnitus, blurred vision, and delirium. Thiocyanate toxicity should especially be watched for when large doses of the drug are used, if duration of treatment is long, and/or the patient has renal failure.

NIFEDIPINE

How Dispensed: 10-mg capsules
Indication: Hypertensive urgency

Dose and Route of Administration

For hypertensive urgency—Split a 10-mg capsule longitudinally, and place the contents under the patient's tongue for several minutes. Alternatively a patient may be asked to chew a capsule with several puncture holes in it to express its contents.

> The dose may be repeated in 20–30 minutes if an adequate blood pressure response is not seen by this time.
>
> Nifedipine will also acutely lower blood pressure

when given orally, but onset of action may be delayed for 30–60 minutes. (However, having the patient swallow the remains of the capsule after sublingual administration will provide a more sustained effect.)

Blood pressure should be checked every few minutes initially and less frequently thereafter.

Comments

Of the three calcium channel blocking agents currently available, nifedipine is the one with the most potent vasodilating effect on the peripheral vasculature. Consequently, the drug is very useful in treatment of hypertension and hypertensive urgency (Ferguson and Vlasses, 1986). When nifedipine is administered sublingually for this indication, blood pressure begins to fall within minutes and remains depressed for 1 to several hours (Young, 1984).

> Compared to other agents used to treat acute elevations in blood pressure, sublingual nifedipine offers the advantages of being easy to administer, well tolerated, and rapidly effective. Treatment may be initiated in the office or emergency department without the continuous need for moment-to-moment blood pressure monitoring that is essential when nitroprusside is used.

For patients with true *hypertensive emergency,* nitroprusside is the drug of choice. However, nifedipine may be an effective agent to consider when blood pressure elevation is less marked and cardiac and/or neurologic complications are absent *(hypertensive urgency).*

ANTIARRHYTHMIC AGENTS

DIGOXIN

How Dispensed:

For IV use: 0.25 mg/ml (2-ml ampule = 0.5 mg)

For Oral use:

Lanoxin—tablets of 0.125 mg, 0.25 mg, and 0.5 mg

Lanoxicaps—capsules of 0.05 mg, 0.1 mg, and 0.2 mg

Indications: Limited in the acute care setting—atrial fibrillation/flutter with a rapid ventricular response, PSVT (2nd drug of choice after verapamil)

Dose and Route of Administration

For patients not previously digitalized—Load with 0.25–0.50 mg IV. This may be followed with 0.125- to 0.25-mg IV increments every 2–6 hours until a total of 0.75–1.50 mg has been given over the first 24 hours. Then follow with daily maintenance dose.

> The above schedule is intended as a rough guideline. It may be varied according to patient tolerance and the resultant ventricular reponse.
>
> The effects of IV digoxin occur much more rapidly than is generally appreciated. Onset of action begins within 5–10 minutes! An initial peak of action is seen at about 30 minutes and continues to maximum peak action in 4–6 hours.
>
> Digoxin given orally may also be effective. Lanoxin has a bioavailability of 68%. When using this oral preparation, one should therefore prescribe about one third less of the drug than the IV dose. (In contrast, bioavailability of the less commonly used Lanoxicaps is ≈ 90%, so that minimal correction is needed when switching from this oral form to IV administration.)

Comments

Digitalis has been a mainstay in the treatment of congestive heart failure since William Withering's first description of the foxglove in 1785.

> The drug has several actions. It increases the force and velocity of myocardial contraction (positive inotropic effect). When used in patients with congestive heart failure, heart size decreases and overall cardiac performance is improved.
>
> The drug also prolongs the refractory period of the AV node and, in so doing, slows the ventricular response to supraventricular tachyarrhythmias.

Despite these beneficial effects, indications for the use of digoxin in the emergency care setting remain limited. This is because the increase in cardiac contractility that the drug produces tends to be offset by an increase in myocardial oxygen consumption. Other medications (IV nitroglycerin, dobutamine, diuretics) are preferable for treating congestive heart failure in the setting of acute ischemia (Genton and Jaffe, 1986). On the other hand, digoxin is a drug of choice when supraventricular tachyarrhythmias complicate acute myocardial infarction.

Special Considerations

> Use digoxin cautiously (and in lower doses) in patients with chronic obstructive pulmonary disease (who may be hypoxemic), hypokalemia, or hypercalcemia and in the setting of acute ischemia.
>
> Be alert to the possibility of **digitalis toxicity,** when any of the following occur in patients taking digoxin:
> —recent development of nausea and vomiting or disturbances of color vision (uncommon)
> —recent addition of drugs that increase digoxin levels (quinidine, calcium channel blockers)
> —recent worsening of renal failure
> —development of certain cardiac arrhythmias (frequent and/or multiform PVCs, atrial tachycardia with block, accelerated junctional rhythms, Wenckebach rhythms, atrial fibrillation with a slow or "regular" ventricular response)
>
> Remember that digoxin is *contraindicated* for treatment of atrial fibrillation in patients who have Wolff-Parkinson-White syndrome.

PROCAINAMIDE (PRONESTYL)

How Dispensed:
For IV bolus: 100 mg/ml (10-ml vials)
For IV infusion: 1 g/2-ml vial
Indication: Ventricular arrhythmias (not responding to lidocaine)

Dose and Route of Administration

Give in increments of 100 mg IV *slowly* over a 5-minute period until:

i) The arrhythmia is suppressed
ii) Hypotension occurs
iii) The QRS complex widens by ≥ 50%
iv) A total loading dose of 1000 mg has been given

> (An alternate loading regimen is to mix 500–1000 mg of drug in 100 ml of D5W and infuse this over 30–60 min.)

Following IV loading, a continuous infusion at 2 mg/min (1–4 mg/min range) may be needed to maintain the effect.

Comments

Procainamide is a type IA antiarrhythmic agent with similar properties to quinidine. Consequently, it decreases both conduction velocity and automaticity and is effective in treatment of *both* atrial and ventricular arrhythmias. In the setting of cardiac arrest, procainamide is the second drug of choice (after lidocaine) for treatment of frequent and complex PVCs (including ventricular tachycardia).

PROPRANOLOL (INDERAL)

How Dispensed: 1 mg/1-ml vial

Indications: Extremely limited in the acute care setting—refractory ventricular arrhythmias (especially if due to acute ischemia, increased sympathetic discharge, or digitalis toxicity), supraventricular tachyarrhythmias (drug of 3rd choice after verapamil and digoxin)

The use of propranolol for the acute treatment of supraventricular tachyarrhythmias has dramatically dropped off with the increased popularity of verapamil. Moreover, once IV verapamil has been tried, IV propranolol is *contraindicated* for at least the next 30 minutes, since the combination of these agents may result in marked cardiac slowing or even asystole.

Propranolol is contraindicated in patients with bronchospasm, congestive heart failure, and intraventricular conduction disturbances.

Dose and Route of Administration

Administer 1 mg IV *slowly* over at least a 5-minute period (not exceeding 1 mg/min!). Allow several minutes for the drug to work. Repeat increments of 1 mg may be given up to a total dose of 5 mg.

Comments

Propranolol is a nonselective beta-blocking agent. The drug decreases automaticity, reduces the sinus rate of discharge, and prolongs AV conduction time. Despite these beneficial actions, IV propranolol is rarely used any more in the acute care setting. *However, there may be instances when this agent is actually the drug of choice for the treatment of ventricular tachyarrhythmias!*

Mason et al. (1986) recently reported on three patients with cardiac arrest in whom ventricular fibrillation was preceded by a period of ventricular tachycardia. In each of the patients, evidence of increased *sympathetic* tone (in the form of markedly elevated systolic blood pressure) was present when the subjects were in sinus rhythm and/or sinus tachycardia. Despite the failure of conventional antiarrhythmic therapy, IV propranolol (2–5 mg) allowed successful conversion and maintenance of normal sinus rhythm in each case.

Other case reports have documented striking ST segment changes on Holter monitoring prior to development of ventricular fibrillation. This suggests that in addition to alterations in autonomic tone, ischemia may play a role in precipitating cardiac arrest in certain individuals (Denes et al., 1981). IV propranolol would seem to be an ideal agent for treating ventricular tachyarrhythmias in such individuals.

We are *not* advocating IV propranolol for treatment of all ventricular tachyarrhythmias in the setting of cardiac arrest. Clearly, lidocaine is the drug of first choice for this indication, and either procainamide or bretylium are next in line. However, in certain select circumstances (patients with ventricular tachyarrhythmias refractory to other agents in whom evidence for increased sympathetic activity or underlying acute ischemia exists), a trial of IV propranolol may prove to be lifesaving.

MISCELLANEOUS DRUGS

FUROSEMIDE (LASIX)

How Dispensed: Ampules of 20 mg and 100 mg

Indications: Acute pulmonary edema, congestive heart failure, hypertensive emergencies, other edema states

Dose and Route of Administration

The usual initial dose for pulmonary edema is 40–80 mg IV. Double this dose if there is no clinical response within an hour.

Some patients who have never received furosemide before will be exquisitely sensitive to the effects of the drug. In such individuals, 20 mg IV may be all that is needed to produce a brisk (and profound) diuresis. In contrast, much higher doses (sometimes up to 160 mg) may be needed in patients with poor renal function to achieve diuresis.

Comments

Furosemide is a potent loop diuretic. As such it inhibits tubular resorption of sodium chloride in the ascending loop of Henle.

Following IV administration, diuresis begins within 5–15 minutes, peaks at 30 minutes, and continues for approximately 2 hours. However the drug's initial therapeutic effect in pulmonary edema stems *not* from this diuresis but rather from its ability to rapidly reduce preload by increasing venous capacitance (Genton and Jaffe, 1986).

> In general, furosemide is well absorbed orally and works almost as well as the IV preparation. Diuresis following oral ingestion usually begins within 1 hour, peaks by 1–2 hours, and continues for 4–8 hours. However, if right-sided heart failure predominates, intestinal absorption may be impaired (due to edema of the gut). When such patients are admitted to the hospital, IV furosemide should be administered.

NALOXONE (NARCAN)

How Dispensed: 0.4 mg/ml (1-ml ampules [= 0.4 mg] and 10-ml vials [= 4 mg])

Indications: None in the setting of cardiac arrest (unless narcotic overdose is suspected as a precipitating cause)

Dose and Route of Administration

For suspected narcotic overdose—2.0 mg IV
For shock—?

Comments

Among the most intriguing concepts to come along in recent years is the possibility that the narcotic antagonist naloxone might be beneficial in treatment of cardiac arrest.

> The theory is based on the properties of *endorphins*. These endogenous opiate like substances are produced by the pituitary gland and released in the body in response to physiologic stress states. Because endorphins are known to lower peripheral vascular resistance and exert a myocardial depressant effect, it is thought that they may play a role in

various shock states. By extension they might also be operative in cardiac arrest, since this condition can be viewed as "the ultimate shock state" (Rothstein et al., 1985).

If release of endorphins is at least partially responsible for the myocardial and peripheral vascular depression of cardiac arrest, might these effects not be reversed by administration of naloxone? Although animal studies suggest that this may occur, clinical studies in humans have failed to demonstrate improved survival when patients in shock are treated with naloxone (Reynolds et al., 1980; Wilson, 1985, Benton, 1985).

Most published reports on the use of naloxone in shock are retrospective case studies in which the drug had been used to treat patients with sepsis after conventional therapy had failed. Little prospective work has been done in the setting of cardiac arrest. Rothstein et al. (1985) examined the effects of the drug after inducing ventricular fibrillation in mongrel dogs. Although naloxone was not found to be helpful in facilitating defibrillation, animals who developed EMD recovered after receiving the drug.

At the present time, *there appears to be no indication for the use of naloxone in the setting of cardiac arrest* (unless narcotic overdose is suspected as a precipitating cause). One should be aware that the doses of naloxone used in the study by Rothstein et al. (1985) were massive (5 mg/kg!). Much more work will need to be done in a prospective manner in human subjects in order to validate their findings. Nonetheless the prospect of being able to treat EMD by narcotic antagonism is fascinating indeed.

CORTICOSTEROIDS

How Dispensed:

Methylprednisolone (Solu-Medrol)—available in 40-mg, 125-mg, 500-mg, and 1000-mg packages with diluent attached

Dexamethasone (Decadron)—vials of 1 ml (4 mg), 5 ml (20 mg), and 25 ml (100 mg)

Indications: None in the setting of cardiac arrest (unless other potentially steroid-responsive conditions are felt to be present)

Dose and Route of Administration ???
Comments

The issue of whether high-dose corticosteroids should be administered to patients in shock fuels a controversy that extends well beyond the scope of this book. However, the question of whether they should be used to treat *pulseless idioventricular rhythm (PIVR)* is pertinent to the interests of the emergency care provider managing cardiac arrest.

> The postulated mechanism of action for corticosteroids is stabilization of myocardial membranes, limiting leakage of lysosomal enzymes and ischemic damage. Moreover, it is felt that steroids may facilitate release of ATP from myocardial mitochondria in a manner that makes ATP more available for the sodium/potassium pump, thus restoring membrane polarization and impulse conduction (Carden, 1984).

Clinically, initial enthusiasm for using corticosteroids stemmed from a report by White in 1976 that the drug was successful in resuscitating five patients with PIVR. Although a few additional reports followed, no studies confirming successful treatment of PIVR with steroids have been published since 1979 (Paris et al., 1984; Carden, 1984).

> Retrospective analysis of subjects responding to steroids in earlier studies suggests that other variables (such as septic shock and cerebral hematoma) may have accounted for some of the success in treatment. Only a minority of patients who responded appear to have arrested because of cardiac disease.

In summary, although a theoretical basis for the use of corticosteroids with PIVR may exist, this has *not* been borne out by clinical studies in recent years. Their use for this indication is not recommended.

MAGNESIUM SULFATE

How Dispensed: 5 g/10 ml:

   10% solution—10-ml ampules (5 g) and 20-ml ampules (10 g)

   50% solution—2-ml ampules (1 g) and 10-ml ampules (5 g)

Indications: Cardiac arrhythmias in the acute care setting that occur in patients who are likely to be hypomagnesemic, particularly if conventional measures have failed

Dose and Route of Administration

For life-threatening arrhythmias—Give 4 g (33 mEq of $MgSO_4$) of the 10% solution IV over 4 minutes, followed by an additional 10 g (81 mEq) as 50% solution given IM.

> When giving magnesium IV, 1 ampule of *calcium chloride* (10 ml of a 10% solution) should be available for IV injection should signs of magnesium overdose (hypotension, hyporeflexia, decreased respirations) occur.

Symptomatic non-life-threatening hypomagnesemia—Give 1–2 g (8–16 mEq) of 50% $MgSO_4$ IM, q.d. for several days.

Comments

Magnesium is "the forgotten cation."

> Because serum magnesium levels are not routinely included as part of the automated chemistry profile at most institutions, hypomagnesemia commonly goes unrecognized. It appears to be present much more frequently than is generally appreciated and has been found in more than 20% of hospitalized patients who have another associated electrolyte disorder such as hypokalemia, hypophosphatemia, hyponatremia, or hypocalcemia (Whang et al., 1984). Other patients at increased risk of having hypomagnesemia include those with a history of alcohol abuse, malnourished patients, and patients on digitalis or diuretics (Graber et al., 1981; Whang et al., 1984; Whang et al., 1985).

Clinically, hypomagnesemia may produce similar cardiovascular effects (and arrhythmias) as hypokalemia. However, little has been written about its role in the setting of cardiac arrest. Although, practically speaking, indications for the use of magnesium in such circumstances are rare, one may want to consider the drug for patients at high risk of being hypomagnesemic if they have not responded to more conventional measures.

> Two particular instances in which life-threatening arrhythmias may respond to therapy with mag-

nesium are digitalis-toxic arrhythmias and torsades de pointes (Cohen and Kitzes, 1983; Tzivoni et al., 1984).

REFERENCES

American Heart Association Subcommittee on Emergency Cardiac Care: Standards and guidelines for cardiopulmonary resuscitation (CPR) and emergency cardiac care (ECC). JAMA 255:2905–2992, 1986.

Bernton EW: Naloxone and TRH in the treatment of shock and trauma: What future roles? Ann Emerg Med 14:729–735, 1985.

Carden DL: High-dose corticosteroids in the treatment of pulseless idioventricular rhythm. Ann Emerg Med 13:817–819, 1984.

Cohen L, Kitzes R: Magnesium sulfate and digitalis—Toxic arrhythmias. JAMA 249:2808–2810, 1983.

Colucci WS, Wright RF, Braunwald E: New positive inotropic agents in the treatment of congestive heart failure: Mechanisms of action and recent clinical developments. N Engl J Med 314:290–299; 349–358, 1986.

Denes P, Gabster A, Huang SK: Clinical, electrocardiographic and follow-up observations in patients having ventricular fibrillation during Holter monitoring. Am J Cardiol 48:9–16, 1981.

Ferguson RK, Vlasses PH: Hypertensive emergencies and urgencies. JAMA 255:1607–1613, 1986.

Flaherty JT: Parenteral nitroglycerin: Clinical usefulness and limitations. In Conti CR (Ed): Cardiac Drug Therapy, Cardiovascular Clinics. F.A. Davis, Philadelphia, 1984, pp 111–118.

Frishman WH: Pharmacology of the nitrates in angina pectoris. Am J Cardiol 56:81–131, 1985.

Genton R, Jaffe A: Management of congestive heart failure in patients with acute myocardial infarction. JAMA 256:2556–2560, 1986.

Graber TW, Yee AS, Baker JF: Magnesium physiology, clinical disorders, and therapy. Ann Emerg Med 10:4957, 1981.

Intravenous amrinone for congestive heart failure. Med Lett Drugs Ther 26:104–105, 1984.

Mason JR, Marek JC, Loeb HS, Scanlon PJ: Intravenous propranolol in the treatment of repetitive ventricular tachyarrhythmias during resuscitation from sudden death. Am Heart J 110:161–165, 1985.

Paris PM, Stewart RD, Deggler F: Prehospital use of dexamethasone in pulseless idioventricular rhythm. Ann Emerg Med 13:1008–1010, 1984.

Rajfer SI, Anton AH, Rossen JD, Goldberg LI: Beneficial hemodynamic effects of oral levodopa in heart failure: Relation to the generation of dopamine. N Engl J Med 310:1357–1362, 1984.

Reynolds DG, Gurll NJ, Yargish T, Lechner RB, Faden AI, Holaday JW: Blockade of opiate receptors with naloxone improves survival and cardiac performance in canine endotoxic shock. Circ Shock 7:39–48, 1980.

Rothstein RJ, Niemann JT, Rennie CJ, Suddath WO, Rosborough JP: Use of naloxone during cardiac arrest and CPR: Potential adjunct for postcountershock electricalmechanical dissociation. Ann Emerg Med 14:198–203, 1985.

Tzivoni D, Keren A, Cohen A, Loebel H, Zahavi I, Cheyzbraun A, Stern S: Magnesium therapy for torsades de pointes. Am J Cardiol 53:528–530, 1984.

Whang R, Oei TO, Aikawa JK, Watanabe A, Vannatta J, Fryer A, Markanich M: Predictors of clinical hypomagnesemia, hypokalemia, hypophosphatemia, hyponatremia, and hypocalcemia. Arch Intern Med 144:1794–1796, 1984.

Whang R, Oei TO, Watanabe A: Frequency of hypomagnesemia in hospitalized patients receiving digitalis. Arch Intern Med 145:655–656, 1985.

White BC: Pulseless idioventricular rhythm during CPR: An indication for massive intravenous bolus glucocorticoids. JACEP 5:449–454, 1976.

Wilson RF: Science and shock: A clinical perspective. Ann Emerg Med 14:714–723, 1985.

Young GP: Calcium channel blockers in emergency medicine. Ann Emerg Med 13:712–722, 1984.

CHAPTER 15

DIFFERENTIATION OF PVCs FROM ABERRANCY

A: THEORY

One of the most difficult problems confronting those involved in emergency cardiac care is the differentiation of PVCs from aberrantly conducted beats. The issue is *not* merely academic. Whereas ventricular arrhythmias may be potentially life-threatening if not adequately controlled, supraventricular beats that conduct aberrantly are most often benign and can usually be safely observed without treatment.

How can one distinguish between PVCs and aberrancy? Is this differentiation reliable?

PROBLEM Consider the rhythms shown in **Figures 15A-1** and <u>15A-2</u>, taken from two patients admitted for acute myocardial infarction. Should one (or both) of these patients be treated for ventricular ectopy?

Only one of these patients needs to be treated, as we will see at the end of this chapter.

The purpose of this chapter is to furnish some guidelines with which one should be able to determine whether aberrancy or ventricular ectopy is present *most* of the time. It is important to emphasize that occasionally it may be impossible to make this distinction. In such cases, cor-

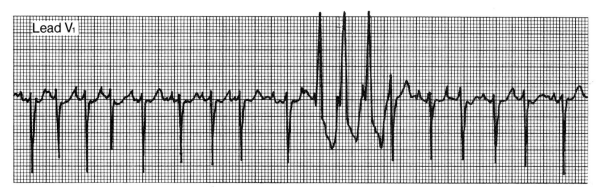

Figure 15A-1

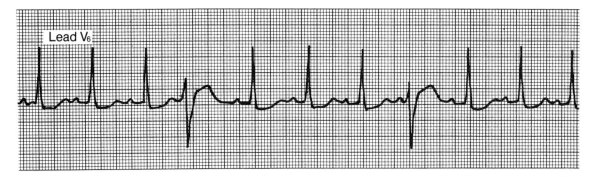

Figure 15A-2

relation of the arrhythmia to the clinical situation becomes critical. For example, the treatment of choice for a hemodynamically significant tachyarrhythmia is synchronized cardioversion *regardless* of whether the arrhythmia is supraventricular or ventricular in nature.

The burden of proof should always lie with demonstrating that an abnormal-appearing QRS complex is aberrant rather than the other way around. *A beat must be judged guilty (a PVC) until proved innocent!!* Application of the basic principles presented in this chapter (and frequent use of a pair of calipers) should make you much more comfortable in exercising this judgement.

Basic Rules for Differentiating PVCs from Aberrancy

The three most helpful findings for diagnosing aberration are the presence of the following:

 i) A *right-bundle branch block (RBBB) pattern* when the anomalous complex is viewed in a right-sided monitoring lead (lead V_1 or MCL_1).
 ii) A *similar initial deflection* of the anomalous and normally conducted beats
 iii) A *premature* P wave preceding the anomalous beat

These features are well illustrated in the aberrantly conducted complex shown in **Figure 15A-3.** Although beat no. 4 in this rhythm strip looks markedly different from the others, it manifests a *typical* RBBB pattern (an rSR′ in this right-sided lead), and its initial QRS deflection is in the same direction as for the normally conducted beats (upward). Inspection of the T wave immediately preceding beat no. 4 reveals extra peaking (compared to the normal T waves) due to a premature P wave.

> It is particularly important to note that with a *typical* RBBB pattern, the second positive deflection of the QRS complex (the R′) is taller than the initial positive deflection (the r)—the QRS has a *taller right rabbit ear*. When the *left* rabbit ear is taller

(when the QRS complex manifests an RSr′ configuration in which the initial R is taller than the r′), ventricular ectopy is suggested.

The reason aberrant beats most often conduct with an RBBB pattern is that the refractory period of the right bundle branch tends to be longer than that of the left bundle branch. Thus a premature impulse arriving at the ventricles will more likely find the right bundle branch still in a refractory state.

> In persons with a normal heart, the overwhelming majority of aberrantly conducted complexes manifest an RBBB pattern (with or without an accompanying hemiblock). Only a minority demonstrate a pure LBBB or isolated hemiblock pattern. Although the RBBB pattern of aberration is still the predominant one in the diseased heart, the other forms become relatively more important.

The initial deflection of aberrant beats frequently is similar to that of the normally conducted beats, since the initial portion of the conduction pathway is usually unaffected—the wave of depolarization is conducted normally until it encounters that part of the conduction system that is still refractory. Statistically one might imagine a 50% chance exists for any ventricular ectopic beat to manifest a similar initial deflection as the normally conducted beats. A beat can be directed in only one of two ways (up or down). Consequently, detection of a similar initial deflection supports the diagnosis of aberrancy but *in no way* rules out the possibility that the anomalous beat could be a PVC. On the other hand, finding that the initial deflection of an anomalous beat is *oppositely* directed to the initial QRS vector of the normally conducted beats favors ventricular ectopy.

> The usefulness of the similar initial deflection applies *only* to aberrant beats that conduct with a *pure* RBBB pattern. This is because the initial vector of conduction may be significantly altered if either an LBBB or mixed pattern of aberration (RBBB and left anterior or posterior hemiblock) is present.

The most convincing finding in favor of aberration is the identification of a *premature* P wave in the T wave preceding the anomalous QRS complex. This premature P wave is often not nearly as obvious as it is in Figure 15A-3,

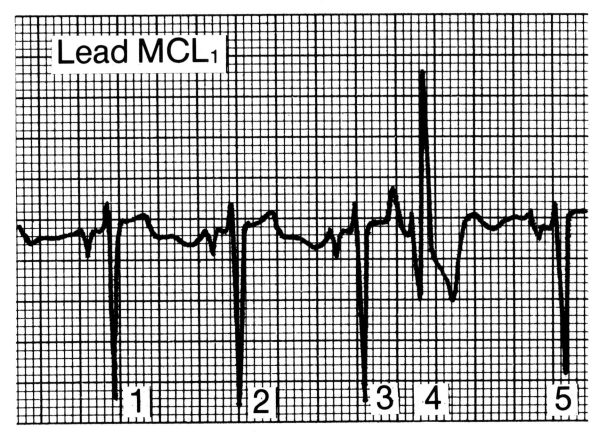

Figure 15A-3

and close scrutiny with careful comparison to the normal T wave may be needed to detect it.

It should be emphasized that *none* of the signs for differentiating between aberration and ventricular ectopy are perfect. Exceptions abound, and one often has to weigh one factor against another in making a judgement about the nature of conduction for any given case. Frequently the result is a *probability* statement rather than a definite determination. Occasionally, no matter how diligent one's efforts are, it will be absolutely impossible from the surface electrocardiogram to determine whether aberrancy or ventricular ectopy is present. *A major purpose of this chapter is to help the reader feel comfortable in knowing when such is the case.* Fortunately, most of the time enough clues *will* be pres-

ent to allow reliable differentiation between PVCs and aberrancy.

EXPLANATION FOR ABERRANCY

Supraventricular impulses arriving at the AV node may or may not be conducted to the ventricles. If the process of repolarization is complete and the conduction system has fully recovered, the impulse will be conducted normally. This would be the case for premature impulse C in **Figure 15A-4** (or for any supraventricular impulse occurring later in the cycle than impulse C).

If on the other hand, the premature impulse occurs very *early* during repolarization, it may

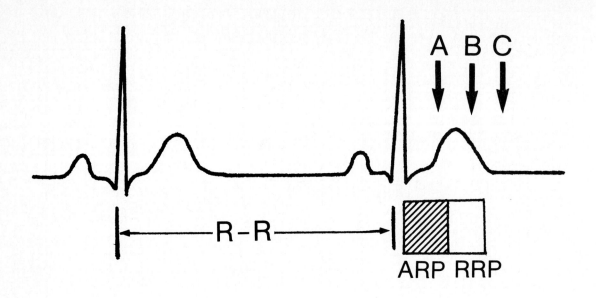

Figure 15A-4

find the ventricles unable to conduct the stimulus. This situation is represented by premature impulse A in **Figure 15A-4,** which occurs during the *absolute refractory period (ARP)*. Conduction is "blocked." Premature impulse B occurs at an intermediate point during the *relative refractory period (RRP)*. It is this impulse that conducts *aberrantly*, because it finds a portion of the conduction system still in a refractory state.

PROBLEM   Examine **Figure 15A-5. Is beat no. 10 a PVC? Why does this beat look different than beat no. 6? How can you explain the pause after beat no. 2?**

ANSWER TO FIGURE 15A-5   The underlying rhythm in this figure is sinus. Premature atrial contractions (PACs) notch the T waves of beats no. 2, 5, and 9. The PAC that occurs *earliest* (A in Fig. 15A-5) is *blocked*. This premature impulse has the shortest *coupling* interval and corresponds to impulse A in Figure 15A-4 (which occurs during the ARP). Beats no. 6 and 10 in Figure 15A-5 are *aberrantly* conducted, with the latter complex manifesting a greater degree of aberrancy. This is because premature impulse B occurs at an earlier point (it has a shorter coupling interval), when the conduction system is more refractory (corre-

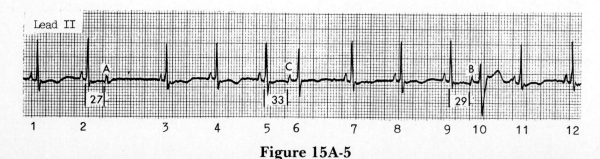

Figure 15A-5

Lead V$_1$

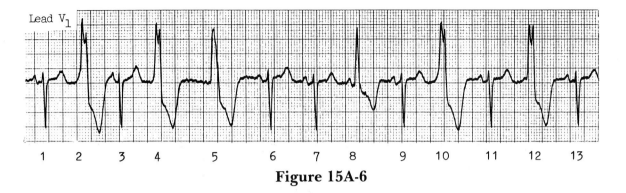

Figure 15A-6

sponding to premature impulse B in Fig. 15A-4). Premature impulse C probably occurs late in the RRP, with the result that beat no. 6 is conducted with only a minimal degree of aberrancy. Were this PAC to occur any later, it would most likely be conducted normally.

In contrast, all of the anomalous QRS complexes in **Figure 15A-6** (beats no. 2, 4, 5, 8, 10, and 12) occur at a later point in the cycle. One would not expect any of these beats to be aberrantly conducted, since they occur well after the T wave (at a time when one would expect the conduction system to have recovered fully). A key point to emphasize whenever one contemplates the diagnosis of aberrancy is the need to determine whether a *reason* exists for the altered conduction. Relatively short coupling intervals

explain the aberrant conduction of beats no. 6 and 10 in Figure 15A-5. Anomalous beats with long coupling intervals (such as those seen in Fig. 15A-6) don't have any "reason" to conduct aberrantly and are much more likely to be PVCs.

Several additional points may be brought out by analyzing Figure 15A-6. Note that beat no. 8 in this figure is preceded by a P wave. If a P wave precedes the beat, then why isn't it aberrant???

The answer is simply that the P wave preceding this beat is not *premature*—it is right on time! The fact that QRS complex no. 8 *is* preceded by a P wave actually represents strong supportive evidence that this beat must be a PVC. The normal PR interval in this tracing for the sinus-conducted beats (beats no. 1, 6, 7, 9, 11 and 13) is 0.14 second. Because the PR interval preceding beat no. 8 is significantly shorter than this, something else *(other than a sinus-conducted complex)* must have oc-

Lead V$_1$

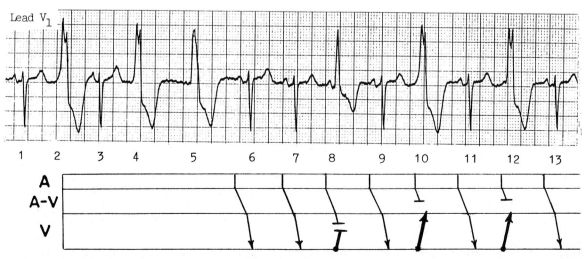

Figure 15A-7

curred *before* this atrial impulse could stimulate the ventricles—namely, a PVC.

Why do you suppose that beat no. 8 looks different from all of the other PVCs in this tracing? (The answer is supplied in the laddergram of **Fig. 15A-7.**)

Beat no. 8 looks different from the other PVCs because it represents the *fusion* of the supraventricular impulse with the PVC. That is, the P wave preceding beat no. 8 is able to conduct partially through the ventricles, but somewhere in its path it meets the wave of depolarization emanating from the PVC. The result (a *fusion* beat) manifests characteristics of both impulses.

Fusion beats are not that commonly seen, but when they do occur they provide overwhelming support for ventricular ectopy.

PROBLEM   **Apply what we have covered up to now to the example shown in Figure 15A-8, taken from a patient in a bigeminal rhythm. There are two abnormal-looking complexes present—beats no. 2 and 6. Are these PVCs, or are they aberrantly conducted?**

—a *premature* P wave (which in this case is a tiny negative deflection with a short PR interval seen just before the onset of the QRS complex)

Beats no. 2 and 6 are premature junctional contractions (PJCs) that conduct aberrantly.

PROBLEM   **Why doesn't beat no. 4 also conduct aberrantly?**

ANSWER   Beat no. 4 conducts normally because it has a longer coupling interval than the aberrantly conducted beats. The coupling interval of beats no. 1–2 and 5–6 is 0.59 second, whereas the coupling interval for beats no. 3–4 is 0.64 second.

Beat no. 4 occurs at a time when the ventricles have recovered, corresponding to premature impulse C in Figure 15A-4. In contrast, beats no. 2 and 6 occur during the RRP. They correspond to premature impulse B in Figure 15A-4 and are conducted to the ventricles with aberrancy.

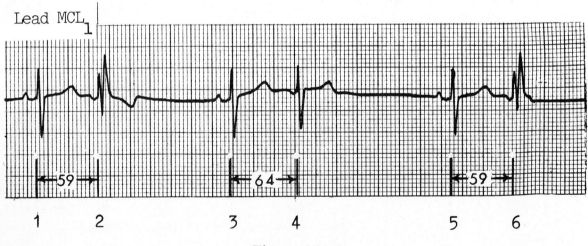

Figure 15A-8

ANSWER TO FIGURE 15A-8:   Beats no. 2 and 6 manifest the three most characteristic features of aberrancy:

—an RBBB pattern in a right-sided monitoring lead
—an initial deflection similar to that of the normally conducted beats

There is thus a *reason* for the aberrancy seen in Figure 15A-8—the premature beats that conduct aberrantly (beats no. 2 and 6) have a shorter coupling interval than the premature beat that conducts normally (beat no. 4).

The type of analysis described above in which one carefully examines coupling intervals to assist in determining if aberration is present is known as *cycle-sequence comparison*. Although the method is not foolproof, it usually works and can be extremely helpful in explaining why some beats in a rhythm strip conduct normally while others conduct with aberration. Use of cycle-sequence comparison in addition to the morphologic features noted above provides *incontrovertible evidence* that beats no. 2 and 6 in Figure 15A-8 are not PVCs!

The Ashman Phenomenon

In addition to the coupling interval, another important determinant of aberrancy is the R-R interval that precedes the anomalous beat in question. This concept is explained in **Figure 15A-9.**

As previously discussed, premature impulses occurring during the ARP are blocked, whereas

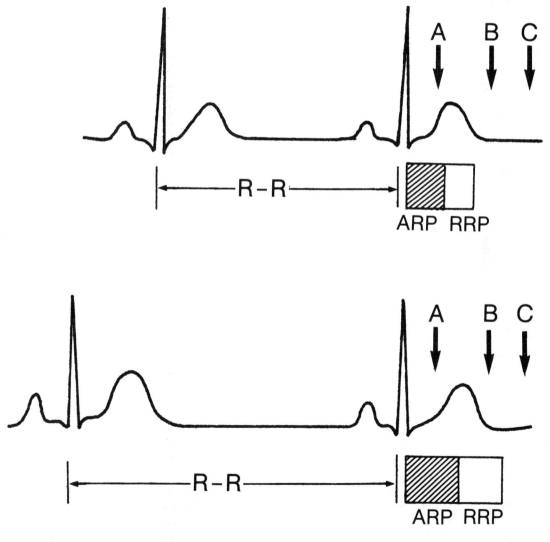

Figure 15A-9

those that occur after repolarization is complete are conducted normally. Premature impulses occurring during the RRP conduct with aberrancy. Thus in the upper panel of Figure 15A-9, premature impulse A is blocked but B and C are conducted normally.

Whether a premature impulse occurs within the RRP and conducts aberrantly is also determined by the length of the R-R interval *preceding* the anomalous beat. *The duration of the refractory period is directly proportional to the length of the preceding R-R interval.* When the heart rate is slowed (as it is in the lower panel of Fig. 15A-9), *both* the ARP and the RRP are prolonged. Premature impulse A is still blocked, and impulse C is still conducted normally. However, impulse B, which previously occurred after the completion of repolarization, now occurs *during* the RRP and is therefore conducted with aberrancy. This is known as the *Ashman phenomenon,* which simply stated says that *the most aberrant beat is most likely to follow the longest pause.*

PROBLEM   **Use the Ashman phenomenon to explain why beat no. 4 in Figure 15A-10 conducts aberrantly, whereas beat no. 6 does not.**

ANSWER TO FIGURE 15A-10   Both of these beats occur prematurely with approximately the same coupling interval, yet the R-R interval preceding beat no. 4 (the R-R interval between beats no. 2-3) is clearly longer than the R-R interval preceding beat no. 6 (the R-R interval between beats no. 4-5). In other words, *the most aberrant beat* (beat no. 4) *follows the longest pause.*

The Ashman phenomenon may be extremely useful diagnostically for patients in sinus rhythm. However, one should be aware that it is of uncertain value for patients with atrial fibrillation. This is because the length of the R-R interval in atrial fibrillation is constantly influenced by *concealed* conduction (variable penetration of atrial impulses through the AV node), so that it no longer accurately reflects the duration of the subsequent refractory period.

Compensatory Pauses

A frequently cited diagnostic criterion for ventricular ectopy is the finding of a full *compensatory pause.* In adults, PVCs usually do not conduct retrograde to the atria. Consequently, the sinoatrial (SA) node most often continues to discharge at its previous rate unaffected by ventricular ectopic activity. The P wave that follows the PVC (P′ in the upper panel of **Fig. 15A-11**) occurs precisely on time, and the pause containing the PVC is *twice* the duration of the normal sinus cycle (58 + 92 = 150 = 75 × 2).

In contrast, a PAC depolarizes the rest of the atria and resets the sinus cycle. Consequently, the pause containing a PAC would not be ex-

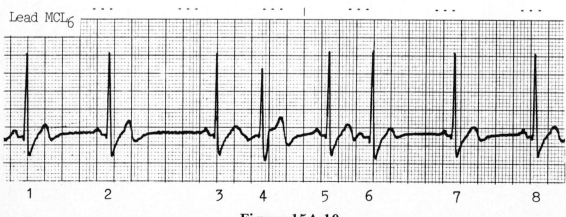

Figure 15A-10

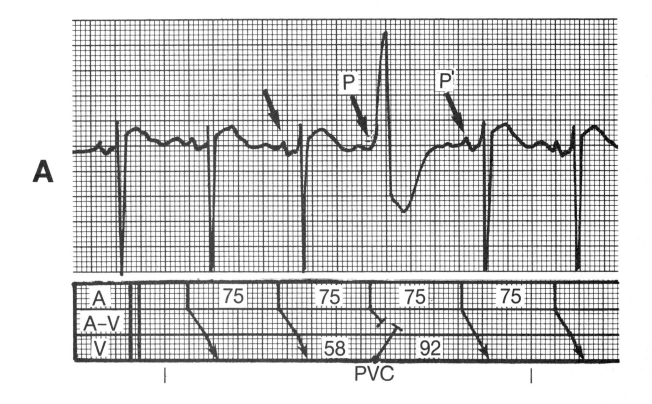

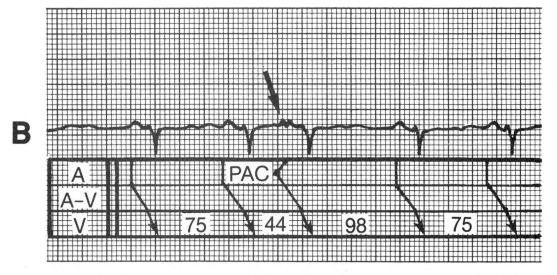

Figure 15A-11

pected to equal twice the duration of the sinus cycle ($44 + 98 = 142 \neq 75 \times 2$ in the lower panel of Fig. 15A-11).

> Determining whether or not a full compensatory pause exists may be an additional helpful point in differentiating PVCs from aberrantly conducted beats. However, caution must be advised! PVCs sometimes *do* conduct retrograde to the atria, in which case they will reset the sinus cycle. Furthermore, a PAC can arise from a site in one of the atria that *by chance* lies at a distance such that the time required to depolarize the atria and reset the SA node coincidentally equals twice the normal R-R interval. Consequently, PVCs *do not always demonstrate a full compensatory pause, whereas PACs may occasionally do so.* One therefore cannot depend solely on the presence or absence of a compensatory pause but rather should use this information in the context of the other characteristics of the abnormal beat before deciding on its etiology.

QRS Morphology

Analysis of QRS morphology may be among the most useful aids in differentiating between PVCs and aberrancy. As discussed earlier, the finding of a *typical* RBBB pattern (rSR′ with taller *right* rabbit ear) in a right-sided monitoring lead strongly suggests aberrancy. Thus in the example shown in **Figure 15A-12,** taken from a

patient in atrial flutter, beats no. 4, 5, 6, and 9 are much more likely to be aberrantly conducted than ventricular ectopics. Each of these beats manifests an rSR′ configuration with a taller right rabbit ear (the R′ of each complex is taller than the initial r).

In contrast, the rabbit ear for beat no. 6 in **Figure 15A-13** is taller on the *left*—this strongly suggests that the beat is a PVC.

These and other morphologic features helpful in differentiating between PVCs and aberrancy are summarized in **Table 15A-1.**

PVCs originate more often from the *left* ventricle than from the right. In general, such left ventricular PVCs tend to manifest a predominant R wave in right-sided monitoring leads. Attention to morphologic features of the QRS complex in leads V_1 or MCL_1 greatly assists in differentiating left ventricular PVCs from aberrantly conducted beats.

> As we have already suggested, the finding of an rSR′ pattern (taller *right* rabbit ear) in a right-sided monitoring lead (V_1, MCL_1) strongly favors aberrancy. A point to emphasize is that for this morphologic clue to be valid, the S wave must *at least* come back down to the baseline (patterns A and B in Table 15A-1). If the S wave does not return to the baseline (pattern G) or if it simply produces a "slur" in the upstroke of the R wave (F), then mor-

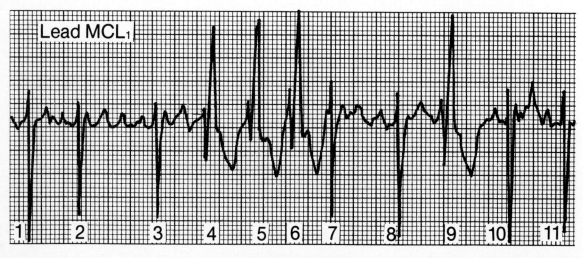

Figure 15A-12

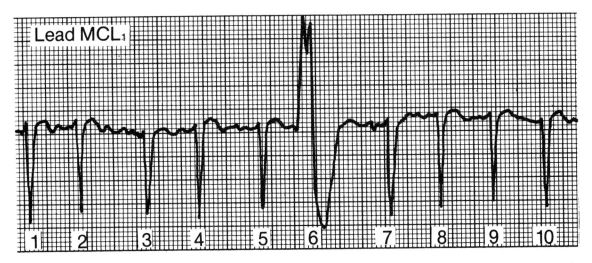

Figure 15A-13

phology is of absolutely no help in differentiation. If on the other hand, the R wave in lead V_1 or MCL_1 is monophasic (pattern C), is preceded by a small q wave (D), or has a taller *left* rabbit ear (E), ventricular ectopy is strongly favored.

Left-sided monitoring leads (leads V_6 and MCL_6) are often neglected in morphologic evaluation of anomalous complexes. This is unfortunate since they may sometimes provide the only clues to the diagnosis.

> The finding of a triphasic qRS pattern (H in the table) in a left-sided monitoring lead represents the *reciprocal* of an rSR′ configuration in a right-sided monitoring lead and carries the same diagnostic implication. (It is extremely unusual for a PVC to manifest a small q wave in a left-sided monitoring lead.) Perhaps even more useful is the finding of a QS (totally negative QRS complex) in lead V_6 or MCL_6 (I). This is almost always due to ventricular ectopy. If instead of being totally negative, a small r wave precedes a deep S wave (J), the finding still suggests ventricular ectopy but is less diagnostic (since patterns such as left anterior hemiblock may produce a similar morphology in lead V_6 or MCL_6). Intermediate patterns when both the R wave and S wave are of substantial amplitude (K) are of no diagnostic benefit.

PVCs that originate from the *right* ventricle are generally less common than left ventricular

PVCs but may pose more of a problem in differentiation. Right ventricular PVCs tend to manifest a predominantly *negative* complex in leads V_1 or MCL_1 that may look surprisingly similar to the normally conducted beats. None of the morphologic clues offered in Table 15A-1 are applicable. Moreover, it may be exceedingly difficult to differentiate between right ventricular PVCs and supraventricular complexes that conduct with the less common LBBB form of aberration. Consider the next two examples.

PROBLEM   Examine **Figure 15A-14**. Are beats no. 3 and 12 PVCs or aberrant?

ANSWER TO FIGURE 15A-14   The underlying rhythm is sinus. Because of a resemblance in the waveform of the anomalous and the sinus-conducted beats (both types of complexes manifest an rS morphology) and a similar initial deflection, one might be tempted to diagnose beats no. 3 and 12 as supraventricular with aberrant conduction. Several factors weigh against this.

First, the setting is *not* ideal for aberrancy, since these beats are not terribly premature (they occur well after the termination of the preceding T wave.) Moreover, they are wide (0.14

TABLE 15A-1   DIFFERENTIATION OF PVCs FROM ABERRANCY

ECG leads	Favors aberrancy	Favors ventricular ectopy	No help in differentiation
Morphologic features Lead V_1 or MCL_1	+++ **A** **B** rSR′ pattern (A, B) with taller right rabbit ear (and S wave at least returning to baseline)	+++ **C** **D** **E** R wave (C), qR (D), or slurred R wave (E) with taller left rabbit ear	+/− **F** **G** Slurred R wave (F) with taller right rabbit ear, or rsR′ (G) where the s wave doesn't return to the baseline
Lead V_6 or MCL_6	++ **H** qRS (H) pattern (the reciprocal of the rSR′ in V_1	+++ **I** + **J** QS (I) or rS (J) pattern	+/− **K** RS (K) pattern

Other features	Favors aberrancy	Favors ventricular ectopy	
Most leads	+ QRS duration ≤0.12	+ QRS duration >0.14	
Any leads	+ Similar initial deflection of anomalous beats to normally conducted beats	++ Opposite initial deflection of anomalous beats to normally conducted beats	
Any leads	+++ Presence of *premature* P wave	+ Absence of any preceding P wave	
Any leads		+++ Presence of preceding P wave that is *not* premature	
Any leads	+ Absence of compensatory pause	+ Presence of compensatory pause	
Any leads		+++ AV dissociation or fusion beats (both are uncommon)	
All of the precordial leads (V_{1-6})		+++ QRS concordance in *all* precordial leads (uncommon)	

+++ Strongly favoring

++ Moderately favoring

+ Slightly favoring

+/− No help in differentiation

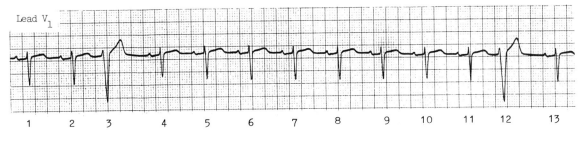

Figure 15A-14

second), are not preceded by a premature P wave, and occur in the middle of a full compensatory pause. Finally, the finding of a similar initial deflection is *only* valid when an RBBB pattern is present in lead V_1! Taken together (and in the absence of any compelling reasons for aberrancy), these factors weigh heavily for ventricular ectopy. Beats no. 3 and 12 are *right* ventricular PVCs.*

An additional subtle clue is present on this tracing. Careful inspection of the initial deflection of the PVC reveals that it is slightly *broader* than the r wave of the normally conducted beats. It is distinctly unusual for an aberrantly conducted complex to alter the initial deflection of the r wave in a right-sided lead in this way.

PROBLEM   **Now examine Figure 15A-15. Do beats no. 7–9 represent a salvo (3 PVCs in a row), or are they aberrantly conducted?**

ANSWER TO FIGURE 15A-15   Once again morphology is of no assistance, as the QRS complex for the anomalous beats is of an LBBB pattern (predominantly negative in lead V_1) and very similar to that of the normally conducted beats. However, a *premature* P wave *is* present (it notches the T wave that precedes

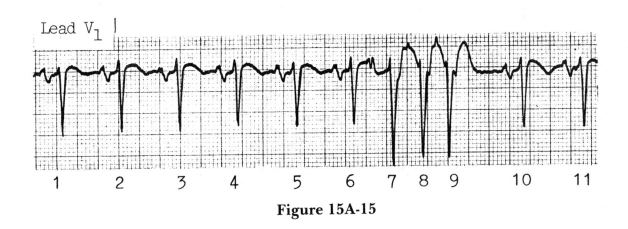

Figure 15A-15

---

*Reference to PVCs as being *left* ventricular or *right* ventricular in origin is helpful in understanding the morphologic appearance of these types of complexes. In general, left ventricular PVCs tend to manifest a predominant R wave in leads V_1 or MCL_1 because these beats originate in the left ventricle and travel in a *rightward* direction (toward leads V_1 and MCL_1). In contrast, right ventricular PVCs tend to manifest a predominantly negative complex in leads V_1 or MCL_1 because after originating in the right ventricle these beats travel *away* from these leads. Strictly speaking, the origin of PVCs cannot always be identified by morphologic appearance.

beat no. 7), and QRS duration of the anomalous complexes does not appear markedly widened (0.11 second in this lead), making it extremely likely that beats no. 7–9 are aberrantly conducted (in this case with an *LBBB pattern of aberration*).

QRS DURATION

Return for a moment to Figure 15A-13. As discussed earlier, morphologic characteristics alone are enough to suggest that beat no. 6 is a PVC. Two other features offer additional support. First, the QRS complex of beat no. 6 begins with a tiny negative deflection that is *opposite* to the initial positive deflection of the normally conducted beats. Second, the QRS duration of beat no. 6 is *at least* 0.16 second. *QRS duration exceeding 0.14 second favors the diagnosis of ventricular ectopy.* Relatively narrow QRS complexes (≤0.11 second) are more likely to be due to aberrancy.

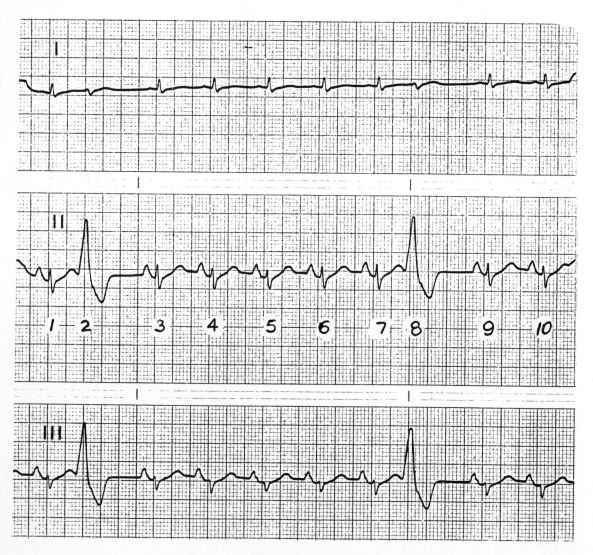

Figure 15A-16

A word of caution is in order. The appearance of a PVC may vary markedly, depending on which lead is used to monitor the patient. Thus a premature beat that looks to be narrow (supraventricular) in one lead may appear much wider and more bizarre (suggesting ventricular ectopy) when viewed from another perspective.

This point is made abundantly clear in **Figure 15A-16,** which shows the simultaneous recording of a rhythm strip from leads I, II, and III. Beats no. 2 and 8 in leads II and III are obviously much wider than the normally conducted beats in these leads. One should have little difficulty in recognizing these as PVCs. However, the same beats in lead I look surprisingly narrow. If this were the only mon-itoring lead available, it would not be at all apparent that beats no. 2 and 8 were PVCs.

The importance of examining an anomalous beat in more than one lead is further emphasized by **Figure 15A-17,** taken from a patient who is in ventricular bigeminy. The arrows indicate the PVCs in each lead. Note that ectopic morphology varies greatly. One certainly would have no difficulty identifying the PVCs in leads I, III, aVR, aVL, V_1, and V_6. The QRS is bizarre in shape and significantly wider than the normally conducted beats in each of these leads.

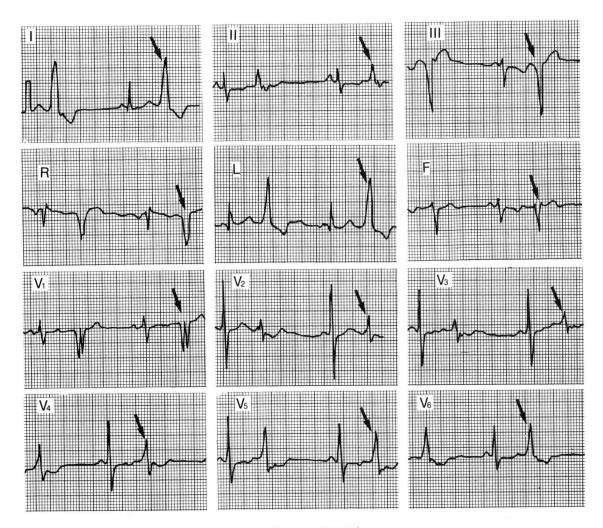

Figure 15A-17

Identification of the bigeminal beats as PVCs is not nearly as apparent from inspection of leads II, aVF, V_2, and V_3. In particular in leads V_2 and V_3, the normally conducted QRS complexes are of much greater amplitude than the beats that follow them and might be mistaken for PVCs if one did not see a preceding P wave. Furthermore in leads V_3 through V_6, notching in the T wave simulates a premature P wave in front of the PVCs.

> Because the anomalous complexes in this example do not manifest an RBBB pattern, attention to the initial deflection is of *no* help in differentiation. It can be seen that in some leads the initial deflection of anomalous beats is in the same direction as the normally conducted beats, whereas it is in the opposite direction in other leads.

Recognition of Aberrancy in Atrial Fibrillation

Differentiation of PVCs from aberrancy is especially difficult in the setting of atrial fibrillation. The reason is twofold. First, because of the loss of organized atrial activity, P waves are no longer evident on the ECG. Consequently, the important differentiating feature of identifying a premature P wave is lost.

Second, the Ashman phenomenon is of uncertain validity in the presence of atrial fibrillation, since the length of the R-R interval is constantly being influenced by concealed conduction. Fortunately, the *irregularity* of the atrial fibrillation itself provides an important clue.

PROBLEM   **Examine the abnormal beats in Figures 15A-18 and 15A-19, taken from two patients who are completely asymptomatic. Is ventricular ectopy likely to be present in one or both of these tracings?**

ANSWER TO FIGURE 15A-18   The string of seven abnormally wide beats toward the end of this rhythm strip at least initially suggests a run of ventricular tachycardia. However, the rhythm remains irregularly irregular throughout the entire strip *irrespective* of the width of the QRS complex. Since *ventricular tachycardia tends to be a fairly regular rhythm,* the gross irregularity present here favors aberrancy, although one cannot be certain from this tracing alone. Analysis of QRS morphology is not helpful in differentiation of PVCs from aberrancy in a standard lead II as was used here. The patient remained asymptomatic and demonstrated wide complexes with a typical aberrant morphology when switched to a right-sided monitoring lead.

ANSWER TO FIGURE 15A-19   Atrial fibrillation is again evident from the lack of P waves and the erratic baseline. A wide and bizarre QRS complex occurs every other beat but, whereas the underlying rhythm is irregularly irregular, the coupling interval of each bigeminal

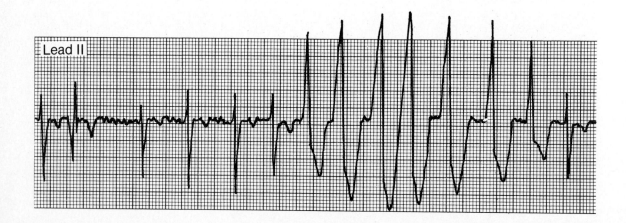

Figure 15A-18

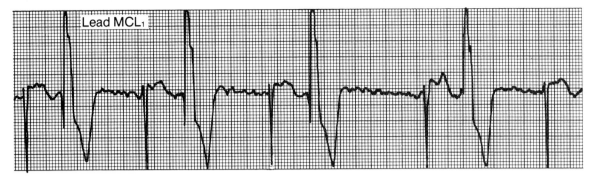

Figure 15A-19

beat is *fixed.* This suggests that these beats are PVCs, since one would expect aberrantly conducted beats to also be irregular when the underlying rhythm is atrial fibrillation. Other factors favoring ventricular ectopy are the width of this QRS complex (which is at least 0.15 second) and a "q-slur-R" configuration of the QRS, with a taller left rabbit ear and an initial negative deflection that is opposite that of the normally conducted beats. The patient was treated with lidocaine.

As a conclusion to this section, return to the question posed at the start regarding whether ventricular ectopy is present in <u>Figures 15A-1</u> and 15A-2.

ANSWER   It should now be clear that the two anomalous beats in Figure 15A-2 are PVCs. Although the initial deflection of these beats is similar to that of the normally conducted complexes, the duration of the QRS complex is greatly prolonged (to ≥0.15 second) and P waves can be seen to walk right through the tracing, resulting in a perfectly compensatory pause. The P wave that precedes the second of these abnormal beats is not a PAC (that conducts aberrantly) since the P wave is *not* premature. The QRS configuration is of an rS pattern that also suggests ventricular ectopy in this left-sided lead.

On the other hand, the three abnormal beats that appear in succession in Figure 15A-1 are aberrantly conducted. The three most helpful features for identifying aberrancy are evident:

an RBBB pattern, an initial deflection similar to that of the normally conducted beats, and a premature P wave that can be seen to produce a notch in the T wave immediately preceding the triplet. The underlying rhythm is multifocal atrial tachycardia (MAT) with an irregularly irregular rhythm but manifesting well-defined (albeit different) P waves in front of most QRS complexes. Finally, the Ashman phenomenon is present (the first aberrant beat in the tracing follows the longest pause).

B: A CHALLENGE In DIAGNOSIS: PVCs or ABERRANCY?

This section will offer you a chance to test your mettle! In it we have included a host of challenging rhythm strips that illustrate principles covered in the first part of this chapter. Many of these rhythms are *not* easy to identify— *we* still are not sure about some of them! Much more important than a yes or no answer—aberrant or not aberrant—is the rationale employed for arriving at one's conclusion. Appropriate management decisions (whether to treat, and if so how) can then be based on the patient's underlying diagnosis and clinical condition. Hemodynamic status permitting, more information (additional leads, reference to previous tracings, response to a vagal maneuver) may then be obtained if needed.

While completing this exercise you may find it impossible at times to be sure of *the answer*. To try and become comfortable at recognizing those times, it may be helpful to formulate your answers in the *relative certainty* you have about a particular diagnosis (definitely PVC, probably PVC, probably aberrant, cannot tell). You are on your own. . . .

PROBLEM   PVCs or aberrant?   **Figure 15B-1**

other beats because it manifests an *incomplete* RBBB pattern. Degree of confidence in diagnosis = 100%!

PROBLEM   Beat no. 4 in **Figure 15B-2** manifests an rsR′ pattern and is preceded by a P wave. Is it also aberrant?

ANSWER TO FIGURE 15B-2   No. Morphology is of absolutely *no* assistance in lead

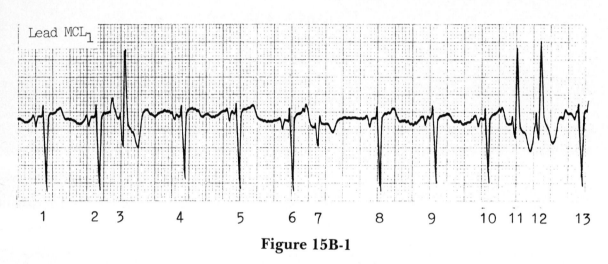

Figure 15B-1

ANSWER TO FIGURE 15B-1   The underlying rhythm is sinus. Beats no. 3, 11, and 12 are all *aberrantly* conducted. All manifest a typical RBBB pattern (rSR′ with a taller right rabbit ear) in this right-sided monitoring lead, with an identical initial deflection and a *premature* P wave (that notches the preceding T wave). Beat no. 7 is also aberrant. It is not as wide as the

II. It is only of use in right-sided (V_1, MCL_1) or left-sided (V_6, MCL_6) leads.

Although a P wave does precede the anomalous beat in Figure 15B-2, it is *not* premature! **Figure 15B-2A** shows that this P wave is on time. The fact that the PR interval preceding beat no. 4 is so much shorter than the normal PR interval (which is 0.24 second in this rhythm strip) is in-

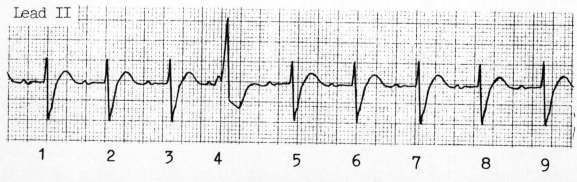

Figure 15B-2

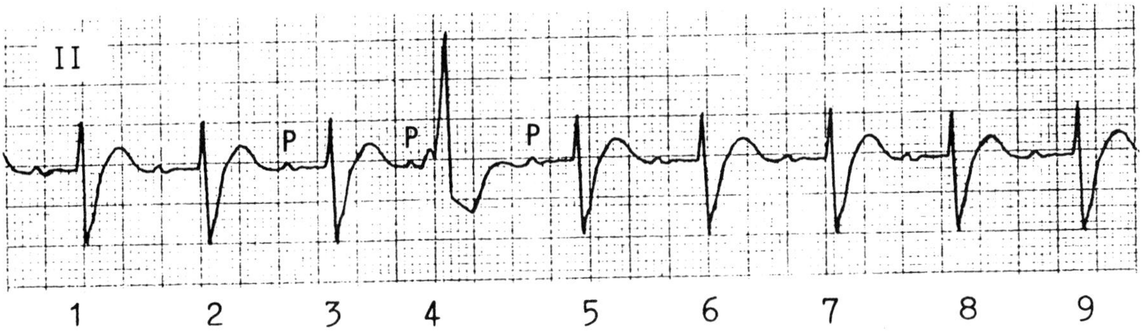

Figure 15B-2A

controvertible evidence that *something* must have occurred before the normal atrial impulse could conduct—*proving* that beat no. 4 is a PVC.

PROBLEM **PVC or aberrant? Figure 15B-3**

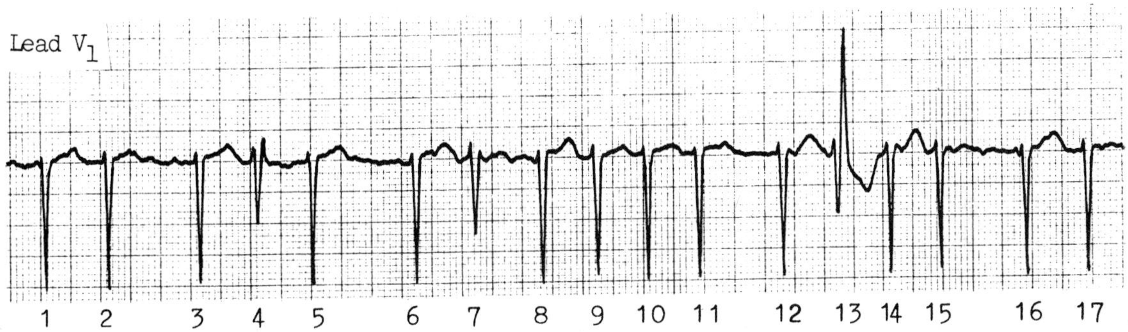

Figure 15B-3

ANSWER TO FIGURE 15B-3 The underlying rhythm here is atrial fibrillation. This eliminates the "premature P wave" as a criterion to look for in differentiating between PVCs and aberrancy. However, the morphology of beat no. 13 is so typical of *aberrancy* that one should feel comfortable making this diagnosis with 95% certainty. Beats no. 4 and 7 also are aberrant (they manifest an incomplete RBBB pattern).

Note the long-short sequence that precedes each of the aberrant beats. This is the Ashman phenomenon *(the funniest beat follows the longest pause)*. Although the Ashman phenomenon is not always reliable in the setting of atrial fibrillation (due to the unpredictable effect of concealed conduction from the numerous atrial impulses that bombard the AV node), it appears to be operative in this example. Cycle-sequence comparison explains why beat no. 17 does not conduct with aberrancy. Although also preceded by a relatively long R–R interval (the R-R interval between beats no. 15–16), the coupling interval of this complex (the distance between beats no. 16–17) is slightly greater than the coupling interval of the aberrantly conducted beats.

While cycle-sequence comparison is not always consistent in the presence of atrial fibrillation, it offers supportive evidence in this case that beats no. 4, 7, and 13 are aberrant.

PROBLEM **PVC or aberrant? Figure 15B-4**

ANSWER TO FIGURE 15B-4 Beat no. 4 is *definitely* a PVC. It is wide, bizarre, and morphologically very suggestive of a PVC. Confirmation of this impression is forthcoming from the P wave that precedes this beat—it is not premature, and the PR interval is too short to con-

Lead MCL₁

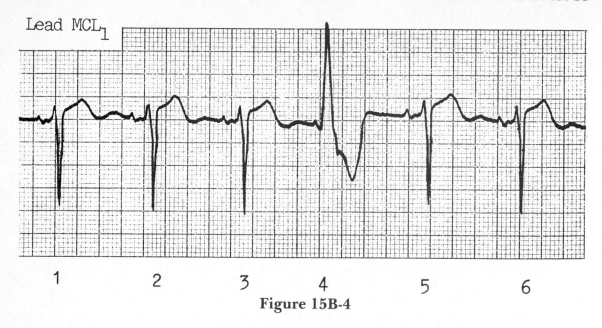

Figure 15B-4

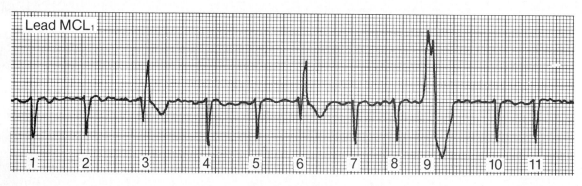

Figure 15B-5

duct. Thus, something must have arisen below the AV node (a PVC) before this atrial impulse could make its way to the ventricles.

PROBLEM **What are beats no. 3, 6, and 9 in <u>Figure 15B-5</u>?**

ANSWER TO FIGURE 15B-5 The underlying rhythm is atrial fibrillation. Beat no. 9 is *definitely* a PVC—it is very wide, bizarre, and manifests an ectopic morphology (taller left rabbit ear in this right-sided lead).

One is unable to be so certain about the etiology of beats no. 3 and 6. Although they manifest a suggestive morphology for aberrancy (rSR′ pattern with taller *right* rabbit ear and similar

initial deflection), confirmatory evidence is lacking because of an inability to identify atrial activity with atrial fibrillation. Of particular concern is that there really is no *reason* for beat no. 3 to be conducted with aberrancy—it occurs so *late* in the cycle, at a time when ventricular repolarization should long be over. We would have expected a beat like no. 11 to conduct aberrantly, as it has a much shorter coupling interval. *We hedge on our interpretation here*, pending more information (for example, additional rhythms strips).

The diagnosis of aberrancy is always made more confidently if a *reason* exists for aberrant conduction to occur. Thus in the previous example of atrial fibrillation reviewed (Fig. 15B-3), each of the anomalous beats (no. 4, 7, and 13) had short coupling intervals—and a reason to be aberrant. This is not the case with beats no. 3 and 6 in Figure 15B-5.

Beat no. 11 is unlike the other aberrantly conducted beats. It is wider and manifests a different morphology (it has an rS configuration)—for lack of evidence supporting aberrancy, one should assume it to be a PVC (*a beat is guilty until proved innocent!*).

PROBLEM PVCs, aberrant, or both? (Figure 15B-6

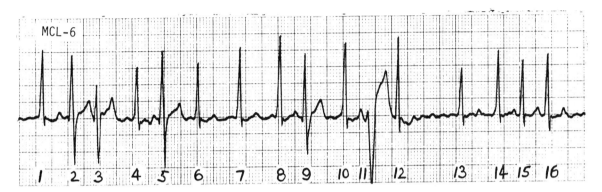

Figure 15B-6

ANSWER TO FIGURE 15B-6 Once again the underlying rhythm is atrial fibrillation, this time with a fairly rapid ventricular response. The normally conducted complexes have an Rs configuration in this *left*-sided monitoring lead. Beats no. 2, 3, 5, and 9 are all probably *aberrant*—they are fairly narrow (<0.12 second) and manifest a qRS configuration (which is the *reciprocal* of an rSR' configuration in a right-sided lead—see Table 15A-1 in the previous section). In addition, there is a *reason* for these beats to conduct aberrantly—they all have short coupling intervals compared to those beats that conduct normally.

The key point in this case is to treat the *underlying* disorder—atrial fibrillation with a fairly rapid ventricular response. Digitalization may be in order. Slowing the ventricular response will probably result in resolution of the anomalous complexes.

PROBLEM Are beats no. 3, 6, and 9 in Figure 15B-7 PVCs? (Note that their initial deflection is opposite that of the sinus beats.)

ANSWER TO FIGURE 15B-7 Despite the fact that the initial deflections of beats no. 3, 6, and 9 are oppositely directed to that of the sinus beats, there is incontrovertible evidence on this tracing that all of these beats are aber-

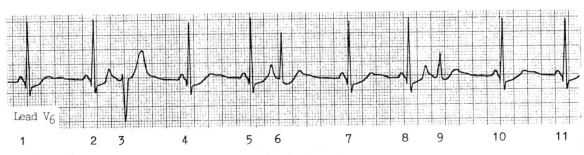

Figure 15B-7

Lead V$_6$

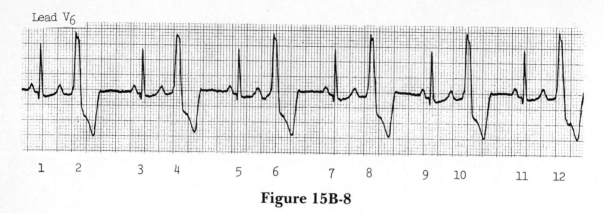

Figure 15B-8

rantly conducted. First is the fact that the QRS complex is not significantly widened. In addition, *each* of these beats is preceded by a premature P wave (that peaks the preceding T wave). Finally, *cycle-sequence comparison* is able to completely explain why beat no. 9 should conduct with a greater degree of aberrancy than beat no. 6 and why beat no. 3 is the most aberrant of all (the premature P wave occurs earliest after beat no. 2 and latest after beat no. 6).

PROBLEM   In **Figure 15B-8**, is a premature P wave hiding in the T wave before each of the anomalous beats?

ANSWER TO FIGURE 15B-8   There is really no way to tell for sure if a premature P wave is buried in the T wave of beats no. 1, 3, 5, 7, 9, and 11. This is because one never sees two sinus beats in a row. The even-numbered beats must be assumed to be ventricular—they are wide and bizarre in shape and manifest an oppositely directed initial deflection. In addition,

there are really no compelling reasons for aberrancy.

Figure 15B-8A was recorded from the same patient a little later. Now that two sinus beats occur in a row, one can compare the T wave preceding anomalous beats with the "normal" T wave. There is no deformity suggestive of premature atrial activity. Thus, Figure 15B-8 represents ventricular *bigeminy,* and Figure 15B-8A ventricular *trigeminy.*

PROBLEM   **Figures 15B-9** and **15B-10** were taken from a patient having an acute myocardial infarction. Based on the anomalous beats seen in these (and numerous other) rhythm strips, the patient was treated with lidocaine. Do you agree?

ANSWER TO FIGURES 15B-9 AND 15B-10   The underlying rhythm is sinus. The morphology of the anomalous beats seen in Figure 15B-9 is not of much assistance in the diagnosis, since the initial r wave is absent from

Lead V$_6$

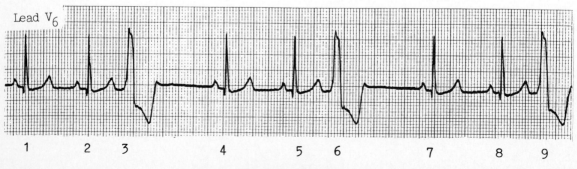

Figure 15B-8A

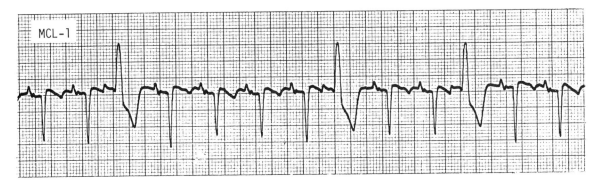

Figure 15B-9

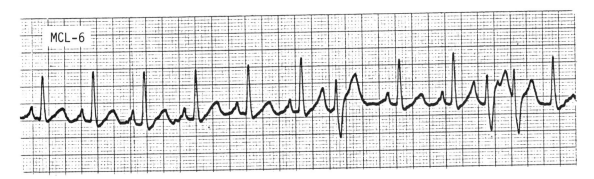

Figure 15B-10

both the sinus-conducted beats and the anomalous beats. A typical RBBB pattern might therefore not occur even in the face of aberrancy. However, *premature* P waves are definitely present and notch the T waves preceding each anomalous beat. This strongly suggests aberrancy.

This conclusion is further supported by notching of the T waves that precede the anomalous beats in the left-sided lead (Fig. 15B-10).

Figure 15B-10A was recorded subsequently. Again, note peaking of the T waves preceding beats no. 3, 7, and 9. Cycle-sequence comparison explains why beat no. 9 conducts nor-

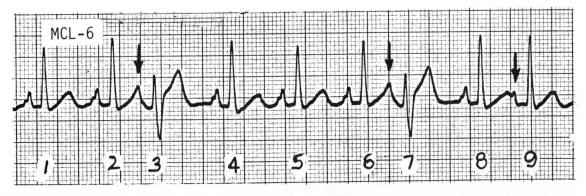

Figure 15B-10A

mally—its P wave occurs later in the refractory period than do the P waves preceding beats no. 3 and 7.

> The importance of differentiating between PVCs and aberrantly conducted beats in the setting of acute myocardial infarction is obvious—the former need to be treated (usually with lidocaine) and the latter do not. However, while premature supraventricular beats (PACs and PJCs) per se do *not* predispose a patient to developing ventricular fibrillation, their frequent occurrence is often a subtle sign of incipient heart failure.

Figure 15B-10B shows what happened shortly after the lidocaine was given.

This patient developed a supraventricular tachycardia shortly after receiving lidocaine. Although not a common response, *lidocaine may occasionally accelerate supraventricular rhythms!*

> Treatment with lidocaine is *not* benign, and the drug should never be given as a "therapeutic trial." In addition to an incidence of adverse reactions that approaches 15%, lidocaine can accelerate supraventricular rhythms (especially atrial fibrillation). The supraventricular tachycardia produced

in this case was totally iatrogenic (the patient should never have received lidocaine), since overwhelming evidence suggesting aberrancy was present on Figures 15B-9, 15B-10, and 15B-10A.

PROBLEM   **PVCs or aberrant? (Figure 15B-11)**

ANSWER TO FIGURE 15B-11   Aberrant. It is hard to tell if the underlying rhythm is sinus with very frequent PACs or multifocal atrial tachycardia. In any event, P waves abound. A premature P wave notches the T wave preceding the first anomalous beat. These beats are not greatly widened (they are ≤0.11 second), and they manifest a typical RBBB pattern with a similar initial deflection in this right-sided lead. Finally, the Ashman phenomenon is present, with aberrant conduction following the longest pause in the tracing. Level of confidence in diagnosing aberrancy = 100%!

PROBLEM   **PVCs or aberrant? (Figure 15B-12)**

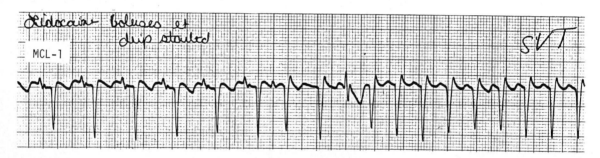

Figure 15B-10B

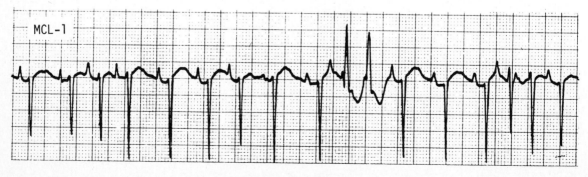

Figure 15B-11

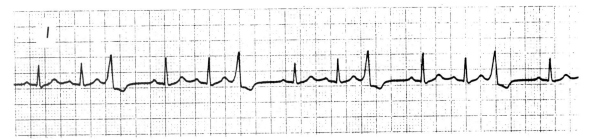

Figure 15B-12

ANSWER TO FIGURE 15B-12 Obviously PVCs (ventricular trigeminy). The anomalous beats are wide and bizarre, and there is no premature P wave. A full compensatory pause is present. Finally, it appears that the sinus-conducted beats manifest a tiny q wave (initial negative deflection) that differs from the initial positive deflection of the wide beats.

PROBLEM PVCs or aberrancy? (**Figure 15B-13**)

Our reason for including this example is once again to emphasize the critical importance of looking at more than one monitoring lead whenever possible.

PROBLEM Why do beats no. 5 and 9 in **Figure 15B-14** look different?

ANSWER TO FIGURE 15B-14 Beats no. 5 and 9 look different because they are PVCs (probably with some degree of *fusion*). The prin-

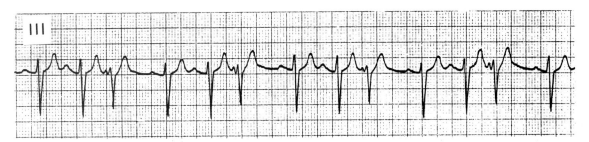

Figure 15B-13

ANSWER TO FIGURE 15B-13 The anomalous beats in this tracing appear to be aberrant. They look very much like the sinus-conducted beats, they are not wide, their initial deflection is similar, and they seem to be preceded by a premature P wave.

Alas, *this is a trick tracing!!!* **Figure 15B-13A** shows that Figures 15B-12 and 15B-13 were recorded *simultaneously on the same patient.*

Note that the notch that looks for all the world like a P wave in lead III (Fig. 15B-13) is really part of the QRS complex!!! The anomalous beats are all PVCs.

cipal clue lies in the atrial rate, which remains perfectly constant throughout the rhythm strip. Thus a regular sinus P wave can be seen to slur the upstroke of the QRS complex of the anomalous beats. Since the PR interval is too short to conduct, an impulse (a PVC) must be arising from below.

The anomalous beats in this example are *end-diastolic PVCs*—they occur toward the end of the R-R interval (at end diastole). As might be imagined, this type of ventricular ectopy commonly produces fusion beats.

Note once again how similar beats no. 5 and 9

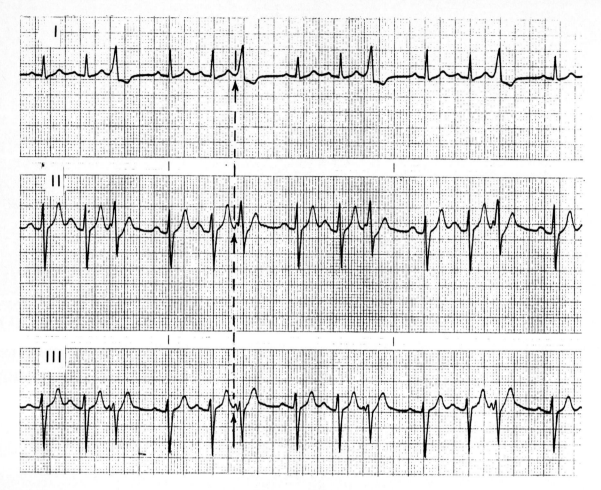

Figure 15B-13A

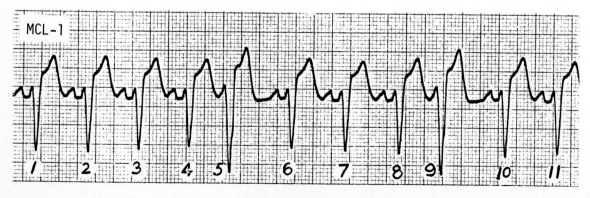

Figure 15B-14

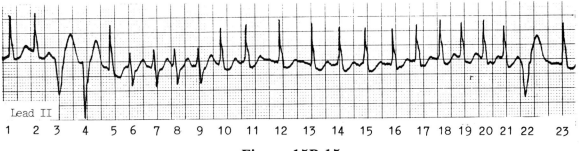

Figure 15B-15

are to the sinus conducted beats. This is a common occurrence with right ventricular PVCs.

PROBLEM   Interpret the rhythm shown in Figure 15B-15.

ANSWER TO FIGURE 15B-15   The underlying rhythm is atrial fibrillation with a moderately rapid ventricular response. Beats no. 3, 4, and 22 are more than likely PVCs—they are wide and oppositely directed to the other beats.

On the other hand, beats no. 6–9 are probably conducted with *aberrancy*. These complexes are not really wide, and their initial deflection is in the same direction as the normally conducted beats. Moreover, this run *maintains the same cadence* as the underlying atrial fibrillation—it begins abruptly with beat no. 6 and ends equally

abruptly with nary a pause before beat no. 10. In contrast, a *postectopic* pause is commonly seen after PVCs in atrial fibrillation (as is noted following beat no. 22).

PROBLEM   Would you treat the rhythm shown in Figure 15B-16 with lidocaine? (The patient was hemodynamically stable.)

ANSWER TO FIGURE 15B-16   The underlying rhythm is atrial fibrillation. Although one might be tempted to call beats no. 3–8 a run of ventricular tachycardia, the morphology of these beats (plus that of no. 10 and 11) demonstrates features suggestive of aberrancy—a similar initial deflection and an RBBB pattern in a right-sided monitoring lead. Statistically, when runs of anomalous beats complicate rapid atrial fibrillation, they are more likely to be aberrantly

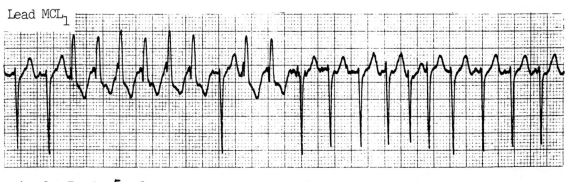

Figure 15B-16

conducted than PVCs. In addition, the irregular irregularity of the underlying rhythm *continues* throughout this run of anomalous beats. The run ends as abruptly as it begins, and there is no postectopic pause after beat no. 8 or 10. Taken together, the sum of these factors strongly favors *aberrancy*—one might do better to try and control the ventricular response (with digoxin) rather than to treat with lidocaine.

Some time after digoxin was given, the rhythm shown in **Figure 15B-16A** was observed. Does this support your previous assumption that the anomalous beats in Figure 15B-16 were aberrant?

The reason beat no. 6 in Figure 15B-16A is conducted aberrantly and beat no. 4 (with an even shorter coupling interval) is not is due to cycle-sequence comparison (the Ashman phenomenon)—the aberrant beat (no. 6) follows the longest pause (the R-R interval between beats no. 4–5 is longer than that between beats no. 2–3).

You are now informed that a run of anomalous beats manifesting still a different QRS configuration has just occurred (beats no. 13–16 in **Fig. 15B-16B**). Should you give the lidocaine now?

Although the presence of atrial fibrillation precludes searching for telltale premature P

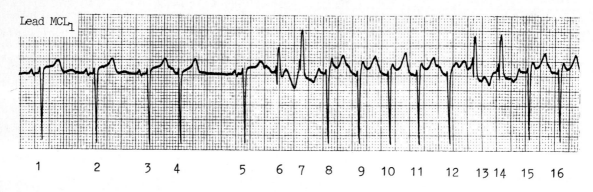

Figure 15B-16A

Sinus rhythm is temporarily restored (beats no. 1, 2, 3, and 5), but the rhythm then reverts back to atrial fibrillation. Beat no. 4 is clearly a PAC—the complex conducts normally, and a premature P wave distorts the preceding T wave. Similarly, a premature P wave produces a notch in the T wave preceding beat no. 6. Note that the morphology of beats no. 6, 7, 13, and 14 in Figure 15B-16A is identical to beats nos. 3–8 and 10 and 11 of Figure 15B-16. In the context of Figure 15B-16A, the premature P wave that precedes beat no. 6, in conjunction with the similar initial deflection to the normally conducted beats and RBBB pattern, establish *beyond doubt* that beat no. 6 is aberrantly conducted. It follows that all of the other similar appearing beats in this figure and Figure 15B-16 must also be aberrant.

waves, several other features suggest that beats no. 13–16 *also* are aberrantly conducted, this time with an LBBB pattern of aberrancy. Note that the underlying irregular irregularity continues unabated throughout the entire rhythm strip in Figure 15B-16B, and that the run of anomalous beats ends as abruptly as it begins. In addition, the QRS complex is not greatly prolonged (0.11 second).

It is not generally appreciated that both RBBB and LBBB aberration commonly alternate in the same patient. This phenomenon of alternating RBBB and LBBB aberration should be suspected particularly when runs of anomalous beats are separated by a single normally conducted beat as they are by beat no. 12 in Figure 15B-16B.

In the context of a hemodynamically stable patient who is having runs of beats that are *def-*

Lead MCL₁

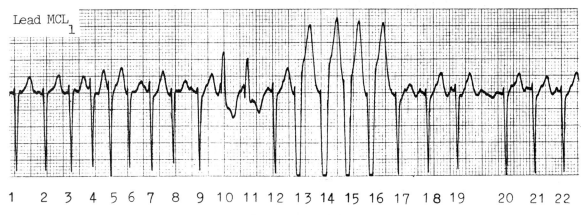

1 2 3 4 5 6 7 8 9 10 11 12 13 14 15 16 17 18 19 20 21 22

Figure 15B-16B

initely aberrant (the anomalous beats with an RBBB configuration), it would be reasonable to assume with a high degree of probability that beats no. 13–16 in Figure 15B-16B also are aberrant. Ultimately the patient converted to sinus rhythm, and no further anomalous beats were seen.

PROBLEM   Aberrancy or ventricular tachycardia? (**Figure 15B-17**)

ANSWER TO FIGURE 15B-17   Ventricular tachycardia. The QRS complex during the tachycardia becomes wide and looks very different from the normally conducted beats. A postectopic pause follows the seven beat run. There is no reason to suspect aberrancy.

PROBLEM   Ventricular   tachycardia? (**Figure 15B-18**)

ANSWER TO FIGURE 15B-18   Following three sinus beats, a long run of anomalous beats occurs. The QRS complex during the run is wide and looks very different from the normally conducted beats. A postectopic pause follows the last beat of the run. This is ventricular tachycardia.

Ventricular tachycardia is often a fairly *regular* rhythm. At times, however, it may exhibit a "warm-up" phenomenon in which it starts off faster (or slower) than its eventual rate. This is the case here—the rate of the tachycardia is extremely fast during the initial part of the run (up to 240 beats/min), before it slows down toward the end of the tracing.

Lead MCL₁

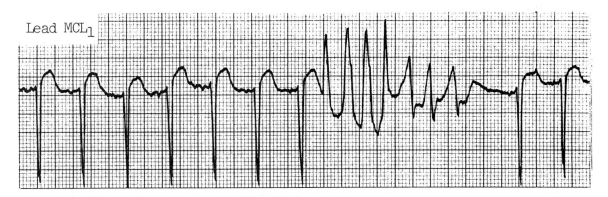

Figure 15B-17

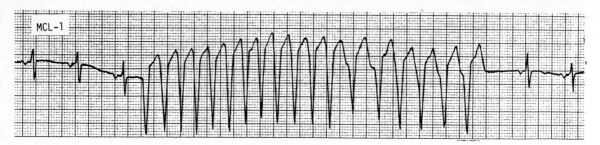

Figure 15B-18

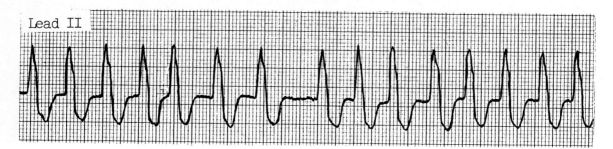

Figure 15B-19

PROBLEM   Ventricular   tachycardia?
(**Figure 15B-19**)

ANSWER TO FIGURE 15B-19   Despite the fact that the QRS complex is wide, the underlying rhythm is grossly irregular. This strongly suggests that the rhythm is atrial fibrillation with a preexisting bundle branch block. Access to a previous 12-lead ECG on this patient would   be   invaluable   in   confirming   this impression.

PROBLEM   Ventricular   tachycardia?
(**Figure 15B-20**)

ANSWER TO FIGURE 15B-20   Sinus rhythm is interrupted by a long run of anomalous beats (no. 5–15). Of note is the fact that a premature P wave initiates the run (notching the T wave preceding beat no. 5) and that the QRS complex during the run is not markedly prolonged (<0.11 second). This strongly suggests *aberrant* conduction. (A premature P wave also is seen in front of beat no. 17.)

It is of interest (but of unknown significance) that P waves can be seen to notch the apex of the T wave during the run of anomalous beats. The reason this finding per se is of little help in deter-

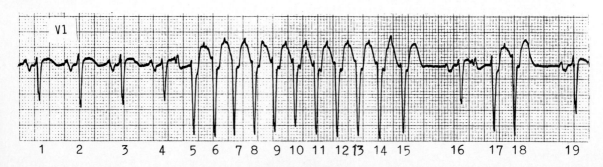

Figure 15B-20

mining if there is aberrant conduction is that ventricular tachycardia may occasionally exhibit retrograde 1:1 conduction and produce a similar finding.

PROBLEM Ventricular tachycardia? (Figure 15B-21)

ative QRS complex. Thus *AV dissociation* exists, with the negative QRS complexes representing runs of ventricular tachycardia that are interrupted by *sinus capture beats* (beats no. 5 and 9). The q waves of these sinus beats and the 1° AV block are manifestations of the patient's acute inferior myocardial infarction.

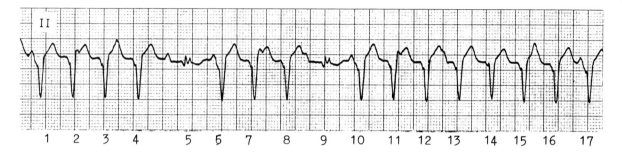

Figure 15B-21

ANSWER TO FIGURE 15B-21 The basic rhythm is composed of QS complexes that are 0.12 second in duration and regular at a rate of 135 beats/min. Two "unusual" complexes (beats no. 5 and 9) interrupt this underlying rhythm. Beat no. 5 is preceded by a P wave that appears to be conducting, although with 1° AV block. Scanning the rest of the tracing for signs of atrial activity, notching and peaking at various points of the QRS complex in many beats are evident. Setting one's calipers to the interval defined by the P wave preceding beat no. 5 and the positive deflection that occurs just before beat no. 6, atrial activity can again be "marched out" throughout the rhythm strip **(Fig. 15B-21A).** This atrial activity is unrelated to the neg-

The finding of AV dissociation during a wide complex tachycardia is extremely useful in identifying the tachyarrhythmia as being ventricular in origin. Although it is theoretically possible for a wide complex tachycardia to manifest AV dissociation as the result of aberrant conduction from an accelerated junctional pacemaker, this is rare. Unfortunately this diagnostic feature is seen in only a minority of cases of ventricular tachycardia.

PROBLEM Figure 15B-22: Ventricular tachycardia? (The patient is hemodynamically stable.)

ANSWER TO FIGURE 15B-22 The underlying rhythm is atrial fibrillation with a rapid ventricular response. Beat no. 5 begins a run of a wide complex tachycardia. Morphology

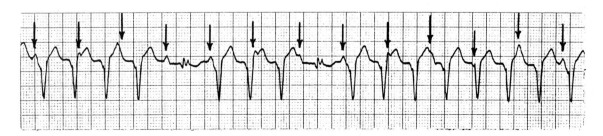

Figure 15B-21A

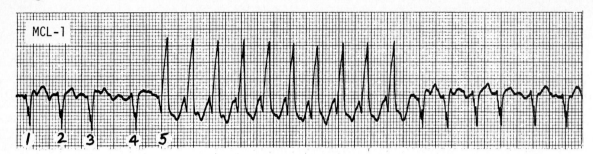

Figure 15B-22

(RBBB pattern in MCL$_1$) suggests that the run may be due to aberrant conduction, although there is no way to know for sure from this one tracing. A long-short (Ashman) sequence precedes the run, but this finding is less reliable in the setting of atrial fibrillation. The string of anomalous beats begins and ends abruptly, and careful measurement of the R-R interval during the run reveals an ever so slight irregularity of the rhythm. Taken together the findings *favor* aberrancy, but this is another one in which we would hedge our bets pending additional information. Obtaining a 12-lead ECG and/or comparison with previous rhythm strips done on this patient might be helpful.

PROBLEM   Ventricular   tachycardia? (**Figure 15B-23**)

ANSWER TO FIGURE 15B-23   Yes! The anomalous beats are wide and bizarre and suggest ventricular tachycardia. AV dissociation during the first two beats of the run (**Fig. 15B-23A**) confirms this suspicion.

PROBLEM   Ventricular tachycardia or **supraventricular tachycardia?** (**Figure 15B-24**)

ANSWER TO FIGURE 15B-24   Neither. Although the arrow in Figure 15B-24 suggests the onset of a tachyarrhythmia, the heart rate during this short burst of anomalous com-

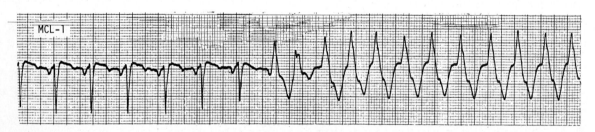

Figure 15B-23

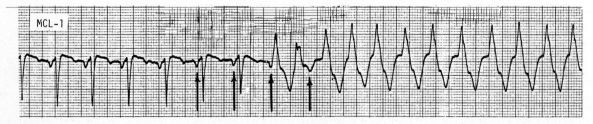

Figure 15B-23A

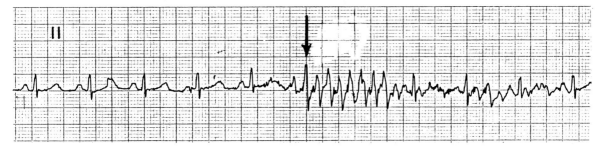

Figure 15B-24

plexes is well over 300 beats/min—much too fast to represent a real rhythm. **Figure 15B-24A** (which demonstrates the simultaneous recording from lead V_5) is revealing.

It can be seen from lead V_5 of Figure 15B-24A that the normal QRS complex is unaffected by the disturbance in the baseline, and regular complexes continue to occur at a rate of 85 beats/min. This patient began seizing as the result of a hypoglycemic reaction at the point indicated by the arrow.

PROBLEM   Ventricular   tachycardia? **(Figure 15B-25)**

ANSWER TO FIGURE 15B-25   Yes! QRS morphology differs greatly from the sinus-conducted beats and of itself suggests ventricular tachycardia. Close analysis of the R-R baseline between beats no. 6–7 provides confirmation **(Fig. 15B-25A)**.

The solid arrows marking the sinus P waves in

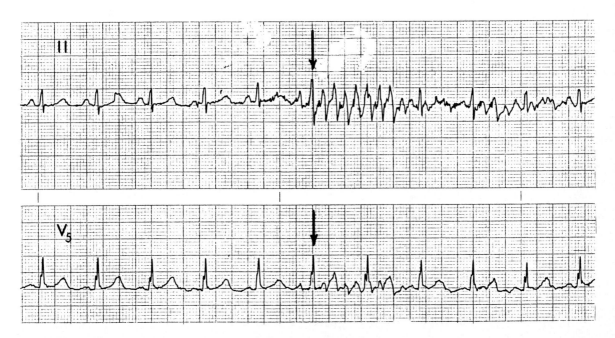

Figure 15B-24A

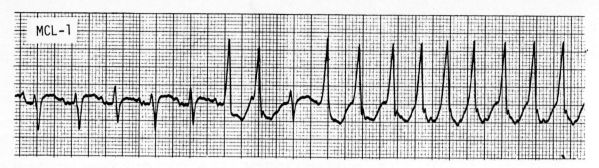

Figure 15B-25

Figure 15B-25A indicate that AV dissociation is present for the first beat of the run!

> The broken arrows indicate notching of the ST segment of beat no. 7 and subsequent beats of the anomalous run. This is most likely due to *retrograde* conduction to the atria during the ventricular tachycardia.

PROBLEM   **Examine Figure 15B-26. How would you explain the QRS widening?**

ANSWER TO FIGURE 15B-26   No atrial activity is evident and the rhythm is irregularly irregular. This suggests atrial fibrillation. QRS widening is the result of an RBBB and left anterior hemiblock.

PROBLEM   **The patient whose rhythm is shown in Figure 15B-27 was treated with verapamil for presumed PSVT. Would you have done the same? (He was hemodynamically stable.)**

ANSWER TO FIGURE 15B-27   All one can say from Figure 15B-27 is that there is a regular tachyarrhythmia at a rate of 170 beats/min. Although the QRS complex in this tracing does not appear to be wide, part of it may lie on a baseline. **Figure 15B-27A** is the 12-lead ECG of this patient. Does it alter your opinion in any way? *(Does the fact that the patient was alert have any bearing on the diagnosis?)*

Figure 15B-27A is the ECG of a patient in ventricular tachycardia! There is no sign of atrial activity, the QRS complex is markedly widened (in virtually every lead *except* V_1), and morphologic clues strongly suggestive of the diagnosis (QS complex in lead V_6 and bizarre frontal plane axis) are present.

> Patients may be awake and alert (as this one was) for minutes, hours (and even *days!*) despite being in ventricular tachycardia. This patient's blood pres-

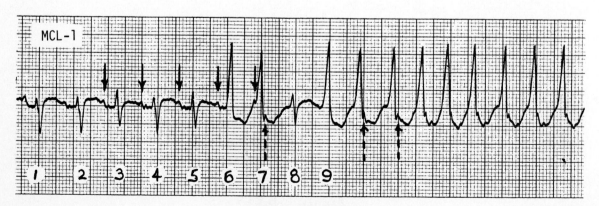

Figure 15B-25A

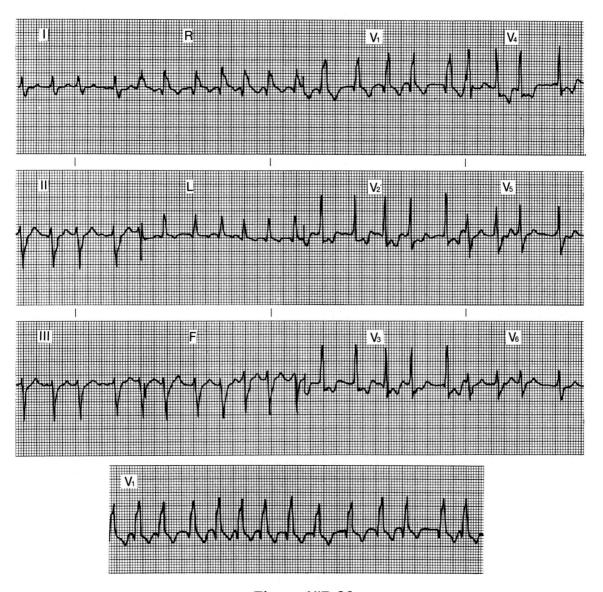

Figure 15B-26

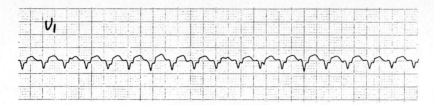

Figure 15B-27

sure dropped after he received verapamil, and he almost decompensated. Fortunately, the correct diagnosis was realized after the 12-lead ECG was obtained. His ECG following synchronized cardioversion is shown in **Figure 15B-27B**.

Verapamil should *not* be given indiscriminately as a therapeutic trial to patients with regular wide complex tachycardias. If the tachyarrhythmia turns out to be ventricular, there is a significant chance that the vasodilatation and negative inotropic effect

of this calcium channel blocking agent will result in acute decompensation of the patient.

PROBLEM   **Ventricular**   **tachycardia?** (**Figure 15B-28**)

ANSWER TO FIGURE 15B-28   There is a regular wide complex tachycardia at a rate of 155 beats/min. Atrial activity is absent. Al-

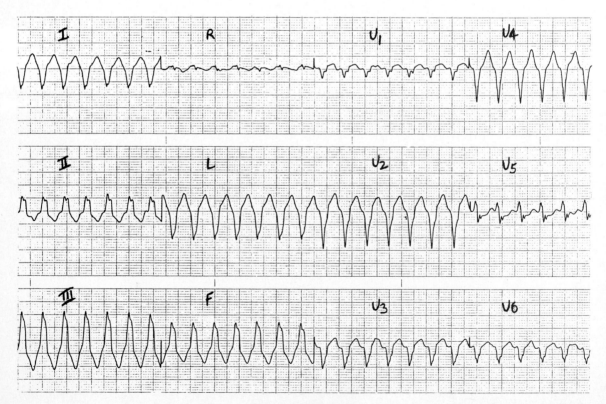

Figure 15B-27A

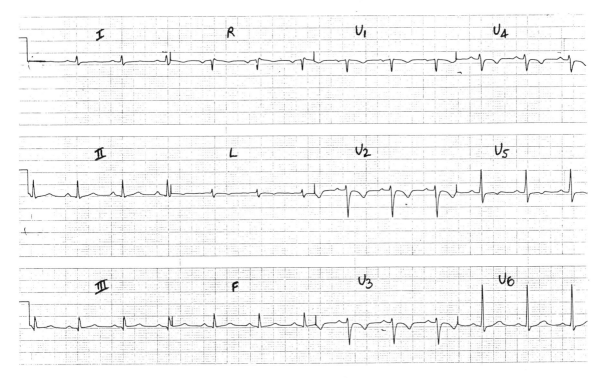

Figure 15B-27B

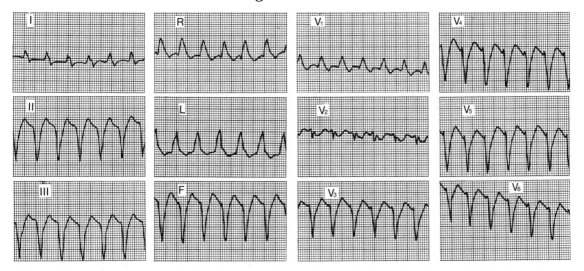

Figure 15B-28

though morphologic analysis of the QRS complex in lead V_1 is of no assistance in the diagnosis, the predominantly negative complex in lead V_6 in conjunction with the bizarre (markedly leftward) frontal plane axis strongly suggest ventricular tachycardia. The patient must be treated as such until this diagnosis is proved otherwise.

PROBLEM This patient was known to have an old LBBB. In view of this, is the ECG shown in <u>Figure 15B-29</u> any cause for concern?

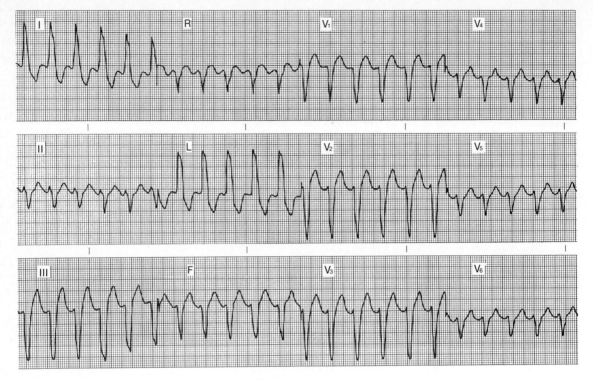

Figure 15B-29

ANSWER TO FIGURE 15B-29   A regular wide complex tachycardia at a rate of 125 beats/min is seen on this tracing. Atrial activity is absent. The ECG superficially resembles LBBB; however, QRS morphology in the precordial leads is *not* typical for this conduction disturbance for two reasons:

   i) The QRS complex is predominantly negative in lead V_6.
   ii) There is concordance (global negativity in this case) of the QRS vectors in the precordial leads.

These findings should strongly suggest that the patient is in *ventricular tachycardia*. This patient remained in ventricular tachycardia for *more than a day* before it was realized that his wide complex tachycardia was not the result of an old LBBB. Following cardioversion the ECG shown in **Figure 15B-29A** was obtained.

   Resumption of sinus rhythm in Figure 15B-29A is marked by the return of atrial activity and

the more "usual" morphology of LBBB—monophasic (upright) R wave in *all* lateral leads.

Although QRS concordance as seen across the precordial leads in Figure 15B-29 is a relatively rare finding, it is extremely helpful if present since it strongly suggests ventricular ectopy (see Table 15-1).

PROBLEM   **As a final exercise examine Figure 15B-30. Do beats no. 3–18 in this rhythm strip represent a run of ventricular tachycardia?**

ANSWER TO FIGURE 15B-30   If one did not see the beginning and end of this run, it would be difficult to rule out ventricular tachycardia since the QRS complex is wide and definite atrial activity is not evident between beats no. 4–18. However, P waves with a normal PR interval precede beats no. 1, 2, 3, and 19. Thus Figure 15B-30 begins and ends with sinus rhythm, and the reason for the QRS widening is a preexisting bundle branch block. Since the

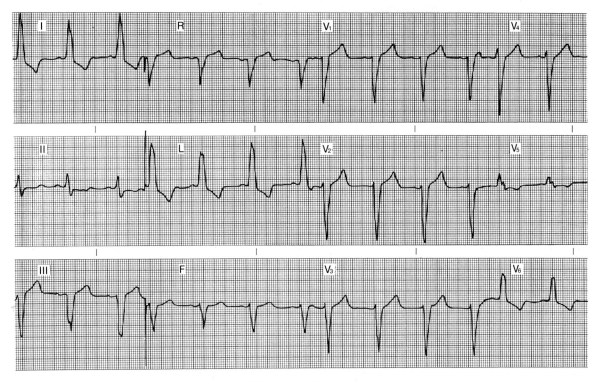

Figure 15B-29A

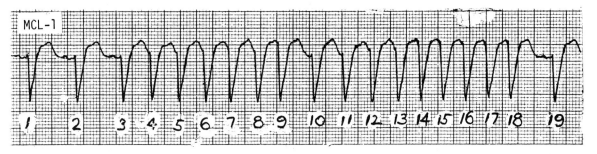

Figure 15B-30

QRS morphology during the run is virtually identical to its morphology during the sinus conducted beats, the tachyarrhythmia that begins with beat no. 3 is most likely *supraventricular.* The irregularity of the rhythm suggests this to be an episode of *paroxysmal atrial fibrillation.*

PROBLEM   **A short while following treatment with digitalis, the ECG shown in Figure 15B-30A was recorded from this patient. What has happened? Has the reason for the QRS widening in Figure 15B-30 become more evident?**

ANSWER TO FIGURE 15B-30A   Digitalis has succeeded in converting the patient to normal sinus rhythm, with the exception of beat no. 5 which is either a PAC or a PJC. Of interest, however, is the fact that the QRS complex is wide for beats no. 2–5 and of normal duration for beats no. 1 and 6–9.

This final example illustrates the phenome-

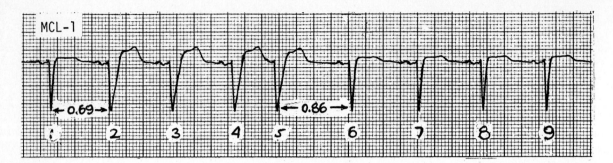

Figure 15B-30A

non known as *rate-dependent bundle branch block (BBB)*. Under certain conditions the refractory period (RP) of one of the bundle branches may become pathologically prolonged. If the heart rate then accelerates to a point where the cycle length (the R-R interval between two successive beats) exceeds the RP of the diseased bundle branch, a rate-dependent BBB will develop and persist until the heart rate slows down enough for normal conduction to occur.

In the case shown in Figure 15B-30A, a left bundle branch block pattern of aberrancy develops with beat no. 2 because of cycle length shortening between beats no. 1–2 (which demonstrate an R-R interval of 0.69 second). Normal conduction does not resume until beat no. 6. The pause following premature beat no. 5 allows the extra time needed for the left bundle branch to recover and conduct normally. Retrospectively in the context of Figure 15B-30A, the QRS widening in Figure 15B-30 may be explained on the basis of cycle shortening that is maintained throughout this rhythm strip.

That rate-dependent BBB does not always come and go at some precise cycle length is evident from Figure 15B-30A since normal conduction persists for beats no. 6–9 despite the fact that the R-R interval of these last few beats is as short as it was when the left bundle branch block aberration developed at the beginning of the rhythm strip.

Although rate-dependent BBB is not a common form of aberration, the importance of recognizing it is obvious from inspection of **Figure 15B-30B,** recorded later from this same patient. Without the knowledge of this patient's tendency to conduct with left bundle branch block aberration at faster rates, it would be easy to misdiagnose beats no. 4–6 and no. 9–11 as salvos of ventricular tachycardia.

REFERENCES

Fox W, Stein E: Cardiac Rhythm Disturbances: A Step-by-Step Approach. Lea & Febiger, Philadelphia, 1983.

Grauer K: Differentiating between aberrantly conducted

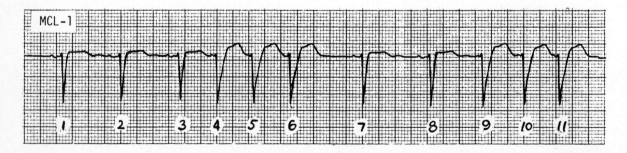

Figure 15B-30B

beats and ventricular ectopy. Cont Ed Fam Phys 19:85–98, 1984.

Langendorf R, Pick A, Winternitz M: Mechanisms of intermittent ventricular bigeminy. I. Appearance of ectopic beats dependent upon length of the ventricular cycle, the "Rule of Bigeminy." Circulation II:422–430, 1955.

Marriott HJL: Practical Electrocardiography. Williams & Wilkins, Baltimore, 1982.

Marriott HJL, Conover MHB: Advanced Concepts in Arrhythmias. The C.V. Mosby Co., St. Louis, 1983.

Swanick EJ, LaCamera F, Marriott HJL: Morphologic features of right ventricular ectopic beats. Am J Cardiol 30:888–891, 1972.

Vera Z, Cheng TO, Ertem G, Shoaleh-var M, Wickramase-karan R, Wadhwa K: His bundle electrocardiography for evaluation of criteria in differentiating ventricular ectopy from aberrancy in atrial fibrillation (abstract). Circulation 45-46 (Suppl 2):90, 1972.

Wellens HJJ, Bar FWHM, Lie KI: The value of the electrocardiogram in the differential diagnosis of a tachycardia with a widened QRS complex. Am J Med 64:27–33, 1978.

CHAPTER 16

MORE ADVANCED CONCEPTS IN ARRHYTHMIA INTERPRETATION

A: TACHYARRHYTHMIAS

Perhaps the greatest challenge faced by the emergency care provider during cardiac resuscitation is the task of interpreting tachyarrhythmias. Institution of the appropriate treatment and the ultimate fate of the patient often hang in the balance. In the previous chapter, we delved into ways of differentiating between aberration and ventricular ectopy, and how to apply such techniques in interpreting wide complex tachyarrhythmias. We expand on this material here and place particular emphasis on diagnosis of supraventricular tachyarrhythmias.

Before turning our attention to electrocardiographic clues in the interpretation of specific arrhythmias, it might be helpful to review an overall approach to the problem.

PROBLEM   **Consider the situation posed by a middle-aged man with the tachyarrhythmia shown in <u>Figure 16A-1</u>. How would you proceed both diagnostically and therapeutically if the patient were tolerating this rhythm?**

ANSWER TO FIGURE 16A-1   A regular tachyarrhythmia with a rate of about 200 beats/min is seen. No distinct P waves can be identified. The critical question is whether this represents a supraventricular or ventricular tachycardia. The answer is *not* forthcoming from analysis of this single rhythm strip. One cannot tell if the QRS complex is widened, since it is virtually impossible to be sure where the QRS complex ends and the ST segment begins. Even if the QRS complex were wide, the possibility would exist that this could be a supraventricular

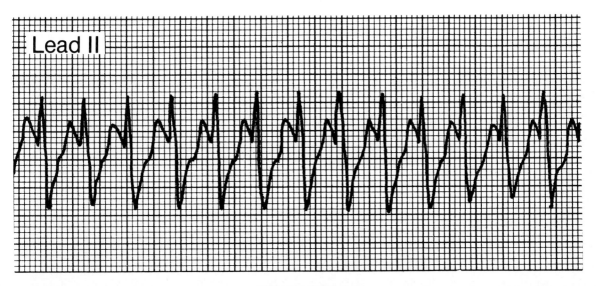

Figure 16A-1

tachycardia with either preexisting bundle branch block or aberrant conduction.

Diagnostic Approach to Tachyarrhythmias

Practically speaking, one is left with three alternatives:

  i) Seek more information.
  ii) Assume the rhythm to be *supraventricular* and treat accordingly.
  iii) Assume the rhythm to be *ventricular tachycardia* and treat accordingly.

Seek More Information

Since the patient is tolerating the tachyarrhythmia, one might consider the following:

a) Obtain a 12-lead ECG to see if P waves are evident in any other leads, or if QRS morphology can aid in differentiation (see Table 15A-1).

b) Determine if rhythm strips on the patient *before* he went into the tachycardia are available. Is the QRS configuration during sinus rhythm similar to that shown in Figure 16A-1? (If so, this implies a supraventricular etiology for the rhythm. If not, the question still remains as to whether Figure 16A-1 represents ventricular tachycardia or a supraventricular arrhythmia with aberrant conduction.)

c) Look at the neck veins and listen to the first heart sound. The presence of irregular cannon waves in the neck and/or variation in the intensity of the first heart sound suggests AV dissociation which almost always means ventricular tachycardia. (Although a wide complex tachycardia may be produced by AV dissociation between an atrial pacemaker and an accelerated junctional rhythm that conducts with aberration, this is rare!)

On the other hand, a lack of variation in the intensity of the first heart sound and either the absence of cannon waves or the presence of regular cannon waves in the neck are evidence against AV dissociation. This suggests a supraventricular etiology of the tachyarrhythmia (but does not rule out ventricular tachycardia with 1:1 retrograde conduction).

d) Consider alternate monitoring lead systems. One of the simplest to apply is the **S5 lead.** With the ECG hooked up to record on standard lead I, the *left* arm (positive) electrode is positioned at the fifth interspace just to the right of the sternum, while the *right* arm (negative) electrode is placed over the manubrium of the sternum. This provides a *bipolar* precordial lead that may elucidate atrial activity.

Assume a Supraventricular Etiology and Treat Accordingly

This would be reasonable, since the QRS complex does not appear to be significantly widened and the patient is tolerating the arrhythmia. In conjunction with a heart rate of about 200 beats/min, these findings favor a supraventricular etiology. (*However, patients with ventricular tachycardia may occasionally remain conscious and alert for extended periods of time.*)

a) Apply **carotid sinus massage (CSM).** Under constant ECG monitoring, turn the patient's head to the left and gently but firmly massage the area of the *right* carotid bifurcation near the angle of the jaw for 5 seconds at a time. After several attempts on the right carotid, the other side may be tried. *Never massage both sides simultaneously.*

The response to CSM varies, depending on the nature of the arrhythmia. Normally, there is a transient decrease of the sinus rate *and* a slowing of AV conduction. (The reason many clinicians prefer to massage the *right* carotid first is that this side is believed to exert a greater influence on the sinus node, while the left carotid is believed to act more on the AV node.)

The most dramatic response occurs with PSVT, in which CSM may abruptly terminate the tachycardia. Alternatively, PSVT may not respond at all to the maneuver. Ventricular tachycardia does not respond to CSM. Consequently, a lack of response to CSM would not differentiate between these two arrhythmias. (See **Table 16A-1** for the expected response of these and other arrhythmias to CSM.)

CSM is *not* a totally benign maneuver, particularly in older individuals. It has been associated with syncope, stroke, sinus arrest, high-grade AV block, prolonged asystole, and ventricular tachyarrhythmias in patients with digitalis intoxication. **Figure 16A-2** demonstrates the response to CSM of an elderly man who was in a supraventricular tachycardia. As can be seen, CSM decreased (almost all too well in this case) conduction through the AV node, revealing *flutter* waves (at 270 beats/min) that had been obscured by the tachycardia.

Because of such responses, CSM should

TABLE 16A-1

Tachyarrhythmia	Response to Carotid Sinus Massage (CSM)
Sinus tachycardia	Gradual slowing with CSM with resumption of the tachycardia after the maneuver
PSVT	Abrupt termination of the tachyarrhythmia with conversion to sinus rhythm or No response to CSM
Atrial flutter or Atrial fibrillation	Increased degree of AV block with resultant slowing of the ventricular rate (CSM often permits diagnosis of atrial flutter by allowing clear visualization of flutter waves as the ventricular rate slows)
Ventricular tachycardia	No response to CSM

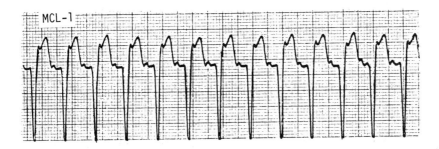

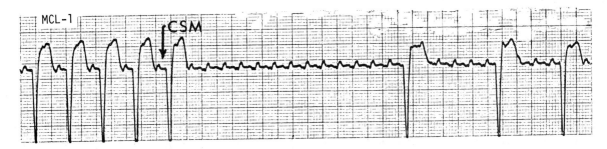

Figure 16A-2

probably *not* be attempted in patients with a history of sick sinus syndrome (SSS), cervical bruits, or cerebrovascular disease, or when the possibility of digitalis intoxication exists.

b) Administer IV **verapamil.** This drug has become the favored treatment for PSVT, successfully converting it to sinus rhythm more than 90% of the time. A dose of 5 mg may be given over a 1-to-2-minute period. Lower doses (3 mg) given more slowly (over 3–4 min-

utes) are advised in the elderly. If there is no response to an initial dose of verapamil in 15–30 minutes, a repeat dose (of 5–10 mg) may be given.

As we have previously emphasized, verapamil should *not* be used indiscriminately as a diagnostic maneuver to differentiate supraventricular tachyarrhythmias from ventricular tachycardia in cases of wide complex tachyarrhythmias.

c) Second-line drugs for treatment of PSVT include *digoxin* and *propranolol*. Digoxin would *not* be recommended in this case, since the possibility still exists that the rhythm in Figure 16A-1 is ventricular tachycardia for which digitalis is contraindicated. Propranolol may be effective for both supraventricular and ventricular tachyarrhythmias, but the IV form of this drug should *not* be given soon after verapamil, since this increases the risk of inducing AV block. (IV verapamil can probably be given safely to patients taking *oral* beta-blockers provided left ventricular function is normal.)

d) If the patient at any time shows signs of hemodynamic decompensation, *immediate* cardioversion should be performed.

Assume a Ventricular Etiology and Treat Accordingly

a) Give the patient a bolus of **lidocaine** and begin an IV infusion.

b) Consider IV **procainamide.** This may be a reasonable approach when the etiology of the tachyarrhythmia is unclear, since procainamide can work for *both* supraventricular and ventricular tachyarrhythmias! Although not nearly as effective as verapamil for the former, at least procainamide is unlikely to precipitate hemodynamic decompensation if the arrhythmia turns out to be ventricular.

c) Proceed with **synchronized cardioversion.** This modality should be effective regardless of whether the rhythm in Figure 16A-1 is supraventricular or ventricular in nature. As long as the patient is tolerating the arrhythmia, cardioversion may be done under *semielective* conditions. The patient may be sedated with 5–10 mg of IV Valium, an anesthesiologist can be called to the bedside, and lower energy levels (20–50 joules) may be tried first.

This case emphasizes the thought process involved in evaluating and treating a tachyarrhythmia when the etiology is unclear.

NARROW COMPLEX TACHYARRHYTHMIAS

Classification of tachyarrhythmias is much easier when the QRS complex is of normal duration. In this case, evaluation of the rhythm's regularity and identification of atrial activity become the important differentiating factors.

Evaluate the following narrow complex tachyarrhythmias:

PROBLEM   **Figure 16A-3 is from an asymptomatic 6-year-old child.**

ANSWER TO FIGURE 16A-3   The rate of this regular supraventricular tachyarrhythmia is 155 beats/min. Each QRS complex is preceded by a P wave with a fixed PR interval. This is *sinus tachycardia.* The PR interval (0.09 second) is normal considering the age of the child.

> Sinus tachycardia needs to be kept in the differential of all supraventricular tachycardias. Although usually easy to recognize (by the presence of an upright P wave in lead II), diagnosis may become difficult with rapid rates as the P wave becomes hidden in the preceding T wave. Clinically there should be a reason for the tachycardia (hyperthyroidism, illness, or exercise). Although sinus tachycardia usually does not exceed 160 beats/min in adults, much faster rates may be recorded in children.

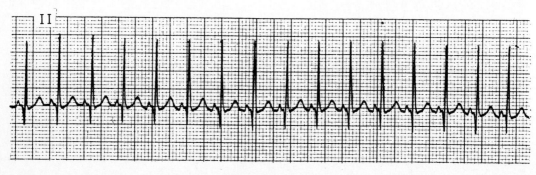

Figure 16A-3

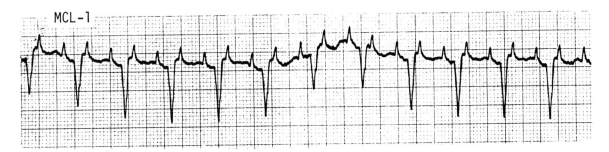

Figure 16A-4

PROBLEM   **Figure 16A-4 is from a middle-aged adult on digitalis.**

ANSWER TO FIGURE 16A-4   The rhythm is regular with a ventricular rate of about 115 beats/min. P waves outnumber QRS complexes by two to one, making the atrial rate about 230 beats/min. The QRS complex is narrow, implying a supraventricular mechanism, and each QRS complex is preceded by a P wave with a constant PR interval. Thus P waves *are* related to the QRS complexes, albeit only one of every two P waves is conducted to the ventricles. This is *atrial tachycardia* with *2:1 AV block.*

> The finding of atrial tachycardia with AV block in a patient on digitalis should prompt the emergency care provider to highly suspect *digitalis toxicity*. Clinically it is important to know if digitalis toxicity is present because if such is the case treatment consists of withdrawing digitalis, whereas treatment of atrial tachycardia not due to digitalis toxicity may entail *administering* the drug!
>
> Treatment of atrial tachycardia with block also entails correction of accompanying electrolyte disturbances (hypokalemia, hypomagnesemia) that might exacerbate the effect of digitalis toxicity. However, hypokalemia in particular must not be

corrected too rapidly because doing so may temporarily worsen the degree of AV block.

PROBLEM   **Examine Figure 16A-4A. What clinical condition is suggested by this tracing?**

ANSWER TO FIGURE 16A-4A   The underlying rhythm is *atrial tachycardia* at a rate of 220 beats/min. *High-grade block* and *ventricular irritability* (PVCs) are present. The combination of these findings is almost pathognomonic for digitalis toxicity.

Differentiating between Atrial Flutter and Atrial Tachycardia with Block

At times it may be extremely difficult to differentiate between atrial flutter and atrial tachycardia with 2:1 AV block. Again the clinical importance of making this distinction is that one condition (atrial flutter) often is treated with digitalis, while the other (atrial tachycardia with

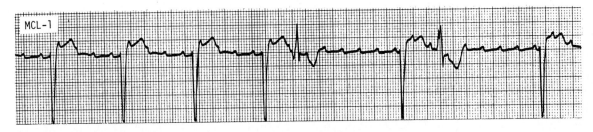

Figure 16A-4A

block) usually is treated by withdrawal of the drug.

Atrial flutter is characterized electrocardiographically by a sawtooth pattern with an atrial rate of between 250 and 350 beats/min *in the untreated adult*. Most commonly there is 2:1 AV conduction, resulting in a ventricular response of between 140 and 160 beats/min. Less commonly there may be 4:1 AV conduction (ventricular response ≈70–75 beats/min) or variable ventricular conduction. Odd AV conduction ratios (such as 3:1 or 5:1) are rare. The point to remember is that if the patient is being treated with a type I antiarrhythmic agent (quinidine, procainamide, disopyramide) or verapamil, the atrial rate of flutter may *decrease,* and a much slower ventricular response may be seen.

The atrial rate with *atrial tachycardia* tends to be slower than for atrial flutter (150–250 beats/min). Electrocardiographically, P waves may or may not be upright in lead II (depending on the site of atrial automaticity). At times *both* P wave morphology *and* the atrial rate may vary, whereas these are constant for atrial flutter (since flutter is believed to be due to reentry within a *fixed* atrial reentrant circuit). In addition, the *baseline* between P waves tends to be *isoelectric* in contrast to the sawtooth pattern of flutter. Although 2:1 AV conduction is common, any conduction ratio may be present.

PROBLEM   Examine **Figure 16A-4B**. Is the rhythm likely to be due to atrial tachycardia with block or atrial flutter?

ANSWER TO FIGURE 16A-4B   The atrial rate is regular at about 170 beats/min, and

If you had difficulty identifying two P waves for each QRS complex in this tracing, try the following. Set your calipers at *exactly* half the ventricular rate. Then position the calipers on the point of the P wave that *is* clearly seen (it occurs right after the T wave). The next advance of the calipers will land on the upstroke of the r wave—this is the other P wave.

The patient in this case was in *atrial flutter.* The atrial rate had been much faster before long-term treatment with quinidine, digitalis, and verapamil was begun.

Type I antiarrhythmic agents (quinidine, procainamide, disopyramide) should *never* be given to patients in atrial flutter who have not already been digitalized. This is because in addition to slowing the atrial rate of flutter (decreased atrial automaticity), these agents may improve AV nodal conduction. A patient who was only able to conduct every other atrial impulse when the rate of flutter was 300/min (2:1 conduction = ventricular response 150/min) may now be able to conduct 1:1 if the atrial rate is slowed to 200/min (= ventricular response of 200/min). Having digitalis on board prevents such increases in the ventricular response from occurring when the type I drug is added.

PROBLEM   Interpret the supraventricular tachyarrhythmia shown in **Figure 16A-5.**

ANSWER TO FIGURE 16A-5   The QRS complex of this tachyarrhythmia is narrow

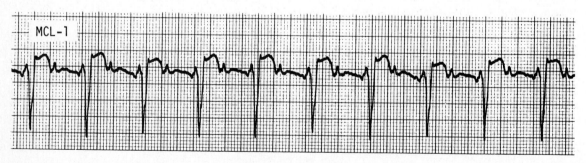

Figure 16A-4B

there is 2:1 AV conduction. Although the atrial rate is much slower than one usually sees with flutter, the baseline is not isoelectric as one would expect for atrial tachycardia. Therefore it is hard to be certain of the diagnosis from this ECG alone.

and regular at about 150 beats/min. *One must therefore be suspicious of atrial flutter with 2:1 AV conduction.* Setting a pair of calipers at precisely half the ventricular rate allows one to walk out atrial activity (the negative deflections) at a rate of 300 beats/min **(Fig. 16A-5A).** A vagal maneu-

Lead MCL₁

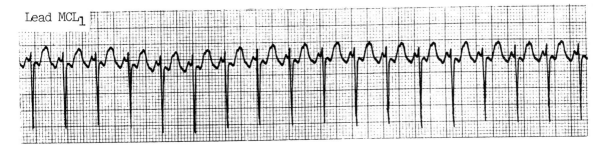

Figure 16A-5

ver could be performed if further confirmation was needed.

Atrial flutter remains one of the most commonly overlooked diagnoses in medicine. Unless one retains a high index of suspicion for flutter (whenever a regular supraventricular tachyarrhythmia at a rate of 140–160 beats/min is seen), the diagnosis will continue to be missed.

As is the case for ventricular fibrillation, atrial flutter may be "set off" by a premature impulse if it arrives at an opportune time during the vulnerable period of repolarization. Consider the interesting tracing shown in **Figure 16A-5B.**

After 5 sinus beats, flutter waves suddenly appear (the first one peaks the T wave of the fifth QRS complex). Initially 4:1 AV conduction is

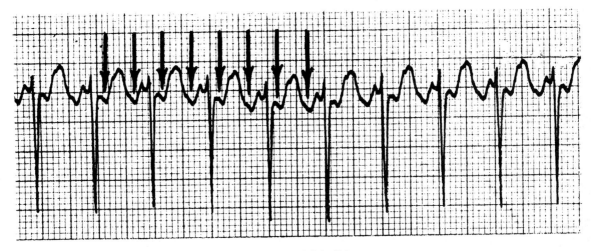

Figure 16A-5A

II

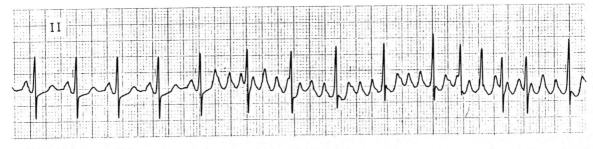

Figure 16A-5B

present, but toward the end of the tracing the ventricular response becomes variable. This particular patient continued to go in and out of atrial flutter numerous times despite aggressive medical therapy.

PROBLEM   A short while later the patient whose rhythm was shown in Figure 16A-5 was observed to be in the rhythm below (Fig. 16A-6). What has happened?

ANSWER TO FIGURE 16A-6   The regular notching in the baseline has disappeared and the rhythm has become ever so slightly ir-

that the rhythm is regular and diagnose PSVT. As mentioned previously, the clinical importance of differentiating between these two rhythms is that treatment may differ. Although digoxin and verapamil are each effective, many clinicians prefer to use verapamil for PSVT and digoxin for atrial fibrillation.

PROBLEM   Apply these concepts to evaluate the supraventricular tachyarrhythmia shown in Figure 16A-6A.

ANSWER TO FIGURE 16A-6A   Once again an ever so slight (but definite) irregular irregularity is evident. Atrial activity is absent. The

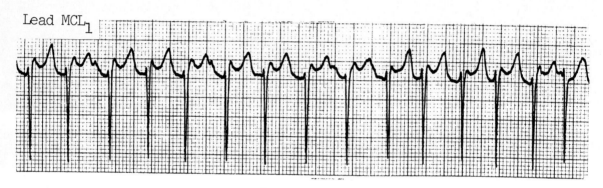

Lead MCL₁

Figure 16A-6

regular. The patient has developed *atrial fibrillation.*

> Although the rhythm still looks regular, *it isn't!* If you missed this—go back and carefully measure the R-R interval with calipers.

Atrial Fibrillation

There often seems to be a reluctance to diagnose atrial fibrillation. Perhaps this is because the entity is diagnosed on *negative* findings (the absence of atrial activity) rather than positive ones. *If the rhythm is irregularly irregular and atrial activity is absent, the diagnosis is atrial fibrillation.* At times, fine undulations may be noted in the baseline *(fibrillatory waves),* but no consistent P waves will be seen.

> The diagnosis of atrial fibrillation is most easily overlooked when the ventricular response is rapid (as it is in Fig. 16A-6). The tendency is to assume

diagnosis is therefore atrial fibrillation with a rapid ventricular response.

Three special situations should be kept in mind with respect to atrial fibrillation. We will present two of them now and save the third for later in this chapter.

PROBLEM   Examine the rhythm shown in Figure 16A-6B. What conditions might cause this?

ANSWER TO FIGURE 16A-6B   The rhythm is irregularly irregular and the ventricular response is slow (between 35 and 55 beats/min). Rapid flutter waves are noted early on but become less well defined toward the end of the tracing *(atrial flutter-fibrillation).* The two conditions that are commonly associated with atrial fibrillation and a slow ventricular response are *sick sinus syndrome* and *digitalis intoxication.*

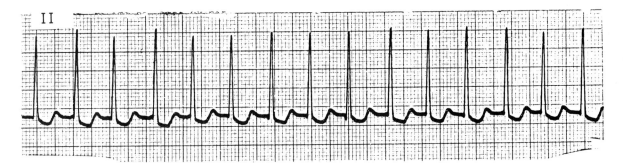

Figure 16A-6A

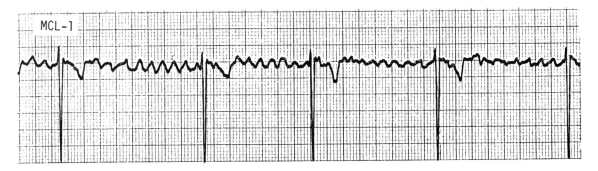

Figure 16A-6B

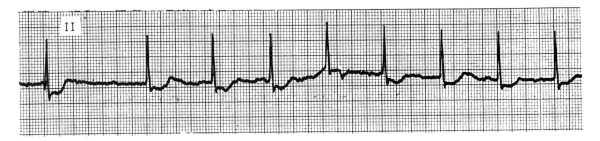

Figure 16A-6C

PROBLEM   **Finally, consider the tracing shown in Figure 16A-6C, taken after treatment from the patient whose rhythm was shown in Figure 16A-6A.**

ANSWER TO FIGURE 16A-16C   Although there are fine undulations in the baseline, no consistent atrial activity is evident. The rhythm becomes regular after the third beat.

Considering that this patient was previously in atrial fibrillation with a *rapid* ventricular response (Fig. 16A-6A) and was treated (presumably with digoxin), *regularization of atrial fibrillation* strongly suggests digitalis toxicity. The mechanism responsible is AV block (from excess digitalis) with resultant escape of a junctional pacemaker (that in this case is slightly accelerated at 75 beats/min).

DIGITALIS TOXICITY

Even today, digitalis toxicity is one of the most common iatrogenic illnesses that results in admission to the hospital. The disorder may present with anorexia, nausea, vomiting, headache, fatigue, depression, confusion, visual disturbances (especially of color vision), or cardiac arrhythmias. Although anorexia and nausea are usually the first signs, at times cardiac arrhythmias may be the *only* manifestation. While almost any cardiac arrhythmia may be seen with digitalis toxicity, the ones listed in **Table 16A-2**

in particular should heighten one's suspicion of the disorder when they occur in a patient taking the drug.

PROBLEM   **The tachyarrhythmia shown in Figure 16A-7 is also irregularly irregular. Is this atrial fibrillation?**

ANSWER TO FIGURE 16A-7   Although the rhythm is irregularly irregular, there *is* atrial activity! Definite P waves precede each QRS complex. Most of these P waves are positive (with either a pointed or notched configu-

TABLE 16A-2

Cardiac Arrhythmias Commonly Associated with Digitalis Toxicity
Inappropriate sinus bradycardia
Sinus pauses or sinus arrest
Sinoatrial block
1° AV block
2° AV block, Mobitz type I (Wenckebach)
Wenckebach-type block with atrial fibrillation or flutter
Atrial tachycardia with block*
Atrial fibrillation if there is:
—a slow ventricular response (<60 beats/min)
—*regularization* of the ventricular response*
AV junctional escape rhythms
AV junctional tachycardia*
Increased ventricular ectopy, especially if there is:
—ventricular bigeminy
—multiform PVCs
*Especially suggestive of digitalis toxicity.

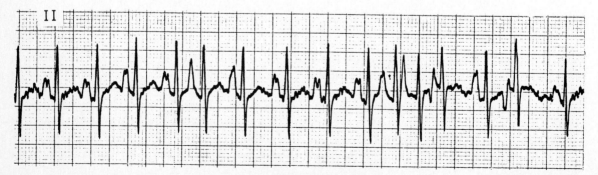

Figure 16A-7

ration), but some are biphasic. P wave morphology constantly varies and no predominant form is noted. This is *multifocal atrial tachycardia (MAT)* or *chaotic atrial mechanism*.

Multifocal Atrial Tachycardia (MAT)

MAT is most often seen in patients with chronic obstructive pulmonary disease (COPD). It is important clinically to distinguish this arrhythmia from atrial fibrillation, since treatment of the two conditions differs dramatically. With rapid atrial fibrillation, digitalization constitutes the medical treatment of choice. In otherwise uncomplicated cases (that is in the absence of acute myocardial infarction, hypoxemia, hyperthyroidism, and hypokalemia), the ventricular response can be used to gauge the amount of IV digoxin that needs to be administered. Following an initial loading dose of between 0.5 and 0.75 mg of digoxin, increments of 0.125–0.25 mg can be given every few hours until the ventricular response is under control.

In contrast, treatment of MAT *must* be directed at correcting the underlying cause of the arrhythmia (hypoxemia). MAT is notoriously resistant to treatment with digoxin. It is easy to imagine what might happen if one fails to recognize this arrhythmia and embarks on a course of vigorous digitalization. Not surprisingly, digitalis toxicity is one of the leading causes of mortality in patients with MAT.

The key to diagnosing MAT is to be aware of the settings in which it most frequently occurs (patients with COPD and hypoxia, or occasionally in extremely ill ICU patients). One may need to look especially close (in more than one monitoring lead) for atrial activity should such individuals present with an irregular rhythm.

P waves in MAT frequently manifest the pattern of *p-pulmonale* (tall and peaked in the inferior leads), suggesting right atrial enlargement. This is to be expected considering that most patients with the rhythm have underlying COPD. For example, note how tall and pointed many of the P waves are in the lead II shown above (Fig. 16A-7).

Although MAT is a rapid rhythm (by definition, heart rate exceeds 100 beats/min), in many cases the overall rate will be less than 120 beats/min and not demanding of antiarrhythmic therapy per se. If rate control is needed, verapamil is the drug of choice. Small doses of digoxin can be used (and may exert a synergistic effect with verapamil); however, this drug *must* not be pushed as it might if atrial fibrillation were present.

A question that frequently arises is how does one sort out a sinus rhythm with frequent PACs from MAT? Consider the example shown in **Figure 16A-7A.**

Like Figure 16A-7, the rhythm here is irregularly irregular and P waves are seen to precede virtually every QRS complex. However, despite the irregularity, *a basic sinus mechanism is present*—similar-appearing P waves with a constant PR interval precede beats no. 1, 2, 5, 6, 7, 9, 10, 14, and 15. This differs from Figure 16A-7 in which no predominant P wave was noted.

Needless to say, at times the distinction between MAT and sinus rhythm with frequent PACs becomes exceedingly difficult and clinically academic.

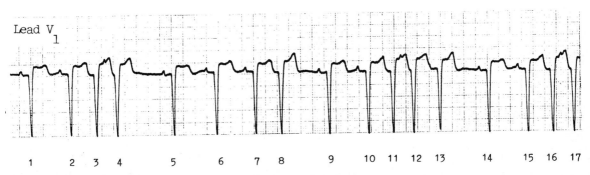

Lead V₁

| 1 | 2 | 3 | 4 | 5 | 6 | 7 | 8 | 9 | 10 | 11 | 12 | 13 | 14 | 15 | 16 | 17 |

Figure 16A-7A

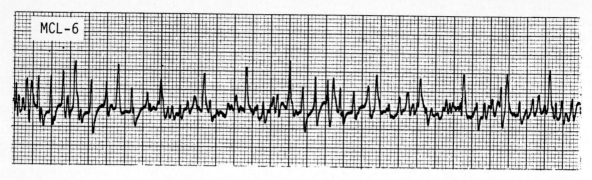

Figure 16A-8

PROBLEM   The woman whose rhythm is shown in <u>Figure 16A-8</u> was coughing at the time this tracing was recorded. Should she be immediately cardioverted?

ANSWER TO FIGURE 16A-8   Although at first glance this tracing may prompt concern, close inspection reveals baseline aber-ration with spurious-looking complexes at a rate of *over* 300 beats/min!!! No real tachyarrhyth-mia is this fast in adults. The *artifact* totally dis-appeared as soon as the patient stopped coughing.

PROBLEM   The tachyarrhythmia shown in **Figure 16A-9** is from a middle-aged woman

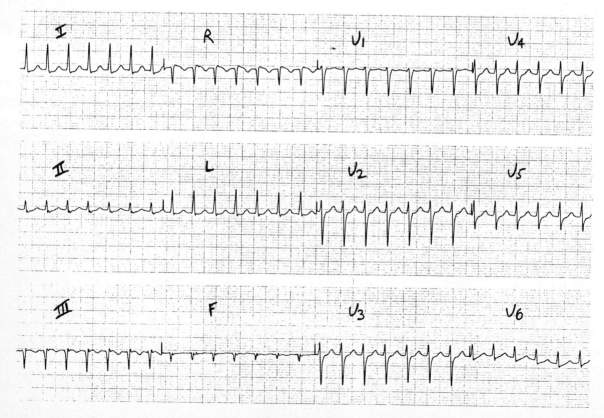

Figure 16A-9

who presented to the emergency department with the sudden onset of palpitations. Diagnosis? Suggested treatment?

ANSWER TO FIGURE 16A-9

A precisely regular supraventricular tachyarrhythmia at a rate of 180 beats/min is seen. Normal atrial activity is absent. The differential includes:

   i) Sinus tachycardia (unlikely at this heart rate)

   ii) Atrial flutter (unlikely as the ventricular response is a bit faster than one usually sees with flutter, and no hint of a sawtooth is present anywhere)

   iii) Atrial fibrillation (ruled out by the precise regularity of the rhythm)

   iv) PSVT (the most likely diagnosis)

Paroxysmal Supraventricular Tachycardia (PSVT)

Confirmation of the clinical impression (PSVT) might be forthcoming from application of a vagal maneuver (Valsalva or carotid sinus massage). If the rhythm were sinus tachycardia or atrial flutter, one would expect the ventricular response to slow and atrial activity to emerge. If on the other hand the rhythm was PSVT, CSM would either convert the tachyarrhythmia or have no effect at all.

CSM had absolutely no effect. The patient was sedated, and on the presumption that the rhythm was PSVT, 5 mg of IV *verapamil* was administered (slowly over a 2-minute period).

In the event that the patient is hemodynamically stable (as is usually the case), a real benefit may be derived from sedation. In addition to relieving the anxiety that so often accompanies this tachyarrhythmia, sedation lowers *sympathetic* tone. Enhanced sympathetic tone appears to play a role in perpetuating PSVT because it shortens the refractory period of AV nodal tissue and speeds conduction through the area. It also attenuates the effects of the vagus nerve on AV conduction, so that a greater degree of vagal tone may be needed to terminate the arrhythmia (Waxman et al., 1980).

PROBLEM   Over the next 20 minutes the rhythms shown sequentially in <u>Figures 16A-9A, -9B, -9C, and -9D</u> were observed. What has happened?

ANSWER TO FIGURES 16A-9A, -9B, -9C, AND -9D

The rate of the tachyarrhythmia progressively decreases from 16A-9A to 9C until conversion to a sinus mechanism (at a rate of 115 beats/min) is observed in Figure 16A-9D. The heart rate is 180 beats/min in 16A-9A, 145 beats/min in 16A-9B, and 135 beats/min in 16A-9C.

As opposed to vagal maneuvers that tend to convert PSVT in a more abrupt manner (if they work), verapamil typically produces a gradual slowing of the ventricular response until a sinus mechanism is restored (Feigl and Ravid, 1979). This is thought to be due to a verapamil-induced progressive slowing of conduction in the pathway contained within the reentry circuit. Occasionally the rhythm may become slightly irregular (with *alternation* of long and short cycle lengths) prior to termination of the tachycardia. At termination, one or more PVCs are sometimes seen before resumption of sinus rhythm.

<u>Figure 16A-9E</u> is taken from a patient whose PSVT was terminated by CSM. During the 10 beats of PSVT that start this tracing, a minimal irregularity develops. Then comes a fusion beat with 2

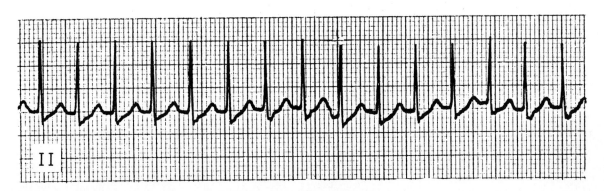

Figure 16A-9A

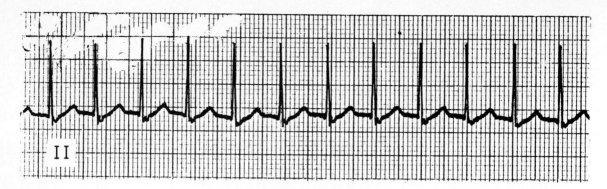

Figure 16A-9B

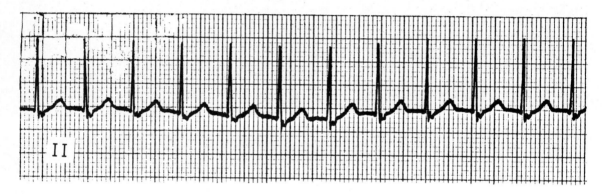

Figure 16A-9C

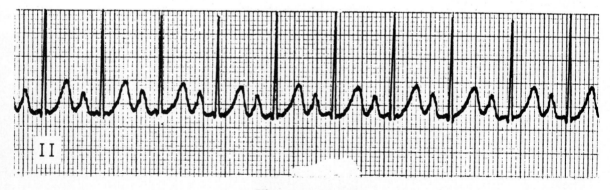

Figure 16A-9D

PVCs, followed by a 1-second pause, a sinus beat, 2 more PVCs, and resumption of sinus rhythm.

PROBLEM Return to the case of the middle-aged woman who presented with the tachyarrhythmia shown in Figure 16A-9. Now that she has been converted to normal sinus

rhythm (Fig. 16A-9D), what should you do next? Why?

ANSWER Obtain a postconversion 12-lead ECG (**Fig. 16A-9F**). One looks for evidence of an accessory pathway (WPW), as well as making sure that no myocardial infarction has oc-

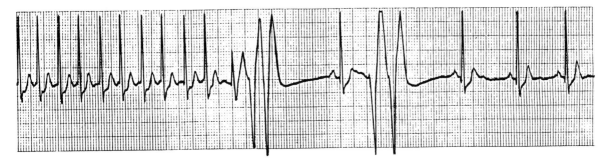

Figure 16A-9E

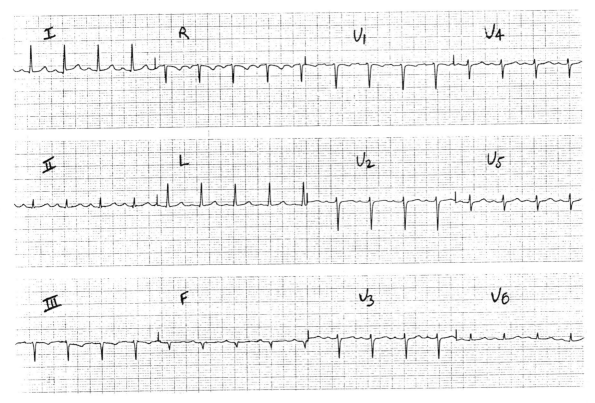

Figure 16A-9F

curred. Occasionally T wave inversion may be seen secondary to the rapid heart rate of the tachycardia.

Note the return of normal upright P waves in lead II. There is no evidence of WPW (no delta waves) and no evidence of infarction. Some of the ST segment depression that had been present in the lateral leads during the tachycardia on Figure 16A-9 was apparently *rate-related,* as it is no longer seen on this postconversion tracing.

Mechanisms of Supraventricular Tachycardias

There are two principal mechanisms of supraventricular tachycardias: increased automaticity and reentry. *Increased automaticity* is the mechanism of atrial tachycardia due to digitalis intoxication. An automatic atrial focus begins to discharge rapidly on its own and takes over the pacemaking function from the SA node. Because the AV node is not involved in perpetuation of the arrhythmia, therapeutic measures designed to decrease AV nodal conduction will not terminate the tachycardia (although occasionally they may slow the rate). Instead, treatment should be directed at the underlying cause of the increased atrial automaticity (often digitalis toxicity).

Reentry as a mechanism of supraventricular tachycardia may occur in a number of sites, including the SA node, the atria, the AV node, and between the atria and ventricles via an accessory pathway. For practical purposes, sinoatrial reentry and intra-atrial reentry are both difficult to recognize electrocardiographically (without electrophysiologic study) as well as being distinctly uncommon in adults. We will not treat them further.

Reentry involving the AV node is by far the most common mechanism of supraventricular tachycardia that the emergency care provider will encounter. Three conditions must be present for a reentry circuit to exist:

  i) Two separate pathways that join to form a closed circuit

  ii) Unidirectional block in one of these pathways

  iii) Slow conduction along the unblocked pathway

These conditions are illustrated in **Figure 16A-9G**. The two pathways are **x** and **y**, and they meet to form a closed loop (panel A in figure). Conduction is slowed down pathway **x**. A zone of *unidirectional* block exists along pathway **y** (lined area in the figure).

When an impulse reaches the circuit, it begins to travel down both pathways. Because of the area of block along the faster pathway, conduction of the impulse is unable to complete the circuit (it is stopped at point y_1 in panel B). However, conduction of the impulse continues along the unblocked pathway (point x_1 in panel B). In order for the reentry circuit to be established, conduction must be slow enough along pathway **x** for the zone of block to have recovered its ability to conduct by the time impulse x_2 arrives (panel C). If this is the case, the impulse will be conducted through this zone and be able to begin traveling around the circuit again (point x_3 in panel D). Along the way, it may give off a retrograde impulse (x_4 in panel D).

The conditions necessary for reentry are felt to exist at the level of the AV node **(Fig. 16A-9H).** Conduction through the AV node is *not* ho-

The Mechanism of Reentry

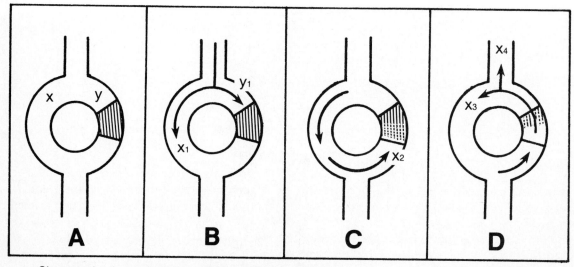

x – Slow conduction pathway   y – Fast conduction pathway

Figure 16A-9G

Reentry in PSVT

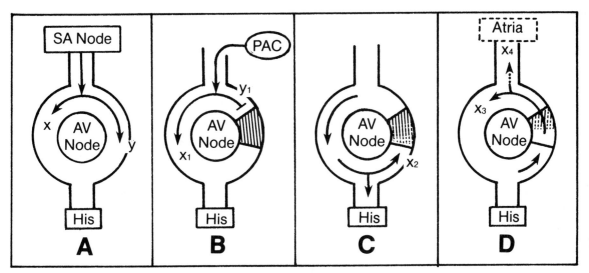

x–slow conduction pathway (with short refractory period)
y–fast conduction pathway (with long refractory period)

Figure 16A-9H

mogeneous (via a single pathway) as one might imagine. Instead there appears to be a *longitudinal dissociation* of conduction fibers, which results in a functional division into two separate conduction pathways. One of these pathways has a long refractory period and conducts *rapidly* (**y** in panel A of Fig. 16A-9H). The other has a short refractory period and conducts *slowly* (**x** in panel A).

Under normal conditions, as one might expect, the impulse arrives at the bundle of His first by conduction along the faster pathway (panel A in Fig. 16A-9H).

In panel B a premature impulse (PAC) occurs. Due to the relatively long refractory period of the fast pathway, the premature impulse is likely to find conduction still blocked down this route when it arrives at the AV node. However, the shorter refractory period of the slow pathway will likely be over, and conduction would then be able to proceed via this route toward the bundle of His (**x₁** in panel B).

If conditions are just right, conduction down the slow pathway will outlast the refractory pe-

riod of the fast pathway. In this case, by the time the impulse reaches point **x₂** (panel C), the fast pathway will have recovered enough to allow *retrograde* conduction. The reentry loop may then be perpetuated if the impulse at point **x₃** is able to be conducted again down the slow pathway (panel D). Along the way the impulse may be returned to the atria (point **x₄**) producing a retrograde P wave on the electrocardiogram (an *echo* beat).

PROBLEM   Consider the ECG shown in Figure 16A-10. Look closely at the QRS complex *during* the tachycardia. Is it different at all from the QRS complex during sinus rhythm (beats no. 1–3)?

ANSWER TO FIGURE 16A-10   Following three beats of sinus rhythm, a PAC occurs (notching the T wave that precedes beat no. 4). This first PAC conducts normally to the ventricles. However, a second PAC (that notches the T wave preceding beat no. 5) sets up the conditions for reentry to occur and precipitates a run of PSVT at a rate of 180 beats/min.

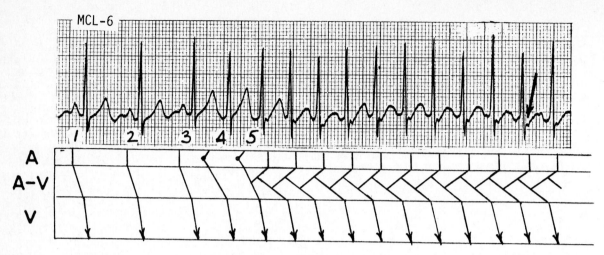

Figure 16A-10

The appearance of the QRS complex *during* the tachycardia is slightly different due to the addition of a notch on the ST segment (arrow). This is the result of retrograde conduction to the atria during the reentry tachycardia.

Several points may be made about this tracing. Note how the reentry cycle is initiated by a PAC (corresponding to panel B in Fig. 16A-9H). Note also that the PR interval of this PAC is *prolonged* compared to the PR interval of the normal sinus beats! This reflects the fact that this impulse is being conducted down the *slow* pathway (corresponding to point x_1 in panel B of Fig. 16A-9H). It is then conducted to the ventricles at the same time as it returns up the fast pathway (panel C). Because conduction goes down the *slow* pathway and back up the *fast* pathway, this type of PSVT is known as the *slow-fast* form. It is by far the most common type in adults. (As we will see momentarily, there is also a *fast-slow* form of PSVT in which conduction first goes down the fast pathway and comes back up the slow pathway.)

Atrial Activity in PSVT

The presence of atrial activity, its polarity, and its location relative to the QRS complex provide important clues to the mechanism of PSVT **(Fig. 16A-10A)**. With normal sinus rhythm, P waves will be upright in lead II (panel A in this figure). They will also be upright and normal in appearance with the uncommon reentry tachycardias in which the reentry circuit is contained within the SA node or the atria, since the impulse arises from the same location as it does for sinus rhythm.

In contrast, for PSVT involving the AV node, P waves will be inverted in lead II, reflecting the fact that they are being conducted in a retrograde manner. Most of the time with the *slow-fast* form of PSVT, the P wave is conducted so rapidly in the retrograde direction (since it is being conducted via the fast pathway) that it coincides with the QRS complex and is not visible on the surface ECG (panel B). If retrograde conduction takes a little longer, however, a retrograde P wave may be seen notching the ST segment (panel C). Patients with accessory pathways (WPW) may demonstrate this pattern when they develop PSVT that conducts down the normal pathway (via the AV node) and retrograde up the accessory pathway. Finally, with the *fast-slow* form of PSVT, the RP' interval will be prolonged (and the inverted P wave will occur only *after* the T wave) due to the very long time required for retrograde conduction to occur over the slow pathway (panel D).

PROBLEM   Examine Figure 16A-11. What type of PSVT is present?

ANSWER TO FIGURE 16A-11   This is the *fast-slow* form of PSVT. Beat no. 3 is sinus conducted. Beat no. 4 is conducted by a P wave with a different morphology. Following this, the tachycardia begins **(Fig. 16A-11A)**. As can be seen, the RP' interval is greatly prolonged, reflecting delayed retrograde conduction over the slow pathway.

Atrial Activity in PSVT

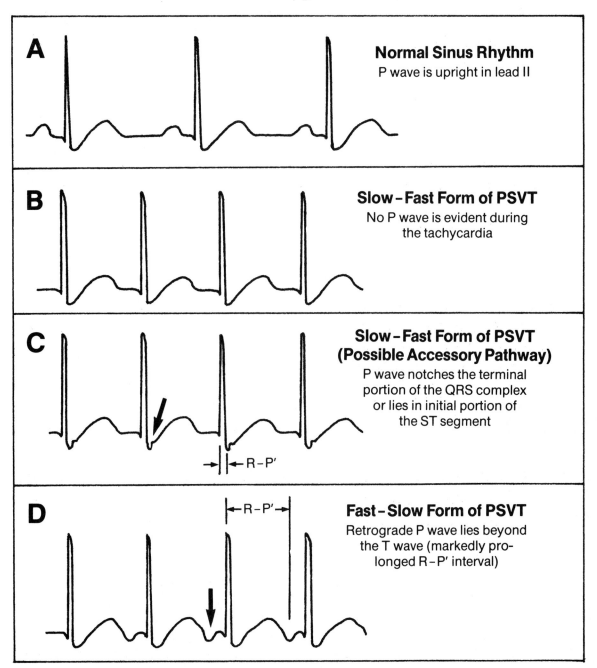

A Normal Sinus Rhythm
P wave is upright in lead II

B Slow – Fast Form of PSVT
No P wave is evident during
the tachycardia

C Slow – Fast Form of PSVT
(Possible Accessory Pathway)
P wave notches the terminal
portion of the QRS complex
or lies in initial portion of
the ST segment

R–P'

D R–P'
Fast – Slow Form of PSVT
Retrograde P wave lies beyond
the T wave (markedly pro-
longed R–P' interval)

Figure 16A-10A

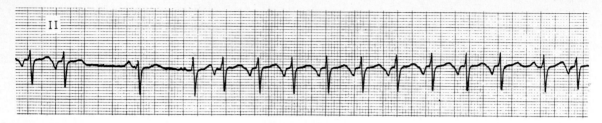

Figure 16A-11

Clinically the significance of the fast-slow form of PSVT is its much greater resistance to therapy than the slow-fast variety. Although the same medications are used to treat both of these entities, recurrences with the fast-slow form are so common that it is often called an *incessant tachycardia*.

PROBLEM   **Return one more time to the case of the middle-aged woman whose presenting ECG was shown in Figure 16A-9. Is there a clue on this tracing to the type of PSVT that she has?**

ANSWER   Close inspection of Figure 16A-9 shows a notch in the terminal portion of the QRS complex in leads II, III, and aVF that is *not* present on the postconversion tracing! This suggests that an *accessory pathway* may be taking part in the reentrant loop. (We will come back to the clinical importance of this finding at the end of section 16A.

PROBLEM   **Try one final example of PSVT—is there a hint to the mechanism in Figure 16A-12?**

ANSWER TO FIGURE 16A-12   Beats no. 1 and 2 are sinus. A PAC peaks the T wave of beat no. 2 and is followed by another PAC that produces a smaller peak in the T wave of beat no. 3. This latter PAC then conducts with a prolonged PR interval to set off the run of PSVT at 200 beats/min. Although the S wave is a bit wider during the run, there is no hint of any retrograde atrial activity. This is the typical slow-fast form of PSVT with no evidence of an accessory pathway (at least not on this monitoring lead).

PROBLEM   **Figure 16A-13 is another example of a narrow complex tachyarrhythmia. Is this PSVT or another type of reentry tachycardia? What clinical conditions are associated with this arrhythmia?**

ANSWER TO FIGURE 16A-13   The rhythm becomes regular after the first beat at a rate of 95 beats/min. The QRS complex is 0.10 second, or at the upper limit of normal. Atrial activity is evident; however, the PR interval constantly varies! At least in the initial part of the

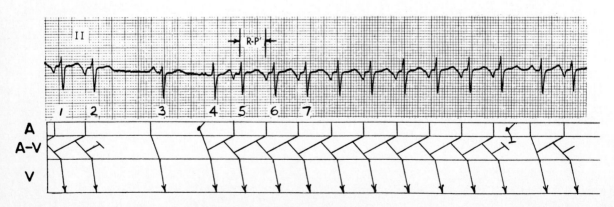

Figure 16A-11A

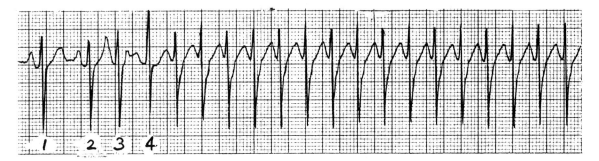

Figure 16A-12

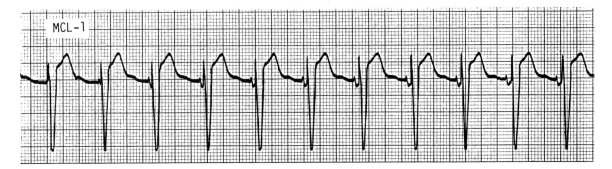

Figure 16A-13

tracing it is too short to conduct—therefore, *AV dissociation is present.* The underlying rhythm is a *junctional tachycardia.* This rhythm most often occurs in the setting of digitalis toxicity, inferior infarction, or after open heart surgery.

> The mechanism of junctional tachycardia is increased automaticity. Because retrograde block in the AV node is frequently seen with this arrhythmia, the SA node is able to continue firing at its own inherent rate. AV dissociation is the usual result. (The presence of AV dissociation per se effectively rules out any type of reentry tachycardia.) Strictly speaking, one might say that Figure 16A-13 would be better termed an *accelerated* junctional rhythm rather than junctional tachycardia since the heart rate is less than 100 beats/min.

WIDE COMPLEX TACHYARRHYTHMIAS

Since we covered the recognition of wide complex tachyarrhythmias in depth in the previous chapter, we will address only a few selected issues.

PROBLEM   The rhythm shown in **Figure 16A-14 was taken from a patient with a known RBBB. What is the likely etiology of the tachyarrhythmia?**

ANSWER TO FIGURE 16A-14   A regular tachyarrhythmia is seen at a rate of 140 beats/min. As noted, the QRS complex is widened. Normal atrial activity is absent, since the P wave is inverted in this lead II monitoring lead. Therefore, the rhythm cannot be sinus tachycardia. Possibilities include:

  i) PSVT—fast-slow form
  ii) Junctional (or low atrial) tachycardia
  iii) Atrial flutter

It is hard to distinguish between these three possibilities based on this tracing alone. CSM increased the degree of AV block and revealed the rhythm to be atrial flutter. The patient reverted to sinus rhythm following treatment (**Figure 16A-14A).**

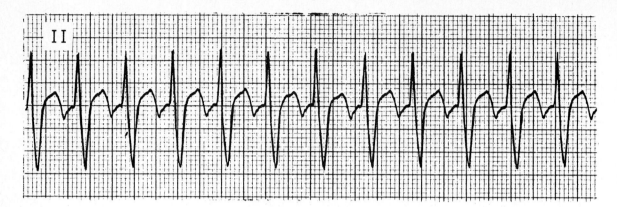

Figure 16A-14

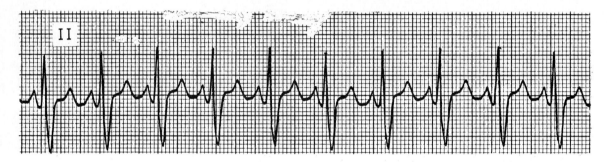

Figure 16A-14A

Note that the P wave is now upright in lead II, as it should be with normal sinus rhythm, and that the QRS complex has not changed.

PROBLEM   The rhythm strip shown in Figure 16A-15 was taken from an elderly lady who presented to the emergency department complaining of a "fluttering" in her chest that had just begun. She was not in any distress, did not complain of chest pain, and had a blood pressure of 90/60 mm Hg at the time this tracing was done. Treatment for PSVT was begun. Do you agree?

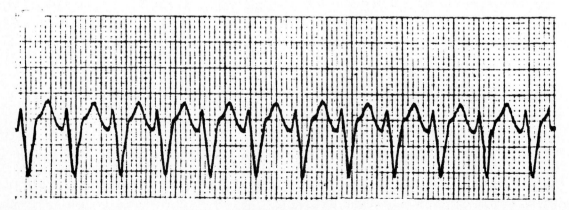

Figure 16A-15

ANSWER TO FIGURE 16A-15

Although QRS morphology does not look grossly abnormal, the QRS complex *is* wide (0.13 second) and no atrial activity is evident. Therefore one must consider the following five entities:

    i) VENTRICULAR TACHYCARDIA
    ii) VENTRICULAR TACHYCARDIA
    iii) VENTRICULAR TACHYCARDIA
    iv) Supraventricular tachycardia with preexisting BBB
    v) Supraventricular tachycardia with aberrant conduction

PROBLEM

Since the patient was tolerating the arrhythmia a 12-lead ECG was obtained (**Fig. 16A-15A**). Does this help in the differential?

ANSWER TO FIGURE 16A-15A

Once again a wide complex tachycardia is seen without evidence of atrial activity. There are two strong clues that this is *ventricular tachycardia:* the taller *left* rabbit ear in lead V$_1$ and the bizarre (markedly rightward) frontal plane axis.

Note that there is notching in the ST segment in leads II, V$_2$, V$_3$, and V$_4$. This may represent 1:1 retrograde VA conduction—it is not really of help in the differential.

PROBLEM

Before any treatment was given, the patient spontaneously converted to the rhythm shown in **Figure 16A-15B**. Does this support your previous suspicion?

ANSWER TO FIGURE 16A-15B

There is now sinus rhythm at 115 beats/min. The anomalous beat toward the end of the tracing is clearly a PVC in the context of this rhythm strip. Since this beat is *identical* in morphology to the wide complex tachycardia seen earlier (in Fig. 16A-15), it *proves* that the patient had been in ventricular tachycardia all along.

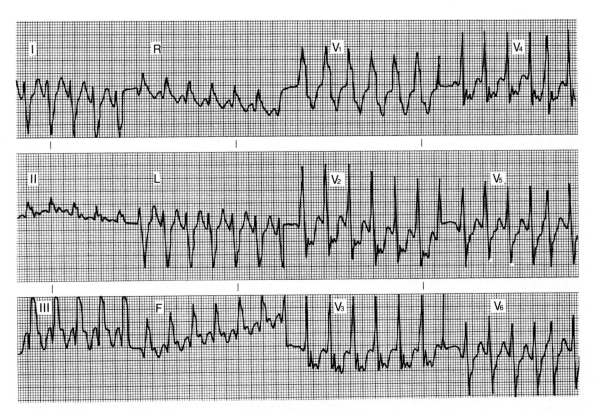

Figure 16A-15A

Lead I

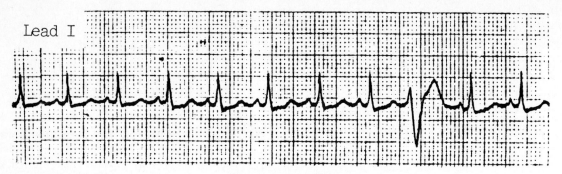

Figure 16A-15B

Lead V$_1$

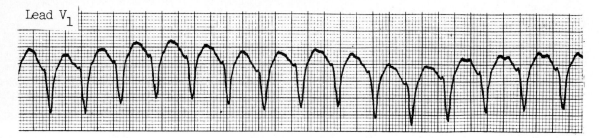

Figure 16A-16

This case is just another example of a patient who remained awake and alert despite being in ventricular tachycardia.

PROBLEM   The rhythm shown in **Figure 16A-16** was taken from a middle-aged man who presented after a syncopal episode. Blood pressure was 100/70 mm Hg at the time this tracing was recorded. Is this ventricular tachycardia?

ANSWER TO FIGURE 16A-16   At first glance the rhythm appears to be fairly reg-

ular at a rate of about 130 beats/min. The QRS complex seems to be somewhat widened, and obvious atrial activity is not seen. However, as the heart rate slows ever so slightly for the last three beats of the strip, P waves begin to emerge from the ST segment **(Fig. 16A-16A)**—this is *sinus tachycardia.*

PROBLEM   Shortly thereafter the pulse weakens and the rhythm shown in **Figure 16A-16B** is observed. How do you interpret this tracing?

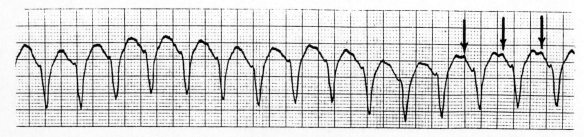

Figure 16A-16A

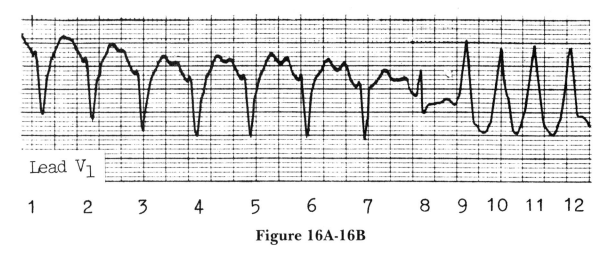

Lead V₁

1   2   3   4   5   6   7   8   9   10 11 12

Figure 16A-16B

ANSWER TO FIGURE 16A-16B

Sinus tachycardia is present for beats no. 1–7. P waves again are initially hidden but become more evident in front of beats no. 5–7 as the rate slows down. Beats no. 9–12 represent a short run of ventricular tachycardia. Beat no. 8 demonstrates a QRS configuration intermediate to the predominantly negative deflection of beats no. 1–7 and the positive deflection of the ventricular ectopic beats—it is a *fusion* beat.

PROBLEM   **From beat no. 12 of Figure 16A-16B the patient goes into the rhythm shown in Figure 16A-16C. What has happened? How is this best treated?**

ANSWER TO FIGURE 16A-16C   The rhythm deteriorates after beat no. 12 in Figure 16A-16C. However, the *polarity* of the QRS complexes during the ventricular tachyarrhythmia alternates from being predominantly positive (beats no. 10–16) to predominantly negative (beats no. 18–25). This changing polarity of ventricular tachycardia has been termed *torsade de pointes* (twisting of the points).

Torsade de Pointes

Originally described by the French physician Dessertenne in 1966, torsade de pointes often goes unrecognized and is treated incorrectly as "ordinary" ventricular tachycardia or ventricular fibrillation. This can have profound consequences for the patient who may be shocked countless times in an attempt to prevent this arrhythmia from recurring. Drugs such as quinidine and procainamide that usually are effective in suppressing ventricular ectopy paradoxically exacerbate the arrhythmia.

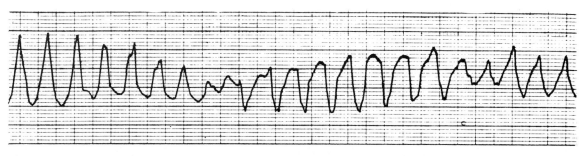

10 11 12 13 14 15 16 17 18 19 20 21 22 23 24 25

Figure 16A-16C

TABLE 16A-3

Causes of QT Prolongation and Torsade de Pointes

Drugs:
- —quinidine
- —procainamide
- —disopyramide
- —phenothiazines
- —tricyclic antidepressants

Electrolyte disturbances (hypokalemia)

Intrinsic heart disease:
- —ischemic heart disease
- —myocarditis

Central nervous system catastrophe:
- —subarachnoid hemorrhage
- —cerebrovascular accident

Liquid protein diet

Congenital QT prolongation syndrome

Torsade de pointes frequently is associated with a long QT interval on the baseline ECG. The arrhythmia is thought to be triggered by the occurrence of a PVC at a relatively late point during the repolarization process. Paroxysms of ventricular tachycardia with alternating polarity ensue. These paroxysms often terminate spontaneously but fre-

quently recur until the underlying predisposing cause of QT prolongation has been corrected. Quinidine, disopyramide, and procainamide are absolutely contraindicated because these agents further prolong the QT interval.

The causes of torsade de pointes are essentially those of QT prolongation **(Table 16A-3).** Of the antiarrhythmic drugs, quinidine is by far the most common precipitating agent. However, toxic levels of this drug need *not* be present for QT prolongation to occur, placing the onus on the physician to periodically check for QT prolongation.

Since the best treatment of torsade de pointes lies in prevention, it is important to be able to recognize QT prolongation. Generally, the QT interval measures less than one half the R-R interval* **(Fig. 16A-16D).** Thus, in panel B of this figure the QT interval is obviously prolonged. Reference to this patient's 12-lead ECG **(Fig. 16A-16E)** shows how striking the QT interval prolongation was in this particular case.

The goal of treatment of torsade de pointes is to eliminate predisposing factors when possible and to suppress the arrhythmia until the QT interval returns to normal. It has already been mentioned how drugs such as quinidine, disopyramide, and procainamide (which prolong the QT interval) are absolutely contraindicated in the treatment of this disorder. *Isoproterenol* shortens the QT interval and is recommended by many as the drug of choice. Use of this drug in the presence of rapid heart rates such as seen in Figure 16A-16 is controversial at best. Lidocaine and phenytoin have little effect on

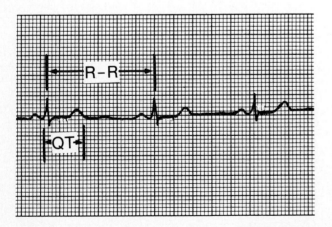
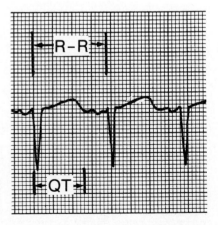

Figure 16A-16D

---

*This rule of thumb is less reliable for heart rates over 100 beats/min.

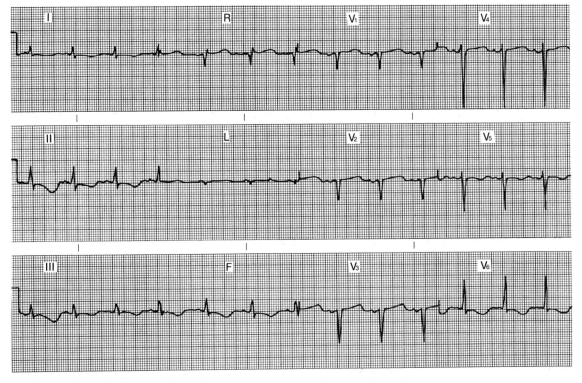

Figure 16A-16E

the QT interval and have met with mixed success. *Cardioversion* may be required for prolonged episodes of torsade de pointes. More often than not this is only a temporary measure because of the arrhythmia's disturbing tendency to recur. *Sequential overdrive pacing* is the generally accepted intervention of choice. Pacing at a rate of 80–120 beats/min usually allows control of the arrhythmia until the precipitating factor is corrected and the QT interval comes back toward normal.

PROBLEM The rhythm shown in **Figure 16A-17** was taken from a middle-aged woman who presented to the emergency department with a blood pressure of 90/60 mm Hg. Is this rapid atrial fibrillation?

ANSWER TO FIGURE 16A-17 Although QRS duration varies in different parts of this tracing, most complexes are widened and

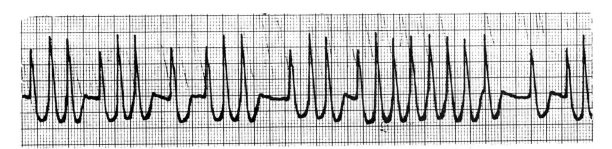

Figure 16A-17

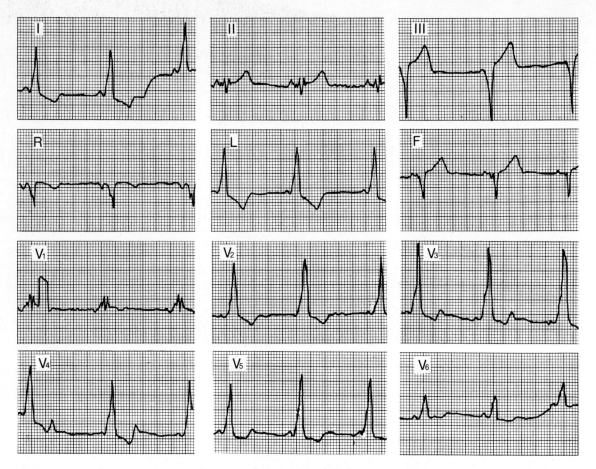

Figure 16A-17A

there is no atrial activity. However, the gross irregularity of this rhythm makes ventricular tachycardia unlikely. Ordinary atrial fibrillation is ruled out by the rapidity of the rate. In certain areas the R-R interval between QRS complexes is just over one large box in duration, which corresponds to a ventricular response of about 250 beats/min. This is too fast for atrial impulses to be transmitted to the ventricles by the normal conduction pathway, since the refractory period of the AV node will not allow so rapid a rate. The only reasonable explanation is that the atrial impulses are *bypassing* the AV node and are being conducted to the ventricles via an *ac-cessory pathway* with a much shorter refractory period.

PROBLEM   **The patient's old chart contained the 12-lead ECG shown in Figure 16A-17A. Is the underlying diagnosis more evident?**

ANSWER TO FIGURE 16A-17A   The diagnosis of *Wolff-Parkinson-White (WPW) syndrome* is now obvious from the short PR interval, QRS widening, and slurring (*delta* waves) of the initial portions of the QRS complex. This ECG was taken when the patient was in sinus rhythm.

Wolff-Parkinson-White (WPW) Syndrome

WPW has an approximate incidence of 2/1000 individuals in the general population. Conduction of the sinus impulse may be via the normal AV nodal pathway, it may be down the accessory tract, or it may alternate between the two. Patients with WPW are prone to develop atrial tachyarrhythmias in which a reentry circuit is set up between the normal AV nodal pathway and the accessory tract. With PSVT this most often results in antegrade conduction down the AV nodal pathway (producing a narrow QRS complex during the tachycardia) and retrograde conduction via the accessory pathway (panel A in **Fig. 16A-17B).** This tachyarrhythmia is by far the most common observed in patients with WPW. It is usually well tolerated by the patient.

In contrast, with atrial fibrillation in WPW, an-tegrade conduction usually occurs down the *accessory* tract with retrograde conduction to the AV nodal pathway. This results in QRS widening during the tachycardia. Because of the short refractory period of the accessory pathway, there may be 1:1 conduction of atrial impulses during atrial fibrillation, resulting in a ventricular response that exceeds 250 beats/min (panel B in Fig. 16A-17B). Such rapid rates may not be well tolerated, and this rhythm can deteriorate into ventricular fibrillation. Similarly, antegrade conduction down the accessory pathway frequently occurs when patients with WPW develop atrial flutter, resulting in a ventricular response that may exceed 300 beats/min.

Although both digoxin and verapamil are extremely effective in slowing the ventricular rate in ordinary atrial fibrillation with a rapid ventricular response, they are *contraindicated* in

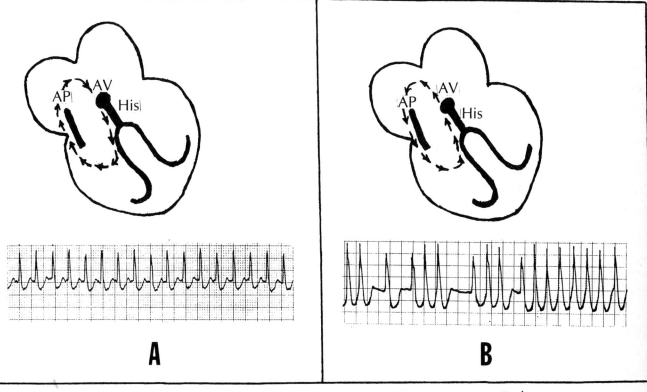

AP - Accessory Pathway
AV - AV Nodal Pathway
His - Bundle of His

Figure 16A-17B

WPW with atrial fibrillation. This is because di-goxin and verapamil *may further accelerate con-duction down the accessory pathway and exacerbate the arrhythmia.*

> The goal of treating rapid atrial fibrillation with WPW is to prevent the 1:1 antegrade conduction of atrial impulses down the accessory pathway. This can be done by lengthening the *antegrade* refrac-tory period of the accessory pathway, an effect shared by procainamide and to a lesser extent li-docaine. Consequently, the medical treatment of choice for this patient is to administer an IV load-ing dose of procainamide (with lidocaine being a second choice). Immediate synchronized cardio-version would be indicated for hemodynamic decompensation.

———————

Let us tie up this section by completing the thought process we were developing for PSVT. As we emphasized in Figure 16A-10A, identifi-cation of atrial activity and its relationship to the QRS complex may provide valuable clues to the mechanism of PSVT. Thus the notching of the ST segment and/or tail end of the QRS complex seen during the PSVT shown in Figures 16A-9 and 16A-10 suggests that an accessory pathway may be participating in the reentry circuit.

> It is not generally appreciated that up to 30% of adults with PSVT have a *concealed* accessory path-way. The term concealed implies that conduction is able to occur only in a *retrograde* fashion. Because there is no antegrade (forward) conduction down the accessory pathway in these individuals, they never manifest ECG evidence of WPW (delta waves, short PR interval, and QRS widening are ab-sent). However, they do maintain the potential to develop reentry tachycardias.
>
> As we have mentioned, *orthodromic* PSVT (con-duction down the normal AV nodal pathway and retrograde up the accessory pathway) accounts for the large majority of observed tachyarrhythmias in patients with WPW. The QRS complex is *narrow* during the tachycardia, and notching may be seen in the terminal portion of the QRS complex or the initial part of the ST segment. *As long as the accessory pathway remains concealed, management of these tachy-arrhythmias is identical to that of the more typical slow-fast PSVT in which the reentry circuit is contained en-tirely within the AV node.* Acute treatment consists of vagal maneuvers, sedation, and verapamil as the drug of choice, with digoxin as a good second line agent. *The problem is that occasionally a patient who*

> *was thought to have purely orthodromic PSVT may spontaneously develop atrial fibrillation during treat-ment with digoxin or verapamil!* Considering that these drugs may accelerate conduction down the accessory pathway, one can see that the conse-quences may be disastrous.

Practically speaking, it will *not* be necessary in most cases to address the supraventricular tach-ycardias with nearly as much sophistication as we have in this chapter. In the acute care set-ting, treatment of PSVT tends to be similar re-gardless of whether the mechanism is the typical slow-fast form of PSVT, the fast-slow form, reentry utilizing an SA nodal or intra-atrial cir-cuit, or orthodromic PSVT in patients with an accessory pathway *with the rare exception of those patients who have an accessory pathway and are pre-disposed to developing atrial fibrillation.* We hope we have at least made you aware of this latter possibility (albeit rare) and of the potential dan-ger of using verapamil or digoxin in such a set-ting. We also hope to have increased your awareness of the different mechanism involved in atrial tachycardia with block and in junctional tachycardia—both of which are commonly as-sociated with digitalis toxicity. Finally, we hope we have increased your enthusiasm for seeking out the subtle clues in arrhythmia recognition that lay before us.

B: AV BLOCKS—AND A STEP BEYOND

In Chapter 3 we introduced basic concepts in the diagnosis of the AV blocks. We would like to pick up from that point and explore some of the difficulties encountered when the arrhythmia "fails to obey all of the rules."

The ability to accurately diagnose the AV blocks (like all other arrhythmias) depends on our systematic four-step approach. One looks for:

i) Regularity of the rhythm (of *both* atrial and ventricular rhythms)

ii) Evidence of atrial activity (P waves)

iii) QRS widening
iv) A relationship between P waves and the QRS complex ("Who's married to whom?")

Identification of atrial activity and its relationship to the QRS complex are particularly important. As a "warmup" to this chapter, pay particular attention to the atrial activity in these first two examples.

PROBLEM   **What happens to the P waves in Figure 16B-1?**

ANSWER TO FIGURE 16B-1   P waves are readily identifiable in this tracing, but their morphology changes. The first two complexes (beats no. 1 and 2) are preceded by a peaked P

wave and are conducted with 1° AV block (PR interval = 0.22 second). P wave morphology then changes and takes on a biphasic configuration for beats no. 3–7, all of which are conducted with a normal PR interval. A negative P wave precedes beat no. 8, followed by resumption of the peaked P wave configuration and acceleration of the rate. This figure illustrates a *wandering atrial pacemaker, sinus bradycardia,* and *sinus arrhythmia*—all components of the *sick sinus syndrome.*

PROBLEM   **Again, what happens to the P waves in Figure 16B-2?**

ANSWER TO FIGURE 16B-2   Initially there is a "regular irregularity" to the rhythm. Sinus rhythm at 70 beats/min is identified by

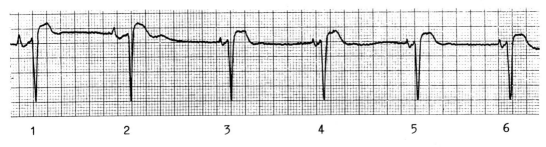

Lead MCL₁

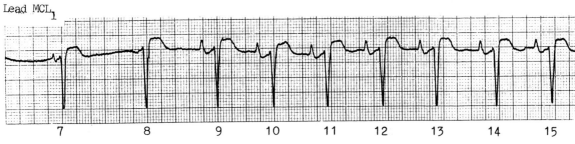

Figure 16B-1

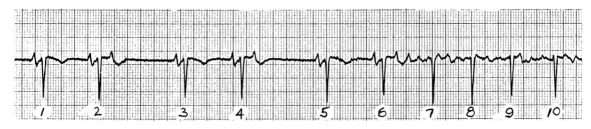

Figure 16B-2

beats no. 1 and 2, 3 and 4, as well as 5 and 6. The third, sixth, and ninth P waves are *early* and peak the T waves of beats no. 2, 4, and 6. Since every third P wave is a PAC, the underlying rhythm is *atrial trigeminy*. The first two premature P waves (the ones that follow in the T wave of beats no. 2 and 4) are *blocked*. The third (that peaks the T wave of beat no. 6) precipitates *atrial flutter* that rapidly deteriorates into *atrial fibrillation* with a controlled ventricular response (beats no. 7–10).

Now on to the AV blocks themselves. . . .

Simplified Classification: Looking for 1° and 3° AV Block

As we indicated in Chapter 3, a way to simplify classification of the AV blocks is the following:

i) Look first to see if 1° AV block is present. (This is usually easy to recognize.)

ii) Look next to see if 3° AV block is present. (This *also* is usually easy to recognize.)

iii) If the block is neither 1° nor 3°, but beats are being dropped *due to AV block,* the block must be 2°.

PROBLEM   **First degree AV block is not *always* easy to recognize. Consider the 12-lead ECG shown in Figure 16B-3. What is the rhythm?**

ANSWER TO FIGURE 16B-3   The rhythm is regular at 95 beats/min, and the QRS complex is of normal duration. It is hard to be sure if atrial activity is present. In lead II (where P waves usually are easiest to identify), all that is seen is an upright deflection at the midpoint of the R-R interval that looks like a T wave. If this were the only monitoring lead available, one

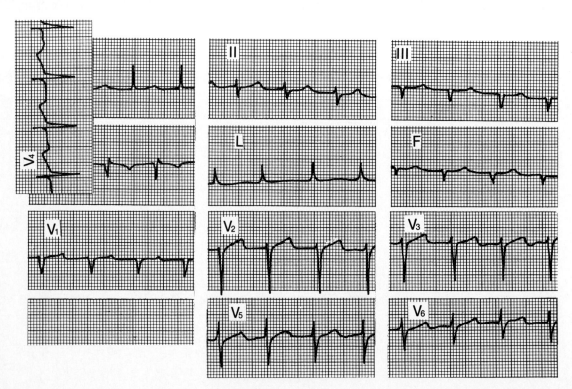

Figure 16B-3

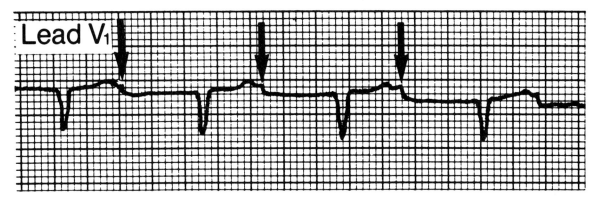

Figure 16B-3A

would have to say that an *accelerated* AV nodal rhythm was present.

However, in lead V_1 (which usually is the next best lead to choose when searching for P waves), the upright deflection in the middle of the R-R interval has much more the appearance of a P wave. Were this the case, then the rhythm would be sinus with 1° AV block. *It is impossible to distinguish between these two entities based on this ECG alone.*

PROBLEM   Some time later, the rhythm strip shown in **Figure 16B-3A** was recorded. Has this clarified the question raised by Figure 16B-3?

ANSWER   The heart rate has decreased, and P waves can now be clearly seen notching each T wave (arrows). The patient had been in 1° AV block all the while!

> First-degree AV block usually is easy to identify, since it is simply a sinus rhythm in which the PR interval is prolonged. The above example illustrates nicely how P waves may occasionally be hidden by

T waves when this PR prolongation is marked. To answer the question "How long can the PR interval be prolonged and still conduct?"—conduction with a PR interval of up to 0.92 second has been observed (Marriott, personal communication).

PROBLEM   Moving up in severity, examine the tracing shown in **Figure 16B-4. Does this represent complete AV block?**

ANSWER TO FIGURE 16B-4   In Chapter 3 we set out the criteria for diagnosing complete (3°) AV block:

i) Atrial regularity (usually)
ii) Ventricular regularity (usually)
iii) Complete AV dissociation *despite adequate opportunity for normal conduction to occur* (usually implying a heart rate of less than 45 beats/min).

All of these conditions are present in Figure 16B-4. The ventricular rate is regular at about 30 beats/min. The atrial rate is regular at 75 beats/min **(Fig. 16B-4A)** and completely dissociated from the QRS despite having more than

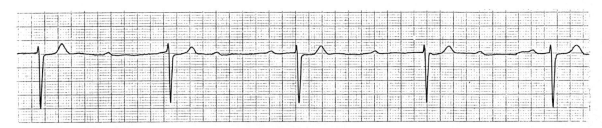

Figure 16B-4

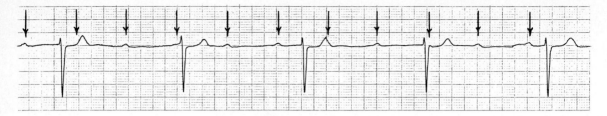

Figure 16B-4A

adequate opportunity to conduct. Thus, the AV block is *unquestionably* complete.

> Although P waves cannot be identified in *every* spot where an arrow is placed in Figure 16B-4A, one can assume that they are there since the regularity of the P waves that are obviously present continues throughout.
>
> One would expect the level of the AV block to be *below* the AV node in this example, since the QRS appears wide (at least 0.11 second) and the ventricular response is so slow.

PROBLEM   Examine **Figure 16B-5. Is this complete AV block?**

ANSWER TO FIGURE 16B-5   The first three beats appear to be sinus conducted with a marked 1° AV block (PR = 0.62 second). *Asystole* (not complete AV block) follows.

AV DISSOCIATION

One of the areas of greatest confusion regarding the AV blocks is diagnosing AV dissociation. We might start with the definition:

> **AV dissociation** is a *secondary* rhythm disturbance (*never* a primary disturbance) that oc-

curs when the atria and ventricles fail to respond to the same impulse and beat independently (Lipman et al., 1984).

Thus, one should *never* say that a rhythm *is* AV dissociation, but rather that AV dissociation is present because of _____ (the primary disorder).

> Common reasons for AV dissociation include:
> i) AV block
> ii) Slowing of the sinus pacemaker (AV dissociation by *default*)
> iii) Acceleration of a junctional or ventricular pacemaker (AV dissociation by *usurpation*)

PROBLEM   Examine **Figure 16B-6. Is this AV dissociation by *default* or *usurpation*? What might the underlying cause of this rhythm disturbance be?**

ANSWER TO FIGURE 16B-6   The QRS complex is narrow and the ventricular rate fairly regular at 115–120 beats/min. P waves precede the first few complexes but become lost in the QRS after beat no. 7. Although the PR interval is short (0.10 second) for beats no. 1–4,

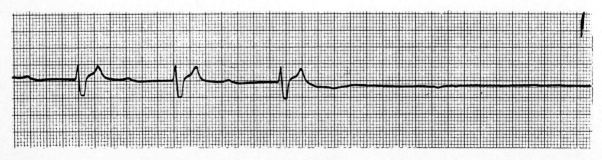

Figure 16B-5

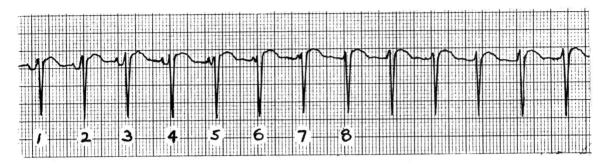

Figure 16B-6

these P waves could possibly still be conducting. However, conduction is definitely *not* possible for the P waves preceding beats no. 5–7 (as the PR interval is just too short). *AV dissociation* therefore is present (P waves are at least temporarily unrelated to QRS complexes), in this case due to *usurpation* of the rhythm by an *accelerated junctional pacemaker* (which technically qualifies as *junctional tachycardia* since the heart rate exceeds 100 beats/min).

> As mentioned earlier, common causes of accelerated junctional rhythm (the *primary* disorder in this case) include digitalis intoxication, inferior myocardial infarction, and the postoperative state following open heart surgery.

It is important to reemphasize that there is no evidence whatsoever of any form of AV block on this tracing! P waves never fail conduction at a time when they would not be expected to do so.

PROBLEM   How would you interpret the rhythm shown in **Figure 16B-7**?

ANSWER TO FIGURE 16B-7   Hopefully you did not answer this question by simply

saying there is AV dissociation. AV dissociation *is* present—however, (as always) it is a *secondary* disorder. The underlying rhythm in Figure 16B-7 appears to be an *AV nodal escape rhythm* at the slow rate of 33 beats/min (as seen from beats no. 2 and 3). Note that sinus conduction had started this tracing (beat no. 1), but that atrial activity then disappeared until just before beat no. 4. This P wave (arrow) is definitely too close to the next QRS complex to conduct—therefore, AV dissociation is present. Note that the sinus pacemaker speeds up at this point (the R-R interval between beats no. 4–5 is less than the R-R interval during the junctional rhythm), and sinus conduction is able to resume with beat no. 5. The correct interpretation of this rhythm is that a slow *AV nodal escape rhythm* is present, arising by *default of the sinus pacemaker* (from marked sinus bradycardia and/or a sinus pause), and produces transient *AV dissociation*.

> We have referred to the escape rhythm here as being *AV nodal* because the QRS complex is narrow and similar in appearance to the sinus-conducted beats. However, one really cannot tell for sure

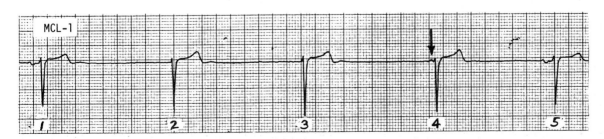

Figure 16B-7

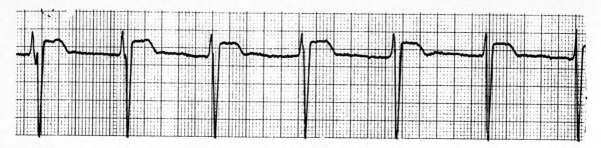

Figure 16B-8

where the focus of the escape pacemaker arises. Potential pacemaking cells exist throughout the myocardium. As long as the impulse arises *from somewhere in the conduction system* (the AV node, the bundle of His, or the bundle branches), the QRS complex may appear similar in morphology to the sinus-conducted beats. In this case, the fact that the rate of the escape pacemaker is slower than the usual rate of an AV nodal rhythm (40–60 beats/min) suggests that its focus is from *below* the AV node.

Although QRS morphology of the escape beats (no. 2, 3, and 4) is similar to that of the sinus-conducted beats (no. 1 and 5), it is *not* identical (it differs in that the S wave is slightly deeper). Such subtle differences in QRS morphology often exist between sinus-conducted beats and escape beats originating from the AV node or slightly lower in the conduction system. As we will see later in this chapter, recognition of such subtle differences may sometimes provide an important clue as to whether a particular P wave is conducting.

PROBLEM   What has happened to the P waves in Figure 16B-8?

ANSWER TO FIGURE 16B-8   A P wave precedes the first complex in this tracing with an extremely short PR interval. After this, atrial activity seemingly disappears. Considering that the first QRS complex in this tracing has a

relatively small (3 mm) r wave, one might suspect that the 6-mm r wave of the other QRS complexes results from *superposition* of the P wave.

PROBLEM   Does **Figure 16B-8A** clarify the situation?

ANSWER TO FIGURE 16B-8A   Atrial activity is much more evident on this tracing. It can now be seen that an underlying *AV nodal rhythm* exists with a regular rate of 53 beats/min. P waves are totally unrelated to the QRS complex—they follow the QRS in the beginning of the tracing (beats no. 1, 2, and 3), then get lost within the QRS (beat no. 4), superimpose on the initial part of the QRS (beats no. 5 and 6), and finally precede the QRS with a short PR interval (beats no. 7 and 8). This confirms our suspicion that P waves were present all along in Figure 16B-8 (and superimposed on the QRS). When atrial and junctional pacemakers are unrelated but operate at nearly identical rates (as they do here), the condition is known as *isorhythmic AV dissociation*.

Occasionally, atrial and junctional pacemakers continue to beat at nearly the same rate for extended periods of time, resulting in a rhythm in which P waves move "in and out" of the QRS com-

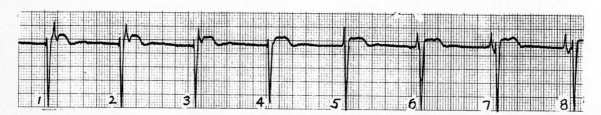

Figure 16B-8A

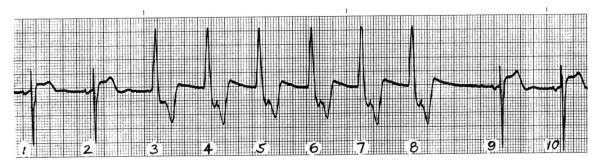

Figure 16B-9

plex. This phenomenon has been colorfully labeled *accrochage* by the French from their verb *s'accrocher* (to cling to). Despite slight variation in rate of one or both competing pacemakers, each remains almost in phase with the other as if some unseen force was acting to keep the two together.

PROBLEM   **Examine <u>Figure 16B-9</u>. Is there AV dissociation?**

ANSWER TO FIGURE 16B-9   Following two sinus beats, the QRS complex widens and changes dramatically in appearance. Beats no. 3–8 represent an *accelerated idioventricular rhythm (AIVR)* which takes over because its intrinsic rate (80 beats/min) is faster than the rate of the sinus pacemaker. In this particular instance, AIVR is *not* an escape rhythm, because the first beat in the sequence (no. 3) begins *before* the next expected sinus beat (that is, the R-R interval of beats no. 2–3 is *less* than the R-R interval of the sinus-conducted beats [no. 1–2]—so that beat no. 3 occurs *early*!).

> Note notching in the ST segment of beats no. 4–8. This represents *retrograde* conduction to the atria from the idioventricular focus. As a result of this retrograde conduction the SA node is suppressed and prevented from discharging during the run of AIVR. Consequently, preservation of retrograde (VA or ventriculoatrial) conduction in this case prevents AV dissociation from taking place. A pause follows the last beat in the run (no. 8), during which time the SA node recovers before resuming the pacemaking function with beat no. 9.
>
> Contrast this situation with one in which retrograde conduction to the atria is blocked (such as occurred with the example of complete AV block we reviewed in Fig. 16B-4). Under such circumstances, the SA node will continue to discharge at

its own inherent rate, and complete AV dissociation will result (Fig. 16B-4A).

The Many Faces of Wenckebach

In Chapter 3 we listed the following as characteristic features of 2° AV block Mobitz type I (Wenckebach):

    i) Regularity of the atrial rate
    ii) Group beating
    iii) Progressive lengthening of the PR interval until a beat is dropped
    iv) Duration of the pause (that contains the dropped beat) of *less* than twice the shortest R-R interval

In addition to the above one might add:

    v) Progressive shortening of the R-R interval within groups of beats.

These features are illustrated in **Figure 16B-10**. Note that as the PR interval lengthens from beats no. 2–4, the R-R interval shortens (the R-R interval between beats no. 2–3 is greater than that between no. 3–4).

> Also note that the pause containing the dropped beat (the R-R interval between beats no. 4–5) is *less* than twice the shortest R-R interval (the R-R between beats no. 3–4). The reason for this is that the greatest *increment* (increase) in the PR interval usually occurs between the first and second beats of the Wenckebach group. When the PR interval remains constant (as it does with Mobitz II), the pause will be *equal* to twice the R-R interval. Finally, with phenomena such as exit block or sinus

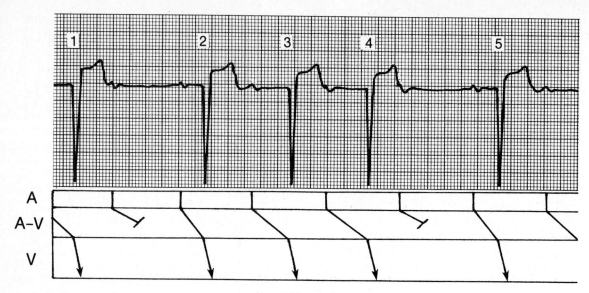

Figure 16B-10

pauses (which both may occur in sick sinus syndrome) and with blocked PACs (that reset and often suppress the SA node), the pause often will be *greater* than twice the shortest R-R interval.

Up to now we have spoken exclusively about Wenckebach that occurs at the level of the AV node (2° AV block Mobitz type I). Actually many other examples of "Wenckebach-like" conduction exist, including:

   i) Sinoatrial (SA) Wenckebach
  ii) Wenckebach AV conduction in the presence of atrial fibrillation or flutter
 iii) Wenckebach AV conduction in the presence of atrial tachycardia
 iv) Junctional rhythm with retrograde Wenckebach

  v) Ventricular tachycardia with Wenckebach exit block
 vi) Others. . . .

Although in depth discussion of these extends beyond the scope of this book, the point to emphasize is that recognition of typical features *(footprints)* of Wenckebach may allow one to suspect this conduction disturbance *even when P waves are absent!*

PROBLEM   **Consider Figures 16B-11 and 16B-12, taken from an elderly woman with known history of *atrial fibrillation* and congestive heart failure. Is she still in atrial fibrillation?**

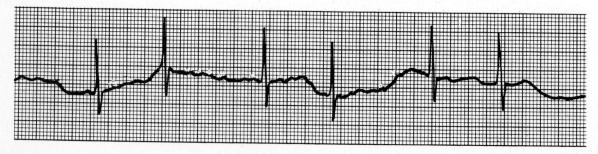

Figure 16B-11

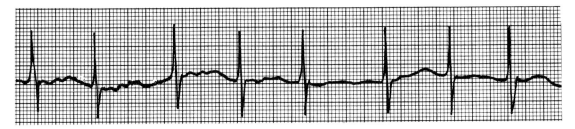

Figure 16B-12

ANSWER TO FIGURES 16B-11 AND 16B-12

Undulations in the baseline and the absence of P waves suggest that underlying atrial fibrillation is still present. One is struck, however, by the *regular* irregularity of the ventricular response *(group beating)*. Long and short cycles alternate in Figure 16B-11, while in Figure 16B-12 typical Wenckebach periodicity is seen (group beating, progressively shortening R-R intervals, pause duration of less than twice the shortest R-R interval). Thus despite atrial fibrillation, Wenckebach conduction emanates from the AV node **(Fig. 16B-12A).**

Clinically the importance of Wenckebach conduction in the setting of atrial fibrillation in a patient on digitalis is the same as that for "regularization" of the ventricular response—it suggests possible digitalis toxicity.

Not all arrhythmias obey all of the rules. For example, an underlying sinus arrhythmia may be present in a patient manifesting Mobitz I 2° AV block. In such a case, the atrial rhythm will no longer be regular (by definition), the R-R interval may not progressively decrease within each Wenckebach group, and the pause may no longer be less than twice the shortest interval. Nevertheless, careful evaluation of the rhythm in the overall context of the clinical situation usually will allow the diagnosis to be made.

We will illustrate some of the "many faces" of Wenckebach over the next few examples in which typical features may not be all that evident.

PROBLEM   **Consider the rhythm shown in Figure 16B-13. Is Wenckebach present?**

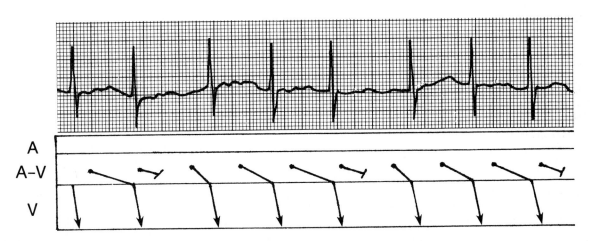

Figure 16B-12A

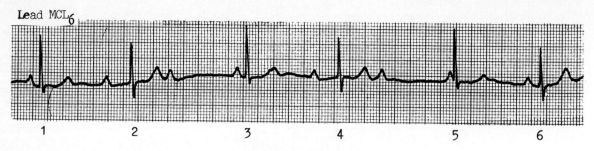

Figure 16B-13

ANSWER TO FIGURE 16B-13   The most striking finding on this tracing is the presence of *group beating*, which should lead you to suspect that a type of Wenckebach *may* be present. P wave morphology is constant but the P-P interval varies, suggesting that *sinus arrhythmia* is the underlying rhythm. Beats *are* being dropped. One would definitely expect the P waves following beats no. 2 and 4 to conduct. Since complete AV block is unlikely (because the ventricular response is so variable), this tracing probably represents a type of 2° AV block. The narrow QRS and the presence of group beating suggest Mobitz I as the prime suspect.

The trick lies with beats no. 1, 3, and 5. On close inspection it can be seen that QRS morphology of these beats differs slightly from that of beats no. 2, 4, and 6. Moreover, the PR interval of beat no. 5 is definitely too short to conduct, implying that this beat and the two others like it (beats no. 1 and 3) are *junctional escape beats.* Supporting this contention is the fact that the R-R interval of the two escape beats seen on this tracing (the R-R interval between beats no. 2–3 and no. 4–5) is the same and corresponds to a junctional escape rate of 38 beats/min.

It is important to appreciate that the emergence of escape beats in this tracing is *appropriate*—without them the ventricular response would be even slower. However, their presence makes definitive diagnosis of the conduction disturbance a difficult task from this tracing alone.

Subsequent rhythm strips on this patient confirmed our suspicion that the block was Wenckebach.

PROBLEM   **Is Wenckebach present in Figure 16B-14?**

ANSWER TO FIGURE 16B-14   Following seven supraventricular beats that manifest a constant R-R interval comes a pause. P waves with a prolonged PR interval *(1° AV block)* are evident in front of beats no. 1–5. Continuation with calipers set at the P-P interval beyond this point reveals a notch in the T wave of beat no. 5, no evidence of atrial activity in the T wave of beat no. 6, peaking of the T wave of beat no. 7, and an undisguised P wave (that is right on time) in front of beat no. 8. Thus the atrial rate is perfectly regular, and the P wave hidden in the T wave of beat no. 7 is not conducted.

The relationship between P waves and the

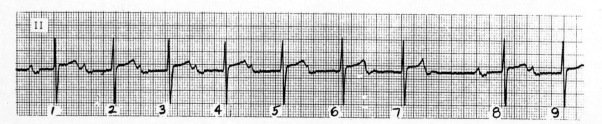

Figure 16B-14

QRS complex is not at all obvious at first glance of the tracing, since it is hard to determine if the PR interval is progressively increasing from beats no. 1–7. However, inspection of the PR interval just *before* the pause and comparing it to the PR interval just *after* the pause reveals a significant difference. Similarly, comparison of the PR interval preceding the first beat in the sequence (beat no. 1) with the PR interval of the last beat in the sequence before the pause (no. 7) suggests that the PR interval must be lengthening until the beat is dropped. Therefore, the rhythm is Mobitz I 2° AV block.

PROBLEM   Interpret the rhythm shown in Figure 16B-15.

ANSWER TO FIGURE 16B-15   The QRS complex is narrow and the ventricular rate is irregular (although group beating is again evident). The atrial rate is fairly regular (assuming that a P wave is hidden within the QRS complex of beat no. 4). Two P waves appear to be "dropped" (the P waves following beats no. 3 and 7), suggesting that 2° AV block is present.

Turning one's attention to the first "group of beats," P waves can be seen to precede each

QRS complex. The PR interval increases until the P wave after beat no. 3 is dropped, suggesting Wenckebach. The next QRS complex (beat no. 4) is not preceded by a P wave. This is a junctional escape beat. The sequence then resumes, as a P wave with a short PR interval precedes beat no. 5. The rhythm is *2° AV block Mobitz I* with (appropriate) *junctional escape beats*.

PROBLEM: Figure 16B-16 was taken from a patient with an acute inferior infarction. Can you explain the irregularity of the ventricular response?

ANSWER TO FIGURE 16B-16   Group beating is seen. The only place where P waves are evident is preceding the QRS complex that terminates each pause. Here the P wave conducts with 1° AV block (PR interval = 0.27 second).

Despite the fact that ST segment elevation from the acute inferior infarction obscures atrial activity, several factors should suggest that Mobitz I may be present:

  i) The setting (acute inferior infarction)
  ii) Group beating

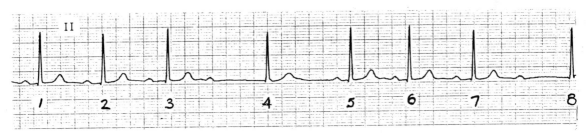

Figure 16B-15

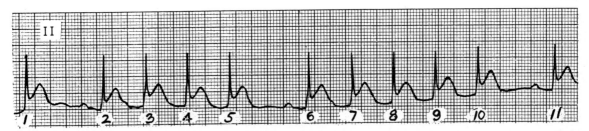

Figure 16B-16

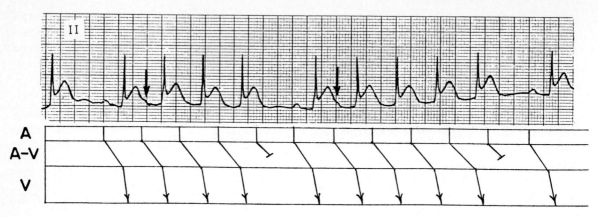

Figure 16B-16A

iii) 1° AV block

iv) Narrow QRS complex

v) Pause duration of less than twice the short-est R-R interval

The explanation of this rhythm is fairly complex. Again we feel it may be best understood by illustration with a laddergram **(Fig. 16B-16A)**. Since atrial activity is not obvious, one must *deductively* determine the P-P interval, which can be done in the following manner. If Mobitz I were present, the atrial rate should be regular and a dropped P wave would have to be contained within the T wave of beat no. 5. If one looks at the entire first Wenckebach cycle (encompassing beats no. 2–6), *five* P waves should therefore be contained inside (one preceding each QRS complex, and the dropped beat). Dividing the entire cycle length (the interval from the R wave of beat no. 2 until the R wave of beat no. 6) by 5 thus gives the P-P interval of the underlying sinus rate. Starting with the P wave that is clearly seen (the one preceding beat no. 2), presumed atrial activity can now be plotted out and the laddergram completed. *That these suppositions are probably accurate is supported by subtle notching of the T wave of beats no. 2 and 6 (arrows) at precisely the place where one would expect the next P wave to occur.*

Although *construction* of this laddergram extends beyond the scope of this text, several important points can be made by this example:

i) Not all of the *footprints* of Wenckebach are always present (or always obvious).

ii) The combination of a high index of suspicion (often raised by the finding of group beating) in the context of an appropriate clinical situation frequently leads to the diagnosis.

WHEN (AND WHY) TO SUSPECT MOBITZ II

Mobitz II 2° AV block is said to occur when atrial impulses are blocked in the setting of *consecutively* conducted beats that manifest a constant PR interval.

PROBLEM   **Almost every other beat in Figure 16B-17 is dropped. Is this Mobitz II?**

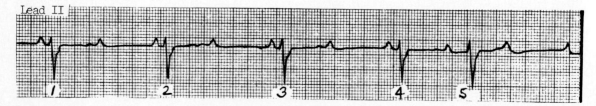

Figure 16B-17

ANSWER TO FIGURE 16B-17 The QRS complex appears to be slightly prolonged in this tracing, although it is hard to be certain of where the QRS ends and the ST segment begins. The atrial rate remains regular throughout at 75 beats/min. There is 2:1 AV conduction and the PR interval remains constant for the first four beats of the tracing. It would be impossible to distinguish between Mobitz I and Mobitz II if the rhythm strip ended here. Moreover, because of QRS widening, one would have to give the nod to Mobitz II.

As we emphasized in Chapter 3, definitive differentiation between Mobitz I and Mobitz II is not possible in the setting of 2° AV block with *pure* 2:1 AV conduction. This is not the case here, however, since the *telltale* sign of Wenckebach surfaces at the end of the tracing (the PR interval of beat no. 5 lengthens with respect to that of beat no. 4). It is extremely unlikely that a patient would switch abruptly from Mobitz I to Mobitz II. Therefore, Figure 16B-17 most probably represents Wenckebach (*not* Mobitz II!) with 2:1 and 3:2 AV conduction.

> The key to making the correct diagnosis in this case is to go back to the definition we gave above for Mobitz II—*consecutive* beats must be conducted with a normal PR interval before one can determine with certainty that any dropped beats are due to Mobitz II.

Clinically, Mobitz II is far less common than Mobitz I. **Figure 16B-18,** taken from a patient with an anterior infarction, illustrates why it is so essential to recognize this conduction disturbance when it does occur.

Initially the patient is in sinus rhythm. Then with nary a warning comes a 4-second period of ventricular standstill that is terminated only by a ventricular escape beat. This behavior is typical of Mobitz II, which sometimes very suddenly and dramatically progresses to either complete AV block or ventricular standstill. The setting in which this conduction disturbance is most likely to occur is acute anterior infarction. As soon as Mobitz II is recognized, a pacemaker should be inserted.

In contrast with acute inferior infarction, conduction disturbances are more often benign. First-degree AV block and Mobitz I are the usual fare. The disorders tend to be transient and associated with an adequate ventricular response so that simple observation (without pacemaker insertion) is often all that is needed. Even when 3° AV block does develop, an escape junctional pacemaker capable of maintaining an acceptable blood pressure and heart rate may result (see Table 3D-3 in Chapter 3). As opposed to the abrupt development of severe conduction disturbances with Mobitz II, a fairly orderly and sequential progression (from 1° AV block, to

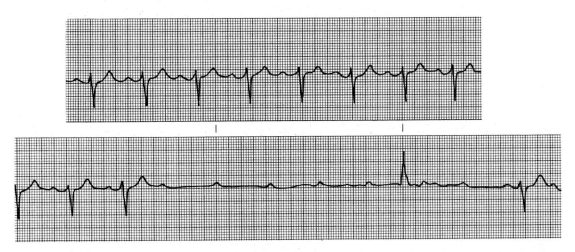

Figure 16B-18

Lead II

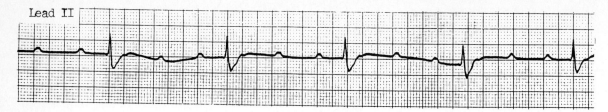

Figure 16B-19

Mobitz I, and finally to 3° AV block) is often seen.

PROBLEM   **Examine Figure 16B-19. What kind of block is present?**

ANSWER TO FIGURE 16B-19   The ventricular rate is regular at just under 40 beats/min. The atrial rate is also regular at 115 beats/min (with a P wave notching the terminal portion of each QRS complex). Despite conduction of only 1 of every 3 P waves, a relationship *does* exist between these P waves and the QRS (as the PR interval remains constant). Although one cannot diagnose Mobitz II with certainty (since *consecutively* conducted beats are never seen before a beat is dropped), QRS widening makes it probable that the anatomic level of the block is low. The interpretation should be:

—*2° AV block with 3:1 AV conduction, probable Mobitz II.*

Mimics of 2° AV Block

In this next section we include examples of rhythm disturbances that are commonly *misdi-*

agnosed as 2° AV block. To keep you honest, we have included a few examples of *real* 2° AV block.

PROBLEM   **In Figure 16B-20 a pause occurs following beat no. 9. Is this the result of 2° AV block?**

ANSWER TO FIGURE 16B-20   The first four beats in this rhythm are sinus. Beat no. 5 is a PAC (with the premature P wave notching the preceding T wave). Following this comes a ventricular couplet, two more sinus beats, and then the pause. . . .

The most common cause of a pause is a blocked PAC! A large percentage of misdiagnosed 2° AV blocks probably stem from inadequate appreciation of this truism. Often the PAC will be obvious (if looked for), but at other times it may be recognizable only as a subtle notching in the preceding P wave. This is the case in this example. Comparing the "normal" T wave (the T wave of beats no. 1, 2, 3, 4, and 8) to the T wave of beat no. 9 reveals this notching.

Note that the PR interval following the pause is short. Beat no. 10 is a junctional escape beat that

Lead V$_1$

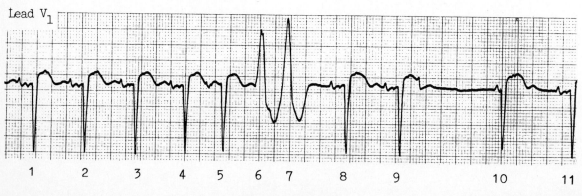

1   2   3   4   5   6   7   8   9   10   11

Figure 16B-20

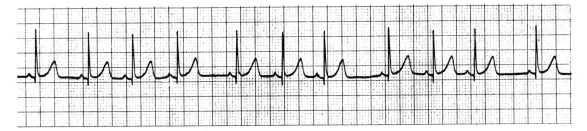

Figure 16B-21

discharged before its preceding P wave was able to conduct.

PROBLEM   Is the group beating shown in Figure 16B-21 due to Mobitz I?

ANSWER TO FIGURE 16B-21   Although the group beating of this tracing may at first suggest Wenckebach, *no P waves are dropped and the atrial rate is irregular.* The QRS complex is narrow and always preceded by a P wave with a normal (and constant) PR interval. This is *sinus arrhythmia.*

PROBLEM   Interpret the rhythm in Figure 16B-22.

ANSWER TO FIGURE 16B-22   Initially there is sinus bradycardia at a rate of about 48 beats/min. There follows a pause which is terminated by a *junctional escape rhythm* (beginning with beat no. 4). Retrograde conduction to the atria occurs with the junctional rhythm. There is no evidence of any AV block.

PROBLEM   Is the group beating in Figure 16B-23 due to Mobitz I?

ANSWER TO FIGURE 16B-23   Yes, although this may not be readily apparent on initial inspection of this tracing. The key lies with mapping out the atrial rate. Many of the T

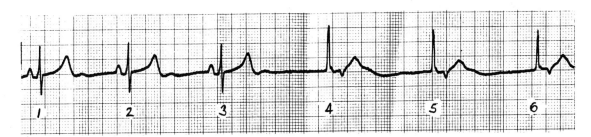

Figure 16B-22

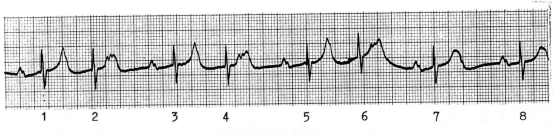

Figure 16B-23

waves have an unusual appearance—either very peaked or notched—suggesting that P waves may be superimposed. If one sets the calipers to the distance between the P wave preceding beat no. 1 and the point at the apex of the T wave of this beat, it is then possible to "walk out" the atrial rate **(Fig. 16B-23A).**

QRS complexes are narrow, and *each* is preceded by a P wave. The PR interval progressively lengthens until a beat is dropped (Fig. 16B-23A). This is 2° AV block, Mobitz I, with 3:2 and 2:1 AV conduction.

PROBLEM   **Is the group beating in Figure 16B-24 due to Mobitz I?**

ANSWER TO FIGURE 16B-24   No. *The most common cause of a pause is a blocked PAC.* The T waves of beats no. 2, 5, and 8 all have an extra notch that the "normal" T waves do not have. This is due to a blocked PAC. Other reasons the rhythm is not Wenckebach are that the atrial rate is irregular and the PR interval does not increase within each group.

Figure 16B-24A was recorded a short while

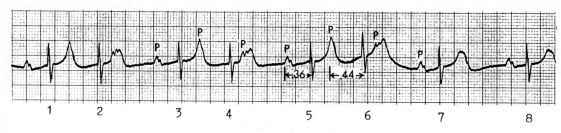

Figure 16B-23A

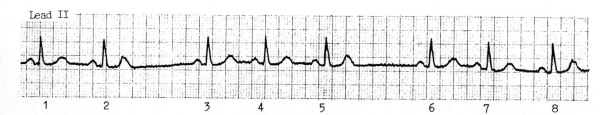

Figure 16B-24

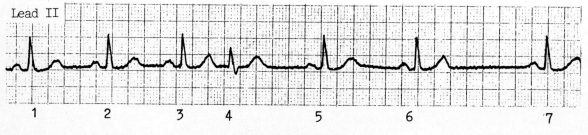

Figure 16B-24A

later on the same patient and again demonstrates PACs. The PAC that peaks the T wave following beat no. 6 is blocked (as were those in Fig. 16B-24), but the one following beat no. 4 is conducted with aberrancy.

> The reason the first premature P wave conducts but the second does not may be explained by cycle-sequence comparison (as was discussed in Chapter 15). Although the coupling intervals of each of these PACs is identical, the R-R interval preceding beat no. 6 is longer than the R-R interval preceding beat no. 3. As a result, the absolute refractory period following beat no. 6 will be slightly longer.

PROBLEM   Interpret   the   arrhythmia shown in Figure 16B-25.

present. Since the QRS complex is widened and each QRS is preceded by a P wave with a *fixed* PR interval, this probably represents *Mobitz II*. Additional support for this diagnosis comes from the fact that two beats in a row are dropped during the longest pause.

PROBLEM   What is the relationship of the "P" waves to the QRS complex in Figure 16B-26?

ANSWER TO FIGURE 16B-26   The rhythm is irregularly irregular in this tracing. Small upright deflections that *simulate* P waves are noted between each R-R interval, but these appear to be related more to the QRS complex

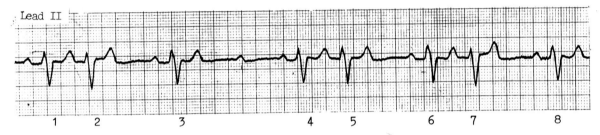

Figure 16B-25

ANSWER TO FIGURE 16B-25   This is a difficult tracing, since at first glance no P waves can be seen in front of beats no. 2, 5, and 7. The key is provided within the long R-R interval—two P waves occur in a row before beat no. 4. If one uses this P-P interval, the atrial rate may be "walked" out across the entire tracing (with the "missing " P waves all corresponding to the apex of the T waves). Thus, several beats are dropped, and a type of 2° AV block must be

that *precedes* them than to the subsequent QRS (the R-"P" interval is fixed). The ventricular response is too irregular for this to be a junctional rhythm with a retrograde P wave. This is *atrial fibrillation* with a controlled ventricular response. The small upright deflections are T waves.

PROBLEM   Does the rhythm in Figure 16B-27 represent 2:1 AV block of the Mobitz I or Mobitz II type?

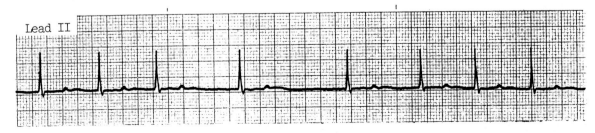

Figure 16B-26

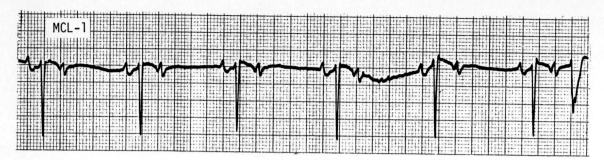

Figure 16B-27

ANSWER TO FIGURE 16B-27   Neither, since there is *no* evidence of any AV block on this tracing. *The most common cause of a pause is a blocked PAC.* The atrial rate here is too irregular for this to be AV block—every other P wave occurs *early*. All of the PACs are *blocked* except for the last one that conducts with an LBBB-type of aberration. Atrial bigeminy with blocked PACs is one of the most common mimics of 2:1 AV block.

PROBLEM   **Interpret the rhythm shown in Figure 16B-28.**

ANSWER TO FIGURE 16B-28   The QRS complex is narrow and the ventricular rate regular at 100 beats/min. The atrial rate is also regular, with 2 P waves occurring for each QRS (atrial rate = 200 beats/min). The relation of P waves to the QRS is constant, with every other atrial impulse being conducted. Rather than a Mobitz I or Mobitz II block here, the problem appears to be *atrial tachycardia* with *2:1 AV block*. The possibility of digitalis toxicity should be considered.

PROBLEM   **Interpret the rhythm in Figure 16B-29.**

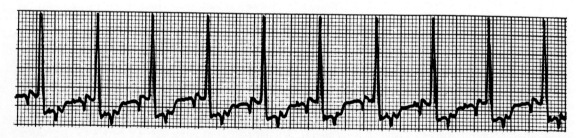

Figure 16B-28

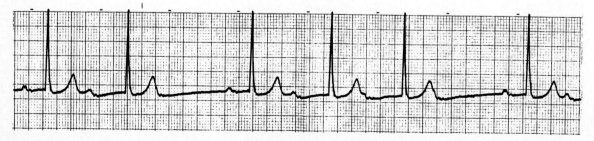

Figure 16B-29

ANSWER TO FIGURE 16B-29   The QRS complex is narrow and the ventricular rhythm irregular. Some P waves are clearly evident—others appear to notch the terminal portion of the T wave. Underlying *sinus arrhythmia* is present, since the atrial rate is slightly irregular. P waves *do* precede each QRS complex, however, and within a group the PR interval lengthens until a beat is dropped. This is *2° AV block Mobitz Type I.* The diagnosis is not initially obvious, due to the sinus arrhythmia, fairly slow atrial rate, and underlying 1° AV block.

In **Figure 16B-29A,** recorded from the same patient, we highlight the P waves. Their relationship to the QRS (progressively lengthening PR interval within a group until a beat is dropped) is now more apparent.

PROBLEM   Is this last example of group beating (Fig. 16B-30) also due to Wenckebach?

ANSWER TO FIGURE 16B-30   No. Once again *the most common cause of a pause. . . .* Premature P waves can clearly be seen to notch the T waves of beats no. 2 and 6. Sinus rhythm is present with blocked PACs.

Let us conclude this chapter with a few clinical vignettes.

PROBLEM   A middle-aged man presents to the emergency department with a several-hour history of severe chest pain. Blood pressure is 100/70 mm Hg, the chest pain has stopped, and he appears fairly comfortable at the time you arrive. His admission ECG is shown in **Figure 16B-31. How do you interpret this tracing?**

ANSWER TO FIGURE 16B-31   There is a bradyarrhythmia with a narrow complex ventricular response of about 48 beats/min. The PR intervals appear to vary in the different leads, indicating *AV dissociation.* The ST segment elevation in leads II, III, and aVF with reciprocal ST segment depression in the anterolateral leads, in conjunction with the history, suggest *acute inferior infarction.*

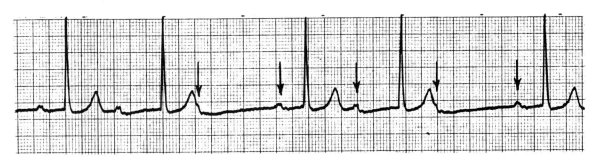

Figure 16B-29A

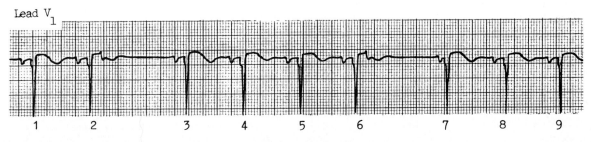

Figure 16B-30

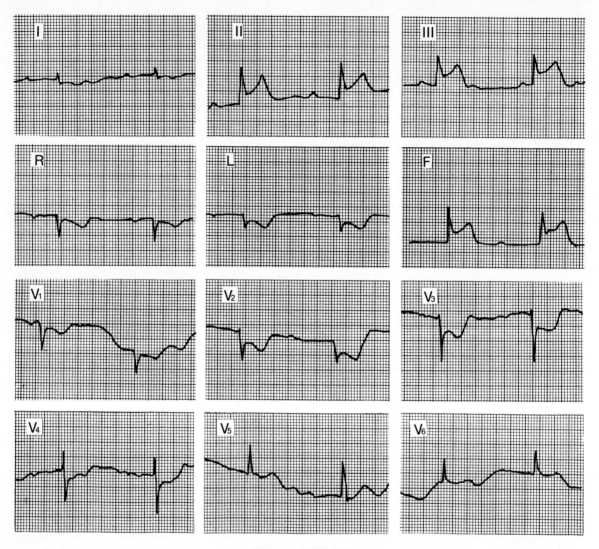

Figure 16B-31

PROBLEM   **Does the rhythm strip shown in Figure 16B-31A clarify the reason for the AV dissociation?**

ANSWER TO FIGURE 16B-31A   The atrial rate is now regular at 80 beats/min, and P waves march through the QRS complexes (**Fig. 16B-31B**). Several of them occur at points during the R-R interval where one would expect conduction if it were possible. Although our criteria for diagnosing 3° AV block are not completely met (the ventricular rate is a bit over 45 beats/min and this rhythm strip is not really long enough to convincingly demonstrate P

waves in *all* phases of the R-R interval), Figure 16B-31A suggests that *3° AV block with a junctional escape pacemaker* may be present.

PROBLEM   **If the patient remained comfortable and hemodynamically stable, what treatment would be indicated? Atropine? Pacemaker insertion?**

ANSWER   AV conduction disturbances in the setting of acute inferior infarction are usually transient and do not require treatment in the asymptomatic, hemodynamically stable patient. At least for the moment, this appears to

Lead II

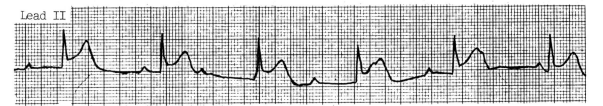

Figure 16B-31A

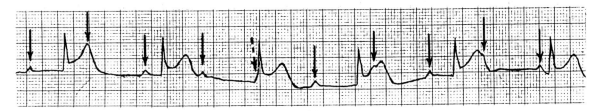

Figure 16B-31B

be the situation in this case. Were the patient to develop chest pain, hypotension, ventricular ectopy, or other signs of hemodynamic compromise, treatment would be indicated. Atropine is the drug of choice. If bradycardia is resistant to therapy, a pacemaker would be required. (Having an *external pacemaker* nearby might make one feel more comfortable about treating this patient conservatively.)

Lead II

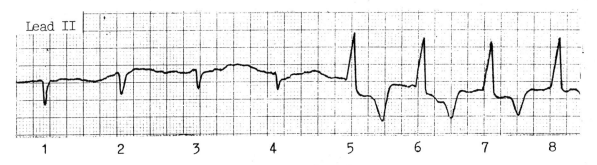

Figure 16B-32

Lead II

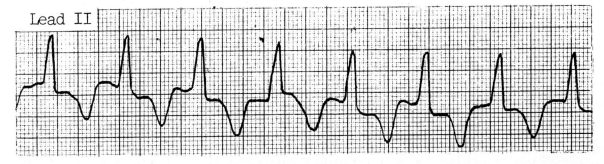

Figure 16B-32A

PROBLEM   The rhythm strips shown in Figures 16B-32 and 16B-32A were recorded sequentially from a patient admitted several hours earlier for suspected myocardial infarction. What has happened? What treatment would be indicated if the patient were asymptomatic and hemodynamically stable?

ANSWER TO FIGURES 16B-32 AND 32A

No P waves are seen in either strip. The QRS complex is narrow for the first four beats in Figure 16B-32, during which time the rhythm is junctional. Beat no. 5 in this strip occurs early and initiates a regular rhythm with a wider QRS complex of a completely different configuration. This is an accelerated idioventricular rhythm (AIVR). It speeds up slightly but continues throughout Figure 16B-32A.

AIVR is commonly observed in the setting of acute myocardial infarction. It is usually a transient disorder that rarely results in adverse hemodynamic effects. The risk of deterioration to ventricular fibrillation is considered to be minimal. Therefore in the asymptomatic, hemodynamically stable patient, the fourth option *(benign neglect)* is usually the treatment of choice.

AIVR may occur when the accelerated ventricular rate overrides the supraventricular pacemaker. This is the case in Figure 16B-32, in which a junctional rhythm at 65 beats/min is superceded by AIVR at 70 beats/min. If hypotension did occur with this rhythm, *atropine* would be the treatment of choice in the hope that this drug would stimulate the supraventricular pacemaker to overtake the ventricular rhythm **(Fig. 16B-32B).**

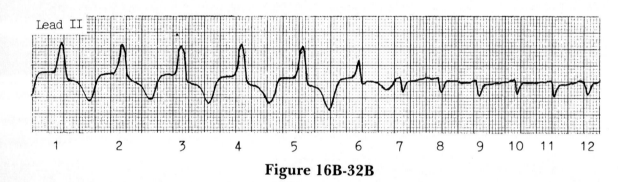

Figure 16B-32B

Four therapeutic options exist for managing AIVR:
  i) Lidocaine
  ii) Defibrillation (or synchronized cardioversion)
  iii) Atropine
  iv) *Benign neglect*

It is important to emphasize that AIVR may also arise as an escape rhythm for a failing SA or AV nodal pacemaker. Under these circumstances, suppression of the ventricular escape rhythm with *lidocaine* may result in ventricular standstill if no supraventricular pacemaker is able to take over. It is for this reason that treat-

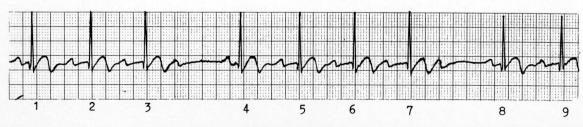

Figure 16B-33

ment of AIVR with lidocaine is generally *not* recommended. Similarly, one would not want to use *countershock* with this rhythm in a patient who is hemodynamically stable.

Two other *footprints* of Wenckebach are present here—decreasing R-R intervals within a group, and pause duration of less than twice the shortest R-R interval.

PROBLEM   This final patient was admitted for an acute inferior infarction. How would you interpret his initial rhythm strip (Fig. 16B-33)?

PROBLEM   The patient is treated with atropine and a while later he is observed in the rhythm shown in Figure 16B-34. Has he gone into a complete AV block?

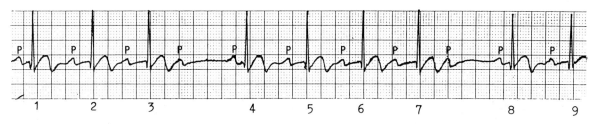

Figure 16B-33A

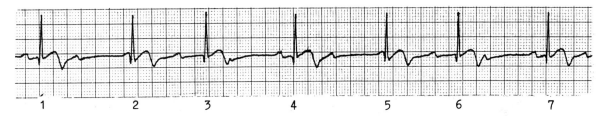

Figure 16B-34

ANSWER TO FIGURE 16B-33   The QRS complex is narrow and the ventricular rate is irregular. There is group beating, raising one's suspicion that Wenckebach may be present. The atrial rate is regular at 80 beats/min (Fig. 16B-33A). Each QRS complex *is* preceded by a P wave, and the PR interval progressively increases within a group until a beat is dropped. This as *2° AV block Mobitz type I.*

ANSWER TO FIGURE 16B-34   Regularly occurring P waves (now at a rate of 85 beats/min) continue. They seem to march through the QRS complex without the slightest relation to it. Yet the R-R interval is *not* regular as one would expect if the AV block were complete. This suggests that some type of 2° AV block is present.

Figure 16B-34A demonstrates the regularity

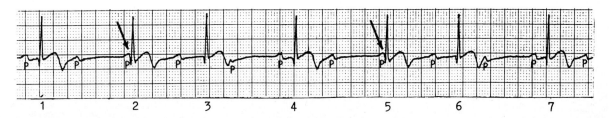

Figure 16B-34A

of the atrial rate in this rhythm. The PR interval preceding beats no. 2 and 5 is definitely too short to conduct (arrows in Fig. 16B-34A). These beats must therefore be *junctional* beats. Since the R-R interval preceding these beats is about the same as the R-R interval between beats no. 3–4 and 6–7, it is likely that this constant R-R interval reflects a *junctional escape rhythm* at 47 beats/min. The reason the R-R interval shortens for beats no. 3 and 6 is that these beats are sinus conducted, albeit with 1° AV

ANSWER   Two-to-one AV conduction is now present, with every other P wave producing a notch in the terminal portion of the QRS complex.

> If you are having difficulty detecting the second P wave, set your calipers at precisely one-half the R-R interval (= 0.58 second). P waves can now be "walked out" on the tracing (**Fig. 16B-35A**).

The degree of AV block has *not* necessarily worsened!!! In effect, the only thing that we know has changed since Figure 16B-33 is the

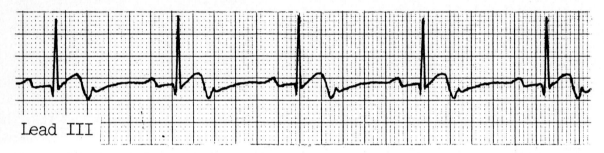

Lead III

Figure 16B-35

block. Thus, *intermittent AV dissociation* rather than complete AV block is present.

> Although the mechanism for this arrhythmia is rather complex, the point to emphasize is that the rhythm in Figure 16B-34 is *not* 3° AV block and does *not* necessarily require a pacemaker (provided that the ventricular response of the junctional escape focus remains adequate to maintain stable hemodynamic status).

PROBLEM   **More atropine is given. The result is the rhythm shown in Figure 16B-35. Has the degree of block "worsened" since Figure 16B-33?**

atrial rate. At an atrial rate of 80 beats/min (as was present in Fig. 16B-33), the patient's AV node is able to conduct most atrial impulses. As the atrial rate increases to 85 beats/min (Fig. 16B-34), fewer impulses are conducted. Finally with atrial tachycardia at 105 beats/min (Fig. 16B-35), only one of every two impulses is conducted. *It is entirely possible that this patient would still be capable of a much more favorable conduction ratio if the atrial rate were still 80 beats/min.*

> Atropine may be a two-edged sword. The drug works by both increasing the rate of the SA nodal pacemaker *and* improving conduction through the

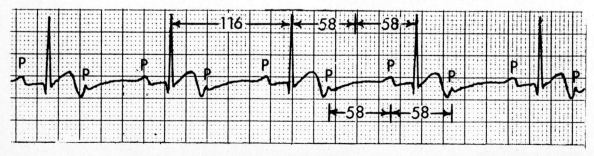

Figure 16B-35A

AV node. This particular case is an example of pre-dominance of the former effect of atropine (increasing the atrial rate) making the patient's condition worse (since the ventricular response decreased as the atrial rate increased!).

Returning to the initial scenario, it can be seen that this patient was asymptomatic and hemodynamically stable in a Wenckebach rhythm with an adequate ventricular response (Fig. 16B-33). *No atropine at all was indicated at that point.*

Finally, one should remember that in addition to classifying the AV blocks by degree, it is important to specify the atrial and ventricular response. The patient in this case manifested Mobitz I 2° AV block throughout. However, clinical implications of 2:1 AV conduction with this disorder may be significantly different from the implications when much more favorable AV conduction ratios exist.

C: PITFALLS IN ARRHYTHMIA INTERPRETATION

1) Forgetting that the most common cause of a pause is a blocked premature atrial contraction (PAC) and *not* AV block.

2) Not distinguishing between AV dissociation and complete AV block.

3) Misdiagnosing 2° AV block with 2:1 AV conduction as Mobitz II.

4) Failure to recognize and appreciate the diagnostic use of group beating (often implies a Wenckebach-type block).

5) Misdiagnosis of accelerated idioventricular rhythm (AIVR) as ventricular tachycardia (and mistreating the arrhythmia with lidocaine or countershock).

6) Falsely assuming a wide complex tachyarrhythmia is supraventricular because the patient is alert and hemodynamically stable.

7) Not suspecting atrial flutter with a supraventricular tachycardia that has a ventricular response of about 150 beats/min.

8) Not recognizing atrial fibrillation when the ventricular response is rapid and only a minor degree of irregularity exists.

9) Falsely assuming anomalous beats are aberrantly conducted without convincingly demonstrating a reason for aberrancy (RBBB pattern in a right-sided monitoring lead, *premature* P wave, relatively narrow QRS complex, etc.).

10) Failure to use more than one monitoring lead (or to obtain a 12-lead ECG) for arrhythmia interpretation, particularly when the patient is hemodynamically stable and the diagnosis is in doubt. Additional monitoring leads are especially valuable for detecting flutter waves, distinguishing fine ventricular fibrillation from asystole, and differentiating between PVCs and aberrantly conducted beats.

D: A BRIEF VIEW AT INTERPRETING PACEMAKER ARRHYTHMIAS

Dysrhythmia interpretation of patients with cardiac pacemakers is a topic unto itself that extends beyond the scope of this text. This has become especially true in recent years with the increased use of programmable dual-chambered pacemakers. As a result, we will not attempt more than introduction of a few basic concepts that may help the emergency care provider determine if a pacemaker is properly functioning.

Demand pacing is the most common mode employed. A pacemaker is set to fire at a fixed rate and does so unless the patient's spontaneous heart rate is faster. For example in **Figure 16D-1** the pacer is set to fire at 72 beats/min (corresponding to an R-R interval of 0.84 second).

The underlying rhythm in this example is atrial fibrillation, and the first three beats are paced. Pacemaker spikes with an R-R interval of 0.84 second precede each of these beats. Beat no. 4 is a spontaneous complex that arises be-

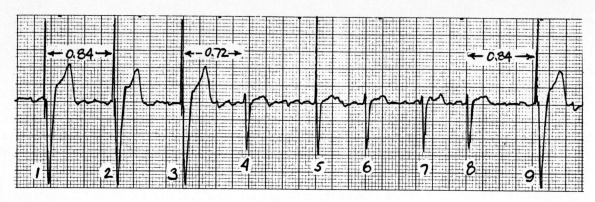

Figure 16D-1

cause the preceding cycle length of 0.72 second is shorter than the inherent rate of the pacemaker (0.84 second). Similarly, beats no. 6–8 are all spontaneous complexes that arise because of their short cycle lengths (the R-R intervals for each of these beats is less than 0.84 second). In contrast, beat no. 9 is paced. Since no spontaneous complex was forthcoming after 0.84 second, the pacemaker fired.

Note that the QRS complex following each of the paced beats (no. 1–3 and 9 is wide and differs in morphology from that of the spontaneous beats (no. 4 and 6–8). Each of the pacemaker spikes *captures* the ventricles.

PROBLEM   **Explain how the QRS complex of beat no. 5 can be narrow despite the fact that this beat is preceded by a pacemaker spike?**

ANSWER   Because the R-R interval between beats no. 4–5 is 0.84 second, a pacemaker spike is produced. However, since the QRS complex of beat no. 5 is narrow and looks like the other supraventricular complexes, a spontaneous beat must have occurred before this pacemaker spike could have been conducted.

From the rhythm strip shown in Figure 16D-1 it appears that this demand pacemaker is functioning normally. It *senses*, appropriately (since pacemaker spikes appear as expected before beats no. 5 and 9 when no spontaneous beat occurs after 0.84 second) and ventricular *capture* (of beats no. 1–3 and 9) is evident.

It should be apparent from this example that *both* paced and spontaneous beats must be present on a particular rhythm strip to adequately assess pacemaker function. If only paced complexes are seen, one will be able to judge only the adequacy of ventricular capture. On the other hand, if there are only spontaneous beats, virtually no information can be learned about pacemaker function.

PROBLEM   **The patient whose rhythm strip is shown in Figure 16D-2 was in cardiac arrest. An emergency transvenous pacemaker was inserted. Is it functioning? What is beat x?**

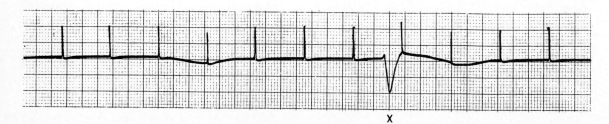

X

Figure 16D-2

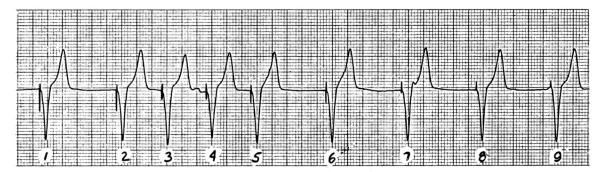

Figure 16D-3

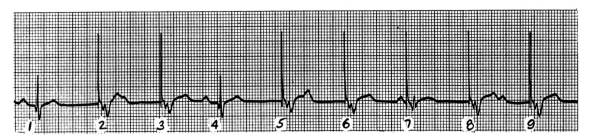

Figure 16D-4

ANSWER TO FIGURE 16D-2   Regular pacemaker spikes at a rate of 95 beats/min are seen. Unfortunately there is no evidence of ventricular *capture,* and the patient remains in asystole. Beat *X* represents an agonal complex that was not sensed by the pacemaker.

PROBLEM   **Are the demand pacemakers shown in Figures 16D-3 and 16D-4 functioning adequately?**

ANSWER TO FIGURE 16D-3   Ventricular capture is adequate since all pacemaker spikes are followed by a widened QRS complex and T wave. The R-R interval between beats no. 1–2, 5–6, 6–7, 7–8, and 8–9 is 0.98 second, corresponding to an inherent pacemaker rate of 62 beats/min. However the pacemaker spikes preceding beats no. 3–5 occur much more rapidly, suggesting malfunction of the pacemaker.

ANSWER TO FIGURE 16D-4   Pacemaker spikes precede beats no. 2, 3, and 5–9. Adequate ventricular *capture* is present, since

QRS complexes follow all pacemaker spikes. The rate of the pacemaker is 72 beats/min (corresponding to an R-R interval of 0.84 second between pacemaker spikes).

Beats no. 1 and 4 represent spontaneous QRS complexes. Each is preceded by a P wave with a constant (albeit slightly prolonged) PR interval. The P waves preceding beats no. 1 and 4 are conducted. The pacemaker appropriately *senses* these QRS complexes and does not fire until 0.84 second after the spontaneous QRS complex.

It is difficult to determine the underlying rhythm (and the reason for pacemaker insertion) from Figure 16D-4. P waves occur throughout this rhythm strip, although the atrial rate is not regular. As noted above, the P waves preceding beats no. 1 and 4 are conducted with 1° AV block. Additional P waves appear to notch the T waves of beats no. 2 and 5, precede the pacemaker spike of beat no. 7, and follow the T wave of beat no. 8. Since one would have at least expected this latter T wave to conduct, some type of 2° AV block must be present.

REFERENCES

Akhtar M: Atrioventricular nodal reentrant tachycardia. Med Clin North Am 68:819–830, 1984.

Barrett PA, Schamroth L, Kelly BJ: Significance of an apparent short return cycle in the mechanism of supraventricular tachycardia. Am J Cardiol 53:361–363, 1984.

Bastulli JA, Orlowski JP: Stroke as a complication of carotid sinus massage. Crit Care Med 13:869, 1985.

Chung EK: Electrocardiography: Practical Application with Vectorial Principles. Harper & Row, New York, 1980, pp 280–304.

Feigl D, Ravid M: Electrocardiographic observations on the termination of supraventricular tachycardia by verapamil. J Electrocardiol 12:129–136, 1979.

Fox W, Stein E: Cardiac Rhythm Disturbances: A Step-by-Step Approach. Lea & Febiger, Philadelphia, 1983.

Grauer K, Curry RW, Benchimol G: ECG of the month: Regularization of atrial fibrillation. CEFP 21:247–250, 1986.

Grogan EW, Waxman LH: Management of Supraventricular Tachycardias. In Dreifus LS, Brest AN (Eds): Cardiovascular Clinics. F.A. Davis, Philadelphia, 1985, Vol 16, No. 1, pp 261–278.

Josephson ME: Paroxysmal supraventricular tachycardia: An electrophysiologic approach. Am J Cardiol 41:1123–1126, 1978.

Kemper AJ, Dunlap R, Pietro DA: Thioridazine-induced torsade de pointes: Successful therapy with isoproterenol. JAMA 249:2931–2934, 1983.

Kim HS, Chung EK: Torsade de pointes: Polymorphous ventricular tachycardia. Heart Lung 12:269–273, 1983.

Kuhn M: Verapamil in the treatment of PSVT. Ann Emerg Med 10:538–544, 1981.

Lipman BS, Dunn M, Massie E: Clinical Electrocardiography. Year Book Medical Publishers, Chicago, 1984.

Marriott HJL, Conover MHB: Advanced Concepts in Arrhythmias. C.V. Mosby, St. Louis, 1983.

Parish C, Wooster WE, Braen GR, Robertson HD: Les torsade de pointes. Ann Emerg Med 11:143–146, 1982.

Schweitzer P, Teichholz LE: Carotid sinus massage: Its diagnostic and therapeutic value in arrhythmias. Am J Med 78:645–654, 1985.

Smith WM, Gallagher JJ: Les torsades de pointes: An unusual ventricular arrhythmia. Ann Intern Med 93:578–584, 1980.

Waxman MB, Wald RW, Sharma AD, Huerta F, Cameron DA: Vagal techniques for termination of paroxysmal supraventricular tachycardia. Am J Cardiol 48:655–664, 1980.

PART VI:

PEDIATRIC RESUSCITATION

CHAPTER 17

PEDIATRIC RESUSCITATION

Dan Cavallaro, NREMT
Jim Hillman, MD
Ken Grauer, MD

A: OVERVIEW OF PEDIATRIC ACLS

Cardiopulmonary arrest is a relatively infrequent event in children. Practically speaking, except for those working in specialized pediatric settings, exposure to cardiopulmonary emergencies in children is likely to be limited. As a result, many emergency care providers are not completely comfortable managing this disorder.

The purpose of this chapter is to present a basic approach for recognition and treatment of cardiac and/or respiratory difficulty in children. In doing this, we will emphasize the differences between adult and pediatric patients as they relate to management of acute cardiac and/or airway related emergencies.

PRIORITIES OF PEDIATRIC RESUSCITATION

Most cardiopulmonary arrests that occur in children are secondary to hypoxemia from respiratory depression. In response to this hypoxemia, the heart slows, and marked bradycardia is frequently seen. Asystole is the most common terminal event. This is in marked contrast to cardiopulmonary arrest in adults, in whom ventricular tachycardia/fibrillation are much more commonly seen.

Unfortunately, meaningful survival from pediatric resuscitation is poor. By the time the pediatric heart arrests, most children will have al-

ready been hypoxic for an extensive period of time. The emphasis in resuscitation of children must therefore be directed at early restoration of ventilation and improvement of oxygenation.

Airway Management and Ventilation

The most important priority in resuscitating children is to effectively manage the airway. Accomplishing this goal alone often improves outcome without the need to resort to pharmacologic intervention.

Effective management of the airway begins with early recognition of the signs of respiratory difficulty. Two entities in particular must be considered early by the emergency care provider: foreign body obstruction and obstruction from upper airway disease.

FOREIGN BODY OBSTRUCTION

Evaluating a patient with suspected foreign body obstruction must be done with extreme care. This is because of the ever-present danger of converting a partial airway obstruction to one that is complete.

In general, children with partial airway obstruction are managed in the same manner as adults—the patient should be allowed to cough in the hope that the foreign body will be expelled. As long as ventilation is effective, there is no need for invasive maneuvers. Instead, the emergency care provider should strive to keep the child as calm as possible (let the parent comfort or hold the child if feasible), protect the patient from further injury, and be ready to intervene at any moment should complete obstruction occur. If partial airway obstruction persists, definitive diagnostic and therapeutic procedures may need to be implemented.

OBSTRUCTION FROM UPPER AIRWAY DISEASE

The term "croup" is applied to a number of infectious processes of the upper airway that produce a brassy *(croupy)* cough, inspiratory stridor, hoarseness, and signs of respiratory distress. Two entities in this syndrome that the emergency care provider must be comfortable differentiating between are acute epiglottitis and laryngotracheobronchitis (LTB). The former is potentially life-threatening while the latter is usually self-limiting.

LTB is a viral form of croup that is most commonly seen between 3 months and 3 years of age. These patients present with a several-day history of low-grade fever, brassy or barking cough, and gradually increasing respiratory difficulty. They rarely appear toxic, and conservative therapy (cool mist) is usually all that is needed.

In contrast, acute epiglottitis is a bacterial infection (most commonly due to *Haemophilus influenzae*). It occurs in a somewhat older age group (2 to 7 years of age) and is much more abrupt in onset. Within hours these children develop high fever, sore throat, dysphagia, and marked respiratory distress. Typically they appear much more distressed than do children with LTB. The child with epiglottitis characteristically sits upright with head and neck protruding forward to assist in breathing (**Figure 17A-1**). Drooling is common because of an inability to swallow secretions. The hoarseness and brassy cough of LTB are not seen. Instead the voice is muffled as if someone had put a pillow over the child's head. As the degree of airway obstruction worsens, air exchange becomes progressively more difficult.

Although LTB is a far more common condition, it is essential that the emergency care provider be able to recognize acute epiglottitis when it does occur. Lateral neck x-rays may sometimes be helpful in this regard. If one is at all suspicious of this entity, *absolutely* no manip-

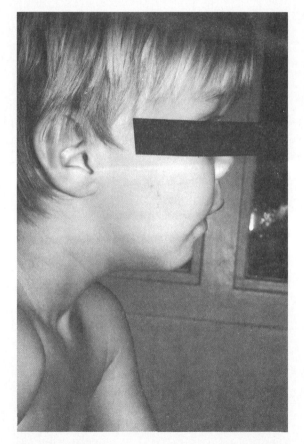

Figure 17A-1.   Characteristic posturing of a child with epiglottitis.

ulation of the airway (not even attempting to visualize the pharynx!) is advised. Instead the child must be kept as calm as possible (no venipunctures!), and emergent consultation with an anesthesiologist for endotracheal intubation is in order. Many clinicians also prefer to call for an otolaryngologist should surgical intervention (emergency tracheostomy) be necessary. Once control of the airway has been achieved, treatment with antibiotics is begun.

OXYGENATION OF THE SPONTANEOUSLY BREATHING PATIENT

All patients with respiratory distress should receive supplemental oxygen. However, pediatric patients may have difficulty tolerating conventional supplemental oxygen devices such as the nasal cannula and oxygen mask. The best method for administering supplemental oxygen to infants (anyone under 1 year of age) is through an *oxygen hood.* The device consists of a clear plastic dome designed to fit securely over the infant's head with ports that allow the infusion of humidified oxygen. Although these hoods are most often found in pediatric or neonatal intensive care units, they should probably also be available in every emergency department.

For older children (those over 1 year of age), the *non-rebreathing oxygen face mask* or *nasal cannula* is preferable. Each of these devices effectively provides supplemental oxygenation and may be tolerated for extended periods of time.

VENTILATION OF THE NONBREATHING PATIENT

More aggressive airway management is required for the patient who is not spontaneously breathing. The first priority is to open the airway. A favored method for doing this is the *jaw thrust,* performed by placing both hands on the patient's head and using the index finger to displace the mandible anteriorly. This lifts the tongue off the hypopharynx (See **Figure 7-3** in the airway chapter).

A second method is to carefully slide a small rolled washcloth (or your hand) under the patient's shoulders. This allows the head to slightly tilt back on its axis until the jaw forms a 90° angle to the long axis of the body (**Figure 17A-2**). The posture is known as the "sniffing position" since the relationship of the head on the neck is similar to that when smelling an object. Anatomically, the epiglottis is lifted off the laryngeal opening, and patency of the airway is restored.

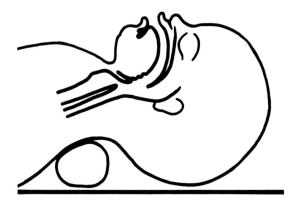

Figure 17A-2. Sniffing position.

Contrary to popular belief, hyperextending the head of a pediatric patient will not assure patency of the airway. All too often it produces the opposite effect, creating soft tissue airway obstruction by allowing the tongue and epiglottis to fall back over and cover the tracheal opening (**Fig. 17A-3**).

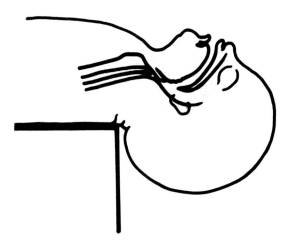

Figure 17A-3. Anatomical airway obstruction created by hyperextension of the head.

Anatomical considerations explain why upper airway obstruction occurs so much more commonly in children than in adults. The tongue and occiput (back part of the head) are relatively larger in children, the epiglottis and larynx both lie more anterior and cephalad, and the airway itself is proportionately smaller. The large occiput causes the head of the unconscious supine child to flex forward. Soft tissue airway obstruction (occlusion of the small pediatric airway by the relatively large tongue and anteriorly lying epiglottis) is the usual result **(Fig. 17A-4).**

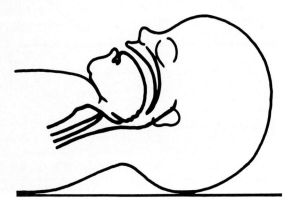

Figure 17A-4. Anatomical airway obstruction created by flexion of the head.

MECHANICAL ADJUNCTS

Of the three mechanical adjuncts for ventilation discussed in the chapter on airway management (Chapter 7), only two are used in children. Our comments here are limited to how these modalities apply to children.

Nasopharyngeal and oropharyngeal airways are the adjuncts of choice for initial management of the pediatric airway. Many clinicians prefer to maintain the airway of the spontaneously breathing patient with a *nasopharyngeal trumpet.* This is particularly valuable for the child with a depressed level of consciousness who still retains a sensitive gag reflex. Caution is advised when using this device in young children, however, since the small diameter and relatively long length of the trumpet may paradoxically increase the risk of airway obstruction.

In the unconscious patient, the *oropharyngeal airway* is the adjunct of choice. Individuals who are obtunded to the point of being able to tolerate an oropharyngeal airway need definitive

management (and protection of the airway) with endotracheal intubation.

> The *esophageal obturator airway (EOA)* is contraindicated in children under 16 years of age. The risk of esophageal and tracheal damage is simply unwarranted when this device is used in the pediatric age group.

ENDOTRACHEAL INTUBATION

The definitive method for managing the *unprotected* airway in the obtunded or unconscious patient is endotracheal intubation. This holds true regardless of whether the patient is still breathing or not.

Advantages of endotracheal intubation are that:

    i) The airway is protected from aspiration

    ii) Positive pressure ventilation may be given without the risk of gastric insufflation

    iii) An alternate route is provided for administering pharmacological agents

The technique for endotracheal intubation of an infant or child is quite similar to that for an adult. Nevertheless, important differences do exist.

Suctioning the patient prior to intubation is an advisable preparatory measure for both adults and children. However, the standard suction tubing currently available in emergency and pre-hospital care settings may be cumbersome when used in the pediatric patient.

> We (J.H., D.C.) have found that slight modification of a Frazier suction device is equally effective and much easier to employ than the standard suction tubing. The Frazier suction device is the kind frequently used in the operating room by neurosurgeons and otolaryngologists. If one cuts off a 6- to 7-cm length of tubing from the distal end of a red rubber Robinson catheter and slips this tubing over the distal tip of the Frazier suction device, intermittent suction of the naso- or oropharynx can much more easily be performed **(Fig. 17A-5).**

In adults, either a straight or curved laryngoscope blade may be used, depending on the personal preference of the operator. In contrast, most clinicians advocate the use of a *straight* blade for intubating very small children or infants. This is because the straight blade is wider

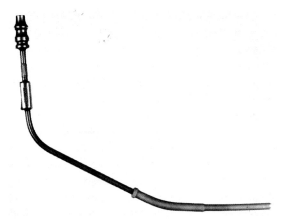

Figure 17A-5. Example of neonatal suction device developed by Dr. Hillman.

and facilitates lifting the tongue out of the way. Clearer visualization of the vocal cords is the result. This consideration becomes less important for older children, for whom either blade may be used.

Sizing of the Endotracheal (ET) Tube

The size of the ET tube varies with age. In general, the appropriate size of the ET tube may be estimated by comparison to the diameter of the patient's little finger. An even easier way to size an endotracheal tube in children is to gauge tube diameter by the size of the child's external nares. A tube that fits well in the nares is almost always the appropriate size for the laryngeal opening.

Premature and full-term newborns require tubes ranging from 2.5 to 3.5 mm in diameter; a 3-year old usually requires a 4.5- to 5.5-mm diameter tube; and a 6-year old a 5.5- to 6.5-mm diameter tube.

Technique for Endotracheal Intubation of Children

The laryngoscope is carefully inserted into the right side of the patient's mouth while the tongue is swept to the left. Insertion continues until the epiglottis is visualized. When using the *straight* blade, the epiglottis is gently lifted anteriorly. The ET tube is then passed from the right corner of the mouth and threaded through the laryngeal opening. The operator should clearly visualize the tube passing *through* the vocal cords.

The procedure is the same with the *curved* blade,

except that the tip of the blade is placed in the valecula instead of underneath the epiglottis. As in adults, the blade must then be lifted *forward and upward* in order to visualize the cords.

Special Considerations for Intubation of Children

The pediatric epiglottis is a much more flimsy structure than its adult counterpart. In addition it is omega-shaped, whereas the curvature of the adult epiglottis is much less pronounced **(Fig. 17A-6).** Therefore the pediatric epiglottis must be manipulated with extreme care.

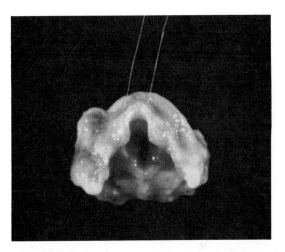

Figure 17A-6. Anatomical specimen demonstrating the omega-shape of the pediatric epiglottis.

Another difference between the pediatric and adult airways is that the laryngeal opening is much smaller in children. As a result, it may be more difficult to pass the tube through the cords. Unlike in adults, the smallest part of the pediatric airway is the *cricoid* cartilage! *Successfully passing the tube through the cords therefore does not necessarily constitute successful intubation.* In view of this, it is always a good idea to have additional endotracheal tubes (0.5 mm smaller and 0.5 mm larger than anticipated) on hand during the intubation phase.

As a result of the small size of the pediatric chest, auscultatory fields lie extremely close to one another. Breath sounds may therefore be easily transmitted from the esophagus to the lung fields. More than simply auscultating the lungs, one must verify that air sounds are not being heard over the stomach. With proper tube placement, the chest should rise symmetrically during ventilaton. If the child had become bradycardic, heart rate will rapidly increase toward normal once the patient is intubated. Ultimately, proper tube placement is confirmed by chest x-ray.

Ventilation of Pediatric Patients

There are two basic methods for ventilating pediatric patients: the self-inflating resuscitation bag and the flow-inflation bag. *Oxygen-powered mechanical breathing devices (Elder/Robert Shaw valves)* such as the manually triggered units used by emergency prehospital care personnel have no role in ventilation of pediatric patients.

The *self-inflating resuscitation bag (bag-valve mask or BVM)* is a unit consisting of a bag, an adapter that can be attached to a mask or endotracheal tube, and a reservoir (See **Fig. 7-14**). In order to provide elevated concentrations of oxygen, the reservoir must be attached to a high-flow supplemental source of oxygen.

> Many different bag sizes exist. The one chosen should depend on the size of the child and the tidal volume you want to deliver.

Pop-off valves (which open when a certain airway pressure is attained) are of no value in the pediatric setting. This is because high airway pressures are needed to ventilate patients through the small endotracheal tubes that are used in children. (Should your equipment contain a pop-off valve, it should be bypassed in this setting.)

The *flow-inflation anesthesia bag (Mapelson-D bag)* requires much more skill to operate than does a BVM. It consists of an anesthesia bag, a piece of plastic tubing (approximately 1 foot long), an exhaust valve, and a multi-purpose adaptor. The adaptor is usually attached to the oxygen source, a manometer, and an endotracheal tube (See **Fig. 7-15**). Advantages of this bag over the standard BVM are that you can apply CPAP (continuous positive airway pressure) or PEEP (positive end-expiratory pressure). In addition, ventilation with close to 100%

oxygen is assured. In contrast, one is never entirely sure of the concentration of oxygen delivered with the BVM because the amount of entrained room air is highly variable.

> It should be emphasized that the Mapelson-D bag should be operated only by individuals highly trained in its use. In the hands of an inexperienced provider, the risk of barotrauma (and tension pneumothorax) is great. In order to prevent this injury, most clinicians place a manometer into the circuit so that airway pressure can be observed during ventilation.

Algorithm for Management of the Pediatric Airway

We have organized the material covered up to now in an Algorithm for Management of the Pediatric Airway (**Fig. 17A-7**). The first step is to simultaneously assess breathing and the level of consciousness. If the patient is conscious, alert, and spontaneously breathing in a normal fashion (**1-2-3**), supplemental oxygen may be all that is needed.

If the patient is not breathing, the rescuer must *open the airway* and reassess ventilation (**4**). If this results in normal ventilation, again all that may be needed is supplemental oxygen (**5**). However, if the patient does not begin to breathe after the airway is opened, *artificial ventilation* (by mouth-to-mouth or BVM) must be attempted (**6**).

> A good rule of thumb is to "ventilate for gentle chest rise," and to check skin color and mucous membranes for improvement.

If artificial ventilation results in adequate ventilation, efforts should be directed toward definitive management of the airway with endotracheal intubation (**4-6-7**). In contrast, if one is unable to successfully ventilate the patient, *complete airway obstruction* must be suspected (**4-6-8**). Reposition the patient's head in an attempt to open the airway. If this is unsuccessful, maneuvers for treating foreign body obstruction should be tried. In the infant under 1 year of age, this includes back blows and chest thrusts.

Pediatric Airway Management

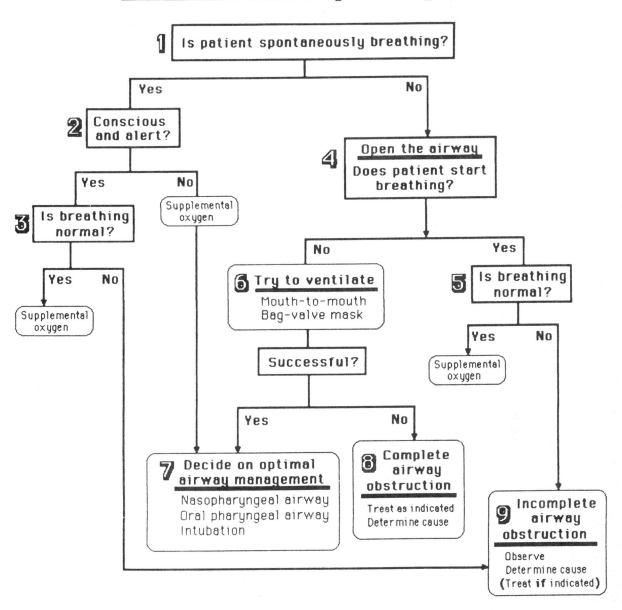

Figure 17A-7. Algorithm for management of the pediatric airway.

For older children, chest thrusts and/or abdominal thrusts should be used.

If the patient begins to breathe after the airway is opened but continues to demonstrate respiratory difficulty, *partial airway obstruction* should be suspected **(4-5-9)**. Similarly, if the patient is conscious and spontaneously breathing but in an abnormal fashion, there may also be partial obstruction **(1-2-3-9)**. Partial airway obstruction may be caused by either soft tissue obstruction (such as the tongue) or a foreign body. In the latter case, coughing should be encouraged in hope that the foreign body will be expelled. *As long as the patient is adequately ventilating, no immediate intervention is required.* However, continued close observation is mandatory since partial airway obstruction may at any time become complete.

Finally, if the patient is spontaneously breathing but not alert, more definitive measures are needed to protect the airway **(1-2-7)**. This would entail at least a nasopharyngeal airway for the *semiconscious* patient who retains a sensitive gag reflex and endotracheal intubation for the *unconscious* individual.

Assessing Circulatory Status

Once control of the **A**irway has been achieved, and adequate ventilation (**B**reathing) assured, attention must be directed toward assessing **C**irculatory status. The two most important parameters to monitor in this regard are *pulse* and *blood pressure.*

PULSE ASSESSMENT

In addition to noting the presence and quality of the pulse, it is essential to accurately determine heart rate. Rates considered normal for adults may represent marked *bradycardia* in children.

> As we discuss later in the section on Pediatric Arrhythmias, normal values for heart rates in infants and children are surprisingly higher than what one might expect. Thus, the mean rate of a 4-month-old child is 140 beats/min. Heart rates of up to 120 beats/min are still considered normal for children 1–2 years of age. Mean heart rate does not drop below 100 beats/min until approximately 8 years of age. Therefore, a heart rate of 80 beats/min in the setting of cardiopulmonary arrest must be interpreted as *relative* bradycardia for most children.
>
> It is particularly important to pay attention to heart rate during attempts at endotracheal intubation. Should one encounter difficulty intubating a patient in respiratory distress, attempts to intubate should be stopped immediately if heart rate drops below 80 beats/min in infants and 60 beats/min in children. In such cases, conventional means of ventilation (BVM) should be resumed *at least* until

heart rate and blood pressure can be restored to more appropriate levels.

The best method for determining the pulse in infants and small children is to palpate for the brachial pulse (Cavallaro and Melker, 1983). This can be done by externally rotating the hand and placing the fingers just below the brachial muscle in the midhumerus area **(Fig. 17A-8)**.

> Because of the short, chubby neck of infants, location of the carotid pulse is extremely difficult in this age group. Infants simply "don't have necks" **(Fig. 17A-9)**. In children more than 1 year of age, either the carotid or brachial pulse may be used.
>
> In the past, the femoral pulse has been used as an alternative site for palpating the pulse. The drawback of this method is that the pulse palpated in the femoral area during external chest compressions may sometimes be the femoral *vein* rather than the artery!

BLOOD PRESSURE ASSESSMENT

Normal blood pressures in children are somewhat lower than those for adults. For example, a systolic blood pressure of 80 mm Hg is *normal* for a 5-year-old child. A simplified method for determining hypotension based on the age of the child has been suggested by the American Heart Association. They define hypotension if systolic blood pressure is less than 70 mm Hg plus 2 times age in years. Thus, the lowest acceptable blood pressure in a 3-year-old child would be 76 mm Hg (70 + [2 × 3]).

> It is difficult to accurately determine blood pressure in infants and young children. This may be due to improper cuff size and/or difficulty hearing Korotkoff sounds. Care must be taken to use a cuff that covers approximately two-thirds to three-quarters of the arm as measured from elbow to axilla. Choosing a cuff too narrow may result in artificially elevated blood pressure readings, while selecting a cuff too wide may have the opposite effect. In the event that Korotkoff sounds are inaudible, use of a *palpable* systolic blood pressure suffices. If available, a Doppler may be invaluable.

External Chest Compressions

If no pulse is present, external chest compressions must be started. The rate recommended

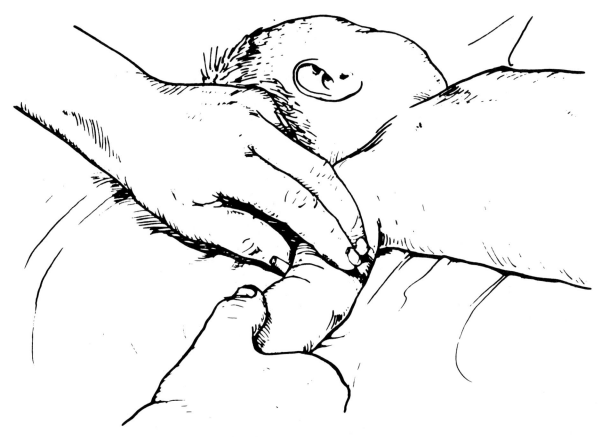

Figure 17A-8. Palpating the brachial pulse.

for compressions is *at least* 100 times per minute for infants, and 80–100 times per minute for children 1 year of age or older. For chest compressions to be effective, the sternum must be depressed at least 0.5–1 inch for infants, 1–1.5 inches for children between 1 and 8 years old, and 1.5–2 inches for children older than 8.

As discussed in Chapter 10 on New Developments in CPR, we now know that compression of the heart between the sternum and vertebral column is not the principal mechanism for blood flow with CPR in adults. Instead, the pressure gradient that develops between the intra-thoracic and extrathoracic compartments appears to be much more important. The opposite is true for infants. Because of the compliance and small size of the infant chest wall, actual compression of the heart *does* occur and probably is the major mechanism for blood flow in this age group. As a result, external chest compressions must be of adequate depth in order to be effective. Direct cardiac compression is also important in older children, although it is still unclear at what age this ceases to be the major mechanism for blood flow.

One interesting change in the new guidelines deals with the recommended hand position for performing external chest compression in infants. In the past it was thought that the infant heart was situated higher in the chest than the heart of older children and adults. Because of this, it was recommended that external chest compressions be delivered over the middle third of the sternum (parallel to the nipple line). Recent data have refuted this recommendation. We now know that the heart of infants lies over the *lower* third of the sternum, just as it does for older children and adults. Consequently, finger position for external chest compression in infants should be 1 fingerbreadth *below* the nipple line.

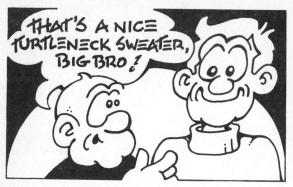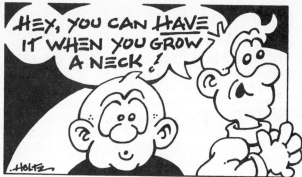

Figure 17A-9.

Intravenous Access

Establishing intravenous access in children is frequently problematic for the nonpediatric oriented health care provider. The task may be made even more difficult in the setting of cardiopulmonary arrest by hypotension and/or endogenous release of catecholamines with resultant vasospasm. Above all, one should remember that the focus in pediatric resuscitation must *never* be on establishment of IV access alone. Instead, early control of the airway so as to be able to adequately oxygenate the child is the key. Accomplishment of this goal is much more likely to bring a child back than is administration of drugs.

CENTRAL LINES

Central venous access is accepted as the ideal method for administering drugs and fluids during cardiopulmonary resuscitation. However, many clinicians are not comfortable with central venous cannulation of the pediatric arrest victim. A major reason for this is the high complication rate seen when placement of central lines is attempted by those not highly skilled with this technique.

The three sites commonly considered for central venous cannulation during resuscitation are the:

  i) Subclavian vein
  ii) Internal jugular vein
  iii) Femoral vein

Special problems are associated with each of these sites when they are used in children.

> The *subclavian vein* is probably the most commonly chosen site for obtaining central venous access in adults. However, cannulation of this vein is fraught with danger (frequent occurrence of pneumothorax) for the inexperienced pediatric care provider. Similarly, the *internal jugular* is not a wise choice for the inexperienced. The short stubby neck of infants and young children make this vein almost inaccessible. Finally, the *femoral vein* is no longer recommended as a site for fluid or drug administration due to decreased subdiaphragmatic venous return during cardiac resuscitation.

PERIPHERAL VENOUS ACCESS

In light of the above, peripheral venous access is most often chosen as the initial route for drug and fluid administration. The three sites most commonly selected are:

  i) External jugular vein
  ii) Antecubital veins
  iii) Long saphenous vein

> The favored site for peripheral venous access in adults and normovolemic children has been the dorsum of the hand. Cannulation of these veins on the chubby hand of a hemodynamically compromised child frequently is impossible.

The *external jugular* vein is commonly overlooked by the non-pediatric-oriented emergency care provider as a site for venous access in children. This is unfortunate since the site is surprisingly easy to cannulate in children over 1 year of age (especially if they are crying). Simply place the child in slight Trendelenburg position and rotate the head to the opposite side. This should distend the vein and make it readily visible. Even though the external jugular is classified as a peripheral vein, fluid and drugs administered by this route reach the central circulation almost as quickly as they do when given through a central line. One should therefore strongly consider this site early in the resuscitation phase.

Antecubital veins are easily accessible in children and are cannulated in the same fashion as for adults. They serve as an effective route for administering fluid and drugs during pediatric resuscitation.

Another frequently forgotten site of venous access is the *long saphenous vein*. The advantage of this site is that the vein is easy to locate, lies superficially, and is simple to cannulate. The long saphenous vein can be found just anterior to the medial malleolus. From there it runs straight up along the medial aspect of the leg. Unfortunately, due to decreased venous return from subdiaphragmatic veins, the value of this route during cardiac arrest has now become questionable.

INTRAOSSEOUS ACCESS

The intraosseous route for fluid and drug administration was first described in the 1940s. With the advent of Teflon and polyvinylchloride catheters, this route was almost forgotten until recently. In view of the difficulty in obtaining intravenous access in hemodynamically compromised infants and small children, interest in the intraosseous technique has recently been revived.

Compelling reasons to consider this route for venous access to the central circulation include:
  i) Minimal complications
  ii) Rapid administration of intravenous fluids, blood products, and drugs (catecholamines, sodium bicarbonate)
  iii) Ease of insertion (With practice, intraosseous access may be established in seconds.)

Practically speaking, it often takes surprisingly long to achieve intravenous access in children during emergency situations. In a study by Kanter et al. (1986), more than $1\frac{1}{2}$ minutes were needed to establish a line in 76% of patients, and greater than 5 minutes were needed in 34% of patients. The authors suggest that if a peripheral line cannot be started within 1–2 minutes, that strong consideration be given to alternative means of achieving intravenous access (such as the intraosseous method).

Unfortunately, the efficacy of the intraosseous route has not been proven during low-flow states such as cardiac arrest.

Technique for Obtaining Intraosseous Access

The preferred site in children less than 3 years of age is the tibia. Prior to cannulation, the area is prepped and draped in the standard fashion. Infiltration with a local anesthetic agent is used. The procedure is performed with an 18-gauge bone marrow needle *with* stylet. The purpose of the stylet is to prevent the needle from becoming clogged with bony fragments. (Although some clinicians suggest using a spinal needle, we have found the procedure easier to perform with a bone marrow needle.)

The needle is inserted 1 fingerbreadth below the tubercle on the anteromedial surface of the tibia. **(Fig. 17A-10)** Direct the needle downward in a slightly caudal orientation until the periosteum is reached **(Fig. 17A-11)**. At this point, application of a boring or screwing motion may be needed to penetrate the bone marrow. A "give" in resistance signals entry into the marrow. Correct placement is confirmed by aspiration of blood and bony debris into a syringe. This is followed by a saline flush to clear the needle of remaining debris. Standard IV tubing can now be connected to the needle, and the site is ready for drug and fluid administration.

A special word of caution is in order. Because of the long length of the needle left exposed, special care is needed in securing the needle and preventing it from being broken off.

ENDOTRACHEAL DRUG ADMINISTRATION

If difficulty is encountered in obtaining venous access, the endotracheal route may provide a very effective alternative for drug administration. Medications that may be given by this route include **a**tropine, **l**idocaine, and **e**pinephrine **(ALE)**.

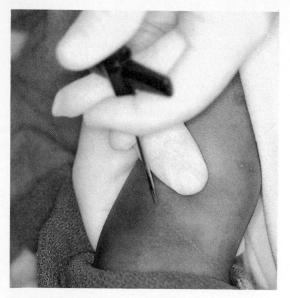

Figure 17A-10. Insertion of the intraosseous needle 1 fingerbreadth below the tibial tubercle of this 2-year-old child's left leg.

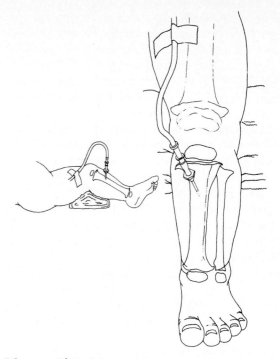

Figure 17A-11. Proper position of intraosseous needle for insertion. (Reproduced with permission from the collection of Rick Wiebly, M.D.)

Useful Drugs in Pediatric Resuscitation

As we have emphasized, most pediatric resuscitations can be successfully managed by improving oxygenation and ventilation without the need for pharmacologic intervention. However, drug therapy may occasionally be needed to accelerate the heart rate, improve perfusion, and correct hypotension. The medications most commonly used in pediatric resuscitation are atropine, epinephrine, and dopamine. As in adults, use of sodium bicarbonate, calcium chloride, and isoproterenol has been strongly deemphasized in pediatric resuscitation. Similarly, lidocaine, procainamide and bretylium are rarely needed, since ventricular tachycardia/fibrillation are so rarely seen in children.

Many nonpediatric emergency care providers are uncomfortable calculating the dosages of drugs used in children, particularly when called on to do so during the stress of a pediatric emergency. For this reason it may be advisable to post a chart of commonly used drugs and dosages for pediatric resuscitation in a readily visible loca-

tion. One way of displaying this information is shown in **Table 17A-1**.

Defibrillation and Cardioversion

Bradycardia or asystole secondary to respiratory arrest is the terminal event in the overwhelming majority of pediatric arrests. Ventricular fibrillation is seldom seen. Consequently, pediatric defibrillation is rarely needed. If defibrillation is necessary, the energy recommended for the initial countershock attempt is 2 joules/kg. If unsuccessful, this energy level should be doubled (to 4 joules/kg) for repeat defibrillation. Thus, for a 1-year-old child weighing 10 kg (22 lb), an energy of 20 joules should be used initially, and additional attempts would be with 40 joules.

TABLE 17A-1   PEDIATRIC DRUG DOSAGES

EPINEPHRINE

Dose = 0.01 mg/kg (Comes in 10-ml syringes [0.1 mg/1 ml] of 1:10,000 soln)

Weight of Patient	Dose for IV Bolus (or ET)
10 kg	0.1 mg (1 ml)
20 kg	0.2 mg (2 ml)
30 kg	0.3 mg (3 ml)
Adult	0.5–1.0 mg (5–10 ml)

IV Infusion Dose of Epinephrine = 0.1–1.0 μg/kg/min
  Mix 0.6 $\times$ body weight (kg) in mg in 100 ml of D5W.
    Then 1 drop/min = 0.1 μg/kg/min; Titrate to effect

Weight of Patient	How to Mix	Initial Rate*	Maximum Rate
10 kg	6 mg in 100 D5W	1 drop/min (= 0.1 μg/kg/min)	10 drops/min
20 kg	12 mg in 100 D5W	1 drop/min (= 0.1 μg/kg/min)	10 drops/min
30 kg	18 mg in 100 D5W	1 drop/min (= 0.1 μg/kg/min)	10 drops/min
Adult	1 mg in 250 D5W	15–30 drops/min (1–2 μg/min)	Titrate up

ATROPINE

Dose = 0.02 mg/kg (Minimum dose = 0.1 mg; maximum single dose = 1.0 mg)
May repeat 0.02 mg/kg q. 5 min up to 1.0 mg (for child) and 2.0 mg (for adolescent)

Weight of Patient	Single Dose (IV or ET)
10 kg	0.2 mg
20 kg	0.4 mg
30 kg	0.6 mg
Adult	0.5–1.0 mg

SODIUM BICARBONATE

Respiratory failure is the most common cause of cardiac arrest in children. The most important treatment priority is to improve ventilation, *not* to administer sodium bicarbonate. Epinephrine is the drug of choice for the arrested heart. Sodium bicarbonate should be considered only if the arrest is prolonged, or if the patient was known to have an underlying metabolic acidosis.

Dose = 1 mEq/kg (50 ml of 8.4% soln = 50 mEq)

Weight of Patient	Dose (IV or Intraosseous)
10 kg	10 mEq ($\frac{1}{5}$ ampule)
20 kg	20 mEq ($\frac{2}{5}$ ampule)
30 kg	30 mEq ($\frac{3}{5}$ ampule)
Adult	50–100 mEq (1–2 ampules)

TABLE 17A-1 PEDIATRIC DRUG DOSAGES (CONTINUED)

LIDOCAINE

Dose = 1.0 mg/kg IV bolus

Weight of Patient	Dose for IV Bolus
10 kg	10 mg
20 kg	20 mg
30 kg	30 mg
Adult	50–100 mg

IV Infusion Dose of Lidocaine = 20–50 μg/kg/min
  Mix 120 mg in 100 ml of D5W = 1200 μg/ml
    Then 1 drop/kg/min = 20 μg/kg/min (Initial rate)
     2.5 drops/kg/min = 50 μg/kg/min (Maximum rate)

Weight of Patient	How to Mix	Initial Rate*	Maximum Rate
10 kg	120 mg in 100 D5W	10 drops/min	25 drops/min
20 kg	120 mg in 100 D5W	20 drops/min	50 drops/min
30 kg	120 mg in 100 D5W	30 drops/min	75 drops/min
Adult	1000 mg in 250 D5W	30 drops/min = 2 mg/min	4 mg/min

DOPAMINE

IV Infusion Dose = 2–20 μg/kg/min
  Mix 6 mg × body weight (kg) in 100 ml of D5W.
    Then 1 drop/min = 1.0 μg/kg/min
       5 drops/min =   5 μg/kg/min (= usual initial rate)
      20 drops/min = 20 μg/kg/min (= maximum rate)

Weight of patient	How to Mix	Initial Rate*	Maximum Rate
10 kg	60 mg in 100 D5W	5 drops/min (50 μg/min)	20 drops/min
20 kg	120 mg in 100 D5W	5 drops/min (100 μg/min)	20 drops/min
30 kg	180 mg in 100 D5W	5 drops/min (150 μg/min)	20 drops/min
Adult (80 kg)	200 mg in 250 D5W	30 drops/min (400 μg/min)	Titrate up

ISOPROTERENOL

IV Infusion Dose = 0.1–1.0 μg/kg/min
  Mix 0.6 mg × body weight (kg) in 100 ml of D5W.
    Then 1 drop/min = 0.1 μg/kg/min; Titrate to effect

Weight of Patient	How to Mix	Initial Rate*	Maximum Rate
10 kg	6 mg in 100 D5W	1 drop/min (= 0.1 μg/kg/min)	10 drops/min
20 kg	12 mg in 100 D5W	1 drop/min (= 0.1 μg/kg/min)	10 drops/min
30 kg	18 mg in 100 D5W	1 drop/min (= 0.1 μg/kg/min)	10 drops/min
Adult	1 mg in 250 D5W	30 drop/min (2 μg/min)	20 μg/min

TABLE 17A-1   PEDIATRIC DRUG DOSAGES (CONTINUED)

DEFIBRILLATION

Dose = 2 J(joules)/kg for initial countershock
If this is unsuccessful, double the dose (to 4 J/kg) and repeat × 2

Weight of Patient	Initial Shock (2nd shock–3rd shock)
10 kg	20 J (then 40 J– 40 J)
20 kg	40 J (then 80 J– 80 J)
30 kg	60 J (then 120 J–120 J)
Adult	200 J (then 300 J–360 J)

OXYGEN

Inadequate oxygenation is the most common cause of cardiac arrest in children!

---

*NOTE—when infusing the small quantities of drug required for pediatric IV infusions, it is essential to use an infusion pump to ensure accuracy.

On rare occasions, synchronized cardioversion may be needed to convert supraventricular or ventricular tachyarrhythmias to normal sinus rhythm. The recommended energy dose for cardioversion of children is 0.2 to 1.0 joules/kg.

> Cardioversion is not an innocuous procedure. Moreover, many children tolerate tachyarrhythmias (of 200 beats/min or more) surprisingly well. As a result, it may be preferable for the adult-oriented emergency care provider to resist the urge to cardiovert a child unless the patient is manifesting signs of profound shock. Help (in the form of an experienced pediatric care provider) will usually be accessible long before this point is reached.

In summary, cardiac arrest in infants and children is rarely due to myocardial ischemia or infarction. Instead, it is usually secondary to a respiratory arrest from some other cause. These include metabolic or electrolyte abnormalities (for example hypoglycemia or hypocalcemia), sudden infant death syndrome, toxic drug ingestion, electrical shock, cardiac arrhythmias, congestive heart failure, poisoning, drowning, allergic reactions, trauma, shock, and cardiac tamponade. Because the outlook for survival once pediatric cardiopulmonary arrest occurs is so dim, a strong emphasis must be on prevention.

B: PEDIATRIC ARRHYTHMIAS: HOW CHILDREN ARE DIFFERENT

Ken Grauer, MD

Children are not just little adults. Nowhere is this more evident than in the area of pediatric dysrhythmia interpretation. Although terminology used to define pediatric and adult arrhythmias is similar, both the spectrum of arrhythmias encountered and the priorities for treatment differ significantly.

Basic concepts in arrhythmia interpretation were presented in Chapter 3. The purpose of this section is neither to duplicate that material nor to attempt to make the reader an expert in pediatric electrocardiography. Instead, our goal is to discuss the more important and clinically relevant differences between pediatric and adult arrhythmias as they pertain to pediatric resuscitation.

Pediatric Norms

Pediatric norms for heart rate and interval (PR and QRS) duration differ markedly from those of adults. This becomes readily apparent on inspection of the rhythm strip shown in **Figure 17B-1** taken from a healthy infant.

Table 17B-1 demonstrates the pediatric norms for heart rate and interval duration. From this table it can be seen that heart rates of up to 180 beats/min are still normal for children during the first year of life. During this time, *mean* heart rate is between 120–140 beats/min, and rates below 90 beats/min constitute sinus *bradycardia.*

It should be emphasized that the values shown in Table 17B-1 represent pediatric norms for heart

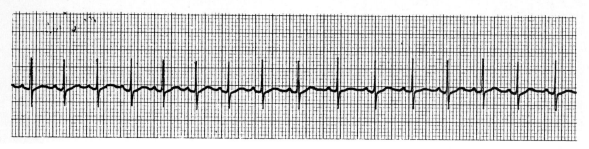

Figure 17B-1

PROBLEM   In what ways is this tracing different from that of a normal adult?

ANSWER TO FIGURE 17B-1   The rhythm is sinus at a rate of about 140 beats/min, the PR interval is 0.11 second, and the QRS is 0.05 second in duration. *All of these parameters are normal for an infant!*

In contrast, for adults the heart rate for normal sinus rhythm varies between 60–99 beats/min, the PR interval is between 0.12–0.20 second, and the QRS complex is usually not so narrow.

rate in children who are *awake.* Heart rates may drop appreciably during sleep—to as low as 60 beats/min for a 2-year old and as low as 40 beats/min for a 12-year old (Garson, 1984).

Normal duration of the PR interval in infants and children is significantly less than for adults. Thus a PR interval of 0.08 second is perfectly normal for a 3-year old, whereas it might suggest an accessory pathway (WPW) in an adult. By the same token, the upper limits of normal for the PR and QRS intervals in children are also less than for adults. Appreciation of this fact is

TABLE 17B-1 PEDIATRIC NORMS*

Age	Heart Rate (beats/min)	PR Interval (sec)	QRS Duration (sec)
Newborn to 1 yr	90–180	0.07–0.16	0.03–0.08
1–3 yr	70–150	0.08–0.16	0.04–0.08
4–10 yr	60–130	0.09–0.17	0.04–0.09
> 10 yr	60–110	0.09–0.20	0.04–0.09

*Adapted from Garson A: The Electrocardiogram in Infants and Children: A systematic Approach, Lea & Febiger, Philadelphia, 1983.

important clinically, since values considered normal for adults are often prolonged for pediatric patients.

Reference to Table 17B-1 makes it evident that a PR interval of 0.18 second is abnormally long for a child under 10 years of age. Such prolongation would constitute 1° AV block in this age group. Similarly, a QRS duration of 0.10 second is also abnormal in a child this age and suggests some type of intraventricular conduction disturbance.

PROBLEM **Interpret the arrhythmia shown in Figure 17B-2. Is this tracing abnormal for a 7-year-old child?**

commonly present with normal sinus rhythm. A difference of *at least* 0.08 second should exist between the shortest and longest R-R intervals before one diagnoses sinus *arrhythmia*.

Escape Rhythms and AV Dissociation

The SA node is the principal pacemaker of the heart. Under usual circumstances, it suppresses all other cardiac tissue with inherent automaticity. In an awake child with normal sinus rhythm,

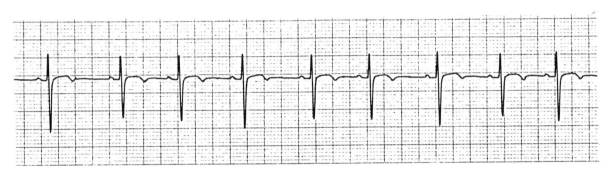

Figure 17B-2

ANSWER Although the rhythm is irregular, each QRS complex is preceded by a P wave with a constant PR interval. This is *sinus arrhythmia*. Note the change in QRS amplitude from beat to beat that reflects the child's respiration.

Sinus Arrhythmia

As discussed in Section A of Chapter 3, sinus arrhythmia is an extremely common normal finding among older children and young adults. Its principal significance is that it not be confused with a disease state. Sinus arrhythmia is thought to be due to variations in autonomic tone and is often related to respiration. Heart rate tends to increase in a gradual manner with inspiration and decrease with exhalation. A repetitive pattern (group beating) is frequently seen (Fig. 17B-2). The arrhythmia does not occur as often in younger children and infants since respiratory variation in autonomic tone is likely to be much less pronounced in the younger age group.

One should be aware that slight irregularity is

the SA node fires at a rate of between 60–180 beats/min depending on the age and activity of the child (Table 17B-1). If for any reason the principal pacemaker slows markedly or fails to fire at all, another *(subsidiary)* pacemaker will have to take over. The resulting rhythm is known as an *escape* rhythm.

Table 17B-2 shows the usual escape rates of subsidiary pacemakers in the atria, AV node, and ventricles.

According to the table, were the sinus rate to slow down in a child less than 3 years of age, a subsidiary pacemaker in the atria should take over at a rate of between 80–100 beats/min. If this did not occur, one would then expect an escape rhythm to arise from the site that was "next-in-line" in the pacemaking hierarchy—the AV node. For a child under 3, the usual rate of a subsidiary pacemaker from this site is between 50–80 beats/min. The lowest escape focus—a site in the ventricles—is left as a final

TABLE 17B-2   USUAL RATES OF SUBSIDIARY PACEMAKERS*

Site of Escape Focus	Up to 3 Yrs (beats/min)	Over 3 Yrs & Adults (beats/min)
Atria	80–100	50–60
AV Node	50– 80	40–60
Ventricles	40– 50	30–40

*Adapted from Garson A: The Electrocardiogram in Infants and Children: A Systematic Approach, Lea & Febiger, Philadelphia, 1983.

safeguard in the event no escape rhythm is forthcoming from either the atria or AV node. The rate of an idioventricular escape rhythm in a child under 3 is usually between 40–50 beats/min. As can be seen from the table, *the rate of subsidiary pacemakers for children after about 3 years of age is similar to that for adults.*

> It is important to emphasize that escape rhythms are extremely common in otherwise healthy children and usually do not represent a disease state. This is particularly true for escape rhythms that occur during sleep, when variations in vagal tone frequently result in sinus slowing. In one study, 45% of healthy teenagers demonstrated sinus slowing and at least three consecutive beats of an AV nodal escape rhythm during Holter monitoring (Scott et al., 1980). In contrast, persistent AV nodal rhythm is distinctly uncommon in otherwise normal children during the waking hours.

Bundle Branch Blocks

As indicated in Table 17B-1, an intraventricular conduction disturbance may be present in a child despite the fact that the QRS complex is not "wide" by adult standards. *Right bundle branch block (RBBB)* is by far the most common type encountered. This conduction disturbance is usually seen in congenital heart disease, after surgical procedures (especially those involving the right ventricle) or associated with inflammatory diseases such as myocarditis or endocarditis.

Left bundle branch block (LBBB) is rare in children. Observation of a tachyarrhythmia with

QRS morphology of an LBBB-type pattern should prompt the emergency care provider to consider ventricular tachycardia or WPW.

AV Block

The atrioventricular (AV) node is under strong influence from the autonomic nervous system. Thus conduction through the AV node may be speeded up or slowed down by alterations in sympathetic or parasympathetic tone.

> As discussed in Chapter 3, the PR interval encompasses the period from initial activation in the SA node until the time of ventricular activation. This includes travel of the depolarization impulse through the atria, AV node, and ventricular conduction system (bundle of His, bundle branches). Because the speed of conduction is by far slowest through the AV node (0.3 m/sec, compared to 1.5 m/sec through the atria and 2–4 m/sec through the His-Purkinje system), a major proportion of the PR interval reflects travel through this structure. Disorders affecting the AV node are therefore the most common causes of PR interval prolongation.

FIRST-DEGREE AV BLOCK

The criteria for *1° AV block* are age related. For example, a PR interval of 0.17 second is prolonged for children under 4 and represents 1° AV block in this age group (Table 17B-1). Clinically, this conduction disturbance is encountered in patients with digitalis intoxication, atrial septal defect (due to alteration of normal atrial anatomy), Ebstein's anomaly, inflammatory cardiac diseases (viral myocarditis, acute rheumatic fever, or Kawasaki's disease), cardio-myopathy, after surgery for congenital heart disease, or as a normal variant. There usually is no functional importance attached to this finding.

> Because of autonomic influence on the AV node, children with high degrees of resting vagal tone (as is so frequently found in the athletically inclined male adolescent) not uncommonly demonstrate 1° AV block. The PR interval may even lengthen and shorten *spontaneously* in such individuals as a normal response to variations in autonomic tone during respiration.

SECOND-DEGREE AV BLOCK

The two types of 2° AV block are Mobitz type I and Mobitz type II. As in adults, *Mobitz type I (Wenckebach)* is by far the most common form.

Clinically, Mobitz I tends to occur with the same conditions that are associated with 1° AV block. Although it may be caused by disease states, normal individuals with increased resting vagal tone frequently manifest this disorder. *The significance of Mobitz I 2° AV block is most strongly related to the clinical setting in which it occurs.* It should therefore be interpreted as a benign normal variant when seen in otherwise healthy, athletically inclined adolescents. In contrast, development of Mobitz I in a patient with underlying cardiomyopathy must be viewed with much more concern.

Mobitz II 2° AV block is distinctly uncommon in children. Rarely, it may be seen postoperatively. Because of the high risk of abrupt cessation of intraventricular conduction, immediate pacemaker insertion is mandatory.

THIRD-DEGREE (COMPLETE) AV BLOCK

Complete (3°) AV block in children may be either congenital or acquired. Both forms are equally common. Clinical manifestations and treatment depend on the type.

The incidence of *congenital 3° AV block* is 1 per 20,000 live births (Roberts, 1983). It occurs in about 5% of all children born with congenital heart disease and is surprisingly common in children born to mothers who have systemic lupus erythematosus. The disorder is thought to be due to abnormal development of the conduction system or intrauterine infection. Because the level of congenital 3° AV block is almost always at the AV node, the QRS complex is narrow and a junctional escape pacemaker (at a rate of between 50–80 beats/min) takes over the pacemaking function. An interesting phenomenon seen in children with congenital 3° AV block is that the ventricular response may increase appropriately with activity. Syncope is rare, especially in those individuals in whom the heart rate does not drop below 50 beats/min. In the absence of other significant cardiac abnormalities, stroke volume and cardiac output may increase as the child grows, allowing many individuals to remain relatively asymptomatic (Roberts, 1983).

The prognosis of congenital 3° AV block depends on the age of the child when the conduction defect is first discovered. Development of congestive heart failure with significantly increased mortality is much more common in children for whom complete heart block is diagnosed at birth. The outlook is much improved when the diagnosis is made after the first year of life. Although still a matter of controversy, asymptomatic children (with no signs of heart failure) who demonstrate a narrow QRS complex escape rhythm with a resting heart rate over 50 beats/min and an appropriate increase in rate in response to exercise may not need to be paced (Garson, 1983; Karpawich et al., 1981).

Acquired 3° AV block tends to occur at a lower level in the conduction system than does the congenital form of this disorder. As a result, the QRS complex is most often wide and the ventricular response slow (under 40 beats/min). Unlike congenital 3° AV block, the ventricular response in the acquired form does not respond to exercise. Syncope is therefore common, and pacemaker insertion is usually essential.

> Although acquired 3° AV block may be due to infection, it much more commonly results from cardiac surgery. In a significant percentage of those patients, the conduction disturbance is transient and only temporary pacing is required. If the conduction defect persists beyond 10 days, it is likely that permanent pacing will be required.

Premature Atrial Contractions

Premature atrial contractions (PACs) are commonly found in otherwise normal children. This is especially true for *newborn* infants who almost uniformly demonstrate at least some PACs if monitored continuously. These premature beats are felt to reflect either increased atrial automaticity or AV nodal reentry from the relative immaturity of the AV node. Although usually of little clinical significance, PACs may predispose to development of supraventricular tachyarrhythmias (PSVT or atrial flutter) in certain infants.

Ten to 20% of older children demonstrate PACs. Although occasionally due to metabolic abnormalities (hypoglycemia, hypokalemia, hypocalcemia), hypoxemia, drugs (digitalis), or cardiac surgery, such PACs usually occur in otherwise healthy children and are most often benign. Unless symptoms are present, neither additional workup nor treatment is indicated.

PROBLEM   **Interpret the rhythm shown in Figure 17B-3, taken from a young child. Are there multiple PACs?**

(with the notable exception of the P wave preceding beat no. 6) have a similar shape (upright and with a *small,* rounded deflection) and a constant PR interval. The underlying rhythm here is *sinus arrhythmia.* P waves *may* vary slightly in morphology with sinus rhythm or sinus arrhythmia as they do here. Beat no. 6 is a *PAC.*

> Practically speaking, it will rarely matter in an asymptomatic child whether an irregularity in a rhythm is due to sinus arrhythmia or sinus rhythm with PACs.

Supraventicular Tachycardia

As discussed in Chapter 3, the term *supraventricular tachycardia* is a general one that encompasses all tachyarrhythmias in which the impulse originates at or above the AV node. As is the case for adults, the types of supraventricular tachycardias in children are many and include:

i) Sinus tachycardia
ii) Junctional tachycardia
iii) Atrial fibrillation or flutter with a rapid ventricular response
iv) Ectopic atrial tachycardia
v) Paroxysmal supraventricular tachycardia (PSVT)

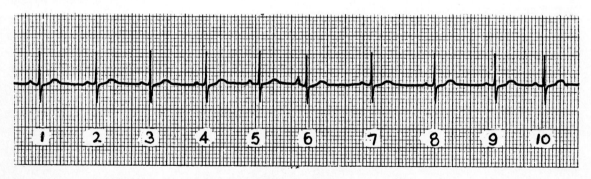

Figure 17B-3

ANSWER   This rhythm illustrates the difficulty one may sometimes have in differentiating between sinus arrhythmia and sinus rhythm with frequent PACs. The rhythm in this figure is not regular. Although P wave morphology varies slightly from beat to beat, all of the P waves

vi) Tachycardias associated with accessory pathways

PROBLEM   **The rhythm in Figure 17B-4, taken from a 4-year old, is quite rapid. In which of the above categories does it fit?**

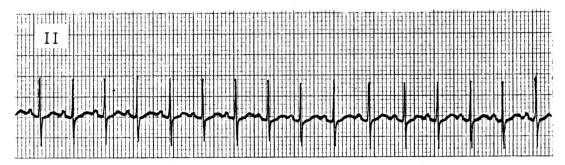

Figure 17B-4

ANSWER   The rhythm is regular at a rate of about 170 beats/min. The QRS complex is narrow and consistently preceded by an upright P wave with a normal PR interval. This is *sinus tachycardia*. The example again illustrates the point that the upper limit for sinus tachycardia in infants and children may be substantially higher than it is for adults.

SINUS TACHYCARDIA

We have previously defined the lower limits for sinus tachycardia in Table 17B-1, in which we gave the usual expected range for heart rate at various ages. Sinus tachycardia should not exceed 200 beats/min in children over 1 year of age; however, rates of up to 260 beats/min have been observed on rare instances (severely ill children with sepsis) in infants (Garson, 1983).

> As in adults, the key to sinus tachycardia is to determine (and correct) the underlying cause. When due to illness, serial changes in heart rate may reflect the status of the patient's clinical condition. That is, further acceleration of the rate is often associated with worsening of the condition, while slowing of the rate toward normal suggests improvement.

JUNCTIONAL (AV NODAL) TACHYCARDIA

The term junctional "tachycardia" is somewhat of an anomaly, since heart rate with this rhythm does *not* exceed the normal maximum sinus rate for age. It would therefore be better to describe these arrhythmias as *accelerated junctional (AV nodal) rhythms*.

Table 17B-2 defines the usual rates of subsidiary pacemakers for children under and over 3 years of age. Thus for an AV nodal rhythm in a 2-year old to be "accelerated," the rate would have to be greater than 80 beats/min. Since these arrhythmias (by definition) do not exceed the normal maximum rate for sinus rhythm at the child's particular age, this means that the heart rate range for this 2-year old with accelerated AV nodal rhythm is between 80–150 beats/min. Similarly, the heart rate range for an accelerated AV nodal rhythm in a 5-year old would be between 60–130 beats/min.

Morphologically, the rhythm is regular in accelerated AV nodal rhythms, and the QRS complex is narrow and similar to the QRS of sinus-conducted beats (unless aberrant conduction is present). Atrial activity is abnormal and reflects the junctional origin of the arrhythmia. Thus, P waves may be inverted (either preceding the QRS with a short PR interval or retrograde), absent (if retrograde P waves occur at the same time as the QRS), or entirely dissociated from the QRS (AV dissociation by *usurpation* [see Section B in Chapter 16]).

> Clinically, *accelerated* AV nodal rhythms are not usually seen in normal children. They most commonly occur in the immediate postoperative period after surgery for congenital heart disease but may also be seen with rheumatic fever, myocarditis, or digitalis toxicity. Treatment is of the underlying condition.

ATRIAL FIBRILLATION

Atrial fibrillation is rare in infants and young children. The rate of the fibrillating atria may be exceedingly rapid (between 400–700 beats/

min), with an accompanying ventricular response of between 120–200 beats/min.

> When atrial fibrillation does occur in the pediatric age group, it is frequently associated with either structurally abnormal heart disease or WPW. This has important clinical implications, since treatment of WPW with either digoxin or verapamil may result in further acceleration of conduction down the accessory pathway with disastrous consequences (Vetter, 1985; McGovern et al., 1986). In contrast, in the absence of WPW, digoxin is the drug of choice for treatment of chronic atrial fibrillation.

ATRIAL FLUTTER

Although it occurs more frequently than atrial fibrillation, *atrial flutter* is still quite uncommon in the pediatric age group. This tachyarrhythmia differs in several ways from its usual appearance in adults.

PROBLEM   **Typical morphologic characteristics of atrial flutter in the pediatric age group are illustrated by the rhythm shown in <u>Figure 17B-5</u>. How does this differ from atrial flutter in adults?**

Atrial flutter in children is distinguished by:
  i) A faster atrial rate
  ii) The frequent occurrence of variable ventricular conduction
  iii) Periods of 1:1 conduction

> While the atrial rate of flutter in children is often around 300 beats/min (as it is in adults), it may be much faster. Rates of up to 450 beats/min have been recorded (Garson, 1984). *It is because of this variability in the atrial rate that atrial flutter in children should be diagnosed by its morphology (sawtooth pattern) and not by its rate.*
>
> Although 2:1 atrioventricular conduction may be seen in children, more commonly the ventricular response is variable (irregular). The point to appreciate is that the ventricular response to atrial flutter may at times be extremely rapid, and periods of 1:1 conduction may occur.

Atrial flutter in children tends to occur in three clinical settings (Garson, 1983):
  i) In hydropic newborns who have had intra-uterine tachyarrhythmias
  ii) In otherwise normal infants less than 6 months of age (especially when frequent PACs were observed during the neonatal period)

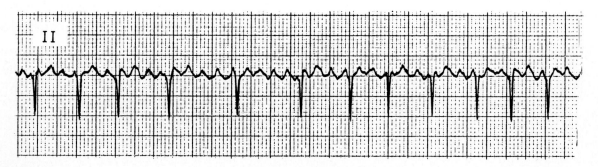

Figure 17B-5

ANSWER   Although the typical sawtooth pattern of atrial flutter is easily recognized in Figure 17B-5, the atrial rate clearly exceeds 300 beats/min (as the R-R interval of each flutter wave is definitely less than one large box). Moreover, the ventricular response (albeit controlled) is irregular.

iii) In children over 1 year of age who have underlying heart disease (cardiomyopathy, congenital heart disease)

The arrhythmia is *not* benign (due to the very rapid ventricular rates that may occur), and it should be treated. Acute therapy entails medications (such as digoxin or verapamil), overdrive pacing, or synchronized cardioversion.

In discussing the remaining supraventricular tachycardias, two principal mechanisms should be considered: *increased automaticity* and *reentry*. Determining which of these mechanisms is operative is instrumental in understanding the behavior of a particular arrhythmia and in predicting its response to therapy.

ECTOPIC ATRIAL TACHYCARDIA

The mechanism of *ectopic atrial tachycardia* is increased automaticity. An ectopic atrial focus begins to fire on its own and overtakes control of the pacemaking function (from the SA node) as it gradually speeds up its rate of discharge.

Electrocardiographically, abnormal P waves (different in morphology from the sinus-conducted P waves) precede each QRS complex. A "warm-up" phase to the tachycardia may be seen, reflecting the fact that the automatic focus gradually accelerated its rate of discharge (**Table 17B-3**). Vagal maneuvers may or may not temporarily slow the tachycardia, but they do not terminate it since the AV node is not involved in perpetuation of the rhythm.

PAROXYSMAL SUPRAVENTRICULAR TACHYCARDIA (PSVT)

In contrast, the mechanism of *PSVT* is reentry. When this mechanism is operative, the im-

Ectopic Atrial Tachycardia	PSVT (Reentry)
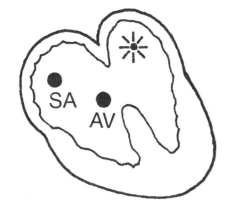	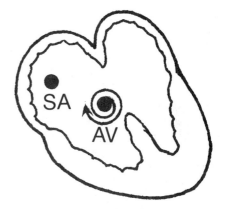
"Warm-up" and "cool-down" phase	Sudden onset and termination
Abnormal P waves precede each QRS	P wave often absent or deform terminal portion of QRS
Not affected by vagal maneuvers	May be converted by vagal maneuvers
Not terminated by a premature beat	Fortuitously timed premature beat may break arrhythmia

TABLE 17B-3

pulse is caught in a perpetual cycle in which it continuously circulates within a reentry circuit (Table 17B-3).

> The site of reentry for PSVT is most commonly the AV node. Occasionally however, reentry may occur elsewhere (in the SA node, the atria, or through an accessory pathway).

As implied in its name, PSVT most often begins abruptly. It frequently is initiated by a PAC that sets up the cycle of continuous circulation within the reentry circuit. P waves are usually not seen during the tachycardia, although occasionally they may deform the terminal portion of the QRS complex.

Because the AV node is intimately involved with perpetuation of the tachycardia, vagal maneuvers (by slowing conduction through the AV node) may be successful in terminating the arrhythmia. Similarly, a fortuitously timed premature impulse (PAC, PJC, or PVC) may momentarily alter conduction properties of the AV node and also terminate the arrhythmia. This is in contrast to the case with ectopic atrial tachycardias in which the automaticity of the ectopic focus is unaffected by premature beats.

PSVT terminates as abruptly as it begins. Once the reentry circuit is interrupted, the cycle is broken and the SA node may resume its normal function. This differs from the situation with ectopic atrial tachycardia which resolves by gradual deceleration ("cool-down") of the ectopic pacemaker.

PROBLEM   Examine Figure 17B-6, taken from a previously well child who suddenly developed palpitations. What is the likely mechanism of this arrhythmia?

ANSWER   The rhythm is regular at a rate of 195 beats/min. The QRS complex is narrow, and no P waves are evident. The differential includes:

 i) Sinus tachycardia
 ii) Atrial flutter
 iii) Ectopic atrial tachycardia
 iv) PSVT

Although the rate seen here is more rapid than one usually expects for sinus tachycardia, one cannot absolutely rule out this possibility, since rates of up to 220 beats/min have been recorded in children. However, this diagnosis is unlikely, since there is no evidence of atrial activity and the child was perfectly well until the sudden onset of this arrhythmia. *Children with rapid sinus tachycardia are almost always ill from some other cause!*

In adults, the diagnosis of atrial flutter must be included in the differential of regular supraventricular tachycardias when the ventricular response is about 150 beats/min. Because the atrial rate of flutter is often greater than 300 beats/min in children (up to 450 beats/min), this rule of thumb does not apply. However, an *irregular* ventricular response is most commonly seen with atrial flutter in children. In this trac-

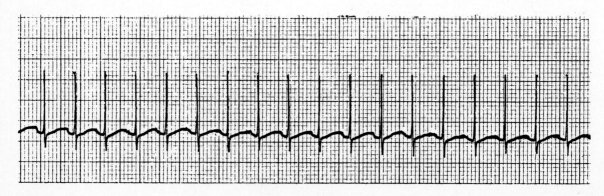

Figure 17B-6

ing the rhythm is regular, and there is not even the slightest hint of atrial actvity. Therefore, it is unlikely that this rhythm represents atrial flutter.

This leaves us with differentiating between ectopic atrial tachycardia and PSVT. In the former, the onset of the rhythm is often gradual, and ectopic (abnormal) P waves are usually clearly visible on the ECG. In contrast, a more abrupt onset is seen with PSVT, and P waves either are not evident or they deform the terminal portion of the QRS complex. *PSVT is the most likely diagnosis of the arrhythmia.*

> *PSVT* is much more common than ectopic atrial tachycardia. This is fortunate because PSVT is much easier to treat. All one has to do is interrupt the reentry circuit (even momentarily), and the arrhythmia is terminated. Measures that may be effective include vagal maneuvers, digoxin, verapamil, and propranolol.
>
> *Ectopic atrial tachycardia*, on the other hand, often is resistant to therapy. Although medications may slow the arrhythmia, they usually will not terminate it. Moreover, episodes of ectopic atrial tachycardia tend to be prolonged, frequently recur, and often become chronic. Whereas in the past the long-term outlook for patients with this arrhythmia was bleak, promising results are now being obtained by definitive therapy with cryoablation and/or surgical excision of the ectopic focus. Considering the disappointing response of ectopic atrial tachycardia to medical therapy and that chronicity of this arrhythmia with persistent tachycardia may lead to development of congestive cardiomyopathy and heart failure, enthusiasm for definitive means of treatment continues to grow (Gillette et al., 1985).

Although PSVT is usually well tolerated by otherwise healthy adults, it is important to appreciate that this arrhythmia is often *not* so benign when it occurs in infants or small children. If allowed to persist, infants in particular face a great risk of developing congestive heart failure. The younger the infant, the higher the ventricular rate (especially if over 180 beats/min), and the longer the duration of the tachycardia (especially if for more than 24 hours), the more likely and the sooner congestive heart failure will develop (Mehta et al., 1983).

> In the newborn, PSVT (with rates of up to 300 beats/min!) is sometimes recognized only after a child becomes listless and stops feeding. The diagnosis is easy to overlook since normal heart rates in children this age are rapid (and increase even more if crying occurs during an examination). *Suspect PSVT if the tachycardia persists when the infant is asleep or at rest.* Develop the habit of routinely *counting* the heart rate on physical examination of infants and young children.

TACHYCARDIAS ASSOCIATED WITH ACCESSORY PATHWAYS

The full-blown syndrome of WPW (delta wave, short PR interval, and prolonged duration of the QRS) is relatively rare in children, with a reported incidence of only 0.15% (Garson, 1984). About two thirds of these individuals have no evidence of underlying cardiac abnormality, while congenital heart disease (especially Ebstein's anomaly or tricuspid atresia) is present in the remainder.

Electrocardiographically, WPW is diagnosed in children in the same manner as for adults, with the exception that the PR interval and the QRS complex may be shorter in duration and the delta wave may be less obvious.

> Despite the fact that outright ECG evidence of an accessory pathway is so uncommon, *concealed* accessory pathways exist in a significant percentage of children. The reason delta waves are not seen on the ECG of such individuals is that conduction is preferentially channeled down the normal pathway (through the AV node, the His, and the bundle branches—panel A of **Table 17B-4**). However, the accessory pathway (AP) is nevertheless able to participate with the AV node in forming a reentry circuit.
>
> With PSVT, the QRS complex during the tachycardia usually remains narrow and the accessory pathway remains *concealed*) since conduction is in an *antegrade* direction (down the normal pathway, and back up the AP—panel B of **Table 17B-4**).
>
> The clinical significance of concealed accessory pathways lies with their potential to conduct in the opposite direction (antegrade down the AP, and back up the normal pathway—panel C of **Table 17B-4**). In this case the QRS complex will be wide during the tachycardia. While antegrade conduction is rare with PSVT, it not uncommonly occurs with atrial fibrillation and atrial flutter. Unknowingly administering digoxin or verapamil in such cases may further accelerate antegrade conduction down the accessory pathway and precipitate ventricular fibrillation!

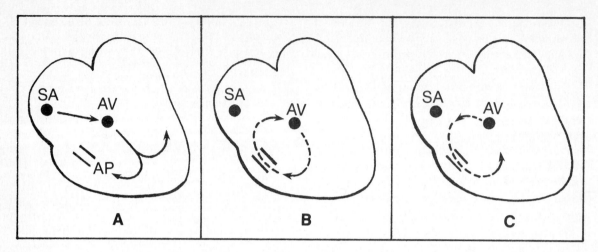

TABLE 17B-4

Ventricular Arrhythmias

As for adults, the significance of PVCs in children is most strongly related to the clinical setting in which they occur. Although occasional PVCs are commonly seen in children, frequent and complex ventricular ectopy is distinctly unusual in the absence of underlying heart disease. The asymptomatic occurrence of isolated PVCs in otherwise healthy children is therefore almost always benign!

ECG diagnosis of ventricular arrhythmias in children differs from diagnosis of such arrhythmias in adults in a number of interesting ways.

PROBLEM   **Examine the rhythm shown in Figure 17B-7, taken from an acutely ill 2-year-old child. Is the sixth complex wide enough to be a PVC?**

ANSWER   The underlying rhythm is sinus tachycardia at a rate of 200 beats/min. The sixth complex differs markedly from all of the other beats in this rhythm strip, and it is not preceded by a P wave. Yet at most it is "only" 0.09 second in duration! Can it be a PVC?

Before answering this question, it may be helpful to once again return to Table 17B-1 presented at the beginning of this chapter. Note that the normal QRS duration for a 2-year old is between 0.04–0.08 seconds, so that the sixth complex in Figure 17B-7 *is* wide considering the child's age. This beat is a PVC.

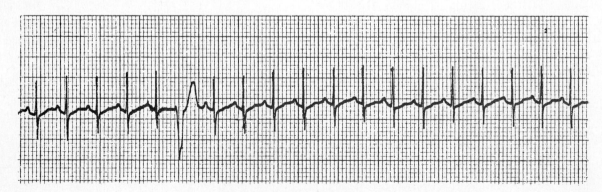

Figure 17B-7

From this example one can easily imagine how ventricular tachycardia in a child might easily be mistaken by an adult-oriented emergency care provider as a supraventricular tachycardia. *Wide* is a relative term, and 0.09–0.10 second represents definite QRS widening in children. (Garson has reported a case of ventricular tachycardia in a 2-day old in which the QRS complex of the tachyarrhythmia was *only* 0.05 second!!!)

DIFFERENTIATION BETWEEN PVCS AND ABERRANCY

One of the most difficult problems in dysrhythmia recognition in adults is differentiating between PVCs and supraventricular premature beats that conduct aberrantly. Features useful in this differentiation were detailed in Section A of Chapter 15. They include:

i) Morphological clues (especially an RBBB pattern in a right-sided monitoring lead)
ii) Similar initial deflection to the normal beats
iii) Recognition of a *premature* P wave
iv) Width of the QRS complex
v) Presence of a full compensatory pause
vi) Rate of the tachycardia
vii) Presence of AV dissociation

Virtually all bets are off in children!!!

As noted above, QRS duration is of little assistance since premature complexes as narrow as 0.09 (or less) may be "wide" in certain age groups. QRS morphology is simply too variable in children for one to place any stock in morphological clues such as an RBBB pattern or a similar initial deflection. Compensatory pauses are meaningless, since a majority of children demonstrate retrograde conduction (which resets the sinus cycle), and the ubiquity of sinus arrhythmia makes it impossible to know which cycle to count. Finally, the rate of a tachycardia is of no help, since ventricular tachycardia as fast as 428 beats/min has been recorded in children!

In reality, aberrant conduction is relatively uncommon in children (Garson, 1983). This helps simplify the problem. If a premature complex is wide (considering the age of the child) and no *premature* P wave can be clearly identified, one must work on the assumption that the beat is a PVC.

As an extension to this, consider the case of the *regular wide complex tachycardia*. In adults the differential for this type of tachyarrhythmia includes:

i) Supraventricular tachycardia with aberrant conduction
ii) Supraventricular tachycardia with preexisting bundle branch block
iii) Ventricular tachycardia

For all practical purposes, this differential can be narrowed even further in children. Intraventricular conduction defects are uncommon in pediatrics except in the postoperative period or in children with congenital heart disease. Since aberrant conduction is also uncommon, this means that *regular, wide complex tachyarrhythmias in children will most often be due to ventricular tachycardia* (especially if a narrow QRS was present during normal sinus rhythm).

At times it may be invaluable to have access to previous rhythm strips on a particular patient to see if the QRS complex had previously been wide during sinus rhythm or to study the morphology of beats that could clearly be identified as PVCs. In the absence of such evidence, one should suspect that wide tachycardias are ventricular in origin.

Overall Perspective of Arrhythmias Encountered in Pediatric Resuscitation

Even though we have greatly simplified our discussion of dysrhythmia recognition in children, we have delved into much greater detail than is necessary for managing the overwhelming majority of cardiac arrests in children. Some general concepts bear repeating:

i) The pediatric heart responds to hypoxemia by slowing its rate. As a result, bradycardia and asystole are far and away the most common arrhythmias associated with cardiopulmonary arrest in children.
ii) Because hypoxemia is the usual precipitating event in pediatric arrest, improving oxygenation (*not* administering drugs) is the most important therapeutic intervention.

iii) Ventricular tachycardia and fibrillation are extremely uncommon terminal events in pediatric arrests. When they do occur, they almost always follow a prolonged period of hypoxemia from a preceding *respiratory* arrest.

iv) Most tachyarrhythmias in children are *supraventricular*. Despite the fact that heart rates may be extremely rapid (150–200 beats/min, or more), these tachyarrhythmias are often well tolerated. Conservative treatment is often best. Rarely will there be a need for immediate intervention, and almost always there should be time to consult with an expert (if needed) regarding optimal therapy for the tachyarrhythmia.

REFERENCES

American Heart Association Subcommittee on Emergency Cardiac Care: Standards and guidelines for cardiopulmonary resuscitation (CPR) and emergency cardiac care (ECC). JAMA:255:2954–2973, 1986.

Cavallaro D, Melker R: Comparison of two techniques for determining cardiac activity in infants. Crit Care Med 11:189–190, 1983.

Eisenberg M, Bergner L, Hallstrom A: Epidemiology of cardiac arrest and resuscitation in children. Ann Emerg Med 12:672–674, 1983.

Garson A: The Electrocardiogram in Infants and Children: A Systematic Approach. Lea & Febiger, Philadelphia, 1983.

Garson A: Arrhythmias in pediatric patients. Med Clin North Am 68:1171–1210, 1984.

Gillette PC, Smith RT, Garson A, Mullins CE, Gutgesell HP, Goh TH, Cooley DA, McNamara DG: Chronic supraventricular tachycardia: A curable cause of congestive cardiomyopathy. JAMA 253:391–392, 1985.

Gillis J, Dickson D, Rieder M, Steward D, Edmonds J: Results of inpatient pediatric resuscitation. Crit Care Med 14:469–471, 1986.

Hoelzer MF: Recent advances in intravenous therapy. In Kobernick MS, and Burney RE (Eds): Emergency Medicine Clinics of North America. WB Saunders, Philadelphia, 1986, pp 487–500.

Kanter RK, Zimmerman JJ, Strauss RH, Stoeckel KA: Pediatric emergency intravaenous access: Evaluation of a protocol. Am J Dis Child 140:132–134, 1986.

Karpawich PP, Gillette PC, Garson AJ, Hesslein PS, Porter CB, McNamara DG: Congenital complete atrioventricular block: Clinical and electrophysiologic predictors of need for pacemaker insertion. Am J Cardiol 48:1098–1102, 1981.

McGovern B, Garan H, Ruskin JN: Precipitation of cardiac arrest by verapamil in patients with Wolff-Parkinson-White syndrome. Ann Med Intern 104:791–794, 1986.

Mehta AV, Casta A, Wolff GS: Supraventricular tachycardia. In Roberts NK, Gelband H (Eds): Cardiac Arrhythmias in the Neonate, Infant and Child. Appleton-Century Crofts, Norwalk, 1983, pp 105–146.

Melker R: CPR in neonates, infants, and children. In Auerbach PS, Budassi SA (Eds): Cardiac Arrest and CPR. Aspen Publications, Rockville, MD, 1983, pp 165–177.

Orlowski JP: Optimum position for external cardiac compression in infants and young children. Ann Emerg Med 15:667–673, 1986.

Roberts NK: Atrioventricular conduction: Disorders of atrioventricular conduction and intraventricular conduction. In Roberts NK, Gelband H (Eds): Cardiac Arrhythmias in the Neonate, Infant and Child. Appleton-Century Crofts, Norwalk, 1983, pp 233–252.

Scott O, Williams GJ, Fiddler GI: Results of 24 hour ambulatory monitoring of electrocardiogram in 131 healthy boys aged 10 to 13 years. Br Heart J 44:304–308, 1980.

Seidel JS, Inkelis SH: Pediatric Resuscitation. In Harwood AL (Ed): Cardiopulmonary Resuscitation. Williams & Wilkins, Baltimore, 1982, pp 134–159.

Spivey WH, Lathers CM, Malone DR, Unger HD, Bhat S, McNamara RN, Schoffstall J, Tumer N: Comparison of intraosseous, central, and peripheral routes of sodium bicarbonate administration during CPR in pigs. Ann Emerg Med 14:1135–1140, 1985.

Vetter VL: Management of arrhythmias in children—Unusual features. Cardiovasc Clin 16:329–358, 1985.

PART VII

MEDICOLEGAL ASPECTS

18

MEDICOLEGAL ASPECTS OF ACLS

Arlene E. Copenhaver, RN
Ken Grauer, MD

Introduction

In this chapter we discuss pertinent medico-legal aspects of cardiopulmonary resuscitation which may be useful to the emergency care provider in addressing ethical and legal issues of management. Numerous changes have occurred during the past 20 years. People are living longer. A majority of deaths in the United States now occur in hospitals and long-term care facilities. Because of continued advances in medical care, the process of dying has become prolonged. In many instances when individuals are no longer able to survive by natural means, sophisticated technology (such as ventilators, dialysis machines, organ transplantation) is called on to preserve vital function—sometimes indefinitely. *Death, once thought of as the final event in a medical process, is now often a process in itself.* Thus the medical predicament has shifted from the question of whether patients *can* be kept alive to whether they *should* be kept alive. Should one continue aggressive treatment for the primary disease process? Should potentially life-threatening complications be treated when they occur? Should one implement/continue mechanical support? Should CPR be performed on all patients? *And how should these decisions be made?*

Patients are demanding a more active voice in the process. Representatives for the incompetent, including deformed newborns and the mentally retarded, want to be sure these individuals are guaranteed rights similar to those of competent individuals. All the while government and the media are demanding cost containment.

However, because the legal system continues to lag behind medical technology, physicians, nurses, paramedics, and other health care providers often find themselves in a precarious situation. Brain-death statutes have been passed in many states, but no national policy yet exists. Despite a number of landmark cases, the courts still cannot agree on what their role should be in determining termination of life support. Health care providers thus face the medicoethical and legal dilemma of having to make life and death decisions on a daily basis without knowing whether the courts will support their actions.

An example of how legal changes have not kept up with medical advances is the *double indemnity clause* (Grey, 1986). Life insurance companies sometimes pay double the amount of a policy for accidental death in which the insured party dies within 120 days of the date of the accident. At the time this rule was made, it seemed logical since the victim of a lethal accident could not possibly survive this long. Times have changed. With advanced life support techniques as are available today, patients have sometimes been kept alive for months and even years following an accident despite remaining in a vegetative state with little chance for meaningful recovery. Should such irreversibly brain damaged patients be kept alive? Should the family be apprised that if life support measures are not withdrawn, the 120-day clause may expire and significant compensation may be lost? More important, should legal technicalities enter into already difficult ethical questions on what constitutes appropriate medical therapy?

GENERAL LEGAL CONCEPTS

Medicolegal Liability

Let us first examine the concept of medicolegal liability as it applies to health care practitioners. To do this, one should appreciate the meaning and implications of the terms criminal and case law. *Criminal law* is the body of law that prohibits conduct harmful to society as a whole. This includes acts of homicide and suicide (Anderson, 1982). In 1973, the AMA passed a resolution stating that "intentional termination of the life of one human being by another (mercy killing) is contrary to that for which the medical profession stands, and is contrary to the policy of the American Medical Association" (Stevens, 1986). Thus for health care professionals, active *euthanasia* is viewed as an act of criminal law.

While criminal law prohibits conduct harmful to society, *civil law* prohibits conduct harmful to individuals. Included in civil law is the broad category of medical malpractice. When a health care professional fails to exercise "reasonable" care and an injury occurs, it is said that a *tort* has been committed. In order for a tort to be successfully prosecuted as an act of malpractice, four conditions must be satisfied:

i) A relationship must have been established between the patient and the health care provider.
ii) Negligence on the part of the health care provider must have occurred.
iii) The patient must have suffered an injury.
iv) A direct *cause-and-effect* relationship between the negligence and the injury that resulted must be proved.

First there must be a duty to care—establishment of a practitioner-patient relationship. This usually is determined by mutual consent between the parties at the time of first meeting. The courts consider such relationships *contractual* and binding. Equally binding is the practitioner-patient relationship between an unresponsive patient who is brought to an emergency facility and the health care provider. Here the contract is *implied* since the courts assume the patient woud request treatment were he/she able to do so. In contrast, if an emergency care provider who is off duty passes the scene of an accident, no medicolegal obligation exists for the practitioner to stop and render assistance. However, a strong moral and ethical obligation to stop and help is still present.

Once a practitioner-physician relationship has been established, it must either be seen through to its conclusion or properly terminated. Failure to do is considered *abandonment*. For a physician in an ambulatory practice, proper termination of a doctor-patient relationship usually entails informing the patient *in writing* of these intentions, continuing to care for acute needs of the patient for a period of at least 30 days, and helping the patient to obtain another source of health care. For the Good Samaritan who decides to help at the scene of an accident, once he/she begins to render care, a medicolegal obligation is formed to continue treatment to the best of one's ability until another capable health care professional arrives on the scene to take over.

A key word in the above description of the ingredients for a malpractice claim is "reasonable." For tort to be proven, it must be shown that *reasonable* care was not exercised by the health care provider. Reasonable is defined legally as using "ordinary skill and diligence (to) apply the means and methods generally used by (health care providers) of *ordinary* skill and learning in the practice of (their) profession" (Levin and Levin, 1979). For example, the courts do not expect a family physician who stops at the scene of an accident to be able to treat a traumatized victim with the skill of a surgeon. However, if the family physician moonlights in an emergency department, patients treated in that facility should receive the same standard of care from the family physician as from a full-time emergency physician.

Once a duty (contract) to provide care has

been established, it must be proved that a *breach of duty (negligence)* occurred. Theoretically, with respect to cardiopulmonary resuscitation, a physician might be tried for failure to attempt resuscitation, for improper resuscitation, or for resuscitation against a patient's will. None of these torts have yet been brought to trial (Hashimoto, 1985).

A case for malpractice cannot be made on the basis of negligence alone. The patient must also suffer some injury, and a *direct causal relationship* must exist between the negligent act and the injury. If all practical precautions were taken, the fact that someone was harmed or injured does not necessarily mean that there was a breach of duty.

The Right to Refuse Treatment

The Bill of Rights adopted by the American Hospital Association guarantees *competent* patients the right to informed consent. The term *informed consent* is used to convey that a patient has been provided with a full explanation (in language that *they* can understand) of the state of their medical condition. In addition, the patient must be advised of potential diagnostic procedures and treatment alternatives along with the purpose, potential benefits, and risks of each.

For a patient to be deemed competent enough by the courts to render informed consent, an understanding of both the situation and the consequences of any actions taken is required. *Clarity* is not necessarily needed for competency. Thus a patient could be considered competent to refuse a treatment despite some temporal disorientation or not knowing the name of the current president of the United States.

The degree of understanding required of a patient to make a decision depends on the clinical situation and the impact on outcome that the decision may have. Traditionally, the severely retarded, unconscious persons, and young children have been considered legally *in-*

competent to give informed consent on their own (Drane, 1984). Acutely ill patients, while potentially impaired by their disease process, are generally considered competent enough to consent to a needed treatment. Little more than a *general awareness* and *assent* may be needed before instituting treatment for an acute life-threatening process for which effective therapy at low risk is available with few other reasonable alternatives (Drane, 1984). In contrast, when patient refusal of treatment will likely lead to severe morbidity or death, much more stringent and demanding standards for competency are required. In such cases, patients may need to demonstrate full appreciation of both the nature of their predicament and the consequences of their decision. They should also be able to present a rationale for making their decision, although their reasons need not necessarily conform to what others (family, the medical profession, or the courts) would do under similar circumstances (Drane, 1984).

For patients who have demonstrated competency by the above-stated criteria, the courts have generally shown that they will honor the right to forego life-prolonging treatment and allow one to "die with dignity" without medical interference. A problem could arise, however, if a competent patient's wishes conflict with the interests of the state. These are preservation of human life, preservation of the interests of innocent third parties, prevention of suicide, and preservation of ethical medical standards (Mueller and Phoenix, 1979). To protect a patient's right to refuse treatment, an increasing number of states have written Natural Death Acts. This legislation officially recognizes patients' rights to determine the course of their own treatment and enables them to do so in writing while still competent. It frees the practitioner from potential liability for withdrawing life support and neither constitutes suicide nor affects a patient's life insurance policy. Unfortunately, Natural Death Acts are not available in every state, and provisions usually have not been made for minors or others who are considered legally incompetent (Raibie, 1977).

Ordinary Versus Extraordinary Means of Prolonging Life Support

Common law dictates that a physician is obliged only to provide *ordinary* care. He or she is not bound to provide *extraordinary* care and may withhold such treatment at any time (Levin and Levin, 1979). The difficulty lies in differentiating between these two types of care. Historically, extraordinary care has meant "all medicines, treatments, and operations which cannot be obtained or used without excessive expense, pain, or other inconvenience, or which if used would not offer a reasonable hope of benefit" (Levin and Levin, 1979). Other definitons of extraordinary care are broader and include "life-sustaining" procedures or those "which involve substantial interference with the bodily privacy of the patient" (Mueller and Phoenix, 1979). Up until recently, ventilators and vasoactive medications were viewed as extraordinary treatments, while oxygen, food, and water were considered ordinary treatments.

During the past few years, the question of whether artificial feedings should still be considered as ordinary or extraordinary care was again brought up. In the 1985 Brophy decision, the judge concluded that once a gastrostomy tube is in place, artificial feedings constitute "ordinary" care.

Paul Brophy was a Massachusetts firefighter who suffered a subarachnoid hemorrhage in March 1983 as the result of a ruptured cerebral aneurysm. He never regained consciousness after surgery and remained in a persistent vegetative state. Despite numerous verbal advance directives by Brophy to family members before the onset of his coma ("No way do I want to live like that" [Karen Quinlan]), the court rejected the family's petition to withdraw nutritional support.

The creation of a stoma for placement of a gastrostomy tube "is an intrusive and invasive surgical procedure" which can be rejected by a patient or the legal guardian. But once the gastrostomy tube is in place, it is "a nursing procedure . . . (that) re-

quires no special knowledge . . . minimal maintenance . . . is neither uncomfortable nor painful . . . is neither invasive nor intrusive . . . and is not likely to produce any major complication" (Annas, 1982; General Counsel of AMA, 1986).

Many have viewed this court decision as an unfortunate setback for patients' rights of self-determination. Despite conceding that if Mr. Brophy were "presently competent (his preference would be) to forego the provision of food and water by means of a G tube and thereby terminate his life," the judge rejected use of the substituted judgement clause and instead demanded that artificial feeding be maintained indefinitely.

Ground was regained in other court decisions. The 1983 Barber case (in which two Los Angeles physicians were indicted for murder after discontinuing IV feedings on a 55-year-old brain-dead individual) resulted in a shifting by the courts from "ordinary-extraordinary" terminology to a *"proportionate-disproportionate"* benefit standard (Paris and Reardon, 1985):

"Even if a proposed course of treatment might be extremely painful or intrusive, it would still be *proportionate* treatment if the prognosis was for complete cure or significant improvement in the patient's condition. On the other hand, the treatment course which is only minimally painful or intrusive may nonetheless be considered *disproportionate* to the potential benefits if the prognosis is virtually hopeless for any significant improvement in condition."

In Florida, the husband of 75-year-old Helen Corbett was able to obtain a court order to discontinue the artificial feeding that was sustaining his wife. In this latter case, the Court of Appeal reversed a previous decision by a lower court and affirmed that "the right to refuse treatment is protected by both state and federal constitutions and cannot be abridged by state statute."

In California, alert and competent Elizabeth Bouvia was granted the right to refuse nasogastric feeding by the Court of Appeal. "Who shall say what the minimum amount of available life must be? Does it matter if it be 15 to 20 years, 15 to 20 months, or 15 to 20 days, if such life has been physically destroyed and its quality, dignity, and purpose gone?" Thus the court supported the tenet that "the decision must ultimately belong to the one whose life is in issue."

Perhaps the greatest amount of publicity regarding this issue was associated with the "Baby Doe" case in Indiana (1982). The involved party was a severely defective newborn who died 6 days after birth when the baby's parents requested that physicians withhold intravenous feeding and forego corrective surgery. Reaction to the case by the public and the Reagan administration resulted in a clamor that led to the Baby Doe regulations. A warning was issued to health care providers that withholding nutritional sustenance to a deformed infant is unlawful (Waldman, 1985). However, in June 1986 the Supreme Court struck down the Baby Doe regulations and ruled that the federal government cannot force hospitals to treat severely handicapped infants over the objections of their parents.

Among the key points brought out by these illustrative cases is that withdrawal of *life-prolonging* medical treatment may be sanctioned in cases in which this measure reflects the desires of a competent patient or is in the best interests of an incompetent patient as determined by the treating physicians, the next of kin, and/or the patient's legal proxy. The premise for withdrawal of life support in both instances must be either that the underlying disease process is irreversible or that the purpose, dignity, and quality of life have been lost. Physicians are not bound (morally or legally obligated) to provide *futile* treatment in cases where no realistic chance exists to reverse the underlying disease process and achieve meaningful survival. Instead the physician's objective (and duty) should be to make the patient as comfortable as possible. These tenets have been summarized in a recently issued opinion from the Council on Ethical and Judicial Affairs (Rouse, 1986):

> For humane reasons, with informed consent, a physician may do what is medically necessary to alleviate severe pain or may cease or omit treatment to permit a terminally ill patient whose death is im-

minent to die. However, he should not intentionally cause death. In deciding whether the administration of potentially life-prolonging medical treatment is in the best interest of the patient who is incompetent to act in his own behalf, the physician should determine what the possibility is for extending life under humane and comfortable conditions and what are the prior expressed wishes of the patient and attitudes of the family or those who have responsibility for the custody of the patient.

> Even if death is not imminent but a patient's coma is beyond doubt irreversible and there are adequate safeguards to confirm the accuracy of the diagnosis and with the concurrence of these who have responsibility for the care of the patient, it is not unethical to discontinue all means of life-prolonging medical treatment.

> Life-prolonging medical treatment includes medication and artificially or technologically supplied respiration, *nutrition*, or *hydration*. In treating a terminally ill or irreversibly comatose patient, the physician should determine whether the benefits of treatment outweigh its burdens. At all times, the dignity of the patient should be maintained.

Thus artificial feeding was equated with respirators and other life-sustaining *(extraordinary)* treatments and could be "withheld or withdrawn from an incompetent patient if it prove(d) disproportionately burdensome and contrary to the patient's values or interests" (Paris and Reardon, 1985).

BRAIN DEATH

Brain death was first identified in 1959 when two French physicians described a condition which they termed "coma depasse" (a state beyond coma) (Pallis, 1982). The best known criteria for determining brain death are contained in the report of the Ad Hoc Committee of the Harvard Medical School. The report states that the characteristics of a permanently nonfunctioning brain are:

1) *Unreceptivity* and *unresponsivity*—"even the most intensely painful stimuli evoke no vocal or other response not even a groan, withdrawal of a limb, or quickening of respiration." The patient is in an irreversible *coma.*

2) *No breathing or movements*

3) *No reflexes*—absence of reflexes includes corneal and pharyngeal reflexes. There is no ocular movement, blinking, swallowing, yawning, vocalization, or evidence of postural activity. The pupils are fixed and dilated.

4) *Flat EEG* (One year after this report, it was decided that an EEG was not essential, but it could provide additional supporting data.)

As brain death criteria became more accepted, criticism was found with the terminology and testing guidelines used in the Harvard proposal. Today, more than half of the states have brain death statutes. Concern for the lack of uniformity in the wording of statutes led several groups to formulate their own proposals for the legal definition of death and to encourage universal acceptance for their proposals. In 1981 these groups met to form the President's Commission for the Study of Ethical Problems in Medicine and Biomedical and Behavioral Research. The purpose of their meeting was to provide a model wording for a statute defining death. Their proposal, the Uniform Determination of Death Act, states:

> "An individual who has sustained either 1) or 2) is dead:
> 1) irreversible cessation of circulatory and respiratory functions, or
> 2) irreversible cessation of all functions of the entire brain, including the brainstem."

Although deceptively simple in its terminology, were this Death Act to become law in every state, much of the confusion on the issue might be resolved (O'Hara, 1983).

Accepted medical standard dictates that when the possibility exists that the brain is viable, and there are no compelling medical or legal reasons to act otherwise, resuscitation should be initiated (McIntyre, 1981). Unfortunately, in practical terms, it often is impossible for a health care provider to know whether compelling reasons for withholding resuscitation might exist at the time a cardiac arrest is first encountered. How can one determine how long the patient was unconscious before help arrived? Can information obtained from bystanders be considered reliable? Are there potentially extenuating circumstances (for example, drug overdose or hypothermia) that might respond to longer attempts at resuscitation? Acute drug intoxication, next to head injury, is probably the most common cause of sudden coma in a previously healthy adult (Pallis, 1982). Because of this and the fact that diagnosis of brain death takes time and expertise, the practitioner usually is obligated to initiate CPR at the scene of a cardiac arrest. It is then up to the physician to decide, based on cardiovascular unresponsiveness, whether or not to continue the resuscitative effort.

RECENT CASE LAW AND STATUTES

The laws in the United States and Canada are of two basic types. These are *statutes* (laws passed by state legislatures or the U.S. Congress to deal with specific problems) and *common* or *judicial law* (based on decisions made by the courts). Natural death acts and state brain death acts are two examples of statutes that we have already discussed. Another important statute is the Durable Power of Attorney Act. This act authorizes a proxy decision maker (family member, significant other, or duly appointed legal guardian) to act on behalf of incapacitated patients. Although this act was originally developed concerning property, it lends itself well to the health care problems of the incompetent patient.

To look for further guidelines for withholding or terminating life support and upholding *do not resuscitate (DNR) orders,* recent court cases must be examined. The most important of these include the cases of Quinlan, Saikewicz, Dinnerstein, Storar, and Spring. *Because each of these cases were argued on the state court level, they can provide only general guidelines.* Nevertheless, they are landmark cases that are still frequently referred to.

The Case of Karen Quinlan

Very few court cases attracted the public attention and media exposure that Karen Quinlan did in 1976. As the result of severe anoxic injury, this 21-year-old woman became comatose and remained in a vegetative state. Purposeful function was nonexistent. However, Karen was not brain dead and continued to exhibit spontaneous, involuntary movements including yawns, facial grimaces, chewing, and eye opening. Karen's father petitioned the court to terminate life support. After much deliberation, the courts finally consented and allowed the ventilator to be turned off. Ironically, Karen did *not* die. It was not until several years after the ventilator was turned off that she finally passed away.

The importance of the Quinlan case is that the courts sanctioned withdrawing life support from a patient despite the fact that brain death by the usual criteria was not present. In addition, by granting Karen's family, her treating physician, and a hospital-appointed ethics committee the right to disconnect her ventilator, the court appeared to be defining a legally acceptable medical standard for future decision-making under similar circumstances (Annas, 1982).

The Case of Joseph Saikewicz

This decision-making standard was jeopardized by the ruling in the case of Joseph Saikewicz. Mr. Saikewicz was a 67-year-old mentally incompetent man who had lived most of his life as a ward of the state of Massachusetts. Severely retarded from birth, Mr. Saikewicz never learned to speak, although he was able to communicate through grunts and gestures. In April 1976, he was found to have acute myeloblastic leukemia. The question arose as to whether full treatment (chemotherapy) should be given.

Mr. Saikewicz would certainly not have understood the reason or potential benefits to be derived from therapy. In addition, he would have had to be restrained to receive such treatment and would be subjected to much pain during the course of therapy. Even with maximal treatment, prognosis for his condition would be poor. As a result, the courts allowed chemotherapy to be withheld, and Mr. Saikewicz died quietly of pneumonia shortly thereafter.

It was the aftermath of the Saikewicz case that stirred tremendous controversy. An opinion rendered by the Massachusetts court after the trial stated:

> We take a dim view of any attempt to shift the ultimate decision-making responsibility away from the duly established courts of proper jurisdiction to any committee, panel or group, ad hoc or permanent. Thus, we reject the approach adopted by the New Jersey Supreme Court in the Quinlan case of entrusting the decision whether to continue artificial life support to the patient's guardian, family, attending doctor, and hospital "ethics committee."

This court opinion astounded the medical community. Physicians and legal advisors now had to question what the true intent of the courts was. Did the legal system want to become involved in all life and death issues of incompetent patients? Could DNR orders ever be written again for incompetent patients without first obtaining a court order?

In spite of the medicolegal uncertainty generated by the Saikewicz decision, a number of positive outcomes did result. Patients' rights to refuse life-sustaining treatment were strengthened and extended to include *incompetent* patients since "the value of human dignity extends to both (the competent and incompetent)" (Annas, 1982). In addition, the theory of *substituted judgement* was introduced by the Quinlan and Saikewicz cases. According to this theory, a proxy decision-maker could speak for an incompetent. In the Quinlan case, Karen's father was appointed her legal guardian and allowed to speak for her. The situation was more difficult in the Saikewicz decision because the patient had never been competent. Under these circumstances, the court decided to speak for the patient. It ruled that if Joseph had been competent he would have decided against the painful side effects of chemotherapy which offered little hope for cure or relief from his illness.

DNR Orders: The Case of Shirley Dinnerstein

The Dinnerstein case of 1978 was important in clarifying some of the confusion raised by the Saikewicz decision. Shirley Dinnerstein was a 67-year-old woman with Alzheimer's disease who subsequently developed a severe stroke that left her paralyzed on the left side. At the time of the trial, she was bedbound, unable to speak, and being fed by nasogastric tube. Mrs. Dinnerstein's husband and physician both felt she should be conferred DNR status. However, in the wake of the Saikewicz decision (which said that *only* the courts could decide if medical care was to be withheld from a patient), the hospital feared legal retribution and refused to allow DNR orders to be written.

The court decision supported the request of Mrs. Dinnerstein's husband and her physician to write the DNR order. This was the first time such an order had ever been asked for. The court noted that the Saikewicz decision had been

> " . . . (mis)interpreted by some in the medical profession as casting doubt upon the lawfulness of an order (from the physician) not to attempt resuscitation of an incompetent, terminally ill patient . . . and that legally requiring resuscitation of all terminally ill patients, without exercise of medical judgement, is a pointless, even cruel, prolongation of the act of dying."

Thus the court affirmed the legitimacy of physicians withholding resuscitation for certain types of patients.

> Withholding resuscitation "presents a question peculiarly within the competence of the medical profession of what measures are appropriate to ease the imminent passing of an irreversibly, terminally ill patient in light of the patient's history and condition and the wishes of her family."

As a result of the Dinnerstein decision, physicians were asked to come to court only if they proposed to withhold therapies designed to restore a patient to a normal, cognitive life. The question of chemotherapy in the Saikewicz case is an example of such a therapy. In contrast, performing CPR on Shirley Dinnerstein would do nothing to restore her to a normal existence.

The Case of John Storar

The decision reached in the John Storar case of 1980 contrasted further with the Saikewicz decision. Storar, like Saikewicz, was a lifelong incompetent. At the age of 52, he was diagnosed as having bladder cancer that soon metastasized widely. As a result of extensive bleeding from the urinary tract, blood transfusions were required. However, within several months his mother requested that the transfusions be stopped since her son's condition was terminal and treatment only seemed to prolong his suffering. Because the director of the state facility where John stayed disagreed, the case came to trial. Although the lower court initially ruled in favor of Mrs. Storar, the New York Court of Appeals reversed this decision. The higher court ruled that since John was incompetent from birth, there was no way that anyone (including his mother) could know for sure what he would have wanted if he were competent. Legally, therefore, he has to be treated as a child and should be given rights commensurate with his mental age of 18 months. This meant that not even his parents could refuse life-saving therapy for him, since patients could not negate life-saving therapy for their children. Thus the emphasis of the court shifted from advocating the right of the patient to refuse therapy (either directly or by substituted judgement) to imposing an obligation on the physician to treat at least lifelong incompetent patients.

The Case of Earle Spring

A return to the importance of the physician in making the decision to withhold resuscitation was brought about by the Earle Spring case of 1980. Mr. Spring was well until his retirement at the age of 65. Within several years after this, he developed end-stage renal failure necessitating dialysis and organic brain disease. Because of the latter condition, by age 78 he was no longer able to recognize even his own family. His wife and son, supported by their father's physician, petitioned the court to terminate dialysis treatments. The court granted this request on the grounds that 1) neither condition (renal failure or dementia) was reversible, 2) both conditions subjected Mr. Spring to unpleasant physical sensations and mental anguish, and 3) the family's strong belief that were Mr. Spring competent he would have requested withdrawal of treatment. The court stated:

> " . . . a competent person has a general right to refuse medical treatment in appropriate circumstances, to be determined by balancing the individual interest against . . . the State interest in the preservation of live. . . . The same right is also extended to an incompetent person, to be exercised through a "substituted judgement" on his behalf. The decision should be that which would be made by the incompetent person, if he were competent, taking into account his actual interests and preferences and also his present and future incompetency."

Summary of Recent Case Law

From the above it would seem that physicians are on firm ground in agreeing to withhold resuscitation from competent consenting individuals or from those who have completed formal advance directives at a time when they were competent. They probably are also supported by the courts in agreeing with a proxy to withhold resuscitation from terminally ill non-lifelong-incompetent patients. As a result of the Storar case, however, legal recourse may be needed when deciding whether to withhold resuscitation from lifelong incompetents. The courts imply that full treatment should be provided in this situation unless a court ruling says otherwise.

Regarding medical liability, the following court statement rendered in the aftermath of the Spring decision should be comforting to clinicians forced to act without prior judicial authorization:

> "Little need be said about criminal liability: there is precious little precedent, and what there is suggests that the doctor will be protected if he acts on a good faith judgement that is not grievously unreasonable by medical standards."

Regarding care of the hopelessly ill, a statement by the Ad Hoc Committee on Medical Ethics is encouraging:

> "The physician has a responsibility to ensure that his hopelessly ill patient dies with dignity and with as little suffering as possible. The preference of the patient in regard to use of life-support measures should be given the highest priority. There may be circumstances in which the physician may elect to support the body when clinical death of the brain has occurred, but there is no ethical standard that dictates he must prolong physical viability in such a patient by unusual or heroic means.
>
> If a physician decides that the disease process or other medical condition that the patient has would not positively be affected by the initiation of resuscitative efforts—in other words, if resuscitative efforts would only prolong the dying process—then a decision to write a DNR order is ethically proper.
>
> When a DNR order has been written the physician must ensure that the patient is as comfortable as possible. A decision to withhold supportive therapy, while ethically sound, may not be acceptable to some families for religious or other reasons. Their wishes must be considered but not necessarily followed. The physician must be the final arbiter in decisions related to a patient, placing the wishes of the patient above all other considerations."

An editorial by Fox and Lipton (1983) summarizes the factors which enter into the decision-making process:

> "Optimal decisions are made when the prognosis is certain, the patient's premorbid preferences are known, his or her view of the quality of life has been expressed, and the family is in complete agreement. However, the realities of clinical practice are such that this is not always the case. Sometimes the physician believes the treatment is futile, the incompetent patient's previous views are unknown, and family members insist that everything possible be done. Sometimes the treatment is futile, yet the physician, for whatever reason, insists on performing it over the objections of the family and nursing staff."

When conflict arises, assistance in the form of consultation with a medical ethicist, hospital ethics committee or legal recourse may need to be sought.

> Differences will exist from one state to another. The emergency care provider would do well to become familiar with the standard of practice in the area where he/she resides.

ALGORITHM FOR DETERMINING CODE STATUS BEFORE THE ARREST

1) Is there Any Reason Not to Resuscitate?

CPR is the standard of care for treating victims of cardiopulmonary arrest. Therefore, unless there are compelling reasons not to initiate CPR, it should always be performed.

2) Is the Patient Now Competent?

If there is reason not to resuscitate, the first question to ask is whether the patient is *now* competent. Does the patient understand the nature of his/her condition? Are the potential consequences of refusing resuscitation fully appreciated?

3) Does the Patient Want to be Resuscitated?

If the patient is now competent and states that he/she does not want CPR performed on them in the event of a cardiac arrest, the medical team is ethically and legally bound to abide by this wish. A DNR ("No Code") order should be written on the chart and all members of the health care team informed of this decision. It should be emphasized that an informed, competent patient has the right to refuse life-sustaining treatment even if the physician and/or family disagree, and even though the patient may not necessarily be in the terminal phase of a terminal illness.

The danger of using terms "DNR" or "No Code" is that once written, the medical care team may become less diligent in providing other aspects of health care (Lipton, 1986). Stevens (1986) has suggested the term "Care and Comfort Only (CCO)" be used instead, as this would remind all that *caring* for and *comforting* the patient continue even if resuscitation is no longer indicated. In addition, other interventions are not necessarily contraindicated simply because a patient is no longer a candidate for resuscitation. It is important to remember that a patient's clinical condition may rapidly change. If this happens, resuscitation status must be reassessed.

The final caveat to mention regarding DNR status is that there is no justification for a *"slow code"*—that is, less than aggressive treatment for patients "not deemed worthy of full resuscitation" and for whom lackadaisical CPR is performed only "for the record" or to reassure the family that "everything was done." Subpar efforts at resuscitation are unnecessarily invasive for the patient, undermine morale, promote cynicism among the staff, and leave one wide open to lawsuit. Sympathetic explanation to the family and active supportive care are probably a much better approach (Lo and Steinbrook, 1983; Perkins, 1986).

In contrast, should a competent patient request to be resuscitated in the event of a cardiac arrest, CPR should *always* be performed since this is the standard of care. This dictum is absolute regardless of the patient's age, underlying disease process, or seemingly low quality of life.

> Ideally the physician will have brought up the possibility of cardiopulmonary resuscitation with the patient *before* the event (and before the patient's illness renders him/her incompetent). Unfortunately this rarely occurs despite common acknowledgement by physicians that patients ought to be involved in the decision to be resuscitated (Davidson and Moseley, 1986). Reasons for avoiding the issue include physician discomfort with the topic, lack of knowledge about the types of advance directives, lack of awareness that many (if not most) patients want to talk about the possibility of resuscitation, and the mistaken belief that informing seriously ill patients about their condition would prove harmful (Davidson and Moseley, 1986; Lo et al., 1986).
>
> A method of eliciting this sensitive information in a compassionate manner from the patient has been suggested by Perkins (1986). He proceeds with a line of questioning that begins in a non-

Algorithm for Determining Code Status Before the Arrest

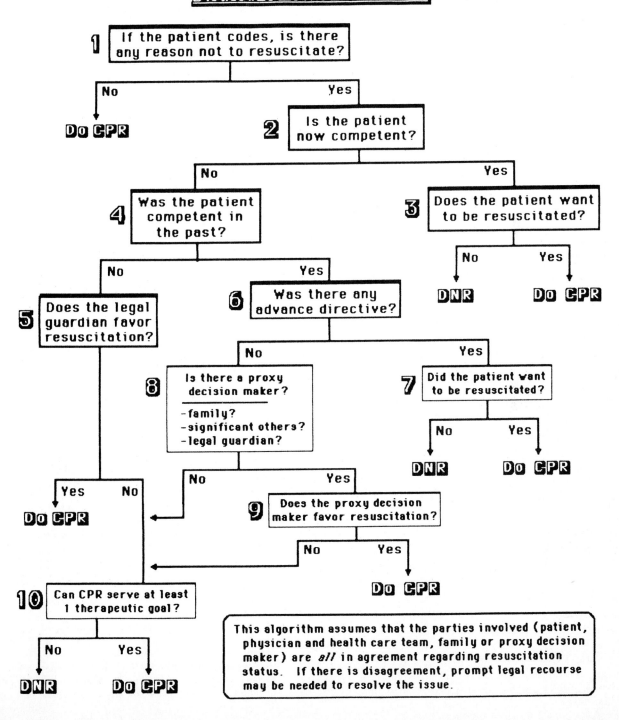

1 If the patient codes, is there any reason not to resuscitate?

No → Do CPR

Yes → **2** Is the patient now competent?

No → **4** Was the patient competent in the past?

Yes → **3** Does the patient want to be resuscitated?

No → DNR
Yes → Do CPR

4 No → **5** Does the legal guardian favor resuscitation?

4 Yes → **6** Was there any advance directive?

5 Yes → Do CPR
5 No →

6 No → **8** Is there a proxy decision maker?
 - family?
 - significant others?
 - legal guardian?

6 Yes → **7** Did the patient want to be resuscitated?

7 No → DNR
7 Yes → Do CPR

8 No →
8 Yes → **9** Does the proxy decision maker favor resuscitation?

9 No →
9 Yes → Do CPR

10 Can CPR serve at least 1 therapeutic goal?

No → DNR
Yes → Do CPR

This algorithm assumes that the parties involved (patient, physician and health care team, family or proxy decision maker) are *all* in agreement regarding resuscitation status. If there is disagreement, prompt legal recourse may be needed to resolve the issue.

threatening manner and gradually leads to more direct inquiry of patient desires:

   i) **Assess the patient's grasp of his/her illness:**
     —What do you think is wrong with you?
     —Have you ever been seriously ill before?
     —What bothers you about being sick?
     —What do you think will happen to you?

   ii) **Define therapeutic goals:**
     —What do you like to do at home?
     —What is important in your life?

   iii) **Probe for treatment refusals:**
     —Would you refuse any particular treatments in the event of critical illness?
     —Have you signed a Living Will (or other advance directive)?

   iv) **Determine patient desires for resuscitation:**
     —Have you thought about whether you would want treatment if your heart suddenly stops beating?
     —How would you want decisions to be made if you became too ill to communicate?

These considerations are particularly important for patients admitted to the hospital in a competent state, whose medical condition places them at risk of becoming incompetent soon after admission.

4) Was the Patient Competent in the Past?

Competent patients enjoy a constitutional right to determine their self-destiny. Is this right lost once the patient becomes incompetent? Obviously not. The question that arises then is once a patient becomes incompetent, *who decides?* The family? A legal guardian? The courts? Or the patient by means of an advance directive completed while he/she was still competent?

Thus, the first thing to determine is whether he/she was ever competent.

5) Does the Legal Guardian Favor Resuscitation?

Patients who have never been competent usually have a legal guardian appointed to make decisions in their behalf. If this guardian favors resuscitation in the event of a cardiac arrest, then CPR should be performed.

6) Was there any Advance Directive?

If the patient was competent in the past but is not competent now, it is essential to determine if an *advance directive* of the patient's wishes was made in the past. Formal advance directives may be *instructional* or by *proxy*. The former includes the *Living Will* and instructs the physician and the family not to use "artificial or heroic measures to prolong the patient's life if he(/she) cannot recover from a physical or mental disability" (Perkins, 1986). Proxy directives involve appointment of a Durable Power of Attorney to decide about resuscitation status for the patient in the event the patient becomes incompetent. Unfortunately, all to often patients are not familiar with advance directives, or they fail to make use of them.

Informal advance directives include physician notation of a patient's treatment wishes and family recollection of what the patient had said in the past (ie, "Please don't ever let them put me on a respirator."). Although better than no directive, informal directives suffer from lack of proof of informed consent (they are not signed by the patient) and the fact that they are unlikely to be legally binding (Davidson and Moseley, 1986).

7) Did the Patient Want to be Resuscitated?

If the patient appropriately filled out an advance directive indicating that he/she did not want to be resuscitated, that wish should be honored.

Occasionally, advance directives will specify limited treatment—"chemical code only" or "defibrillate but don't intubate." If properly documented (and written in the orders), such requests by the patient should also be honored.

   The role of the family in the case where an advance directive has been made should be to help "interpret" the patient's desires ("Yes, that's what my father would have done") and to see that they are carried out. Even if a family member disagrees with their loved one's decision, it is hoped that the patient's wishes will be respected.

   Reasons for involving the family in the decision-making process when the patient is no longer competent are that they usually have the patient's best interests at heart and that they are frequently in the best position to know what the patient would desire if competent. Because potential conflicts of interest may exist, however (due to feelings of guilt, financial concerns, or simply becoming tired of caring for the patient), the physician must always assure to the best of his/her ability that the family is acting in patient's behalf.

8) Is there a Proxy Decision-Maker?

If the patient did not fill out any advance directive, it is important to determine if there is a *proxy decision-maker*. This may be a family member, a significant other, or a duly appointed legal guardian.

9) Does the Proxy Decision-Maker Favor Resuscitation?

If the patient is not now competent and no advance directive was made but the proxy decision-maker favors resuscitation, CPR should be performed.

It should be emphasized that the proxy decision-maker should *never* be asked what he/she personally prefers for the patient. Not only may this question be burdening to the proxy, but it may also produce a conflict of interest. Instead proxy decision-makers must respond with what they feel the patient would want were the patient still able to express his/her desires *(substituted judgement)*.

The role of the physician in the process is to help the family (or proxy) by defining the standards for making their decision ("What would your mother want done if she were able to decide?").

10) Can CPR Serve at Least One Therapeutic Goal?

The question of whether CPR serves at least one therapeutic goal is the final common pathway for several points on the algorithm. This entails the reasonable expectations for rehabilitation of the patient in the event that CPR is successful. Even though the patient may have a terminal disease, CPR would still serve a therapeutic purpose if successful resuscitation allows such a patient to return home to spend meaningful time with their family.

" . . . younger family members, nurses and even physicians have difficulty in appreciating the pleasure an elderly incapacitated patient may derive from very simple experiences and just being alive. . . . An existence that might be intolerable at age 30 may be pleasurable at age 80" (Charlson et al., 1986).

Time is frequently more precious to elders because it is so limited.

In contrast, a patient with a terminal disease who is bedbound, fed by nasogastric tube, and in constant pain would probably not have any therapeutic goal served by receiving CPR in the event of a cardiac arrest.

In general, the courts have indicated that they do not wish to become involved with DNR decisions except under special circumstances. Thus the physician should be on firm ground writing DNR orders for the incompetent patient if CPR will not serve any therapeutic goal and the family, significant others, legal guardian, and medical team all agree that DNR status is in the patient's best interests and is what the patient would have wanted were he/she competent.

Should disagreement exist between any of the involved parties, prompt legal recourse may be needed to resolve the issue. *Full code status should be designated* until either a consensus is reached or a legal decision is forthcoming.

As previously discussed (the case of John Storar), an exception to the above general rule is the procedure for the lifelong incompetent. The difficulty here is the impossibility of knowing what the patient would have wanted, since incompetence has been present since birth. Unless a "reasonable person" standard is invoked by the court ("What would a *hypothetical* reasonable person do under similar circumstances?"), full therapy should be provided for the lifelong incompetent.

THE DNR ORDER

Evans and Brody (1985) have suggested that there are at least two widely understood goals for a hospital policy on resuscitation:

i) To ensure that physicians decide on the medical and ethical appropriateness of resuscitation attempts *before* they are needed, on the assumption that a better decision will be made if it is made by the physician most familiar with the case and if it is made without the stress induced by facing a sudden arrest.

ii) To encourage the physician to consult the patient, or the family of an incompetent patient, to determine their wishes concerning further treatment.

All too frequently, however, both goals fall short. To improve the situation, these same authors have offered a number of suggestions which we present with a few modifications:

1) All hospitals with a heavy load of seriously ill patients should develop formal policies for DNR orders.
2) Such policies should insist that competent patients not be bypassed (as they all too frequently are) in decisions to write a DNR order and that patients and their families be involved in both resuscitation and non-resuscitation decisions.
3) DNR policies should involve methods to help overcome physician reluctance to discuss these decisions with patients or families. (Consideration might be given to bringing up these issues routinely on admission to the hospital.)
4) The medical and ethical appropriateness of partial resuscitative efforts should be addressed.
5) The order sheet for each DNR patient must indicate in very concrete terms which medical and supportive efforts will be maintained and which will not. Documentation should also be made in the progress notes of relevant discussions held with the patient and/or family and of the rationale for such orders.
6) A mechanism must be in place for cooperatively resolving disagreements between housestaff, attending physicians, nursing staff, and families regarding DNR orders.
7) A mechanism should also be in place to assure that decisions regarding the resuscitation of any particular patient are frequently (daily or every other day) reviewed.

ALGORITHM FOR RESUSCITATION AFTER ARREST

1) Is there a DNR Order on the Chart?

Practically speaking, about the only reason for not performing CPR once a cardiac arrest is called would be the serendipitous discovery of a heretofore unseen "DNR" order hidden *(written)* in the chart. Verbal recollections of what the patient said (informal directives) are unacceptable in this setting.

2) Is the Patient Responding to Resuscitation?

If the patient is responding to efforts at resuscitation, CPR should continue.

3) Is there a Reason Not to Continue?

If the patient does not respond to initial attempts at resuscitation, but no reason exists for stopping CPR, resuscitation should continue until there is firm evidence of cardiovascular unresponsiveness to competently delivered BLS and ACLS.

> With respect to when CPR should be terminated in the emergency department, Eliastam has suggested a number of guidelines (1979):
>
> i) Apnea and pulselessness known to have exceeded 10 minutes
> ii) No response after more than 30 minutes of ACLS, including that administered in the prehospital setting
> iii) No ventricular ECG activity (asystole) after more than 10 minutes of ACLS
> iv) Preexisting terminal illness
>
> In contrast, Chipman et al. (1981) feel it preferable not to use specific criteria for deciding when to stop CPR because there are "too many uncertainties—clinical, ethical, and emotional—to subject this situation to standardized criteria."
>
> Note should be made of the special situation of *hypothermia*, for which CPR should continue until the patient is "warm and dead" (Chipman et al., 1981). Case reports exist of children who have made full recovery without neurologic deficit following cold water submersion for periods of well beyond 20 minutes.

4) Additional Sources of Information

As noted above, once a code has started, resuscitation efforts must continue unless compelling reasons exist for stopping. While in most instances nothing short of cardiovascular unresponsiveness will dissuade the code director from proceeding with resuscitation, additional sources of information (as available from the patient's chart and discussion with the family or at-

Algorithm for Resuscitation After the Arrest

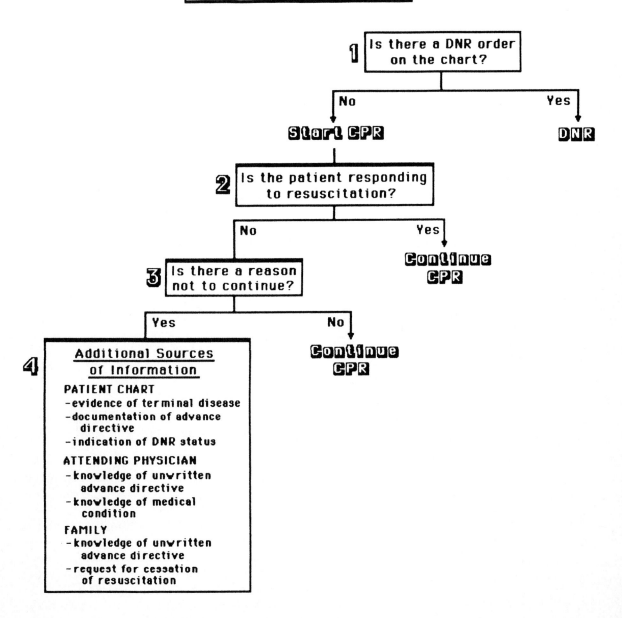

1 — Is there a DNR order on the chart?

No → Start CPR

Yes → DNR

2 — Is the patient responding to resuscitation?

No

Yes → Continue CPR

3 — Is there a reason not to continue?

Yes

No → Continue CPR

4 — **Additional Sources of Information**

PATIENT CHART
- evidence of terminal disease
- documentation of advance directive
- indication of DNR status

ATTENDING PHYSICIAN
- knowledge of unwritten advance directive
- knowledge of medical condition

FAMILY
- knowledge of unwritten advance directive
- request for cessation of resuscitation

tending physician) may sometimes prove invaluable in helping to decide whether to continue.

MEDICOLEGAL CASE STUDY

At the Scene

Imagine you are part of the paramedic team dispatched to the scene of a cardiac arrest. On arrival you find CPR being performed by the patient's son. The monitor reveals ventricular fibrillation. There is no spontaneous pulse. The son tells you that it took him "about 5 minutes" to arrive after his mother called and that he has been doing CPR ever since. As you prepare to defibrillate the patient, the mother (the patient's wife) grabs your arm and pleads with you to stop. Her husband has already suffered three myocardial infarctions and "never wanted them to work on me again." How would you proceed?

> ANSWER   CPR is the standard of care for treating victims of cardiopulmonary arrest. As long as there is the slightest possibility that the brain may be viable, resuscitation must be started.
>
> With the exception of decapitation or rigor mortis, there is no expedient, reliable method for determining brain death at the scene of a cardiac arrest. The history that it took "about 5 minutes" before the son was able to start CPR is not extremely helpful since one has no way of knowing what the rhythm was during this period (partially perfusing ventricular tachycardia? ventricular fibrillation?), and time estimation by the lay public during the stress of an emergency is notoriously inaccurate.
>
> Finally, despite the wife's pleas and description of an *informal* advance directive (he "never wanted them to work on me again"), EMS was summoned, and there is no evidence of any formal advance directives. Furthermore, despite the history of three prior infarctions, there is no evidence that the patient's pre-arrest condition is terminal.

In the Emergency Department

The patient is successfully defibrillated into a supraventricular rhythm with a pulse. He is in-

tubated, an IV line is started, and the appropriate emergency drugs are given. The patient is rushed to the emergency department where the resuscitation effort is continued. Further discussion with the family reveals that the patient's health had deteriorated rapidly since his last admission. The wife states that her husband had told her time and time again how he no longer wished to continue living. She again begs you to stop the resuscitation. Although the son agrees that his father had been depressed of late, he still feels that "everything should be done" at this point. How would you proceed if you were the physician in charge?

> ANSWER   "Once a physician-patient relationship exists, the physician has an obligation to initiate (continue) CPR when medically indicated and when DNR status is not in force" (JAMA Suppl, 1986). Thus you must continue aggressive attempts at resuscitation.
>
> Once you have started, the decision to discontinue resuscitation should be based on cardiovascular unresponsiveness. In this particular case, the patient has responded to your therapy.
>
> While morally you may feel otherwise, "when the resuscitation decision must be made in an emergency, the decision must be made in favor of life" (Fox and Lipton, 1983). Despite disagreement among the family (and any personal empathy that you may feel for the wife), without a written DNR order or a formal advance directive from the patient indicating otherwise, you are legally bound to treat in the acute setting.

In the Coronary Care Unit the Day After

The patient's vital signs stabilize, but he remains comatose. The wife continues to beg the staff to "let him go." The son remains cautiously optimistic that there may still be hope. A neurologist is consulted on the case. Although the patient is not yet "brain dead," the outlook appears dim. However, because of the conflicting feelings among family members, no DNR order is written.

Imagine yourself as the nurse assigned to the patient's care. As the medical resident in charge leaves, he informs you that the patient is "not a full code. Should he arrest, we will just go through the motions." Nothing is written regarding this on the chart. Moments later you note that the patient has gone into ventricular fibrillation. How should you proceed?

ANSWER   Unless specific interventions to be carried out are clearly spelled out on the order sheet and in the progress notes (that is, "lidocaine for ventricular tachycardia" or "defibrillate but do not intubate"), no justification exists for a *"slow code."* Thus in this case you are once again bound to resuscitate the patient in a vigorous manner despite instructions to the contrary from the medical resident.

If a patient suffers irreversible brain damage and shows no sign of recovery, withholding resuscitation and withdrawing life support are reasonable options provided that the family, significant others, and the medical team all agree. Should a conflict arise, involving a hospital medical ethics committee (and if necessary, seeking legal council) may be helpful.

In this particular case, although the overall outlook for the patient is extremely poor, brain death was not present, and adequate time had not yet passed for irreversibility to be diagnosed with certainty. Therefore continued supportive care of the patient was indicated. In addition, a sympathetic approach toward the family combined with frequent updates on the patient's medical condition, and involvement of a hospital social worker and/or psychologist would be invaluable in helping the family work through their grief. Should disagreement between mother and son persist over patient disposition, legal recourse may be needed.

As a final note, it is important to emphasize that policies and protocols may differ significantly from state to state, and even from hospital to hospital within the same state. As a result, health care providers are urged to become familiar with the policies in practice within their own institution.

REFERENCES

Ad Hoc Committee of the Harvard Medical School to Examine the Definition of Brain Death: Landmark article: A definition of irreversible coma. JAMA 252:677–679, 1984.

American Heart Association Subcommittee on Emergency Cardiac Care: Standards and guidelines for cardiopulmonary resuscitation (CPR) and emergency cardiac care (ECC). VIII. Medicolegal considerations and recommendations. JAMA 255:2979–2984, 1986.

Annas GJ: Reconciling Quinlan and Saikewicz: Decision-making for the terminally ill incompetent. In Doudera E, Peters JD (Eds): Legal and Ethical Aspects of Treating Critically and Terminally Ill Patients. Aupha Press, Ann Arbor, 1982, pp 28–62.

Annas GJ: Do feeding tubes have more rights than patients? Hastings Center Report 16:26–28, 1986.

Anderson RD: Legal Boundaries of Florida Nursing Practice. RD Anderson Publishing Company, Sacramento, 1982, pp 1–2.

Braithwaite S, Thomasma DC: New guidelines on foregoing life-sustaining treatment in incompetent patients: An anti-cruelty policy. Ann Intern Med 104:711–715, 1986.

Charlson ME, Sax FL, MacKenzie R, Fields SD, Braham RL, Douglas RG: Resuscitation: How do we decide? A prospective study of physicians' preferences and the clinical course of hospitalized patients. JAMA 255:1316–1322, 1986.

Chipman C, Adelman R, Sexton G: Criteria for cessation of CPR in the emergency department. Ann Emerg Med 10:11–17, 1981.

Davidson KW, Moseley R: Advance directives in family practice. J Fam Pract 22:439–442, 1986.

Dickey NW: Withholding or withdrawing treatment (letter). JAMA 256:469–471, 1986.

Drane JF: Competency to give an informed consent: A model for making clinical assessments. JAMA 252:925–927, 1984.

Eisenberg M: Termination of CPR in the prehospital arena. Ann Emerg Med 14:1106–1107, 1985.

Eliastam M: When to stop cardiopulmonary resuscitation. Topics in Emergency Medicine 1:109–114, 1979.

Evans AL, Brody BA: The do-not-resuscitate order in teaching hospitals. JAMA 253:2236–2239, 1985.

Farber NJ, Bowman SM, Major DA, Green WP: Cardiopulmonary resuscitation (CPR): Patient factors and decision making. Arch Intern Med 144:2229–2232, 1984.

Fox M, Lipton HL: The decision to perform cardiopulmonary resuscitation (editorial). N Engl J Med 309:607–608, 1983.

Grey L: Death and dying: Medicine and the law collide. Generics 1:19–27, 1986.

Hashimoto DM: A structural analysis of the physician-patient relationship in no-code decision-making. Specialty Law Digest: Health Care 7:7–28, 1985.

Haynes BE, Niemann JT: Letting go: DNR orders in prehospital care (editorial). JAMA 254:532–533, 1985.

Levin DL, Levin NR: DNR: An objectionable form of euthanasia. Specialty Law Digest: Health Care 3:5–17, 1979.

Lipton HL: Do-not-resuscitate decisions in a community hospital: Incidence, implications and outcomes. JAMA 256:1164–1169, 1986.

Lo B, Jonsen AT: Clinical decisions to limit treatment, Ann Intern Med 93:764–768, 1980.

Lo B, Steinbrook RL: Deciding whether to resuscitate. Arch Intern Med 143:1561–1563, 1983.

Lo B, McLeod GA, Saika G: Patient attitudes to discussing life-sustaining treatment. Arch Intern Med 146:1613–1615, 1986.

McIntyre KM: Medicolegal aspects of CPR and ECC. In McIntyre KM, Lewis AJ (Eds): Textbook of Advanced Cardiac Life Support. American Heart Association, Dallas, 1981, pp 275–291.

Meisel A, Grenvik A, Pinkus RL, Snyder JV: Hospital guidelines for deciding about life-sustaining treatment: Dealing with health "limbo." Crit Care Med 14:239–246, 1986.

Mueller RA, Phoenix GK: A dilemma for the legal and medical professions: Euthanasia and the defective newborn. Specialty Law Digest: Health Care 4:5–22, 1979.

Office of the General Counsel of the AMA: Hospital enjoined from discontinuing artificial feeding of comatose patient. The Citation, Vol 52, No. 8 (Feb 7, 1986).

O'Hara PJ: Medical-legal agreement on brain death: An assessment of the uniform determination of death act. Specialty Law Digest: Health Care 5:7–32, 1983.

Pallis C: From brain death to brain stem death. Br Med J 285:1487–1489, 1982.

Pallis C: Diagnosis of brain stem death. Br Med J 285:1558–1567, 1982.

Paris JJ, Reardon FE: Court responses to withholding or withdrawing artificial nutrition and fluids. JAMA 253:2243–2245, 1985.

Perkins HS: Ethics at the end of life: Practical principles for making resuscitation decisions. J Gen Med Intern 1:170–176, 1986.

President's Commission for the Study of Ethical Problems in Medicine and Biomedical and Behavioral Research: Deciding to Forego Life-Sustaining Treatment Decisions: Ethical, Medical, and Legal Issues in Treatment Decisions. Superintendent of Documents, U.S.G.P.O., 1983 pp 15–40.

Raibie JA: The right to refuse treatment and natural death legislation. Medicolegal News 5:6–8, 1977.

Smith JP, Bodai BI: Guidelines for discontinuing prehospital CPR in the emergency department: A review. Ann Emerg Med 14:1093–1098, 1985.

Stephens RL: "Do not resuscitate" orders: Ensuring the patient's participation. JAMA 255:240–241, 1986.

Stevens MB: Withholding resuscitation. AFP 33:207–212, 1986.

Suber DG, Tabor WJ: Withholding of life-sustaining treatment from the terminally ill, incompetent patient: Who decides? JAMA 248:2250–2251, 1982 (Part I); 248:2431–2432, 1982 (Part II).

Tagge GF: Decisions on prolonging life. Crit Care Med 13:692, 1985.

Wagner A: Cardiopulmonary resuscitation in the aged: A prospective survey. N Engl J Med 310:1129–1130, 1984.

Waldman JS: Termination of life-support for newborns: Whose choice is it anyway? Florida Bar Journal, October 1985.

COURT CASES

In the matter of Karen Quinlan, 70 NJ 10, 335 A 2d 647, 1976.

Superintendent of Belchertown State School vs Saikewicz 370 NE 2d 417, 1977.

In re Dinnerstein, 380 NE 2d 134, 1978.

In re Spring, 399 NE 2d 493, 1979.

In re Spring, 405 NE 2d 115, 1980.

New York State Court of Appeals opinions concerning: In the matter of John Storar. New York Law J 185 (63):1, 4–6, 1981.

Barber v Superior Court, 195 Cal Rptr 484, 491, 1983.

FLASH CARD NO. 1

Ventricular Fibrillation (V Fib)
Countershock × 3 (200 J–300 J–360 J)
CPR
Establish IV/intubate
Epinephrine (1 mg IV or ET)
Consider sodium bicarbonate (if the period of arrest has been long or pre-existing metabolic acidosis is suspected)
Countershock at 360 J
Lidocaine (50–100 mg IV bolus; consider IV infusion)
Countershock at 360 J
Repeat epinephrine (1 mg IV or ET)
Reconsider sodium bicarbonate
Repeat lidocaine bolus (up to 225 mg) or give bretylium (500 mg IV)
Repeat bretylium (100–1000 mg IV)
Countershock at 360 J
Continue to repeat epinephrine and countershock as needed

> Give lidocaine bolus and infusion (if not already done) as soon as patient converts to stable rhythm

Ventricular Tachycardia
No pulse:
— treat as V Fib
Hypotensive:
— cardiovert with 100–200 J
Alert, good BP:
— lidocaine (may repeat)
— procainamide
— bretylium
— cardiovert with 50–200 J

> Do *not* use IV verapamil as a "therapeutic trial" for patients with regular, wide complex tachycardia.

Asystole
CPR
Epinephrine (1 mg IV or ET)
Atropine (1 mg; may repeat)
Sodium bicarbonate (if appropriate)
Repeat epinephrine frequently
Pacemaker therapy

Bradyarrhythmias
Atropine (0.5–1 mg IV, up to 2 mg)
Infusion of dopamine, epinephrine, or isoproterenol (as a temporizing measure)
Pacemaker therapy

Electromechanical Dissociation
CPR
Epinephrine (1 mg IV or ET)
Look for underlying cause:
— right mainstem bronchus intubation
— tension pneumothorax
— cardiac tamponade
— acidosis, ↑ K$^+$, ↓ K$^+$
— pulmonary embolus
— ruptured aortic aneurysm
— cardiogenic shock
— hypovolemic shock
Consider fluid challenge and/or treatment of other underlying cause
Consider sodium bicarbonate
Repeat epinephrine frequently

PSVT/Rapid Atrial Fibrillation/Flutter
Verapamil (vagal maneuver for PSVT)
Digoxin
Propranolol
Cardioversion

> Do *not* administer IV propranolol soon after treatment with IV verapamil

FLASH CARD NO. 2

DRUGS IN CARDIAC ARREST

Epinephrine (1 ampule = 10 ml = 1 mg): 0.5–1.0 mg (5–10 ml of 1:10,000 solution) by IV or ET tube; may repeat at least every 5 minutes as needed.

Sodium bicarbonate (1 ampule = 50 mEq): 1 mEq/kg initially; $\frac{1}{2}$ dose every 10 minutes; *in general the drug has been deemphasized and is probably not indicated unless the period of arrest has been long (over 5–10 minutes) or pre-existing metabolic acidosis is suspected–if the drug should be given at all.*

Atropine: 0.5–1.0 mg IV (or by ET tube) every 5 minutes up to 2 mg. (May dose more frequently if needed)

Lidocaine: 1 mg/kg (50–100 mg) initial IV bolus; may repeat 50- to 75-mg boluses every 5–10 minutes up to a total loading dose of 225 mg.

Procainamide: 100-mg increments IV slowly over a 5-minute period until a) the arrhythmia is suppressed; b) hypotension occurs; c) the QRS complex widens by $\geq 50\%$, or d) a total loading dose of 1000 mg has been given. (Instead, may add 500–1000 mg of drug to 100 ml of D5W and infuse this over 30–60 minutes.)

Bretylium (1 ampule = 500 mg): 5–10 mg/kg ($\approx$ 500 mg) IV bolus initially. Defibrillate. If patient is still in ventricular fibrillation, give a second dose of 10 mg/kg (1–2 ampules). This may be repeated in 15–30 minutes up to a total loading dose of 30 mg/kg.

    For VT, dilute 500 mg bretylium in 50 ml D5W and infuse over 10 min.

Verapamil: 3–5 mg IV to be given over a 1- to 2-minute period (or over 3–4 minutes in the elderly). May give up to 10 mg in a dose and repeat once in 30 minutes if needed.

IV INFUSION RATES

Lidocaine **Bretylium** **Procainamide**	Mix 1 g in 250 ml D5W (= 2 g in 500 ml); begin drip at 15–30 drops/min (= 1–2 mg/min)
Isoproterenol **Epinephrine**	Mix 1 mg in 250 ml D5W; begin drip at 15–30 drops/min (= 1–2 μg/min)
Dopamine	Mix 200 mg (= 1 ampule) in 250 ml D5W; begin drip at 15–30 drops/min ($\approx$ 2–5 μg/kg/min)
Sodium nitroprusside **Nitroglycerin**	Mix 50 mg in 250 ml D5W (= 200 μg/ml); begin drip at 3 drops/min (10 μg/min); may increase infusion rate by 3 drops/min (= 10 μg/min) every 5 minutes

FLASH CARD NO. 1

Ventricular Fibrillation (V Fib)
Countershock × 3 (200 J–300 J–360 J)
CPR
Establish IV/intubate
Epinephrine (1 mg IV or ET)
Consider sodium bicarbonate (if the period
    of arrest has been long or pre-existing
    metabolic acidosis is suspected)
Countershock at 360 J
Lidocaine (50–100 mg IV bolus; consider IV
    infusion)
Countershock at 360 J
Repeat epinephrine (1 mg IV or ET)
Reconsider sodium bicarbonate
Repeat lidocaine bolus (up to 225 mg) or
    give bretylium (500 mg IV)
Repeat bretylium (100–1000 mg IV)
Countershock at 360 J
Continue to repeat epinephrine and coun-
    tershock as needed

> Give lidocaine bolus and infusion (if not al-
> ready done) as soon as patient converts to sta-
> ble rhythm

Ventricular Tachycardia
No pulse:
    —treat as V Fib
Hypotensive:
    —cardiovert with 100–200 J
Alert, good BP:
    —lidocaine (may repeat)
    —procainamide
    —bretylium
    —cardiovert with 50–200 J

> Do *not* use IV verapamil as a "therapeutic
> trial" for patients with regular, wide complex
> tachycardia.

Asystole
CPR
Epinephrine (1 mg IV or ET)
Atropine (1 mg; may repeat)
Sodium bicarbonate (if appropriate)
Repeat epinephrine frequently
Pacemaker therapy

Bradyarrhythmias
Atropine (0.5–1 mg IV, up to 2 mg)
Infusion of dopamine, epinephrine, or iso-
    proterenol (as a temporizing measure)
Pacemaker therapy

Electromechanical Dissociation
CPR
Epinephrine (1 mg IV or ET)
Look for underlying cause:
    —right mainstem bronchus intubation
    —tension pneumothorax
    —cardiac tamponade
    —acidosis, ↑ K⁺, ↓ K⁺
    —pulmonary embolus
    —ruptured aortic aneurysm
    —cardiogenic shock
    —hypovolemic shock
Consider fluid challenge and/or treatment
    of other underlying cause
Consider sodium bicarbonate
Repeat epinephrine frequently

PSVT/Rapid Atrial Fibrillation/Flutter
Verapamil (vagal maneuver for PSVT)
Digoxin
Propranolol
Cardioversion

> Do *not* administer IV propranolol soon after
> treatment with IV verapamil

FLASH CARD NO. 2

DRUGS IN CARDIAC ARREST

Epinephrine (1 ampule = 10 ml = 1 mg): 0.5–1.0 mg (5–10 ml of 1:10,000 solution) by IV or ET tube; may repeat at least every 5 minutes as needed.

Sodium bicarbonate (1 ampule = 50 mEq): 1 mEq/kg initially; $\frac{1}{2}$ dose every 10 minutes; *in general the drug has been deemphasized and is probably not indicated unless the period of arrest has been long (over 5–10 minutes) or pre-existing metabolic acidosis is suspected–if the drug should be given at all.*

Atropine: 0.5–1.0 mg IV (or by ET tube) every 5 minutes up to 2 mg. (May dose more frequently if needed)

Lidocaine: 1 mg/kg (50–100 mg) initial IV bolus; may repeat 50- to 75-mg boluses every 5–10 minutes up to a total loading dose of 225 mg.

Procainamide: 100-mg increments IV slowly over a 5-minute period until a) the arrhythmia is suppressed; b) hypotension occurs; c) the QRS complex widens by $\geq$ 50%, or d) a total loading dose of 1000 mg has been given. (Instead, may add 500–1000 mg of drug to 100 ml of D5W and infuse this over 30–60 minutes.)

Bretylium (1 ampule = 500 mg): 5–10 mg/kg ($\approx$ 500 mg) IV bolus initially. Defibrillate. If patient is still in ventricular fibrillation, give a second dose of 10 mg/kg (1–2 ampules). This may be repeated in 15–30 minutes up to a total loading dose of 30 mg/kg.

For VT, dilute 500 mg bretylium in 50 ml D5W and infuse over 10 min.

Verapamil: 3–5 mg IV to be given over a 1- to 2-minute period (or over 3–4 minutes in the elderly). May give up to 10 mg in a dose and repeat once in 30 minutes if needed.

IV INFUSION RATES

Lidocaine **Bretylium** **Procainamide**	Mix 1 g in 250 ml D5W (= 2 g in 500 ml); begin drip at 15–30 drops/min (= 1–2 mg/min)
Isoproterenol **Epinephrine**	Mix 1 mg in 250 ml D5W; begin drip at 15–30 drops/min (= 1–2 μg/min)
Dopamine	Mix 200 mg (= 1 ampule) in 250 ml D5W; begin drip at 15–30 drops/min ($\approx$ 2–5 μg/kg/min)
Sodium nitroprusside **Nitroglycerin**	Mix 50 mg in 250 ml D5W (= 200 μg/ml); begin drip at 3 drops/min (10 μg/min); may increase infusion rate by 3 drops/min (= 10 μg/min) every 5 minutes

INDEX